Core Curriculum for Oncology Nursing

ONCOLOGY
NURSING
SOCIETY

Core Curriculum for Oncology Nursing

THIRD EDITION

Joanne K. Itano, RN, PhD, OCN
Associate Professor
University of Hawaii at Manoa
School of Nursing
Honolulu, Hawaii

Karen N. Taoka, RN, MN, AOCN
Clinical Nurse Specialist, Oncology
The Queen's Medical Center
Honolulu, Hawaii

W.B. SAUNDERS COMPANY
A Division of Harcourt Brace & Company
Philadelphia   London   Toronto   Montreal   Sydney   Tokyo

W.B. SAUNDERS COMPANY
A Division of Harcourt Brace & Company

The Curtis Center
Independence Square West
Philadelphia, Pennsylvania 19106

Library of Congress Cataloging-in-Publication Data

Core curriculum for oncology nursing / Oncology Nursing Society. --
3rd ed. / editors, Joanne Itano, Karen Taoka.

p.   cm.

Includes bibliographical references and index.

ISBN 0–7216–7156–X

1. Cancer--Nursing.   2. Cancer.   I. Itano, Joanne.   II. Taoka,
   Karen.   III. Oncology Nursing Society.

[DNLM: 1. Oncologic Nursing--outlines.   WY 18.2 C797 1998]

RC266.C67   1998   616.99′4′0024613--dc21

DNLM/DLC   97–14399

CORE CURRICULUM FOR ONCOLOGY NURSING   ISBN 0–7216–7156–X

Printed in the United States of America.

Last digit is the print number: 9   8   7   6   5   4   3   2   1

Contributors

Doris Ahana, RN, MSN, OCN
Oncology Clinical Nurse Specialist/Case
  Manager, St. Francis Medical Center,
  Honolulu, Hawaii
  *Symptom Management and Supportive
  Care: Rehabilitation and Resources*

Joyce Alexander, RN, MSN, AOCN
Clinical Nurse Specialist, Bone Marrow
  Transplant and Oncology, Halifax
  Medical Center, Daytona Beach, Florida
  *Nursing Care of the Client With
  Lymphomas and Multiple
  Myeloma*

Barbara W. Ashley, RN, MSN, CANP
Nurse Practitioner, The Johns Hopkins
  Breast Center, Baltimore, Maryland
  *Prevention of Cancer; Screening and
  Early Detection of Cancer*

Catherine Bender, RN, PhD
Assistant Professor, University of
  Pittsburgh School of Nursing/University
  of Pittsburgh Cancer Institute,
  Pittsburgh, Pennsylvania
  *Nursing Implications of Antineoplastic
  Therapy*

Marilynn C. Berendt, RN, EdM, OCN
Director of Infusion Services, In Home
  Health Care Service West, Inc.,
  Downers Grove, Illinois
  Alterations in Nutrition

Marge Bernice, RN, MS, OCN
Clinical Assistant Professor, University of
  Hawaii at Manoa, School of Nursing,
  Honolulu; Women's Health Care Nurse
  Practitioner, The Queen's Medical
  Center, Honolulu, Hawaii
  *Nursing Care of the Client With Breast
  Cancer*

Marva Bohen, RN, MS
Neuro-Oncology Program Coordinator,
  Fairview University Hospital,
  Minneapolis, Minnesota
  *Nursing Care of the Client With
  Cancer of the Neurologic System*

Jeannine M. Brant, RN, MS, AOCN
Assistant Affiliate Professor, Montana
  State University, Bozeman; Oncology
  Clinical Nurse Specialist and Pain
  Consultant, Saint Vincent Hospital and
  Health Center, Billings, Montana
  Comfort

Lynne Brophy, RN, MSN
Quality Improvement Coordinator, Interim
  Health Care, Durham, North Carolina
  Immunology

Kathleen A. Calzone, RN, MSN
Nursing Coordinator, Cancer Risk
  Evaluation Program, University of
  Pennsylvania Cancer Center,
  Philadelphia, Pennsylvania
  Genetics

**Dawn Camp-Sorrell, RN, MSN, FNP,
AOCN**
Adjunct Faculty, University of Alabama at
  Birmingham, School of Nursing,
  Birmingham; Oncology Nurse
  Practitioner, University of Alabama at
  Birmingham Hospital, Birmingham,
  Alabama
  Myelosuppression

Ellen Carr, RN, MSN, AOCN
Clinical Nurse Manager, Alaris Medical
  Systems, San Diego, California
  *Nursing Care of the Client with Bone
  and Soft Tissue Cancers; Changes in
  Oncology Health Care Settings*

Mary Ann Crouch, RN, MSN
Clinical Associate, Duke University School
of Nursing, Durham; Assistant Chief
Operating Officer, Duke University
Hospital, Durham, North Carolina
*Cancer Economics and Health
Care Reform*

Margaret J. Crowley, RN, MS Ed, CRNH
Director of Patient Services, Wissahickon
Hospice, Philadelphia, Pennsylvania
*Symptom Management and Supportive
Care: Dying and Death*

Coni Ellis, RN, MS, OCN, C, CETN, CS
Clinical Instructor, General Instruction,
Adjunct Faculty, University of Texas
Health Science Center, School of
Nursing, Houston; Nursing Outreach
Coordinator, The University of Texas
M.D. Anderson Cancer Center,
Houston, Texas
Professional Issues in Cancer Care

Nina Entrekin, RN, MN, OCN
Director, Medical Affairs and Program
Planning, American Cancer Society,
Florida Division Inc., Tampa, Florida
*Nursing Care of the Client With Breast
Cancer*

Susan A. Ezzone, RN, MS, ANP
Auxiliary Clinical Instructor, The Ohio
State University College of Nursing,
Columbus; Clinical Nurse Specialist,
Arthur G. James Cancer Hospital and
Research Institute, The Ohio State
University Medical Center, Columbus,
Ohio
*Nursing Care of the Client With
Leukemia*

Joanne Peter Finley, RN, MS
Clinical Nurse, The Johns Hopkins
Oncology Center, Baltimore,
Maryland
Metabolic Emergencies

Marie Flannery, RN, MS, AOCN
Senior Associate, University of Rochester,
School of Nursing, Rochester; Oncology
Nurse Practitioner, University of
Rochester Cancer Center, Rochester,
New York
*Nursing Care of the Client with
Genital Cancer*

Beth A. Freitas, RN, MSN, OCN
Nurse Manager, Oncology Unit, The
Queen's Medical Center, Honolulu,
Hawaii
*Coping: Altered Body Image and
Alopecia*

Patricia M. Grimm, RN, PhD, CS-P
Associate Professor, The Johns Hopkins
University School of Nursing, Baltimore;
Psychiatric Consultation Liaison Nurse,
The Johns Hopkins Oncology Center,
Baltimore, Maryland
Coping: Psychosocial Issues

**Mary Magee Gullatte, RN, MN, ANP,
AOCN**
Clinical Associate Faculty, Nell Hodgson
Woodruff School of Nursing, Emory
University, Atlanta; Director of Nursing,
Oncology and Transplant Services,
Emory Hospitals, Atlanta, Georgia
Legal Issues Influencing Cancer Care

Robin R. Gwin, RN, MN, FNP
Nurse Practitioner, Emory University,
Department of Radiation Oncology,
Atlanta, Georgia
*Selected Ethical Issues in Cancer
Care*

James Halloran, RN, MSN, ANP
Clinical Director, Clinical Partners,
Houston, Texas
*Nursing Care of the Client With HIV-
Related Cancer*

Jane C. Hunter, RN, MN, OCN
Clinical Nurse Specialist, Breast Health
Sciences, Presbyterian Cancer Center,
Charlotte, North Carolina
Structural Emergencies

Joanne K. Itano, RN, PhD, OCN
Associate Professor, University of Hawaii
at Manoa, School of Nursing, Honolulu,
Hawaii
Cultural Issues

Ryan R. Iwamoto, RN, ARNP, MN, AOCN
Clinical Instructor, School of Nursing,
University of Washington, Seattle;
Clinical Nurse Specialist, Department of
Radiation Oncology, Virginia Mason
Medical Center, Seattle, Washington
*Nursing Care of the Client With Head
and Neck Cancer*

Judith (Judi) L. Johnson, RN, PhD, FAAN
Nursing Consultant, Minneapolis,
Minnesota
The Education Process

Mary B. Johnson, RN, PhD, OCN, HNC
Associate Professor, Nursing Department,
Minnesota Intercollegiate Nursing
Consortium, St. Olaf College, Northfield;
Nursing Instructor/Board Member,
Abbott Northwestern Hospital,
Minneapolis, Minnesota
The Education Process

Annette W. Kuck, RN, MS, OCN
Adjunct Faculty, University of Minnesota,
Minneapolis; Oncology Nurse
Practitioner, Minnesota Oncology
Hematology PA, Minneapolis,
Minnesota
Alterations in Elimination

Susan Leigh, RN, BSN
Cancer Survivorship Consultant, Tucson,
Arizona
*Coping: Survivorship Issues and
Financial Concerns*

Julena Lind, RN, MN
Assistant Professor of Clinical Nursing,
University of Southern California, Los
Angeles, California
*Nursing Care of the Client With
Cancer of the Urinary System; Nursing
Care of the Client With Lung Cancer*

Alice J. Longman, RN, EdD, FAAN
Professor Emeritas, The University of
Arizona, College of Nursing, Tucson,
Arizona
*Nursing Care of the Client With Skin
Cancer*

Carolyn S. J. Ma, PharmD
Clinical Pharmacy Specialist in Oncology
and Pain Management, The Queen's
Medical Center, Honolulu, Hawaii
*Symptom Management and Supportive
Care: Pharmacologic Interventions*

Leslie V. Matthews, RN, MS, ANP, AOCN
Clinical Nurse Specialist, Hematology and
Oncology, Winthrop-University
Hospital, Mineola, New York
Alterations in Ventilation

Jan Hawthorne Maxson, RN, MSN, AOCN
Clinical Faculty, Frances Payne Bolton
School of Nursing, Case Western
Reserve University, Cleveland; Care
Manager, Women's Surgical Oncology,
University Hospitals of Cleveland,
Cleveland, Ohio
*Principles of Preparation,
Administration, and Disposal of
Antineoplastic Agents*

Molly J. Moran, RN, MS, CNP, OCN
Clinical Nurse Specialist, Arthur G.
James Cancer Hospital and Research
Institute, The Ohio State University
Medical Center, Columbus, Ohio
*Nursing Care of the Client With
Leukemia*

Candis H. Morrison, RN, PhD, CANP
Assistant Professor, The Johns Hopkins
University, School of Nursing,
Baltimore; Nurse Practitioner, The
Johns Hopkins Oncology Center,
Baltimore, Maryland
*Prevention of Cancer; Screening and
Early Detection of Cancer*

Mary Mrozek-Orlowski, RN, MSN, AOCN
Adjunct Instructor, Massachusetts General
Institutes of Health, Boston,
Massachusetts; Clinical Nurse Specialist,
Comprehensive Breast Care Program,
Norris Cotton Cancer Center,
Dartmouth-Hitchcock Medical Center,
Lebanon, New Hampshire
Alterations in Circulation

Patricia W. Nishimoto, RN, MPH, DNS
Associate Professor, University of Hawaii,
School of Nursing, Honolulu; Adult
Oncology Clinical Nurse Specialist,
Tripler Army Medical Center, Honolulu,
Hawaii
Sexuality

Sharon J. Olsen, RN, MS, AOCN
Instructor, The Johns Hopkins University,
School of Nursing, Baltimore; Clinical
Director, Cancer Prevention and
Screening Services, The Johns Hopkins
Oncology Center, Baltimore, Maryland
*Prevention of Cancer; Screening and
Early Detection of Cancer*

Jennifer Douglas Pearce, RN, MSN, OCN
Associate Professor, University of
  Cincinnati Raymond Walters College,
  Department of Nursing, Cincinnati,
  Ohio
  *Alterations in Mobility, Skin Integrity,
  and Neurologic Status*

Jan Petree, RN, MS, FNP
Staff Nurse IV, Nurse Practitioner,
  Stanford Health Systems, Stanford,
  California
  *Symptom Management and Supportive
  Care: Therapies and Procedures*

Elisa Ricciardi, RN, MS, CETN
Clinical Nurse Specialist, Abbott
  Northwestern Hospital, Minneapolis,
  Minnesota
  Alterations in Elimination

Joan Exparza Richters, RN, MN, CRNH
Senior Consultant, MontEagle Inc.,
  Atlanta, Georgia
  Selected Ethical Issues in Cancer Care

**Paula Trahan Rieger, RN, MSN, ANP, CS,
OCN**
Cancer Detection Specialist, Human
  Clinical Cancer Genetics Program, The
  University of Texas M.D. Anderson
  Cancer Center, Houston, Texas
  Nursing Implications of Biotherapy

Paul J. Ross, RN, MA
Adjunct Instructor, Department of
  Anthropology, University of Hawaii at
  Manoa, Honolulu; Staff RN, Oncology,
  The Queen's Medical Center, Honolulu,
  Hawaii
  *Issues and Challenges: Alternative
  Therapies*

Teresa Wikle-Shapiro, RN, MSN, CFNP
Pediatric and Adult Nurse Practitioner,
  Bone Marrow Transplant Program,
  University of Arizona, University
  Medical Center, Tucson, Arizona
  *Nursing Implications of Bone Marrow
  and Stem Cell Transplantation*

Ellen Sitton, RN, MSN, OCN, RT(T)
Clinical Nurse Specialist, Radiation
  Oncology, University of Southern
  California, Kenneth Norris Jr. Cancer
  Hospital, Los Angeles, California
  *Nursing Implications of Radiation
  Therapy*

Roberta Anne Strohl, RN, MN, AOCN
Clinical Associate Professor and Clinical
  Nurse Specialist, University of
  Maryland, Department of Radiation
  Oncology, Baltimore, Maryland
  *Nursing Care of the Client With
  Cancer of the Gastrointestinal Tract*

Thomas J. Szopa, RN, MS, AOCN, CETN
Clinical Nurse Specialist, Oncology and
  Ostomy/Wound Management, Optima
  Health–Elliot Hospital, Manchester,
  New Hampshire
  *Nursing Implications of Surgical
  Treatment*

Karen N. Taoka, RN, MN, AOCN
Clinical Assistant Professor, University of
  Hawaii at Manoa; Clinical Nurse
  Specialist, Oncology, The Queen's
  Medical Center, Honolulu, Hawaii
  *Symptom Management and Supportive
  Care: Pharmacologic Interventions*

Deborah Lowe Volker, RN, MA, OCN
Nursing Education Coordinator, The
  University of Texas M.D. Anderson
  Cancer Center, Houston, Texas
  *Carcinogenesis; Application of the
  Standards of Practice and Education*

Jean Ellsworth Wolk, RN, MS, AOCN
Clinical Faculty, Frances Payne Bolton
  School of Nursing, Case Western
  Reserve University, Cleveland;
  Oncology Nurse Educator, Independent
  Consultant, Cleveland, Ohio
  *Principles of Preparation,
  Administration, and Disposal of
  Antineoplastic Agents*

Reviewers

Frances A. Cecere, RN, MS, CNS, OCN
Clinical Nurse Specialist, Hematology/
Oncology, Syracuse Veterans
Administration Medical Center,
Syracuse, New York

Sharon Cook, RN, MS
Patient/Family Care Administrator,
Hospice of Southwest Florida,
Bradenton, Florida

Patrick J. Coyne, RN, MSN, CS, CRNH
Clinical Nurse Specialist, Oncology/Pain
Management, Medical College of
Virginia Hospitals, Richmond,
Virginia

Vickie K. Fieler, RN, MS, AOCN
Advanced Practice Nurse, University of
Rochester Cancer Center, Rochester,
New York

Monica Fox, RN, MS OCN
Cancer Care Specialist, West Florida
Cancer Institute, Columbia West
Florida Regional Medical Center,
Pensacola, Florida

Brenda K. Hodge, RNC, MSN, OCN
Clinical Staff Nurse, Hahne Regional
Cancer Center, DuBois Regional
Medical Center, DuBois, Pennsylvania

Glenda Lady Kaminski, RN, MS, AOCN, CRNI
Advanced Practice Specialist, Oncology,
Lakeland Regional Medical Center,
Lakeland, Florida

Jamie S. Myers, RN, MN, AOCN
Oncology Clinical Nurse Specialist,
Research Medical Center, Kansas City,
Missouri

Beverly Nicholson, RN, MS
Clinical Nurse Specialist, University of
California, Davis Cancer Center,
Sacramento, California

Elaine B. Owen, RNCS, MSN, AOCN
Clinical Specialist, Medical Oncology,
Mountain Medical, Montpelier, Vermont

Rose M. Perreault, RN, C, MS, OCN
Oncology Nurse Staff Development
Specialist, Roswell Park Cancer
Institute, Buffalo, New York

Mary Garlick Roll, RN, MS
Oncology Nurse Educator, Ortho Biotech,
Cheektowaga, New York

Elizabeth W. Swap, RN, MSN, CETN, CDE, OCN
Clinical Nurse Specialist and Instructor,
DePaul Medical Center and School of
Nursing, Norfolk, Virginia; Enterostomal
Therapy Nurse, Sentara Southside
Hospitals, Norfolk, Virginia

Marge Whitman, RN, MS, AOCN
Oncology Case Manager, Utah Valley
Regional Medical Center, Provo, Utah

Preface

The third edition of the *Core Curriculum for Oncology Nursing* continues to describe and refine the essential content for the generalist in cancer nursing. It establishes the knowledge base from which nurses at the generalist level support their practice.

The impetus for this third edition is the continued expansion of knowledge and technologic development in cancer nursing. In addition, the test blueprint of the *Generalist Oncology Nursing Certification* examination was revised based on the Role Delineation Study by the Oncology Nursing Certification Corporation. This study identified the expected competencies of the generalist nurse from a survey of practicing registered nurses and nurse educators. In the same year (1995) the *Standards for Oncology Nursing Practice* was also revised.

The test blueprint directed the organization of the book with the addition of chapters relevant to cancer nursing practice today. Similar to the second edition, most chapters begin with a theory section that outlines the knowledge necessary to understand a content area and provides the foundation from which the practice of cancer nursing is based. Subsequent sections on assessment, nursing diagnoses, outcome identification, planning and implementation, and evaluation reflect the nursing process and the *Standards for Oncology Nursing Practice*. With the added emphasis on outcomes, the outcome identification section provides the benchmarks that may be used to determine the degree of outcome achievement.

New chapters on genetics, culture, immunology, and cancer economics have been added. The generalist test blueprint also directed the reorganization and inclusion of new information, resulting in chapters on Alterations in Ventilation; Alterations in Circulation; Alterations in Mobility, Skin Integrity and Neurologic Status; and new sections on electrolyte imbalances, staff education, and patient advocacy.

Chapters that have been expanded include Pharmacologic Interventions, Cancer of the Gastrointestinal Tract, Soft Tissue and Bone Cancer, and Genital Cancer, and the inclusion of multiple myeloma in the chapter on Lymphomas.

The book is a valuable resource for generalist and advanced practice cancer nurses. With its outline format, it is an easy to use reference tool when faced with questions in practice. Many nurses will utilize this text to prepare education materials. A bibliography is presented at the end of each chapter for additional sources of information. The book is a handy reference to prepare for the certification examination for the generalist level in oncology nursing.

We are excited about the currency and relevancy of the chapters. Contributors brought their expertise to the text, representing the best in cancer nursing from throughout the United States. Reviewers assisted by critically critiquing the chapters. We feel the final product reflects the most current information for the generalist in cancer nursing.

Our mahalo to the Oncology Nursing Society for providing us the opportunity to edit this book. It has been our privilege to work with the contributors and reviewers. We have gained in our own knowledge and have had the marvelous opportunity to collaborate with our cancer nursing colleagues on a significant task.

Aloha,

Joanne K. Itano
Karen N. Taoka

Contents

PART ONE

Quality of Life

Comfort

Jeannine M. Brant, RN, MS, AOCN

PAIN

Theory

I. Overview.
- A. Definition.
  1. Unpleasant sensory and emotional experience associated with actual or potential tissue damage or described in terms of such damage.
  2. Pain is whatever the person says it is existing whenever he/she says it does.
- B. Temporal characteristics of pain.
  1. Acute pain.
     - a. Usually lasts less than 6 months.
     - b. Etiology of the pain is often known.
     - c. Objective pain behaviors are more frequently exhibited.
  2. Chronic pain.
     - a. Usually lasts longer than 3 months.
     - b. Etiology of the pain is often unknown.
     - c. Often does not respond to multiple treatment regimens.
     - d. Fatigue and depression are common.
  3. Cancer pain.
     - a. Includes acute cancer-related pain caused by the cancer or cancer therapy.
     - b. Includes chronic cancer-related pain from tumor progression or cancer therapy.
     - c. Increased pain may precipitate fear of cancer progression; increased pain worsens anxiety, hopelessness, depression.

II. Types of pain.
- A. Nociceptive pain—result of activation of nociceptors (pain fibers) in deep and cutaneous tissues.
  1. Somatic pain—usually well-localized and characterized by an aching or gnawing sensation.
  2. Visceral pain—result of nociceptor activation in thoracic or abdominal tissue.
     - a. Usually poorly localized.
     - b. Characterized by an aching sensation.

B. Neuropathic pain— result of compression or injury to peripheral, sympathetic, and/or central nervous system.
  1. Peripheral neuropathic pain—often characterized by a numbness and tingling sensation.
  2. Sympathetically-generated pain—often referred to as reflex sympathetic dystrophy (RSD) or causalgia.
  3. Centrally-generated pain—characterized by radiating and shooting sensations with a background of burning and aching.

III. Barriers in pain management.
  A. Misunderstood definitions that lead to barriers in pain management:
    1. Drug tolerance—after repeated administration of a narcotic, a given dosage begins to lose its effectiveness with a shorter duration of action and subsequently less analgesic action.
      a. Physiologic phenomenon that clients cannot control.
      b. When tolerance occurs, it is necessary to administer more frequent doses and/or a higher dose to obtain the same effect.
    2. Physical dependence—after repeated administration of an opioid drug, withdrawal symptoms occur when the drug is not taken.
      a. Physiologic phenomenon that clients cannot control.
      b. Will occur if long-term opioid drugs are stopped for any reason.
    3. Addiction—overwhelming involvement with obtaining and using a drug for psychic effects, not for approved medical or social reasons.
      a. Psychological phenomenon.
      b. Clients, health care workers, and society often confuse "addiction" with "tolerance."
      c. Incidence of addiction in clients taking prescribed opioid substances is less than 1%!
  B. Societal barriers.
    1. School programs aimed at drug abuse prevention.
      a. Positive programs for America's school systems.
      b. May cause confusion in distinguishing between legitimate and illegitimate use of opioid drugs.
    2. Practitioners fear prescribing opioid drugs because of discrimination by opioid regulatory agencies.
  C. Knowledge deficits—inadequate curricula in pain management in nursing and medical schools across the nation.
  D. Client barriers.
    1. Clients reluctant to take opioid drugs for fear and misunderstanding of "tolerance" and "addiction."
    2. Clients fear that pain may be a sign of progressive disease; denial prevents them from taking adequate analgesia.
    3. Clients do not want to burden the physician and desire to be a "good patient."

IV. Risk factors.
  A. Disease-related factors.
    1. Bone metastases are the most common source of cancer pain.
      a. Breast, prostate, and lung cancer, and multiple myeloma, have the greatest incidence of bone metastases.
      b. Pain is the result of bone destruction or compression of the bone on nerves and soft tissue.

2. Nerve compression or injury to peripheral, sympathetic, and/or central nerves.
   a. Spinal cord compression (see Chapter 18).
   b. Plexopathies—pain is often a first sign followed by extremity weakness and sensory loss.
   c. Peripheral neuropathies—characterized by painful numbness, tingling, weakness, sensory loss; may progress similar to Guillain-Barré syndrome.
3. Abdominal visceral pain—may be caused by tumor obstruction of the small or large bowel, liver metastasis, omental metastasis, blood flow occlusion to visceral organs, and other causes.
B. Treatment-related factors.
   1. Chemotherapy-related pain.
      a. Mucositis (see Chapter 13).
      b. Peripheral neuropathies.
         (1) Vincristine, cisplatin, and taxol have the highest incidence.
         (2) Characterized by burning and numbness on the hands and feet.
      c. Herpetic neuralgia.
         (1) Often occurs from the immunosuppression of chemotherapy.
         (2) Characterized by burning, aching, and shocklike pain in the area of the lesions.
   2. Radiation therapy–related pain.
      a. Mucositis may occur with radiation therapy to head and neck.
      b. Radiation may induce peripheral nerve tumors characterized by a painful, enlarging mass in a previously irradiated area.
      c. Radiation skin burns.
   3. Pain related to cancer surgery.
      a. Postmastectomy pain—characterized by tightness in the axilla, medial upper arm, and/or the chest; often exacerbated with movement, extending, reaching, lifting, pulling, and pushing.
      b. Postthoracotomy pain—characterized by aching and sensory loss in the incisional area.
      c. Postradical neck dissection—characterized by tightness or burning or shocklike pain.
      d. Postnephrectomy pain—characterized by flank, groin, or abdominal heaviness or numbness.
      e. Postlimb amputation:
         (1) Stump pain—a burning sensation exacerbated with movement.
         (2) Phantom pain—characterized by cramping, throbbing, and burning in the former anatomic location of the amputated limb.
V. Principles of medical management.
   A. Treat underlying cause of pain—chemotherapy, radiation therapy, biotherapy.
   B. Pain management (Fig. 1–1).
      1. Step 1—nonopioid analgesics.
         a. Use for mild pain or as adjuvants to opioid drugs.
         b. Examples: acetaminophen, aspirin, nonsteroidal antiinflammatory agents.
      2. Step 2—weak opioid analgesics.
         a. Use for moderate pain or if pain persists or increases from Step 1 of the World Health Organization (WHO) ladder.

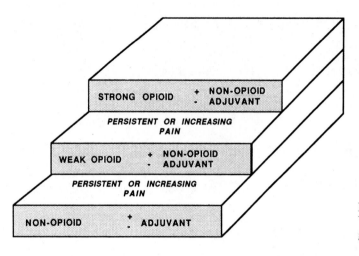

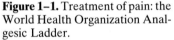

Figure 1–1. Treatment of pain: the World Health Organization Analgesic Ladder.

     b. Examples: propoxyphene, hydrocodone, oxycodone.

     c. Beware of acetaminophen combinations; dose should not exceed 4000 mg of acetaminophen in 24 hours.

     d. Agonist-antagonists (pentazocine, nalbuphine, butorphanol) are not recommended for cancer pain management.

  3. Step 3—strong opioid analgesics.

     a. Use for severe pain or if pain persists or increases from step 2 of the WHO ladder.

     b. Examples: morphine, hydromorphone, fentanyl, meperidine, levophoranol.

     c. Used most commonly for cancer pain management.

     d. Avoid meperidine for cancer pain management; the metabolite normeperidine may accumulate and cause central nervous system toxicity.

  4. Adjuvant analgesics: use on each step of the WHO ladder to enhance analgesia, relieve concurrent symptoms that exacerbate pain, and/or relieve side effects associated with opioid drugs (Table 1–1).

  5. Miscellaneous pharmacologic and radiopharmaceutic interventions.

     a. Strontium 89 for pain relief in disseminated metastatic bone cancer.

     b. Bisphosphonates (e.g., pamidronate) for relief of pain in osteolytic bone metastases.

  6. Surgical interventions.

     a. Peripheral neurectomy—destruction of peripheral nerves; example: chest wall pain.

     b. Dorsal rhizotomy—ablation of sensory nerve root fibers; examples: lung, head, and neck cancer pain; visceral pain.

     c. Anterolateral cordotomy—ablation of pain-conductive tracts involving sensory and thermal fibers; examples: visceral, somatic, unilateral pain.

     d. Commissural myelotomy—ablation of a polysynaptic pain pathway involving sensory and thermal fibers; examples: bilateral, midline pelvic, and perineal pain.

     e. Sympathectomy—interruption or partial removal of the sympathetic nervous system; example: visceral pain.

7. Nonpharmacologic interventions
   a. Transcutaneous electrical nerve stimulation (TENS).
   b. Occupational and physical therapy, cancer rehabilitation.
   c. Complementary therapies—distraction, music, guided imagery, hypnosis, massage, or relaxation.

Assessment

I. Special populations.
   A. Elderly population.
      1. Obtain a comprehensive medication history because many elderly patients are taking numerous medications.
      2. Start with lower doses of opioid and nonopioid substances and titrate up slowly because advanced age results in a prolonged half-life of the drug.
      3. Consider presence of confusion and poor vision, availability of home supervision, and cost when planning analgesics for the elderly.
   B. Pediatric population.
      1. Developmental age rather than chronologic age provides the basis for pain assessment.
      2. Pain faces are usually used in children ages seven years and younger.
      3. The poker chip pain assessment tool is used primarily in school-aged children.
      4. The "0 to 10" scale is sometimes used for school-aged and older children.
   C. Clients with a history of addiction.
      1. Assess current history—client may be actively involved in illicit drug use, may be on a methadone maintenance program, or may not have used drugs for several years.
      2. Undertreatment of pain occurs frequently because reported pain may be confused with drug-seeking behavior.
   D. Clients with dementia.
      1. Client may be unable to respond to verbal pain assessment.
      2. Observe for signs of pain—increased agitation, increased confusion, pain behaviors such as grimacing.
   E. Clients with a psychiatric history.
      1. Client may have difficulty expressing the pain experience.
      2. Observe for signs of pain—withdrawal, exaggerated psychiatric behaviors (i.e., delusions, increased agitation).
II. Clinical pain assessment.
   A. Location, intensity, quality, and temporality (Table 1–2).
   B. Affective or emotional dimension—how pain affects the client's mood and affect (i.e., depression, anxiety, hopelessness, and fear).
   C. Behavioral dimension—how pain prevents specific behaviors (i.e., mobility); how the client uses self-care behaviors to relieve pain.
   D. Cognitive and mental dimension—what pain means to the client, how pain medications affect cognitive and mental functioning (i.e., inability to concentrate, disorientation).
   E. Social evaluation—how pain affects finances, roles in and outside the home, family dynamics.
III. History and physical examination.
   A. Evaluation of computerized transaxial tomography (CT), magnetic resonance imaging (MRI), and tumor markers.

TABLE 1–1. Adjuvant Drugs Used in Cancer Pain Management

Drug Classifications	Indications	Side Effects
Analeptics		
Dextroamphetamine	Counteract opioid-induced sedation and psychomotor retardation	Nervousness, sleep disorder, hypertension, palpitations, anxiety
Methylphenidate		
Anticonvulsants		
Phenytoin	Neuropathic pain, trigeminal neuralgia, postherpetic neuralgia	Sedation, bone marrow depression, nausea, rash, confusion
Carbamazepine		
Valproate		
Clonazepam		
Gabapentin		
Antidepressants		
Amitriptyline	Neuropathic pain, postherpetic neuralgia	Dry mouth, sedation, constipation, agitation, delirium, tachycardia
Desipramine		
Imipramine		
Nortriptyline		
Antihistamines		
Hydroxyzine	Pruritic pain, anxiety associated with pain	Dry mouth, sedation, dizziness, blurred vision, tachycardia
Diphenhydramine		
Orphenadrine		
Antispasmodics		
Belladonna and opium supprettes	Gastrointestinal spasm, bladder spasm	Dry mouth, sedation, constipation
Scopolamine		
Dicyclomine		

Drug class / Agents	Indication	Side effects
Benzodiazepines Diazepam Lorazepam Alprazolam	Anxiety associated with pain, panic attack, muscle spasm	Sedation, dementia, delirium, motor incoordination, hypotension, dizziness, respiratory depression
Corticosteroids Dexamethasone Prednisone Methylprednisone	Nerve compression (brachial and lumbosacral plexopathies), lymphedema and visceral distention, increased intracranial pressure	Gastritis, fluid retention, insomnia, hypertension, hyperglycemia, psychosis, candidiasis
Muscle relaxants Diazepam Baclofen Methocarbamol Cyclobenzaprine	Muscle spasm	Sedation, nausea, weakness, confusion, dizziness
Neuroleptics Haloperidol Prochlorperazine Chlorpromazine	Continuous neuropathic pain, agitation and restlessness associated with pain	Sedation, confusion, extrapyramidal symptoms, orthostatic hypotension
Nonsteroidal Antiinflammatory Agents Ibuprofen Indomethacin Ketorolac Flurbiprofen Diflunisal Naproxen Choline magnesium Trisalicylate Sulindac	Bone metastases, soft tissue infiltration, tumor fever	Inhibition of platelet aggregation, gastritis, renal toxicity, hepatotoxicity

Data from Levy, M. (1993). *American Society of Clinical Oncology Conference on Cancer Pain: Cancer Pain Assessment and Treatment Curriculum Guidelines Teaching Syllabus and Slide Sets.* Pittsburgh: ASCO.

TABLE 1–2. **Components of Pain Assessment**

Pain Assessment Component	Description	Advantages
Location	Patient points to exact location of pain or draws pain location on a body diagram	Useful to assess multiple pain syndromes, exact locations of pain, and focal versus referred patterns
Intensity	Patient rates individual pain intensity on a 0–5 or a 0–10 pain scale with 0 being no pain and 5 or 10 being the worst possible pain	Allows caregivers the ability to objectively determine the amount of pain and to assess effectiveness of current medication regimen
Quality	Patient describes how the pain feels (i.e., constant, burning, radiating)	Provides information for the identification of specific pain syndromes
Temporality	Patient describes the onset, duration, exacerbating and relieving factors, and how pain changes over time	Provides data on the nature of pain (i.e., acute episodic versus chronic constant pain); assists in developing the pain management plan

Modified from Brant, J., Brumit, J., Forseth, J., et al. (1996). *Pain and Symptom Management in the Terminally Ill.* Billings, MT: Big Sky Hospice.

    B. Physical and neurologic examination—assess pain behaviors and changes in muscle tone, vital signs, and pupillary dilation.

IV. Evaluation and reassessment of pain.

    A. Pain should be assessed in each client with cancer.

    B. Pain should be assessed with each new report or increase in pain.

    C. Pain should be reassessed after appropriate intervals following pain interventions.

Nursing Diagnoses

    I. Acute or chronic pain.

    II. Activity intolerance.

    III. Hopelessness.

    IV. Knowledge deficit.

    V. Self-care deficit.

    VI. Sleep pattern disturbance.

    VII. Social isolation.

Outcome Identification

    I. Client recognizes importance of preventing and controlling pain.

    II. Client communicates pain intensity and temporality using standardized measures.

    III. Client uses appropriate pharmacologic and complementary interventions to control pain.

    IV. Client states that the pain is reduced or relieved to his or her satisfaction.

    V. Client participates in the usual daily lifestyle with appropriate modifications, as needed.

Planning and Implementation

I. Measures to increase client and family knowledge.
  A. Prevention of pain.
    1. Encourage the client to take analgesics early in the pain experience to avoid severe pain.
    2. Communicate with the client and family the need to prevent pain to maximize sleep, self-care, quality-of-life parameters.
    3. Begin a bowel regimen upon initiation of opioid analgesics.
  B. Safety.
    1. Inform high-risk clients with potential spinal cord compression to notify the health care team if signs occur.
    2. Assess for alterations in the following systems:
      a. Respiratory status—decreased rate, increased level of carbon dioxide, decreased ventilatory volume.
      b. Central nervous system changes—sedation, euphoria, coordination, and mood.
      c. Cardiovascular system—hypotension.
      d. Gastrointestinal system—constipation, inability to evacuate stool, nausea.
      e. Genitourinary system—urinary retention, difficult urination.
      f. Dermatologic system—cutaneous reactions, diaphoresis, facial flushing, pruritus.
    3. Reposition immobile clients every 2 hours as needed to prevent skin breakdown.
  C. Myths and misperceptions.
    1. Discuss a positive philosophy of pain management with the client and family, including the state-of-the-art technology available to control pain.
    2. Differentiate between tolerance, physical dependence, addiction, and other pain terms as needed.
  D. Pain assessment and management.
    1. Educate clients and families regarding the use of standardized pain rating scales to communicate the pain experience.
    2. Educate clients and families about the need to communicate alterations in comfort.
    3. Educate the client and family about use of nonopioid, opioid, and adjuvant analgesics and complementary therapies to control pain.
II. Measures to facilitate coping.
  A. Complementary therapies.
    1. Use adjunct therapies such as bubbles, pop-up books, magic gloves, and puppets to decrease pain perception in the pediatric population.
    2. Discuss the use of humor, reading, arts and crafts, and music as measures to distract from pain.
    3. Provide information about additional complementary therapies including relaxation, hypnosis, guided imagery, and deep breathing as appropriate.
  B. Incorporate self-care behaviors and cultural and spiritual preferences into the plan of care.
III. Measures to promote physical comfort.
  A. Use of analgesics.
    1. Administer long-acting analgesics around the clock for constant pain.
    2. Administer and offer analgesics for breakthrough pain.

3. Administer analgesics at appropriate intervals before anticipated pain-inducing activities (incident pain).
4. Begin with the least invasive route of administration (oral, transdermal, rectal), and change routes if intolerable side effects or intractable pain occur despite escalating doses.
5. Implement strategies to minimize side effects of analgesic therapy: antacids, antiemetics, H_2 antagonists, analeptics.

B. Use of a team approach.
   1. Include the client and family in the plan of care.
   2. Use consistent pain assessment tools to assess the client's pain experience (Fig. 1–2).
   3. Recommend analgesic changes: changes in medication, dosage, frequency of administration, and route as needed.
   4. Collaborate with family leaders, a minister or other spiritual leader, or a healer as needed.

IV. Measures to promote maximum mobility.
   A. Use special equipment as needed: assistive devices, toilet lifts, special beds.
   B. Maintain comfort to promote mobility and minimize skin breakdown.

Evaluation

The oncology nurse systematically and regularly evaluates the client's and/or family's responses to interventions to determine progress toward the achievement of expected outcomes. Relevant data is collected and actual findings are compared with expected findings. Nursing diagnoses, outcomes, and plans of care are reviewed and revised as necessary.

FATIGUE

Theory

I. Definition—tires easily and a diminished ability to maintain adequate performance.
II. Risk factors.
   A. Disease-related factors.
      1. Most frequently experienced symptom of cancer.
      2. Precedes and accompanies most malignancies; dependent on stage and duration of illness.
   B. Treatment-related factors.
      1. Chemotherapy.
         a. Most common side effect of chemotherapy.
         b. Fatigue generally peaks 3 to 4 days following the nadir.
      2. Biotherapy.
         a. Common side effect of interferon, interleukin-2, and tumor necrosis factor.
         b. Rare reports of fatigue with hematopoietic growth factors such as granulocyte-macrophage colony-stimulating factor and interleukin-3.
      3. Radiation therapy.
         a. Fatigue affects almost 100% of patients.
         b. Effects from ionizing radiation on cells.
         c. Cumulative over the course of treatment.

Pain Assessment Chart (For Admission and/or Follow-up)

1. Patient _____ **2.** DX _____

Assessment on Admission

Date _____/_____/_____   Pain ☐   No Pain ☐   Date of Pain Onset _____/_____/_____

  1. Location of Pain (indicate on drawing)

  2. Description of Predominant Pain (in patient's words) _____

_____

_____

  3. Intensity [Scale 0 (no pain) — 10 (most intense)] _____

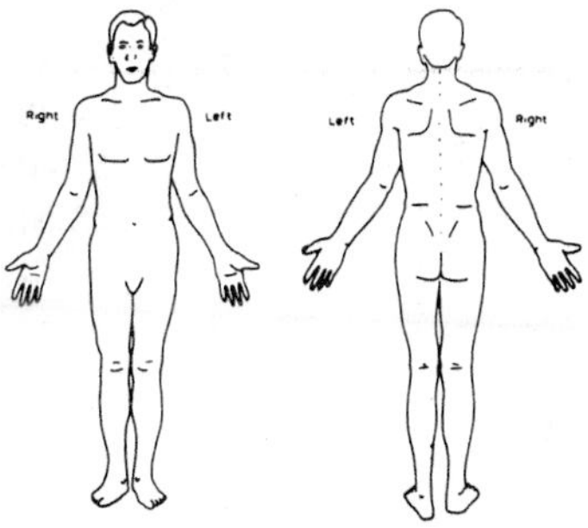

_____

  4. Duration & when occurs _____

_____

  5. Precipitating Factors _____

_____

  6. Alleviating Factors _____

_____

  7. Accompanying Symptoms

    GI: Nausea ☐   Emesis ☐   Constipation ☐   Anorexia ☐

    CNS: Drowsiness ☐   Confusion ☐   Hallucinations ☐

    Psychosocial: Mood _____ Anger _____

    Anxiety _____ Depression _____

    Relationships _____

_____

  8. Other Symptoms

    Sleep _____ Fatigue _____

    Activity _____ Other _____

  9. Present Medications _____

_____

_____

    Doses and times medicated last 48 hours _____

_____

  10. Breakthrough Pain _____

_____

Signature: _____

Figure 1–2. Pain assessment chart. Modified from the Initial Pain Assessment Tool and Flow Sheet. (From McCaffery, M., & Beebe, A. (1989). *Pain: Clinical Manual for Nursing Practice.* St. Louis: C.V. Mosby, p. 21.)

    4. Surgery.
      a. Altered cardiovascular function, nutritional status, and neuromuscu-
         lar function contribute to postoperative fatigue.
      b. Fear, anticipation of surgery, and surgical outcomes contribute to
         preoperative and postoperative fatigue.
      c. Postoperative fatigue lasts on average 3 months.
  C. Lifestyle-related.
    1. Stress.
    2. Employment.
    3. Social and daily activities.
    4. Accompanied with caregiver burden.
III. Principles of medical management.
  A. Treatment of the malignancy or the underlying cause.
  B. Treatment of fatigue-related anemia.
    1. Erythropoietin (rEPO).
      a. Stimulates the production of red blood cells.
      b. Starting dose 150 units/kg SQ three times per week.
      c. May significantly improve quality of life with fewer side effects than
         red blood cell transfusions.
    2. Red blood cell transfusions.
    3. Oxygen therapy.
    4. Proper nutrition.

Assessment

  I. Clinical fatigue assessment (Fig. 1–3).
    A. Temporal assessment.
      1. Assess for various patterns of fatigue including circadian pattern, timing,
         onset, and duration.
      2. Methods of assessment.
        a. Client's self-report.
        b. Adjective lists describing fatigue: constant, intermittent, transient.
    B. Sensory dimension.
      1. Assess the client's individual symptoms.
      2. What makes the fatigue feel worse or better?
      3. Methods of assessment.
        a. Client's self-report.
        b. Symptom checklists.
    C. Affective and emotional dimension.
      1. How has fatigue affected the overall mood of the client?
        a. Depression, social isolation.
        b. Less motivation.
      2. How distressing is the fatigue to the client?
      3. Methods of assessment.
        a. Client's self-report.
        b. Symptom distress scales.
        c. Depression scales.
    D. Behavioral dimension.
      1. Has the fatigue affected the client's ability to perform the usual basic
         activities of daily living?
        a. Bathing.

        b. Grooming and hygiene.
        c. Dressing.
        d. Mobility.
    2. Has the fatigue affected the client's ability to perform advanced activities of daily living (ADLs)?
        a. Housekeeping.
        b. Shopping and meal preparation.
        c. Laundry.
        d. Child care.
        e. Work and leisure.
    3. Are there activities that take longer to perform or are there activities the client can no longer perform?
    4. Methods of assessment.
        a. Client's self-report.
        b. Functional and performance scales.
        c. Physical and observational examination.
  E. Cognitive and mental dimension.
    1. Has the fatigue affected the client's mental abilities?
        a. Concentration.
        b. Memory.
        c. Alertness.
    2. Methods of assessment.
        a. Client's self-report.
        b. Neurocognitive screening.
           (1) Recall of words.
           (2) Orientation (name, date, place, time).
           (3) Attention (count backward by threes).
           (4) Memory (repeat words given in recall).
II. History and physical examination.
  A. Potential laboratory findings.
    1. Decreased red blood cell, hemoglobin, hematocrit levels.
    2. Decreased oxygen or increased carbon dioxide levels on the arterial blood gas report.
    3. Hypoglycemia, hyponatremia, hypercalcemia, hypothyroidism.
    4. Increased melatonin.
  B. Potential physical examination findings.
    1. General appearance is fatigued.
    2. Review radiology scan data for progressive disease.
    3. Surface electromyogram (EMG) results are abnormal.

Nursing Diagnoses

   I. Activity intolerance.
  II. Fatigue.
 III. Knowledge deficit.
  IV. Hopelessness.
   V. Self-care deficit.
  VI. Social isolation.

Outcome Identification

   I. Client recognizes fatigue as a manifestation of cancer and a side effect of cancer treatment.

Piper Fatigue Questionnaire

Instructions: Many individuals may become more tired/fatigued as they become sick or recover from the effects of treatment and illness. In order to better plan your care should you experience increased tiredness/fatigue, please complete the left side of this questionnaire and return the completed form to your nurse. Thank you very much.

To be completed by:
☐ Patient   ☐ Family Member   ☐ Nurse

To be completed by:
☐ Nurse

Name: _____

Name: _____

Date: _____

Date: _____

If you are a family member, please state your relationship to the patient.

_____

1. Are you experiencing any feelings of tiredness/fatigue now?

	No*	Yes
	☐	☐

* If You Answered No To #1, You Do Not Need To Complete Any More Questions On This Form.

2. Overall, how severe is this tiredness/fatigue for you right now? (Circle the best number in the toxicity rating scale below.)

1a. ☐ Action not needed at this time.
  b. ☐ Fatigue teaching plan given.

2.   ☐ More complete assessment is needed.

3. Signs and symptoms of fatigue. (Circle all that are being experienced by the patient.)

Tired eyes, legs, arms   Whole body fatigue
Lack of energy   Lack of endurance
Lack of stamina   Loss of strength
Weakness   Other _____

Fatigue Toxicity Rating Scale

0	1	2	3	4
• I am not at all tired/fatigued	• I am mildly tired/fatigued	• I am moderately tired/fatigued	• I am severely tired/fatigued	• I am experiencing overwhelming tiredness/fatigue
• I can do all my usual activities without any effort or assistance from someone else	• I can do all my usual activities but it takes some effort on my part	• I can do some of my usual activities, but it takes moderate effort on my part	• I have difficulty carrying out many of my usual activities, it takes so much effort on my part	• I am totally unable to carry out my usual activities, it just takes too much effort on my part
	• I do not need any assistance at this time to help me with my usual activities	• I need occasional assistance from someone else at this time to help me with my usual activities	• I often need assistance from someone else at this time to help me with my usual activities	• I almost always need help from someone else at this time to assist me with my usual activities

Copyright © 2/16/96 Barbara F. Piper, DNSc, RN, FAAN   Revised 6/13/96

Figure 1–3. Piper fatigue questionnaire. (From the University of Rochester Cancer Center. Rochester, New York, 1993.)

Piper Fatigue Questionnaire (continued)

To be completed by: ☐ Patient ☐ Family Member ☐ Nurse	To be completed by: ☐ Nurse

To be completed by:
☐ Patient   ☐ Family Member   ☐ Nurse

3. How long have you been tired/fatigued?

____ Hours   ____ Months

____ Days   ____ Years

____ Weeks

4. Is the tiredness/fatigue causing problems in your:

                                                    No   Yes

a. Ability to carry out your usual   ☐   ☐
   activities of daily living?

b. Ability to think clearly/to concentrate?   ☐   ☐

c. Motivation?   ☐   ☐

d. Mood(s)?   ☐   ☐

e. Relationship with others?   ☐   ☐

5. What does this tiredness/fatigue mean to you?
   Please describe: _____

   _____

   _____

   _____

6. What makes your tiredness/fatigue worse?

   a. _____

   b. _____

   c. _____

   d. _____

7. What makes your fatigue better?

   a. _____

   b. _____

   c. _____

   d. _____

8. Are you experiencing any other   No   Yes
   symptoms at this time?   ☐   ☐
   If yes, please describe:

   _____

   _____

   _____

To be completed by:
☐ Nurse

4. Determine what specific area of activities of daily living (ADL) have been negatively affected.
   (Circle all that apply.)

   a. Bathing, dressing, shopping, cooking

   b. Social relationships, sexual patterns

   c. Employment, work patterns

   d. Physical activities, exercise patterns

   e. Sleep, rest, nap patterns

   f. Eating patterns

   g. Hobbies, interests, other patterns

   h. Taking longer to do certain activities

   i. Certain activities no longer can be performed because of tiredness/fatigue

5. If ability to think clearly or concentrate has been affected, complete this cognitive screen.
   Total Score: 20 points

   a. Recall   *4 Points*
      Repeat these words after me.
         Table, Lion, Orange, Glove.
      I will ask you to recall these four words later.
      (1 point for each correct word repeated at this time)

   b. Orientation   *5 Points*
      What's your name?   (1 point)
      What place is this?   (2 points)
      What time is it?   (1 point)
      What is today's date?   (1 point)

   c. Attention   *7 Points*
      Count backwards from 20 by three's.
         20, 17, 14, 11, 8, 5, 2
      (1 point for each correct response.)

   d. Memory   *4 Points*
      Please repeat the four words that I asked you to remember earlier.
         Table, Lion, Orange, Glove.
      (1 point for each word remembered.)

6. If motivation has been negatively affected, explore this further.

   _____

   _____

   _____

   _____

Piper Fatigue Questionnaire (continued)

To be completed by: ☐ Patient ☐ Family Member ☐ Nurse	To be completed by: ☐ Nurse

Thank you for answering these questions. Please return this completed questionnaire to your nurse.

7. If moods have been negatively affected, explore this further.

_____

_____

_____

8. If relationships have been negatively affected, explore this further.

_____

_____

_____

9. Rate the effectiveness of each self-initiated intervention by circling the appropriate number. (Refer to patient's response to Question #7 on page 2)

		Not Very Effective										Completely Effective
a.	_____	0	1	2	3	4	5	6	7	8	9	10
b.	_____	0	1	2	3	4	5	6	7	8	9	10
c.	_____	0	1	2	3	4	5	6	7	8	9	10
d.	_____	0	1	2	3	4	5	6	7	8	9	10

10. Determine how intense/severe these symptoms are by circling the appropriate number. (Refer to patient's response to Question #8 on page 2)

		Not At All Severe										Very Severe Overwhelming
a.	_____	0	1	2	3	4	5	6	7	8	9	10
b.	_____	0	1	2	3	4	5	6	7	8	9	10
c.	_____	0	1	2	3	4	5	6	7	8	9	10
d.	_____	0	1	2	3	4	5	6	7	8	9	10

(continued)

Piper Fatigue Questionnaire (continued)

To be completed by: ☐ Patient ☐ Family Member ☐ Nurse	To be completed by: ☐ Nurse

11. Any significant findings pertinent to tiredness/fatigue from:

		No	Yes
a.	Medical History	☐	☐
b.	Physical Exam	☐	☐
c.	Laboratory Data	☐	☐
d.	Radiology/Scan Data	☐	☐
e.	Other Measures	☐	☐

What are these significant findings:

_____

_____

_____

_____

12. Referrals initiated:
    - ☐ Medicine/Symptom Control
    - ☐ Nutrition/Dietary
    - ☐ Physical Therapist
    - ☐ Occupational Services
    - ☐ Social Services
    - ☐ Discharge Planner
    - ☐ Pain Service
    - ☐ Other: Specify _____

II. Client describes self-care measures for the management of fatigue.

III. Client performs ADLs and participates in desired activities at his or her level of ability or adapts to decreased energy levels.

IV. Client copes with fatigue using individual and community support resources.

Planning and Implementation

I. Measures to increase knowledge of client and family.
  A. Discuss the potential for fatigue at the time of diagnosis and at treatment initiation.
  B. Inform the client and family of therapies known to cause the greatest amount of fatigue.
  C. Educate the client and family about the management of fatigue including medical interventions, energy conservation, exercise, nutrition, restoration of attention, and sleep and rest (Fig. 1–4).

II. Measures to facilitate client and family coping.
  A. Encourage the client and family to discuss fatigue and its impact on ADLs.
  B. Consult with psychosocial services when fatigue may be related to psychological and social factors such as depression, stress, or difficulty coping with the disease.

III. Measures to facilitate client comfort.
  A. Include the client and family in the fatigue management plan using consistent fatigue assessment tools.
  B. Encourage the client to participate in interventions that assist in the management of fatigue.
    1. Energy conservation—assist the client in prioritizing needs, planning, using proper body mechanics, pacing the daily schedule, and modifying plans if needed.
    2. Exercise—maintain adequate activity to promote the body's energy regulatory system.
    3. Nutrition—maintain adequate nutrition to promote ideal weight and body energy.
    4. Restoration of attention—reduce environmental demands (information, stimuli, distractions) to conserve attention for priority needs.
    5. Sleep and rest—maintain adequate sleep and rest.
  C. Administer medical interventions in a timely and appropriate manner.

IV. Measures that address sexuality.
  A. Acknowledge the potential for fatigue to interfere with sexuality.
  B. Encourage the client and a significant other to discuss the impact that fatigue has on sexuality.
  C. Discuss satisfactory alternative methods for expressing sexuality.

V. Measures that assist client ventilation.
  A. Provide information about medical interventions used to treat fatigue-related anemia that interferes with ventilation, including erythropoietin, red blood cell administration, and oxygen therapy.
  B. Discuss self-care interventions that maximize energy conservation.

Evaluation

The oncology nurse systematically and regularly evaluates the client's and/or family's responses to interventions to determine progress toward the achievement of expected outcomes. Relevant data is collected and actual findings are compared

Fatigue/Tiredness

The purpose of this sheet is to provide you with information to help you manage any fatigue you may experience as a result of the radiation. Fatigue may begin in the second week of treatment, would then continue throughout treatment, and disappear about three to six weeks after your treatment has ended. The information and suggestions listed below are based on information people similar to you have given us about their fatigue while receiving radiation treatments and what was helpful to them. Fatigue will be easier to deal with if you know about it and how you can manage it.

Tiredness or feeling fatigued is a common side effect of radiation therapy. The degree of tiredness varies greatly from person to person and is thought to be caused by three main factors. First, the body is working hard to rid itself of the cancer cells that have been destroyed by the radiation. Secondly, the normal cells that have been destroyed are constantly in the process of repairing themselves. Finally, coming to the radiation department on a daily basis disrupts your routine and may add to your tiredness.

Patients have found the following tips to be helpful:

1. Rest when you feel tired. Naps during the day, sleeping later in the morning or going to bed earlier at night may be helpful.

2. Maintain your usual lifestyle activities, as much as possible, but pace activities according to your energy level. Plan on doing your most important activities first or when you are feeling best.

3. Many patients continue to work or attend school while receiving radiation treatments. If your fatigue becomes great, you may find that you need to reduce your hours or stop temporarily.

4. Ask friends and family members to help with daily chores, shopping, child care or driving.

5. Good nutrition will help your energy level. Additional protein and calories are needed to help the normal cells repair themselves.

    Good sources of protein are: meat, poultry, fish, cheese, yogurt, milk shakes, Carnation Instant Breakfast™, Ensure™, Sustacal™.

6. Mild exercise such as walking, golf, swimming or stretching may actually increase your feelings of energy. Heavy exercise, however, should be avoided.

© University of Rochester Cancer Center, 1993

Figure 1–4. Fatigue and tiredness. (From Barbara F. Piper, D.NSc., R.N.: *Fatigue Initiative Through Research and Education.* Co-sponsored by Orthobiotech Pharmaceutical Corporation and the Oncology Nursing Society, 1995.)

with expected findings. Nursing diagnoses, outcomes, and plans of care are reviewed and revised as necessary.

PRURITUS

Theory

I. Definition—itching.

II. Risk factors (Table 1–3).
   A. Disease-related factors.
      1. Cancer-related—leukemia, multiple myeloma, adenocarcinoma, Hodgkin's disease, non-Hodgkin's lymphoma, melanoma, central nervous system tumors, perineal Paget's disease.
      2. Unrelated to the cancer—thyroid disease, diabetes, anemia, polycythemia.
      3. Hepatic and renal disease.
      4. Fluid and electrolyte imbalances—dehydration, hypercalcemia.
      5. Infection.
      6. Allergic reactions—medications, food, clothing.
   B. Treatment-related factors.
      1. Chemotherapy—most commonly L-asparaginase, cisplatin, and cytarabine; the client may experience allergic reaction and pruritus with most chemotherapeutic agents.
      2. Radiation—skin reactions and pruritus are most common when radiation dosage is greater than 20 to 28 Gy.
      3. Biotherapy—interferon, high-dose interleukin-2, local tissue response at injection sites.
      4. Surgery—postsurgical wound healing.
   C. Lifestyle-related factors.
      1. Stress and anxiety.
      2. Dry atmospheric conditions.
III. Principles of medical management.
   A. Treatment of the underlying cause if it is disease-related.
   B. Drug or allergic reaction: antihistamines, corticosteroids.
   C. Opioid intraspinal reaction—treat with an agonist/antagonist such as nalbuphine.
   D. Biliary obstruction—cholestyramine.
   E. Comfort—antihistamines, corticosteroids, tranquilizers.

Assessment

I. Clinical assessment (see Table 1–3).
   A. Review medication history and potential allergies.
   B. Presence of underlying disease.
   C. Temporal patterns.
      1. Patterns of pruritus including circadian occurrence (pruritus typically increases at night), timing, onset, and duration.
      2. Aggravating and alleviating factors.
      3. Impact of pruritus on daily activities.
      4. Methods of assessment.
         a. Client's self-report.
         b. Adjective lists describing pruritus: constant, intermittent, transient, burning, numbness.
II. History and physical examination.
   A. Potential laboratory findings.
      1. Complete blood count—elevated white count.
      2. Blood chemistries—hyperglycemia, hyperuricemia, elevated blood urea nitrogen (BUN) or creatinine levels, abnormal liver function test results.

   B. Physical and psychosocial findings.
     1. Skin assessment—scratch marks, erythema, excoriation, thickening, dryness.
     2. Vaginal discharge.
     3. Presence of urea or bilirubin on the skin.
     4. Presence of stress and anxiety.

Nursing Diagnoses

   I. Impaired tissue integrity.
  II. Ineffective coping.
 III. Knowledge deficit.
 IV. Pain.
  V. Sleep pattern disturbance.

Outcome Identification

   I. Client states the potential for pruritus with specific cancers and cancer therapies.
  II. Client and the family describe appropriate interventions to manage pruritus and maximize comfort.
 III. Client and the family contact an appropriate health care team member when pruritus interrupts protective mechanisms.
 IV. Client reports alleviation of pruritus and increased comfort.

Planning and Implementation

   I. Measures to increase the client and family knowledge base.
    A. Educate about therapies that may cause pruritus.
    B. Inform about the signs and symptoms of infection related to pruritus: fever, erythema, edema, pain, purulent drainage.
    C. Educate about self-care interventions to decrease the severity of pruritus.
  II. Measures to facilitate client and family coping.
    A. Teach behavioral interventions that may distract from the pruritus: imagery, television, reading, crafts.
    B. Encourage relaxation and stress reduction.
    C. Refer to psychosocial services if coping is impaired.
 III. Measures to maximize comfort (see Table 1–3).
    A. Modify the environment to prevent and minimize pruritus.
      1. Keep the room humidity at 30 to 40%.
      2. Keep the room temperature cool to prevent vasodilation.
      3. Use cotton clothing and sheets.
      4. Use hypoallergenic soaps.
    B. Minimize vasodilation.
      1. Encourage cool baths, showers, and environmental conditions.
      2. Avoid alcohol and caffeine intake.
      3. Reduce stress and anxiety.
    C. Promote skin integrity.
      1. Encourage fluid intake of 3000 mL/day.
      2. Encourage a diet high in iron, zinc, and protein.
      3. Avoid tight-fitting clothing.
      4. Avoid scratching.

TABLE 1–3. **Cutaneous Reactions Associated With Pruritus**

Cutaneous Reaction	Nursing Assessment	Management
Acral Erythema A painful, erythematous, edematous, and potentially pruritic rash on the palmar surfaces of the hands and plantar surfaces of the feet General progression to bulla formation, desquamation, and reepithelialization	Assess for risk factors: high-dose cytarabine, bleomycin, fluorouracil, doxorubicin, cyclophosphamide, methotrexate, and mercaptopurine Inspect palmar and plantar surfaces each shift for sensation, color, and movement Monitor for signs and symptoms of infection Assess for pain, pruritus, discomfort	Apply cold compresses to affected areas to relieve pain Elevate the affected areas to reduce edema Apply steroid creams Administer pyridoxine 50 mg TID as ordered
Inflammation of Keratoses Inflammation of actinic keratoses Pruritus and erythema may be noted adjacent to previous actinic keratoses.	Assess for risk factors: history of actinic keratoses; chemotherapy (fluorouracil, dacarbazine, dactinomycin, doxorubicin, pentostatin) Assess skin of potentially affected areas: face, arms, hands, and upper chest Assess for pain, pruritus, discomfort.	Report skin changes to the physician. Apply skin care products for comfort.
Radiation Enhancement A synergistic effect of concurrent radiation therapy and chemotherapy, which augments the effects of the radiation May involve cutaneous edema, erythema, blisters, erosions, ulceration, or hyperpigmentation in radiated field	Assess for radiation enhancement risk factors: may only occur if chemotherapy administered within 1 week of radiation therapy, associated with dactinomycin, doxorubicin, bleomycin, hydroxyurea, fluorouracil, and methotrexate Assess for radiation recall risk factors: combined chemotherapy and radiation therapy, most frequently associated with doxorubicin and dactinomycin Observe for dry desquamation (dry, scaling skin) in former irradiated sites	Instruct patient to avoid trauma and irritation to the affected area Apply cool wet compresses with acute reactions. Apply topical steroids (usually 0.25%) BID or TID as ordered Use water-soluble lubricants and aloe-based products over area Use mild astringent soaks such as Domeboro solution (Miles Laboratories). Débride ulcerated areas and apply an antimicrobial ointment and a nonadherent dressing over the area

Radiation Recall

An inflammatory reaction occurring in previously irradiated tissue

May occur in the skin, lung, gastrointestinal tract and heart

See Radiation Enhancement.

Drug Reaction

Characterized by a generalized macular, papular rash

Rash may appear on the trunk, extremities, face, and/or hands

Review cancer treatment regimen to assess for potential cause: chemotherapy (aminoglutethimide commonly causes a pruritic rash), biologic therapy (most commonly interleukin-2)

Review supportive therapy: antibiotics, antifungals, opioids

Discontinue suspected drug as ordered. Note: more common to manage pruritic rash with cancer therapy; more common to discontinue antibiotics and antifungals

Administer antihistamines as ordered

Administer corticosteroids as ordered

Increase medications at bedtime because pruritus typically increases at night

See Radiation Enhancement.

Modified from Powel, L., Fishman, M., Mrozek-Orlowski, M. (eds.). (1996). *Cancer Chemotherapy Guidelines and Recommendations for Practice*. Pittsburgh: Oncology Nursing Society.

    D. Use skin care products that promote comfort.
       1. Medicated baths with antipruritics.
       2. Local anesthetic creams.
       3. Emollient lotions.
IV. Measures to protect client from potential sequelae.
    A. Use massage, pressure, and rubbing as alternatives to scratching.
    B. Cut the fingernails short and file smooth.
    C. Instruct others about the importance of good handwashing.
    D. Assess the pruritic areas for signs of infection.

Evaluation

The oncology nurse systematically and regularly evaluates the client's and/or family's responses to interventions to determine progress toward the achievement of expected outcomes. Relevant data is collected and actual findings are compared with expected findings. Nursing diagnoses, outcomes, and plans of care are reviewed and revised as necessary.

SLEEP DISORDERS

Theory

   I. Definition.
    A. Sleep—natural suspension of consciousness during which the processes of the body are restored.
    B. Sleep disorder—interruption in the amount or quality of sleep: inability to go to sleep, stay asleep, sleep long enough, and feel restored and relaxed upon awakening.
  II. Risk factors.
    A. Disease-related factors.
       1. Presence of concurrent symptoms such as pain, pruritus, fever, nausea, night sweats, shortness of breath, and fatigue.
       2. Hodgkin's disease, lymphomas in association with night sweats.
       3. Paraneoplastic syndromes with an associated increase in corticosteroid production.
       4. Electrolyte disturbances.
       5. Delirium, confusion, and altered mental status.
       6. Patients with brain tumors commonly experience sleep disorders.
    B. Treatment-related factors.
       1. Post-treatment pain syndromes.
       2. Chemotherapy—approximately 55% of patients experience a sleep disorder 2 days after chemotherapy administration.
       3. Medications—antimetabolites, steroids, analeptics used as adjuvants in pain management, dopamine antagonists (associated with extrapyramidal side-effects), and sedatives.
       4. Perimenopause and menopause that may be related to treatment; sleep disorder caused by a decreased estrogen level.
       5. Hospitalization—interruption of normal routine, increased intravenous or oral fluids, increased frequency of voiding.
    C. Lifestyle-related factors.
       1. With depression, early morning awakening is common.
       2. Stress and anxiety.

   3. Physical inactivity.
   4. Alcohol intake.
III. Principles of medical management.
   A. Medications to induce and maintain sleep: psychotropics, analgesics, sedatives, hypnotics, and antidepressants.
   B. Medications to provide pain and symptom management: analgesics, antihistamines, and muscle relaxants.

Assessment

   I. Clinical assessment.
   A. Usual pattern of sleep.
      1. Time when retiring to bed.
      2. Amount of time needed to fall asleep.
      3. Time(s) of awakening.
         a. Reason for awakening.
         b. Ability to return to sleep.
      4. Quantity and quality of daytime naps.
      5. Exercise patterns.
   B. Sleeping environment.
      1. Light and noise factors.
      2. Room temperature.
      3. Presence of a bed partner and potential disturbances.
   C. Bedtime routine.
      1. Exercise versus relaxation within 2 hours of retiring.
      2. Caffeine and alcohol intake in afternoon or evening.
      3. Food and fluid intake before retiring.
      4. Use of sleeping aids: medications, warm milk.
   D. Impact of insomnia on daily living: self-care, concentration, cognitive functioning, fatigue, mood, depression, restlessness, irritability, and anxiety.
   E. Family perception and involvement with the sleep disorder.
   F. Relationships with others, role performance alterations, and perceived reasons for inability to sleep.
   II. History and physical examination.
   A. Client observation—dark circles under the eyes, expressionless face, nystagmus, ptosis of the eyelids, frequent yawning, slurred speech, incorrect word usage.
   B. Sleep studies—polysomnography.

Nursing Diagnoses

   I. Sleep pattern disturbance.
   II. Fatigue.
   III. Anxiety.
   IV. Ineffective coping.

Outcome Identification

   I. Client states the risk factors of disease and treatment that may alter sleep patterns.
   II. Client identifies pharmacologic strategies to facilitate sleep.
   III. Client describes specific behavioral and cognitive interventions to promote sleep.
   IV. Client reports adequate sleep patterns.

Planning and Implementation

I. Measures to increase the knowledge base of the client and family.
   A. Inform the client about the need to report sleep disorders.
II. Measures to facilitate client and family coping.
   A. Teach the client and family stress management techniques.
   B. Provide the client with cognitive strategies to sleep.
      1. Counting and word games.
      2. Loading Noah's Ark with animals.
      3. Prayer.
      4. Turning thoughts into gray and black images.
   C. Educate the client about relaxation techniques such as progressive muscle relaxation and imagery for sleep induction.
   D. Encourage a restful environment beginning approximately 2 hours before bedtime.
III. Measures to maximize client comfort.
   A. Plan nursing interventions succinctly to prevent unnecessary interruption of sleep.
   B. Implement pain and symptom management interventions in a timely and appropriate manner to control pain and concurrent symptoms.
   C. Administer sleeping medications in a timely and appropriate manner (see Chapter 10).
   D. Provide a restful environment.
      1. Decrease light and noise factors.
      2. Maintain the client's preferred room temperature.
      3. Straighten and provide clean bed linens.
      4. Encourage the practice of a normal bedtime routine when the client is hospitalized: sleepwear, reading before bedtime, warm milk, medications.
   E. Provide or promote relaxation before bedtime.
      1. Bathing, massage, relaxation techniques, reading, television, small snack, and warm milk.
      2. Avoid eating large amounts of food, drinking caffeine and stimulants and excessive fluids.

Evaluation

The oncology nurse systematically and regularly evaluates the client's and/or family's responses to interventions to determine progress toward the achievement of expected outcomes. Relevant data is collected and actual findings are compared with expected findings. Nursing diagnoses, outcomes, and plans of care are reviewed and revised as necessary.

BIBLIOGRAPHY

Brant, J., Brumit, J., Forseth, J., et al. (1996). *Pain and Symptom Management in the Terminally Ill.* Billings, MT: Big Sky Hospice.
Breitbart, W., Bruera, E., & Lynch, M. (1995). Neuropsychiatric syndromes and psychological symptoms in patients with advanced cancer. *J Pain Symptom Manage 10*(2), 131–141.
Bruera, E., & Watanabe, S. (1994). Psychostimulants as adjuvant analgesics. *J Pain Symptom Manage 9*(6), 412–415.
Bunn, P.A., & Ridgway, E.C. (1993). Paraneoplastic syndromes. In V.T. DeVita, Jr., S. Hellman, & S.A. Rosenberg (eds.). *Cancer: Principles and Practice of Oncology* (4th ed.). Philadelphia: JB Lippincott, pp. 2026–2017.
Clark, J.C., McGee, R.F., & Preston, R. (1992). Nursing management of responses to the cancer experi-

ence. In J.C. Clark & R.F. McGee (eds.). *Core Curriculum for Oncology Nursing* (2nd ed.). Philadelphia: WB Saunders, pp. 80–91.

Collins, J.J., Grier, H.E., Kinney, H.C., et al. (1995). Control of severe pain in children with terminal malignancy. *J Pediatr 126,* 653–657.

DeSpain, J.D. (1992). Dermatologic toxicity. In M.C. Perry (ed.). *The Chemotherapy Source Book.* Baltimore: Williams & Wilkins, pp. 531–547.

Glaus, A. (1993). Assessment of fatigue in cancer and non-cancer patients and in healthy individuals. *Supportive Care in Cancer 1*(6), 305–315.

Goodman, M., Ladd, L.A., & Purl, S. (1993). Integumentary and mucous membrane alterations. In S.L. Groenwald, M.H. Frogge, M. Goodman, & C.H. Yarbro (eds.). *Cancer Nursing: Principles and Practice* (2nd ed.). Boston: Jones & Bartlett, pp. 734–799.

Graydon, J.E., Bubela, N., Irvine, D., & Vincent, L. (1995). Fatigue-reducing strategies used by patients receiving treatment for cancer. *Cancer Nurs 18*(1), 23–28.

Hill, S., Sheidler, V., Foley, K., et al. (1993). *American Society of Clinical Oncology Conference on Cancer Pain: Cancer Pain Assessment and Treatment Curriculum Guidelines Teaching Syllabus and Slide Sets.* Pittsburgh: ASCO.

Irvine, D.M., Vincent, L., Graydon, J.E., et al. (1994). The prevalence and correlates of fatigue in patients receiving treatment with chemotherapy and radiotherapy. *Cancer Nurs 17*(5), 367–378.

McCaffery, M., & Beebe, A. (1989). *Pain: Clinical Manual for Nursing Practice.* St. Louis: C.V. Mosby.

Nail, L.M., & Winningham, M.L. (1993). Fatigue. In S.L. Groenwald, M.H. Frogge, M. Goodman, & C.H. Yarbro (eds.). *Cancer Nursing: Principles and Practice* (2nd ed.). Boston: Jones & Bartlett, pp. 608–618.

Paice, J.A., Jacox, A., Ferrell, B., et al. (1994, September/October). The AHCPR cancer pain clinical practice guidelines: Implications for oncology administrators. *J Oncol Manage 4,* 37–42.

Powel, L., Fishman, M., & Mrozek-Orlowski, M. (eds.). (1996). *Cancer Chemotherapy Guidelines and Recommendations for Practice.* Pittsburgh: Oncology Nursing Society.

Reddy, S., & Patt, R.B. (1995). The benzodiazepines as adjuvant analgesics. *J Pain Symptom Manage 9*(8), 510–514.

Richardson, A. (1995). Fatigue in cancer patients: A review of the literature. *Eur J Cancer Care 4*(1), 20–32.

Robinson, R., Preston, D., Schiefelbein, M., & Baxter, K.G. (1995). Strontium 89 therapy for the palliation of pain due to osseous metastases. *JAMA 274*(5), 420–424.

Shannon, M.M., Ryan, M.A., D'Agostino, N., & Brescia, F.J. (1995). Assessment of pain in advanced cancer patients. *J Pain Symptom Manage 10*(4), 274–278.

Skalla, K.A., & Rieger, P.T. (1995). Fatigue. In P.T. Rieger (ed.). (1995). *Biotherapy: A Comprehensive Overview.* Boston: Jones & Bartlett, pp. 221–242.

Stevens, P.E., Dibble, S.L., & Miaskowski, C. (1995). Prevalence, characteristics, and impact of postmastectomy pain syndrome: An investigation of women's experiences. *Pain 61,* 61–68.

Stewart, A., Hays, R., Wells, K., et al. (1994). Long-term functioning and well-being outcomes associated with physical activity and exercise in patients with chronic conditions in the medical outcomes study. *J Clin Epidemiol 47,* 719–730.

Watson, C.P.N. (1994). Antidepressant drugs as adjuvant analgesics. *J Pain Symptom Manage 9*(6), 392–405.

Winningham, M.L., Nail, L.M., Burke, M.B., et al. (1994). Fatigue and the cancer experience: The state of the knowledge. *Oncol Nurs Forum 21*(1), 23–36.

2

Coping: Psychosocial Issues

Patricia M. Grimm, RN, PhD, CS-P

EMOTIONAL DISTRESS

Theory

I. Definition—a pattern of expected changes in thinking, feelings, and behaviors that occur in response to the diagnosis, prognosis, treatment, and events that occur in the clinical course of cancer.
   A. Changes are related to a specific stressor or stressors and to diagnosis and treatment of cancer.
   B. Duration of feelings not as long and intensity of feelings not as severe as with clinical anxiety or depression.
II. Risk factors—issues influencing emotional response to cancer.
   A. Disease-related and treatment-related.
      1. Site, stage, and clinical course.
      2. Nature of dysfunction and symptoms produced.
      3. Treatment required (i.e., surgery, chemotherapy, radiotherapy, combined modalities, bone marrow transplant [BMT], biologic response modifiers).
      4. Rehabilitative options.
      5. Psychological management by the health care team.
   B. Situational.
      1. Social attitudes about cancer, its stigma, and the meaning attached.
      2. Nature and availability of social supports: family, friends, affiliated groups.
      3. Changes in family communication, roles, functional responsibilities.
   C. Developmental.
      1. Age-specific developmental life tasks threatened or disrupted by cancer.
      2. Personality, prior coping ability in response to major life stresses.
III. General treatment approaches.
   A. Individual or family psychotherapy.
   B. Spiritual counseling.
   C. Cognitive and behavioral interventions, such as support groups, relaxation training, guided imagery.
   D. Occupational or recreational therapy.
   E. Pharmacologic management of symptoms with sedatives, anxiolytics, and/or antidepressants.
IV. Potential sequelae of emotional distress.
   A. Chronic emotional distress.

B. Development of major psychiatric disorders: anxiety or depression, with risk for suicide.

C. Somatic symptoms such as gastrointestinal disturbances, headaches, dizziness, chest pain, and insomnia.

D. Interference with performance at home, school, or work.

E. Decreased compliance with the recommended treatment regimen.

Assessment

I. History.
  A. Presence of risk factors.
  B. Presence of discomforting thoughts, feelings and behaviors—nervousness, worry, jitteriness, tearfulness, hopelessness, difficulty concentrating, social withdrawal, difficulties with school and work.

II. Pattern of emotional distress.
  A. Onset; frequency; intensity; associated symptoms; precipitating, aggravating, and alleviating factors.
  B. Duration—not considered major psychiatric disorder if it is assessed as a normally expected response to current stressors and it is episodic in nature.

III. Perceived effect on client and family functioning—physical, lifestyle, interpersonal, work, or school.

Nursing Diagnoses

I. Impaired adjustment.
II. Ineffective individual coping.
III. Fear.
IV. Altered role performance.
V. Self-esteem disturbance.
VI. Impaired social interaction.

Outcome Identification

I. Client verbalizes knowledge of cancer diagnosis and treatment.
II. Client identifies expected symptoms and side effects of the disease and its treatment.
III. Client verbalizes emotional responses to cancer diagnosis and treatment.
IV. Client identifies personal strengths and support systems available for managing emotional distress.
V. Client makes decisions and follows through with appropriate interventions to manage emotional distress.

Planning and Implementation

I. Interventions to minimize risk and severity of emotional distress.
  A. Discuss concerns that may be precipitating emotional distress.
  B. Discuss the meaning of disease and treatment to client.
  C. Provide teaching regarding cancer diagnosis, treatment, and expected outcomes to reduce fear of the unknown.
  D. Explore past coping responses to stressful events and support use of those responses that have been successful in the past.

E. Inform of appropriate resources for emotional distress management—psychotherapy, support groups, relaxation training.

F. Support use of support groups, relaxation, psychotherapy.

II. Interventions to maximize comfort during emotional distress.

A. Provide a comfortable, supportive environment.

B. Allow the client to ventilate thoughts, feelings, and fears.

C. Listen attentively, conveying honesty and empathy.

D. Encourage use of self-help interventions, such as relaxation, distraction, or exercise.

III. Interventions to monitor for complications related to emotional distress.

A. Observe for somatic symptoms and discuss treatment with the health care team.

B. Observe for indications of major psychiatric disorders: anxiety, depression, risk for suicide.

C. Observe for untoward effects of pharmacologic management of symptoms—sedatives, anxiolytics, and/or antidepressants.

D. Report indications of psychiatric disorders and untoward effects of medications to the appropriate member of the health team.

E. Monitor compliance with the recommended treatment regimen.

IV. Interventions to enhance adaptation and rehabilitation.

A. Provide ongoing teaching regarding the client's treatment plan and expected responses.

B. Promote ongoing discussion of the client's thoughts, feelings, and fears regarding diagnosis and treatment.

C. Provide positive feedback for use of alternative coping approaches that lessen emotional distress, such as relaxation, distraction, exercise.

D. Implement strategies to manage symptoms and side effects of cancer and treatment, and psychotropic medications.

V. Interventions to increase client and family involvement with care.

A. Assist family members to identify experiences and thoughts that result in emotional distress.

B. Provide teaching regarding the client's and family's role in the client's care—encourage a sense of control over these aspects of the treatment plan.

C. Instruct the client and family in recreational and diversional outlets for emotional energy.

D. Provide information on educational materials and community resources available through the American Cancer Society, National Cancer Institute, and other hospital programs and community agencies (See Chapter 8).

Evaluation

The oncology nurse systematically and regularly evaluates the client's and/or family's responses to interventions to determine progress toward the achievement of expected outcomes. Relevant data is collected and actual findings are compared with expected findings. Nursing diagnoses, outcomes, and plans of care are reviewed and revised as necessary.

ANXIETY

Theory

I. Definition—a state of feeling uneasy and apprehensive in response to a vague, nonspecific, or unidentifiable threat.

II. Risk factors.
   A. Disease-related.
      1. Uncertainty of prognosis and/or social stigma of diagnosis.
      2. Inadequate symptom control—pain, insomnia, nausea and/or vomiting.
      3. Abnormal metabolic states—hypoxia, pulmonary embolus, sepsis, delirium, hypoglycemia, bleeding, heart failure.
      4. Hormone-secreting tumors.
      5. Recurrence of disease.
      6. Progression of disease—paraneoplastic syndrome, cachexia.
   B. Treatment-related.
      1. Prolonged treatment regimen and hospitalization.
      2. Intensive therapy—mutilative surgery, combination therapy, bone marrow transplantation.
      3. Anxiety-producing drugs—corticosteroids, neuroleptics used as antiemetics, thyroxine, bronchodilators, β-adrenergic stimulants.
      4. Untoward effects or side effects—alopecia, immunosuppression.
      5. Failure or termination of therapy.
   C. Lifestyle and situational.
      1. Disease-related losses—health, status, finances, family relationships and roles, social interaction.
      2. Exposure to the new situations and relationships of cancer treatment.
      3. Excessive intake of caffeine and nicotine.
      4. Withdrawal from alcohol and narcotic or sedative-hypnotic drugs.
   D. Developmental.
      1. Preexisting anxiety disorder—generalized anxiety, phobias, panic attacks, post-traumatic stress.
      2. Low self-esteem or intense fears in childhood.
      3. Blocked age-specific expectations, needs, or goals.
III. General treatment approaches.
   A. Individual or family psychotherapy.
   B. Pharmacologic management with anxiolytics such as benzodiazepines, antidepressants (see Chapter 10).
   C. Cognitive and behavioral interventions—biofeedback, relaxation training, guided imagery, support groups.
   D. Occupational or recreational therapy—diversional activities, exercise.
IV. Potential sequelae of anxiety.
   A. Somatic symptoms—nausea, vomiting, headaches, gastrointestinal distress.
   B. Behavioral—substance use, eating disturbances, self-destructive activities.
   C. Cognitive changes—problems with concentration and decision making, memory difficulties, disorientation.
   D. Chronic anxiety disorders—generalized anxiety, panic attacks, phobias, obsessive-compulsive disorder.
   E. Psychosomatic illnesses—gastric ulcers, colitis, migraine headaches.
   F. Interference with performance at home, school, or work.

Assessment

I. History.
   A. Presence of risk factors.

    B. History of defining characteristics of anxiety.
      1. Physical—flushing, sweating, tenseness, tremors, pacing, overactivity or immobility, changes in weight (loss or gain), changes in sleep patterns (insomnia, hypersomnia), shortness of breath, vomiting, diarrhea, muscle aches, feelings of heaviness, headaches, dry mouth, palpitations, decreased hearing or visual acuity.
      2. Emotional—irritability, feeling "keyed up," cries easily, self-doubting and blaming.
      3. Cognitive and behavioral—changes in perceptual field (hypervigilant or narrowly focused), difficulty with problem solving and decision making, compulsiveness, anger, withdrawal.
    C. Patterns of anxiety—past experiences; onset; frequency; severity; associated symptoms; precipitating, aggravating, and alleviating factors.
    D. Previous responses to anxiety, perceived effectiveness of these responses (constructive, destructive).
    E. Anxiety management strategies used—medication, relaxation, biofeedback, psychotherapy.
    F. Perceived effect of anxiety on client and family functioning—physical, lifestyle, interpersonal, work or school.
  II. Symptoms and signs
    A. Appearance and behavior—flushed face, tense or worried expression, restlessness, signs of nail-biting, sweating.
    B. Neurologic—poor concentration and memory, decreased interest in usual activities, irritability, dizziness, weakness, exhaustion, fine tremors, insomnia, nightmares, headaches, drowsiness.
    C. Other physical symptoms and signs—palpitations, elevated blood pressure, hyperventilation, dyspnea, anorexia, heartburn.
  III. Laboratory findings.
    A. Increased blood sugar level.
    B. Increased epinephrine level.

Nursing Diagnoses

  I. Anxiety.
  II. Ineffective individual coping.
  III. Fatigue.
  IV. Altered nutrition: less than, or more than, body requirements.
  V. Pain.
  VI. Sleep pattern disturbance.

Outcome Identification

  I. Client identifies anxiety-provoking situations and responses.
    A. Identifies sources of anxiety.
    B. Ventilates feelings of anxiety to others.
    C. Identifies effective and ineffective coping responses.
    D. Discusses the disease and treatment accurately.
  II. Client participates in anxiety-reducing interventions.
    A. Describes methods to decrease feelings of anxiety.
    B. Omits or limits alcohol, caffeine, and nicotine intake.
    C. Complies with pharmacologic and/or behavioral interventions.
    D. Identifies support systems within the family and community.

Planning and Implementation

I. Interventions to minimize risk and severity of anxiety.
  A. Use of interpersonal skills related to management of anxiety.
    1. Use a calm, reassuring approach.
    2. Listen attentively.
    3. Help the client identify situations that precipitate anxiety.
    4. Seek to understand the client's perspective of a stressful situation.
    5. Encourage verbalization of feelings, perceptions, and fears.
    6. Explore similarities between the present situation and successful resolution of problems in the past.
  B. Institute measures to enhance management of anxiety.
    1. Provide factual information concerning diagnosis, treatment, and prognosis.
    2. Explain all procedures, including sensations likely to be experienced during the procedure.
    3. Use diversional activities or relaxation techniques as appropriate.
    4. Administer prescribed medications to reduce anxiety.
II. Interventions to maximize client safety with anxiety.
  A. Assess the level of the client's anxiety.
  B. Provide a safe, supportive, and predictable environment.
  C. Stay with the client to promote safety and reduce fear.
  D. Assist with self-care as needed.
  E. Refrain from asking the client to make decisions during high anxiety states.
  F. Set limits to minimize risks to the client.
  G. Report critical changes in the results of client assessment to the appropriate health team member.
    1. Panic attacks.
    2. Withdrawal, noncompliance with cancer therapeutic regimen.
    3. Untoward effects of anxiolytic drug therapy.
    4. Abrupt discontinuance of anxiolytics.
    5. Suicidal attempts or ideation.
III. Interventions to monitor for complications related to anxiety and its treatment.
  A. Observe for severe anxiety reactions—panic attacks, decreased level of orientation, concentration, hallucinations, "fight or flight" responses of anger, hyperactivity.
  B. Observe for untoward effects of anxiolytic medications—dry mouth, drowsiness, dizziness, memory losses.
  C. Observe for symptoms of withdrawal if use of anxiolytics is abruptly discontinued.
IV. Interventions to enhance adaptation and rehabilitation.
  A. Discuss possible secondary gains of anxious behavior.
  B. Discuss interference with daily functioning regarding use or ineffective coping responses—overeating, overactivity.
  C. Limit or discontinue intake of alcohol, caffeine, and nicotine.
  D. Promote sleep, with comfort measures and/or medications, balanced diet, and regular physical exercise.
  E. Implement strategies to manage side effects of anxiolytic and/or antidepressant medications.
    1. Dry mouth—fluid intake increase, frequent mouth care, use of sugarless gum or hard candies.
    2. Constipation—fluid intake increase, high-fiber diet, exercise.

    3. Blurred vision—will improve over time; new glasses should not be needed.
    4. Drowsiness—take medication at bedtime; symptom usually improves with time; caution about operating an automobile or other machinery.
    5. Dizziness—avoid rapid movements of the head and change positions slowly.
  V. Interventions to incorporate the client and family in care.
    A. Assist the client and family to identify feelings of anxiety, to discuss these feelings, and to seek support in their management.
    B. Instruct the client and family in the importance of recreational and leisure activity outlets for emotional energy.
    C. Provide information on resources for support in managing anxiety—individual and/or family therapy, crisis intervention hotlines, emergency rooms, support groups and programs such as I Can Cope, or CanSurmount.

Evaluation

The oncology nurse systematically and regularly evaluates the client's and/or family's responses to interventions to determine progress toward the achievement of expected outcomes. Relevant data is collected and actual findings are compared with expected findings. Nursing diagnoses, outcomes, and plans of care are reviewed and revised as necessary.

DEPRESSION

Theory

  I. Definition—a state of feeling sad, discouraged, hopeless, and worthless, which may vary from transient emotional distress to a major psychiatric illness with possible suicidal ideation.
    A. Primary symptoms are depressed mood and loss of interest or pleasure.
    B. Symptoms have persisted over the same 2-week period.
    C. Symptoms represent a change from the previous level of functioning.
    D. Important to differentiate from delirium, which has an acute onset, induces impaired cognitive function, and typically waxes and wanes.
  II. Risk factors.
    A. Disease-related.
      1. Type of cancer—lung, pancreas, central nervous system.
      2. Differences in prognosis with different types of cancer—lung and pancreas versus skin and cervical.
      3. Status of cancer—stage, recurrence, progression.
      4. Inadequate symptom control, particularly pain.
    B. Treatment-related.
      1. Prolonged or difficult treatment.
      2. Medications—corticosteroids, chemotherapeutic agents, antihypertensives, benzodiazepines, β-blockers (propranolol), opiates, estrogens.
    C. Other medical conditions—anemia, alcoholism, hypertension, electrolyte abnormalities.
    D. Situational and developmental:
      1. History of depression (client or family).
      2. History of suicide attempts (client or family).
      3. History of, or concurrent, substance abuse.
      4. Perceived or actual loss of personal control.

  5. Cumulative crises in family or crises related to illness.
  6. Perceived, or actual, lack of social support.
  7. Changes in family and social roles and relationships.
III. General treatment approaches.
  A. Treatment of underlying medical conditions.
  B. Modification of pharmacologic influences.
  C. Individual or family psychotherapy.
  D. Pharmacologic management of depression with antidepressants, stimulants; management of other symptoms (insomnia, restlessness) with anxiolytics, sedatives.
  E. Cognitive and behavioral interventions, such as support groups, relaxation, cognitive restructuring.
  F. Occupational or recreational therapy: diversional activities, exercise.
IV. Potential sequelae of depression.
  A. Somatic problems related to changes in appetite and sleep patterns.
  B. Severe psychological regression, loss of function, somatic delusions.
  C. Suicidal ideation and/or attempts.
  D. Interference with the role of the client functioning at home, work, or school.
  E. Decreased compliance with the recommended medical regimen.

Assessment

  I. History
  A. Presence of risk factors.
  B. Presence of five or more of the defining symptoms of depression.
    1. Depressed mood (feeling sad or tearful).
    2. Decreased interest or pleasure in activities.
    3. Weight loss or gain, increased or decreased appetite.
    4. Insomnia or hypersomnia.
    5. Psychomotor agitation or retardation.
    6. Fatigue, loss of energy.
    7. Sense of worthlessness or excessive guilt.
    8. Decreased concentration, indecisiveness.
    9. Recurrent thoughts of death.
  C. Presence of delirium as the etiology of depression-like symptoms.
  D. Patterns of symptoms of depression—previous history, onset, frequency, severity, associated symptoms, and precipitating, aggravating, and alleviating factors.
  E. Presence of suicidal ideation, suicide plan, means to accomplish the plan.
  F. Perceived effectiveness of strategies to relieve symptoms.
  G. Perceived meaning of depression for the client and family.
  H. Perceived effect of depression on client and family functioning—physical, lifestyle, interpersonal, work, or school.
  II. Symptoms and signs.
  A. Appearance and behavior—flat affect, lack of spontaneity, changes in eye contact (consider cultural differences), slowed speech or minimal verbalizations, inactivity or agitation.
  B. Emotional and cognitive—crying, labile emotions; verbalization of self-reproach, pessimism, guilt, hopelessness; problems with concentration and decision making.

III. Laboratory or measurement findings.
  A. Changes in cortisol levels.
  B. Mental status examination changes may be indicative of delirium, not depression.

Nursing Diagnoses

  I. Individual ineffective coping.
  II. Fatigue.
  III. Hopelessness.
  IV. Altered nutrition: less than, or more than, body requirements.
  V. Pain.
  VI. Altered role performance.
  VII. Self-esteem disturbance.
  VIII. Sleep pattern disturbance.
  IX. Social isolation.

Outcome Identification

  I. Client describes personal risk factors for depression.
  II. Client lists strategies to decrease risks or complications of depression.
  III. Client identifies signs and symptoms of depression.
  IV. Client and family discuss the impact of depression on patient and family functioning—physical, emotional, and social; at home, work or school.
  V. Client and family identify personal, family, community, and professional resources to meet the crises of cancer experience that result in a depressed state.
  VI. Client and family discuss situations that require professional interventions.
  A. Acute changes in ability to control physical and psychological responses.
  B. Rapid deterioration of physical status.
  C. Indications of suicidal ideation or attempts.
  VII. Client participates in recommended treatment interventions for depression.

Planning and Implementation

  I. Interventions to minimize risk of symptom occurrence and severity of depression.
  A. Enhance client and family sense of control by informing them of the diagnosis and treatment or of changes in diagnosis and treatment and by offering choices in treatment and self-care when possible.
  B. Spend time with the client—listen, communicate acceptance.
  C. Validate thoughts, feelings, and self-perceptions as needed.
  D. Encourage the client to express feelings and ask for help when needed.
  E. Foster communications between client, family, and health team by formulating a list of concerns, facilitating care conferences, or other strategies.
  F. Initiate appropriate symptom management—pain (Chapter 1), sleep disturbances (Chapter 1), nausea and vomiting (Chapter 13).
  G. Assist the client and family to redefine their goals and self-beliefs in terms of the reality of the disease, treatment, and resources,
  H. Initiate referrals to spiritual, occupational, and psychological resources, when appropriate.
  II. Interventions to maximize client safety and comfort.
  A. Assess the client's mental status to rule out delirium as the causative factor for symptoms.

B. Attend to dietary needs and activities of daily living if the client is extremely withdrawn or apathetic.

C. Consider all discussions of suicide as serious and report them to appropriate members of the health team.

D. Review medications for any contribution to depressive symptoms—corticosteriods, chemotherapeutic agents, antihypertensives, benzodiazepines, β-blockers, opiates, estrogens.

E. Monitor and report reactions to antidepressants, sedatives, and anxiolytics.

F. Caution the client against abrupt discontinuance of antidepressants, and caution against use of alcohol while taking these drugs.

G. Report critical changes in client behaviors to appropriate health care members.

   1. Marked changes in mood or interactions, either withdrawal or agitation.

   2. Weight changes—loss or gain of 10% or more of body weight.

   3. Cognitive and physiologic changes related to insomnia that impede functioning or progress.

III. Interventions to monitor responses to depression and its treatment.

A. Monitor physiologic changes that may explain somatic complaints.

B. Monitor for side effects or adverse reactions to antidepressants.

C. Observe for symptoms of withdrawal of antidepressants.

D. Monitor behavioral changes that indicate improvement or persistence of depression.

IV. Interventions to enhance adaptation and rehabilitation.

A. Assist with problem solving and information gathering.

B. Provide positive reinforcement for behaviors that approximate goal achievement.

C. Accept verbalized anger or negative feelings; try to avoid personalizing.

D. Teach and assist the client to manage side effects of antidepressants.

   1. Dry mouth—fluid intake increase, frequent mouth care, use of sugarless gum or hard candies.

   2. Constipation—increase fluid intake, high-fiber diet, exercise.

   3. Blurred vision—will improve over time; new glasses should not be needed.

   4. Drowsiness—take medication at bedtime, symptom usually improves with time; caution about operating an automobile or other machinery.

   5. Dizziness—avoid rapid movements of the head, and change positions slowly.

V. Interventions to increase client and family involvement with care.

A. Teach the client and patient to recognize the signs and symptoms of depression.

B. Initiate referral to self-help and support groups as appropriate.

C. Inform the client and family of telephone hotlines for crisis intervention.

D. Teach alternative coping strategies such as relaxation, music, or recreational activities.

E. Assist the client to focus energy constructively by participating in health care, verbalizing feelings, and instituting health promotion activities—sleep, diet, and exercise.

Evaluation

The oncology nurse systematically and regularly evaluates the client's and/or family's responses to interventions to determine progress toward the achievement

of expected outcomes. Relevant data is collected and actual findings are compared with expected findings. Nursing diagnoses, outcomes, and plans of care are reviewed and revised as necessary.

SPIRITUAL DISTRESS

Theory

  I. Definition—state of experiencing a disturbance in one's belief or value system that provides strength, hope, and meaning in life.
- A. Presence of a spiritual self allows transcendence of immediate circumstances, such as cancer and treatment.
- B. Cultural or ethnic background influences client and family perceptions of spiritual distress.
- C. May be misdiagnosed as psychological distress when it more correctly stems from a spiritual crisis of loss of faith or meaning.

  II. Risk factors.
- A. Disease-related and treatment-related.
  1. Site, stage, and clinical course.
  2. Nature of dysfunction and symptoms produced.
  3. Treatment required (i.e., surgery, blood transfusions, dietary restrictions, isolation).
- B. Situational.
  1. Conflict between client and family spiritual beliefs and prescribed treatment regimen.
  2. Hospital and treatment barriers to practicing spiritual rituals.
     - a. Restrictions of setting (e.g., isolation, intensive care).
     - b. Confinement to the bed or room, lack of privacy.
     - c. Lack of availability of special foods and usual diet.
     - d. Lack of understanding of, or opposition to, beliefs by family, peers, health care providers.
  3. Embarrassment at practicing spiritual rituals.
  4. Availability of spiritual resources.

  III. General treatment approaches.
- A. Spiritual counseling.
- B. Performance of spiritual rites or services by an appropriate spiritual leader.
- C. Maintenance of dietary restrictions.

  IV. Potential sequelae of spiritual distress.
- A. Decreased compliance with the recommended medical regimen.
- B. Loneliness and social isolation.
- C. Development of major psychiatric disorders: anxiety or depression, with a risk for suicide.

Assessment

I. History.
- A. Presence of risk factors.
- B. Presence of defining characteristics.
  1. Expresses concern with the meaning of life and death, suffering, or a belief system.
  2. Verbalizes inner conflict about beliefs and the relationship with a deity.
  3. Questions meaning of his or her own existence.
  4. Expresses anger toward religious representatives, God.

5. Questions moral or ethical implications of the treatment regimen.
6. Alterations of behavior or mood: anger, crying, withdrawal, preoccupation, anxiety, apathy.
C. Pattern of spiritual distress: onset; frequency; intensity; precipitation, aggravating, and alleviating factors.
D. Perceived effect of spiritual distress on client and family functioning—lifestyle, interpersonal, work, or school.

Nursing Diagnoses

I. Spiritual distress.
II. Hopelessness.
III. Potential for enhancement of spiritual well being.

Outcome Identification

I. Client continues spiritual practices not detrimental to health.
II. Client expresses decreased feelings of guilt, fear, and anxiety.
III. Client expresses satisfaction with spiritual condition.
IV. Health team states acceptance of the client's moral and ethical decisions.
V. Client experiences positive meaning of his or her existence within the present circumstances.

Planning and Implementation

I. Interventions to minimize risk and severity of spiritual distress.
   A. Eliminate or reduce barriers to spiritual practice.
      1. Provide privacy and quiet for daily prayers or other rituals.
      2. Contact the client's spiritual leader to clarify practices.
   B. Encourage spiritual practices not detrimental to health.
      1. Facilitate contacts with spiritual leaders and folk healers.
      2. Maintain the diet within spiritual restrictions when not contraindicated.
      3. Encourage spiritual practices and rituals.
      4. Contact the spiritual leader to meet with client.
   C. Be open to expressions of loneliness and powerlessness.
      1. Be available to listen and express empathy.
      2. Use values clarification to help the client identify beliefs and values.
      3. Assure the client that the nurse and others will be available to support the patient in time of suffering.
      4. Be open to the client's discussion of illness and/or death.
II. Interventions to maximize safety and comfort.
   A. Provide privacy and quiet for daily prayers and rituals and visits with spiritual leaders.
   B. Provide spiritual articles according to client preferences.
   C. Facilitate the client's use of meditation, prayer, and other religious traditions and rituals.
III. Interventions to monitor complications of spiritual distress.
   A. Encourage verbalization of thoughts and feelings regarding spiritual comfort.
   B. Assess the client for lessening or continuation of feelings of fear, guilt, or anxiety.
   C. Evaluate the client for development of major psychiatric disorders—anxiety, depression, and suicidal ideation.

    D. Report critical changes in emotional state to appropriate health team members—make appropriate referrals.

IV. Interventions to increase client and family involvement with care.

    A. Seek opinions and suggestions about spiritual needs from the client and family.

    B. Encourage the client and family to participate in spiritual practices together.

    C. Encourage the family to continue usual spiritual practices in the health care setting as much as possible.

    D. Discuss the treatment regimen with the client and family to identify potential areas of difficulty resulting from conflicts with spiritual beliefs.

    E. Encourage the family to participate in care of client in keeping with spiritual beliefs and practices.

    F. Discuss with the client and family the spiritual meaning illness has for them.

Evaluation

The oncology nurse systematically and regularly evaluates the client's and/or family's responses to interventions to determine progress toward the achievement of expected outcomes. Relevant data is collected and actual findings are compared with expected findings. Nursing diagnoses, outcomes, and plans of care are reviewed and revised as necessary.

LOSS OF PERSONAL CONTROL

Theory

    I. Definition—perception that one's own actions will not significantly affect an outcome; a perceived lack of control over certain events or situations that affect outlook, goals, and lifestyle.

    A. Each individual has a desire for control.

    B. Response to loss of personal control depends on the meaning of loss, the individual patterns of coping, personal characteristics, and the response of others.

   II. Risk factors.

    A. Disease-related.

      1. Lack of knowledge about the disease process or health status.

      2. Physiologic and psychological demands of disease.

      3. Perceived loss of part of the self.

      4. Progressive, debilitating disease.

    B. Treatment-related.

      1. Lack of knowledge about the treatment course, demands, and expected outcomes.

        a. Physiologic and psychological demands of treatment.

      2. Uncontrolled symptoms and side effects of treatment (i.e., pain, nausea and vomiting, fatigue).

      3. Loss of ability to perform daily activities and roles.

    C. Situational.

      1. Loss of ability to manage one's own health care.

      2. Loss of control in decision-making matters.

      3. Hospital or institutional limitations—control relinquished to others, no privacy, altered personal space, relocation for treatment.

      4. Ineffective interpersonal interactions.

   D. Developmental.
      1. Control highly valued as part of personality.
      2. Lifestyle of dependency.
      3. Age-specific considerations.
         a. Adolescent—dependence on peers, independence from family.
         b. Young adult—marriage, parenthood.
         c. Adult—adolescent children, signs of aging, career pressures.
         d. Elderly—retirement, sensory and motor deficits, losses.
III. General treatment approaches.
   A. Inclusion of the client and family in decision making about medical treatment and care.
   B. Individual or family psychotherapy.
IV. Potential sequelae of prolonged loss of personal control.
   A. Lowered self-esteem.
   B. Helplessness.
   C. Hopelessness.
   D. Development of depression.

Assessment

I. History.
   A. Presence of risk factors.
   B. Presence of subjective characteristics of loss of personal control.
      1. Expression of dissatisfaction over inability to control a situation—work, illness, prognosis, care, recovery.
      2. Expression of dissatisfaction or frustration with the negative impact of the inability to have control on outlook, goals, and lifestyle.
   C. Presence of objective characteristics of loss of personal control.
      1. Refusal or reluctance to participate in decision making.
      2. Refusal or reluctance to participate in activities of daily living.
      3. Refusal or reluctance to express emotions.
      4. Emotional responses may include apathy, resignation, withdrawal, uneasiness, anxiety, aggression.
      5. Responses to limitations on personal control may include attempts to circumvent limits, increased attempts to exercise control, ignoring of limits.
      6. Noncompliance with the medical treatment regimen.
   D. Perceived impact of loss of personal control on client and family activities of daily living, lifestyle, relationships, role responsibilities, work, or school.

Nursing Diagnoses

   I. Ineffective individual coping.
  II. Hopelessness.
 III. Personal identity disturbance.
  IV. Powerlessness.
   V. Altered role performance.
  VI. Self-esteem disturbance.

Outcome Identification

   I. Client describes personal risk factors for loss of personal control.
  II. Client participates in measures to minimize the risk, occurrence, severity, and complications of loss of personal control.

  III. Client identifies factors that can be controlled by self.
  IV. Nurse reports signs, symptoms, and complications of a loss of personal control to a member of the health care team.
   V. Client lists changes in his or her condition that require professional assistance in management.
     A. Lack of motivation to participate in self-care activities and the treatment regimen.
     B. Verbal expressions of intention to harm self.

Planning and Implementation

   I. Interventions to minimize the risk of occurrence, severity, or complications of a loss of personal control.
     A. Provide the client with information regarding disease, treatment, responses and hospital or clinic routines.
     B. Provide the client and family with opportunities to participate in decision-making about care.
     C. Identify factors that contribute to loss of personal control for the client.
     D. Provide consistent communications about changes in health status and the treatment regimen.
     E. Encourage client and family to express feelings related to living with cancer.
     F. Maintain personal articles, a call light, and a telephone within reach of client.
     G. Provide successful management of symptoms—pain, nausea and vomiting, sleep disturbances.
     H. Encourage the client to identify areas over which control can be maintained and to exercise decision-making skills in these areas.
  II. Interventions to monitor for complications related to loss of personal control.
     A. Elicit subjective responses of the client and family about satisfaction with amount of information received, interpersonal communications, and opportunities to participate in decision-making.
     B. Assess the client's level of participation in decision-making and information-seeking activities.
     C. Assess for outcomes of loss of personal control—hopelessness, depression, suicidal intentions.
     D. Report critical changes in assessment data to appropriate health team members—inability to participate in decision-making and health care, verbal expressions of despair, or suicidal intentions.
  III. Interventions to incorporate the client and family in care.
     A. Seek opinions and suggestions about care from the client and family members.
     B. Reinforce participation in decision making by the client and family members.
     C. Encourage the client and family to be responsible for portions of care, as appropriate for condition.

Evaluation

The oncology nurse systematically and regularly evaluates the client's and/or family's responses to interventions to determine progress toward the achievement of expected outcomes. Relevant data is collected and actual findings are compared with expected findings. Nursing diagnoses, outcomes, and plans of care are reviewed and revised as necessary.

LOSS AND GRIEF

Theory

I. Definitions.
  A. Loss—an experience in which an individual relinquishes a connection to a valued person, object, relationship, or situation.
    1. Loss can occur without death.
    2. Any loss can result in grief and mourning.
  B. Grief is the emotional response to loss; grief work is the adaptive process of mourning. Grief work is a process.
    1. Expressed as changes in thoughts, feelings, and behaviors experienced as a natural human response to an actual or perceived loss of a loved person, relationship, object, function, status, or identity.
    2. Affected by many factors—personality, loss history, intimacy of the lost relationship, and personal resources.

II. Risk factors.
  A. Disease-related and treatment-related.
    1. Diagnosis of cancer, poor prognosis, uncertain outcome, likelihood of recurrence.
    2. Perceived or actual changes in body structure and function—amputation, mastectomy, colostomy, alopecia, cachexia, cognition.
    3. Chronic pain.
  B. Situational and social.
    1. Loss of persons through death, divorce, or separation.
    2. Loss of objects such as pets, home, or possessions.
    3. Nature of the relationship with the lost person or object.
    4. Multiple losses or crises and unanticipated losses.
    5. Perceived or actual loss of, or inadequate, support system.
    6. Employment losses—demotion, firing, retirement, or bankruptcy.
  C. Developmental.
    1. Aging—loss of friends, occupation, function, home.
    2. Symbolic losses—hope, dreams, autonomy or independence, loss of normalcy owing to illness.
    3. History of psychiatric illness.

III. General treatment approaches.
  A. Individual or family psychotherapy.
  B. Spiritual counseling.
  C. Pharmacologic management of symptoms—anxiolytics, antidepressants, sedatives (see Chapter 10).
  D. Behavioral and cognitive interventions—support groups, relaxation training.
  E. Occupational or recreational therapy.

IV. Potential sequelae of loss and grief.
  A. Anticipatory grief—the experiencing of grief in response to an anticipated loss.
  B. Dysfunctional grief responses.
    1. Failure to resolve grief, resulting in detrimental activities.
      a. Prolonged denial of loss, preoccupation with images of the lost person or object, refusal to mourn.
      b. Lasting loss of normal patterns of behavior.
      c. Somatic symptoms—gastrointestinal disorders, shortness of breath, muscle tension.

2. Behavioral—abuse of substances; obsessive-compulsive behavior; phobias; difficulties with concentration, attention, and decision-making.
C. Development of psychiatric disorder—depression, suicidal ideation or attempts.

Assessment

I. History.
   A. Presence of risk factors.
   B. Presence of defining physical and emotional characteristics of loss and grief.
      1. Shock and disbelief—emotional and physical immobility and denial of loss.
      2. Developing awareness—crying, angry outbursts, shortness of breath, choked feelings, sighing, flashes of anguish, retelling the story, painful dejection, and changes in eating, sleeping, and sexual interest.
      3. Bargaining and restitution—idealizing the loss and contracting for reprieval or deliverance.
      4. Accepting the loss—reliving past experiences, preoccupation with thoughts of loss, painful void in life, crying, somatic symptoms, dreams or nightmares.
      5. Resolving the loss—establishing new relationships, planning for the future, recalling rich memories or past experiences, affirming oneself, and resuming previous roles.
II. Patterns of loss and grief response.
   A. Duration.
   B. Previous losses and patterns of resolution.
   C. Presence or potential for cumulative losses.
   D. Sociocultural factors that influence the grief response—ethnicity, spiritual beliefs, religion.
   E. Potential strengths and weaknesses that may facilitate or impede the grief process such as coping patterns, family patterns of interaction, social support system, availability of community resources.
III. Client and family knowledge and understanding of expected thoughts, feelings, and behaviors involved with loss and grief.
IV. Perceived meaning of the losses for the client and family.
V. Perceived effect of losses and grief on client and family functioning—roles, relationships, activities of daily living, work, or school.

Nursing Diagnoses

I. Anticipatory grieving.
II. Dysfunctional grieving.
III. Altered role performance.
IV. Altered family processes.
V. Sleep pattern disturbances.
VI. Risk for loneliness.

Outcome Identification

I. Client identifies perceived losses, significance of losses, and adaptive coping strategies.
II. Client and family discuss stages of the normal grief response.

III. Client and family describe personal strengths and resources for dealing with loss and grief.
IV. Client and family identify institutional and community resources to deal with loss and grief.

Planning and Implementation

I. Interventions to minimize risk of occurrence and severity of dysfunctional grief.
  A. Use interpersonal relationship skills appropriate to the stage of the grief process.
    1. Encourage talking about perceived or actual losses.
    2. Actively listen to subjective responses to losses.
    3. Provide a supportive, nonjudgmental atmosphere to facilitate expression of negative emotions and minimize feelings of guilt.
    4. Validate perceptions of responses.
    5. Give the client permission to grieve and to resolve the loss.
  B. Institute measures to facilitate coping.
    1. Assist the client to identify effective personal coping strategies.
    2. Teach relaxation techniques.
    3. Encourage participation in support groups.
    4. Refer for counseling as indicated.
    5. Give the client permission to resume past roles and establish new relationships.
  C. Identify a means to channel energy constructively.
II. Interventions to maximize client safety and comfort.
  A. Encourage the client to implement cultural, religious and social customs and rituals associated with loss and grief.
  B. Advocate avoidance of conditions that block resolution of the grief process: oversedation, closed communications, and social isolation.
  C. Report critical changes in behavior to appropriate members of the health care team:
    1. Oversedation.
    2. Withdrawal or social isolation.
    3. Extreme emotional reactions—guilt, anger, hostility, depression.
    4. Substance abuse—alcohol or other drugs.
    5. Expression of suicidal ideations.
III. Interventions to monitor for complications related to loss and grief.
  A. Monitor for weight changes—gain or loss.
  B. Monitor changes in sleep, rest, eating patterns.
  C. Assess for a decline in physical and psychosocial functioning.
  D. Observe for withdrawal from social relationships.
IV. Interventions to enhance adaptation and rehabilitation.
  A. Encourage expression of anticipatory grief.
  B. Allow the client and family to experience the discomforts of the loss within a supportive environment.
  C. Assist in identifying modifications that will be needed in lifestyle.
  D. Provide bereavement care to assist in resolving secondary losses, attend to unfinished business, and incorporate loss into life.
  E. Support progression through the personal grieving stages.
  F. Encourage referral for support groups or psychotherapy as indicated.

V. Interventions to incorporate the client and family in care.
  A. Use teaching aids on loss and grief.
  B. Encourage the client and family to discuss their thoughts and feelings with each other.
  C. Include the family in discussion and decisions as appropriate.
  D. Provide or refer the client and family to family counseling and bereavement care.

Evaluation

The oncology nurse systematically and regularly evaluates the client's and/or family's responses to interventions to determine progress toward the achievement of expected outcomes. Relevant data is collected and actual findings are compared with expected findings. Nursing diagnoses, outcomes, and plans of care are reviewed and revised as necessary.

SOCIAL DYSFUNCTION (CLIENT AND FAMILY)

Theory

  I. Definition—a state of being unable to interact effectively with one's social environment—family, work or school, and community.
    A. Effective reality testing, ability to solve problems, and various coping skills are necessary for the client and family to be socially functional.
    B. The client, or family, and the environment may contribute to social dysfunction. One may be able to function in one environment or situation but not in others.
    C. Family members interact in a variety of roles that result from individual and group needs: spouse, parent, sibling, teacher, friend. Illness of one member may cause significant changes, putting the family at risk for social dysfunction.
 II. Risk factors.
    A. Disease-related and treatment-related.
      1. Perceived or actual change in body structure or function.
      2. Untoward effects and side effects of treatment.
      3. Inadequate symptom control of pain, nausea and vomiting, fatigue.
      4. Chronicity of cancer.
    B. Situational.
      1. Social isolation, living alone.
      2. Language and/or cultural differences from the community and the health care environment.
      3. Prolonged treatment and hospitalization.
      4. History of substance abuse, violence, legal difficulties.
    C. Developmental.
      1. Poorly developed social and interpersonal skills.
      2. Age-related issues:
        a. Child and adolescent—altered appearance, separation from family.
        b. Adult—loss of ability to be employed.
        c. Elderly—retirement, death of spouse, friends.
      3. History of psychiatric disorder—anxiety, depression, antisocial personality, psychotic disorders, prior difficulties within the family or other interpersonal relationships.

   D. Family.
      1. Dysfunctional responses to the changing health status of family member.
      2. Dysfunctional responses to the role changes resulting from illness.
      3. Limited social support, a pattern of isolation from community, extended family, friends.
      4. Disruption of family routines due to illness.
      5. Changes in income—loss of a job, inadequate income.
      6. History of psychiatric illness or family dysfunction—depression, psychosis, violence, substance abuse, conflicting relationships, inadequate decision making and problem solving, legal difficulties.
III. General treatment approaches.
   A. Management of disease and treatment symptoms and their side effects.
   B. Individual, family, and group psychotherapy.
   C. Spiritual counseling.
   D. Social and financial counseling.
   E. Cognitive and behavioral interventions—behavior modification, relaxation training, support groups.
   F. Occupational and recreational therapy.
IV. Potential sequelae of social dysfunction.
   A. Caregiver burden—inability of family member to care for the client, changes in health of the caregiver.
   B. Social and emotional isolation of the client and family.
   C. Noncompliance with the medical treatment regimen.
   D. Interference with the client and family role while functioning at home, work, or school.
   E. Development of social deviant behavior—substance abuse, violence.
   F. Development of psychiatric disorders—anxiety, depression, suicidal ideation and/or attempts.
   G. Disruption of family relationships—separation, divorce.

Assessment

   I. History
   A. Presence of client risk factors.
   B. Presence of family risk factors.
  II. Presence of client behaviors or characteristics indicative of social dysfunction.
   A. Interpersonal patterns and skills.
      1. Egocentricity.
      2. Lack of self-care.
      3. Superficial relationships, blames others for interpersonal difficulties.
      4. Social isolation.
      5. Employment difficulties.
   B. Response to cancer diagnosis and treatment—anxiety, dependency, hopelessness.
   C. Support system.
      1. Living alone, alienation from family and friends.
      2. Lack of compliance with the treatment regimen.
   D. Coping skills
      1. Poor problem-solving and decision-making skills.
      2. Aggression, violence, substance abuse, legal difficulties.
      3. Psychiatric history—depression, suicidal ideation and/or attempts, antisocial personality, psychoses.

III. Presence of family characteristics or behaviors indicative of social dysfunction.
  A. Identification of family—developmental level, health status of members, caregiving abilities, current roles and relationships.
  B. Understanding of the cancer experience.
    1. Perceived threat of pain, disability, or death.
    2. Understanding of treatment and side effects.
    3. Beliefs regarding prognosis and the client's potential for regaining health.
  C. Meaning of the cancer experience.
    1. Perceived impact of cancer on family roles and relationships—role conflict, role strain, conflict, family violence.
    2. Perceived emotional impact of cancer—frustration, helplessness, guilt, grieving.
    3. Perceived impact on family decision-making and problem-solving—evaluation of effectiveness.
  D. Family resources.
    1. Limited or threatened financial resources—unemployment, social service agency involvement, insurance limitations.
    2. Limited social and emotional resources.
      a. Socially isolated.
      b. Estranged or troubled relationships with extended family.
      c. Minimal connection with community support systems (i.e., churches, social service agencies, neighborhood activities).
    3. Ineffective family coping.
      a. Family conflict and/or violence, substance abuse.
    4. Legal difficulties, involvement of social service agencies.

Nursing Diagnoses

  I. Ineffective individual coping.
 II. Ineffective family coping: compromised.
III. Altered family processes.
IV. Altered role performance.
 V. Impaired social interaction.

Outcome Identification

  I. Client describes the impact of disease and its treatment on the ability to function socially.
 II. Client identifies problematic effects that interfere with social functioning.
III. Client discusses strategies to promote more effective social functioning.
IV. Family verbalizes thoughts and feelings to health care team and each other regarding the illness of the family member and its effects on the family.
 V. Family participates in care of the ill family member in keeping with their desire and ability.
VI. Family discusses the stresses of caregiving and strategies to reduce such stress.
VII. Family maintains a functional system of support for each member of the family.
VIII. Family uses appropriate health agency, community, and other resources as needed.

Planning and Implementation

I. Interventions to minimize risk and severity of social dysfunction.
  A. Client-centered interventions.
    1. Instruct regarding disease, treatment regimen and expected responses, symptoms and side effects.
    2. Discuss effects of disease and treatment on the ability to function socially.
      a. Assist the client in managing disease-related and treatment-related stresses, including symptom management.
    3. Help the client identify how stress precipitates problems with social functioning.
    4. Encourage an increase in awareness of strengths and limitations in communicating to others, analyzing which approaches work best.
    5. Support appropriate interpersonal communication.
    6. Encourage respect for the rights of others—family members, friends, health team members.
    7. Encourage involvement in already established relationships.
    8. Encourage involvement in social and community activities.
    9. Refer to appropriate agencies and services for support of optimal social functioning—financial counseling, social services, community activities, support groups, psychiatric services, substance abuse programs.
  B. Family-focused interventions.
    1. Instruct regarding the disease, treatment regimen, and expected client responses—symptoms and side effects.
    2. Discuss the effect of the client's illness and treatment on family functioning—physical; emotional; role; activities at home, work, or school.
    3. Assist the family in managing stresses stemming from the client's illness.
    4. Encourage family members to discuss thoughts and feelings regarding the illness and its effects with each other and with the client.
    5. Encourage the family to continue relationships with others, including those who are extended family and friends, and to continue community activities.
    6. Support the family in maintaining functional family routines as much as possible.
    7. Refer the family to appropriate resources—support groups, financial counseling, social services, individual or family psychiatric services, substance abuse programs.
II. Interventions to maximize safety and comfort related to social function or dysfunction.
  A. Communicate empathy and understanding regarding the impact of diagnosis and treatment on social functioning.
  B. Establish limits on problematic client and family behaviors that interfere with social functioning.
    1. Social isolation, withdrawal.
    2. Lack of self-care, lack of compliance with treatment regimen.
    3. Inappropriate expressions of anger and violence.
    4. Substance abuse.
    5. Suicidal attempts and/or ideation.
  C. Provide positive feedback for compliance with limits on socially dysfunctional behavior.
  D. Report changes in behavior that threaten client and family social functioning to the appropriate health team members.

   III. Interventions to enhance adaptation and rehabilitation.
      A. Create a private and supportive care environment for the client and family.
      B. Assist the client and family in identifying their strengths in managing the demands of illness and its treatment.
      C. Discuss with the client and family the family's limitations in providing care for the client—risk of caregiver burden, available resources to assist with care.
      D. Identify, with the client and family, cultural and spiritual beliefs and practices that may be judged by others as interfering with social functioning.
      E. Educate the health care team as to cultural and spiritual beliefs and practices.
      F. Support family cohesiveness.
      G. Make appropriate referrals to needed agency and community resources.
   IV. Interventions to incorporate the client and family in care.
      A. Provide the client and family with knowledge and skills required for provision of day-to-day care.
      B. Facilitate family strengths related to care of the client.
         1. Acknowledge the family's ability to care for the client.
         2. Involve the family in care of the client as desired.
         3. Involve the family in the decision-making process with health team members regarding care.
      C. Encourage the client to participate in self-care within limits of the physical condition.
      D. Assess outcomes of caregiving activities—effects on caregiver, effects on social functioning of client and family members.

Evaluation

   The oncology nurse systematically and regularly evaluates the client's and/or family's responses to interventions to determine progress toward the achievement of expected outcomes. Relevant data is collected and actual findings are compared with expected findings. Nursing diagnoses, outcomes, and plans of care are reviewed and revised as necessary.

BIBLIOGRAPHY

American Psychiatric Association. (1994). *Diagnostic and Statistical Manual of Mental Disorders* (4th ed.). Washington, DC: American Psychiatric Association.
Carpenito, L.J. (1993). *Nursing Diagnosis: Application to Clinical Practice* (5th ed.). Philadelphia: JB Lippincott.
Carson, V. (1989). *Spiritual Dimensions of Nursing Practice.* Philadelphia: W.B. Saunders.
Chochinov, H. (1993). Management of grief in the cancer setting. In W. Breitbart & J. Holland (eds.). *Psychiatric Aspects of Symptom Management in Cancer Patients.* Washington, DC: American Psychiatric Press.
Chochinov, H., & Holland, J. (1990). Bereavement: A special issue in oncology. In J. Holland & J. Rowland (eds.). *Handbook of Psychooncology: Psychological Care of the Patient With Cancer.* New York: Oxford University Press.
Fincannon, J. (1995). Analysis of psychiatric referrals and interventions in an oncology population. *Oncol Nurs Forum 22*(1), 87–92.
Furhmann, J., & Carson, V. (1996). Shared attributes of every traveler: The mosaic of self-concept. In V.B. Carson & E.N. Arnold. *Mental Health Nursing: The Nurse-patient Journey.* Philadelphia: W.B. Saunders.
Germino, J., & O'Rourke, M. (1996). Cancer and the family. In B. McCorkle, M. Grant, M. Frank-Stromborg, & S. Baird (eds.). *Cancer Nursing: A Comprehensive Textbook.* Philadelphia: W.B. Saunders.
Given, B., & Given, W.C. (1996). Family caregiver burden from cancer care. In R. McCorkle, M. Grant, M. Frank-Stromborg, & S. Baird (eds.). *Cancer Nursing: A Comprehensive Textbook.* Philadelphia: W.B. Saunders.

Holland, J. (1990). Clinical course of cancer. In J. Holland & J. Rowland (eds.). *Handbook of Psychoon-cology: Psychological Care of the Patient With Cancer.* New York: Oxford University Press.

McCloskey, J.C., & Bulechek, G.M. (eds.). *Nursing Interventions Classification (NIC),* (2nd ed.). Balti-more MD: C.V. Mosby.

Massie, M.J. (1990). Depression. In J. Holland & J. Rowland (eds.). *Handbook of Psychooncology: Psychological Care of the Patient With Cancer.* New York: Oxford University Press.

Massie, M.J. (1990). Anxiety, panic and phobias. In J. Holland & J. Rowland (eds.). *Handbook of Psychooncology: Psychological Care of the Patient With Cancer.* New York: Oxford University Press.

Townsend, M. (1996). *Psychiatric Mental Health Nursing: Concepts of Care* (2nd ed.). Philadelphia: F.A. Davis.

Valente, S., Saunders, J., & Cohen, M. (1994). Evaluating depression among patients with cancer. *Cancer Prac 2*(1), 65.

Wise, M., & Rundell, J. (1994). *Concise Guide to Consultation Psychiatry* (2nd ed.). Washington, DC: American Psychiatric Press.

3

Coping: Altered Body Image and Alopecia

Beth A. Freitas, MSN, OCN

BODY IMAGE

Theory

I. Body image is an individual's self-perception of physical, personal, social, and moral-ethical self. It is a component of an individual's self-concept that affects sexuality.

II. Risk factors.
   A. Actual or perceived changes in body reality.
      1. Altered physiology—cachexia, cognitive dysfunction, sterility.
      2. Treatment and side effects—surgical scars or amputation, alopecia, weight gain, hormone changes, central lines.
      3. Pain and discomfort.
      4. Normal development—growth spurts, dependency with aging.
      5. Loss of control and unpredictable illness course—length of time since diagnosis and treatment and not returned to "normal."
   B. Actual or perceived changes in coping strategies.
   C. Actual or perceived changes in social network.
   D. Degree of visibility of body image change.

III. Principles of medical management.
   A. Preventive and reconstructive procedures to minimize disease or treatment effects (e.g., lumpectomy and radiation versus mastectomy, functional replacement of bladder versus ileal conduit).
   B. Prosthetic devices.
   C. Medications such as antianxiety drugs or antidepressants.
   D. Behavioral interventions such as self-help groups or relaxation therapy.
   E. Psychotherapy either as an individual or a group.

IV. Potential sequelae of disturbed body image.
   A. Depression.
   B. Suicide.
   C. Role abandonment or ineffectiveness.
   D. Social isolation and loneliness.
   E. Sexual dysfunction.
   F. Emotional distress-anxiety.

Assessment

I. Presence of risk factors.

II. Pertinent personal history.
   A. Number of stressful events preceding cancer diagnosis.
   B. History of depression.
   C. Perception of client before body image change regarding overall attractiveness, self-confidence, self-concept, and sexuality, and responses of significant others and work and social contacts regarding body image changes.
III. Physical, cognitive, and psychosocial assessment of defining characteristics of body image changes.
   A. Physical changes.
      1. Neglect or compulsive attention to self-care or grooming.
      2. Weight gain or loss.
      3. Insomnia or hypersomnia.
   B. Cognitive changes.
      1. Decreased attention span.
      2. Problems with concentration.
      3. Difficulty with problem solving and decision making.
   C. Psychosocial changes.
      1. Anorexia or increased appetite.
      2. Dysfunctional grieving (see Chapter 2).
      3. Expressions of self-doubt, self-negation, or fear of rejection.
      4. Hesitancy or discomfort in social interactions—avoidance of intimacy or social contact.
      5. Self-destructive behaviors such as self-neglect or alcoholism.
      6. Sexual dysfunction such as impotence or frigidity.
      7. Refusal to look at or assume responsibility for the changed body part or function (e.g., to view the mastectomy incision, care for a stoma, or wear a prosthesis).

Nursing Diagnoses

   I. Ineffective individual coping.
  II. Ineffective family coping.
 III. Personal identity disturbance.
  IV. Self-esteem disturbance.
   V. Altered sexuality patterns.
  VI. Social isolation.

Outcome Identification

   I. Client identifies losses, significance of losses, and adaptive coping strategies.
  II. Client discusses plans for reintegration of roles and social interactions.
 III. Client utilizes community resources to deal with changes and achieve maximal functioning.
  IV. Client identifies emergency resources to manage self-destructive behaviors.
   V. Client identifies opportunities for personal growth and self-help.

Planning and Implementation

   I. Interventions to minimize risk of occurrence or severity of body image disturbance.
   A. Provide an opportunity to discuss perceived losses and meaning to self and significant others.

    B. Give permission to grieve and to resolve losses.

    C. Allow the client to ventilate negative emotions such as anger and guilt.

    D. Monitor responses of professionals and significant others that imply rejection of the client or negative reactions to body changes.

    E. Educate the client about potential body image changes and reactions before treatment.

    F. Educate the client and family as to concerns related to body image changes approximately 6 to 10 months after surgical intervention. These concerns come after the issues of life and death are faced.

    G. Stress the temporary nature of some side effects.

II. Interventions to enhance adaptation and rehabilitation—prepare the client and family for changes in structure or function.

    A. Ensure participation in the informed consent and treatment decision-making processes.

    B. Initiate referral to client and family services such as United Ostomy Association, Reach to Recovery, or International Association of Laryngectomees before surgery.

    C. Assess readiness to view changes and assume responsibility for self-care.

    D. Adapt teaching to client readiness.

    E. Support the client and family during the initial viewing of changes:

        1. Provide literature, educational videos, audio tapes, resource referrals such as *I Can Cope, National Cancer Institute Information Line, American Cancer Society,* and *Look Good Feel Better Program,* and peer support resources such as *Reach to Recovery.*

        2. Initiate discharge planning that facilitates integration back into work or the school system.

        3. Provide resources for product and prosthesis sources.

III. Interventions to incorporate the client and family in care.

    A. Teach use of restorative devices and rehabilitation procedures.

    B. Observe client and family return demonstrations of self-care.

    C. Initiate home care referrals as needed for follow-up and rehabilitative care.

    D. Teach the client and family strategies to detect and manage self-destructive behaviors.

    E. Use active listening and nonjudgmental acceptance to facilitate discussion of concerns such as intimacy, resumption of sexual activity, and explanations to significant others.

    F. Encourage positive family coping behaviors: open communication, distraction, and humor.

Evaluation

    The oncology nurse systematically and regularly evaluates the client's and/or family's responses to interventions to determine progress toward the achievement of expected outcomes. Relevant data is collected and actual findings are compared with expected findings. Nursing diagnoses, outcomes, and plans of care are reviewed and revised as necessary.

ALOPECIA

Theory

    I. Alopecia is the loss of hair (scalp, facial, axillary, pubic, eyebrows, eyelashes, nasal, and body).

II. Risk factors.
  A. Treatment methods that have an affinity for rapidly dividing cells damage hair follicles, causing temporary or permanent hair loss.
  B. Radiation therapy dosage greater than 30–35 Gy may cause temporary hair loss, and dosage greater than 40 Gy may cause permanent hair loss in the area being treated.
  C. Hair loss associated with chemotherapy generally is temporary.
  D. Chemotherapeutic agents that cause alopecia are actinomycin, bleomycin, cyclophosphamide, dactinomycin, daunorubicin, doxorubicin, etoposide, 5-fluorouracil, hydroxyurea, methotrexate, mitomycin, mitoxantrone, melphalan, paclitaxel, vinblastine, and vincristine.
  E. Administration of multiple chemotherapy agents increases the chances of total alopecia.
III. Principles of medical management.
  A. No significant data exists that scalp hypothermia or scalp tourniquets decrease hair loss.
  B. Scalp hypothermia or scalp tourniquet increases the risk of scalp metastases.
IV. Potential sequelae of alopecia.
  A. Increased heat loss through scalp.
  B. Impaired self-concept.
  C. Decreased sexual and social interaction.
  D. Loss of eyelashes and nasal hair decreases the body's natural resistors.

Assessment

I. Pertinent personal history.
  A. Patterns of hair growth.
  B. Picture of current style and snip of hair to match color.
II. Physical examination.
  A. Thinning of hair or complete hair loss.
  B. Location of hair loss.
III. Psychosocial examination.
  A. Perceptions of client before and after hair loss about self-concept; body image; perceived sexuality; and responses of significant others, social and work acquaintances to hair loss.
  B. Decreased social interaction.

Nursing Diagnoses

I. Altered sexuality patterns.
II. Social isolation.
III. Ineffective individual coping.
IV. Body image disturbance.
V. Situational low self-esteem.

Outcome Identification

I. Nurse identifies the client's risk factors for alopecia.
II. Client describes potential patterns of hair loss and potential for hair regrowth.
III. Client discusses potential effects of alopecia on self-concept, body image, sexuality, and social interaction.

IV. Client identifies measures to prevent, minimize, and/or adapt to alopecia.

V. Client identifies community resources and insurance benefits available.

Planning and Implementation

I. Interventions to minimize the risk of symptom occurrence and severity of alopecia.
  - A. Provide anticipatory guidance related to hair loss.
    1. Provide information related to hair loss and regrowth.
       a. Hair loss occurs 2 to 3 weeks after treatment begins.
       b. Loss occurs over a period of days to weeks.
       c. Regrowth usually starts 6 to 8 weeks after completion of therapy.
       d. Color and texture of regrown hair may be different from hair growth before loss.
    2. Encourage clients to obtain scarves, turbans, caps, (cotton products let scalp breathe), and/or wigs before hair loss.
    3. Encourage clients to experiment with new hair styles and colors before hair loss.
  - B. Initiate measures to decrease hair loss.
    1. Wash hair less frequently with mild (pH-balanced) or dry shampoo, use cream rinse and a soft bristle brush.
    2. Avoid the use of permanents, hair coloring, hair spray, and excessive use of blow dryers, curling irons, and heated rollers.
  - C. Other measures to decrease side effects of hair loss.
    1. Shower cap to catch shedding hair.
    2. Ski cap or other head cover to prevent heat loss in cold climates.
    3. Large-brimmed hat or sun screen on the scalp, SPF 15 or greater, to protect from the sun.

II. Implement strategies to enhance adaptation and rehabilitation.
  - A. Identify community and personal resources such as insurance companies and the American Cancer Society for financial assistance with head coverings.
  - B. Refer to the *Look Good, Feel Better Program* of the American Cancer Society.
  - C. Encourage discussion of responses to alopecia among clients, significant others, and members of the health care team.
  - D. Fictional character helps children cope by the caregiver's placing a sample of hair under the pillow and during the night replacing it with a gift.

Evaluation

The oncology nurse systematically and regularly evaluates the client's and/or family's responses to interventions to determine progress toward the achievement of expected outcomes. Relevant data is collected and actual findings are compared with expected findings. Nursing diagnoses, outcomes, and plans of care are reviewed and revised as necessary.

BIBLIOGRAPHY

Bello, L.K., & McIntire, S.N. (1995). Body image disturbances in young adults with cancer. *Cancer Nurs* *18*(2), 138–143.
Bjerre, B.D., Johansen, C., & Steven, K. (1995). Health-related quality of life after cystectomy: Bladder substitution compared with ileal conduit diversion. A questionnaire survey. *Br J Urol* 75(2), 200–205.
Burt, K. (1995). The effects of cancer on body image and sexuality. *Nurs Times* 91(7), 36–37.
Clark, J.C., McGee, R.F., & Preston, R. (1992). Nursing management of responses to the cancer experi-

ence. In J.C. Clark & R.F. McGee (eds.). *Core Curriculum for Oncology Nursing* (2nd ed.). Philadelphia: W. B. Saunders, pp. 67–155.

Dow, K.H. (1995). A review of late effects of cancer in women. *Semin Oncol Nurs 11*(2), 128–136.

Fawzy, F.I., & Fawzy, N.W. (1994). A structured psychoeducational intervention for cancer patients. *Gen Hosp Psychiatry 16,* 149–192.

Freedman, T.G. (1994). Social and cultural dimensions of hair loss in women treated for breast cancer. *Cancer Nurs 17*(4), 334–341.

Held J.L., Osborne D.M., Volpe H., & Waldman, A.R. (1994). Cancer of the prostate: Treatment and nursing implications. *Oncol Nurs Forum 21*(9), 1517–1529.

Hubner, W.A., & Pfluger, H. (1995). Functional replacement of bladder and urethra after cystectomy for bladder cancer in a female patient. *J Urol 153,* 1043–1046.

Lamb, M.A., & Sheldon, T.A. (1994). The sexual adaptation of women treated for endometrial cancer. *Cancer Pract 2*(2), 103–113.

Mock, V., Burke, M.B., Sheehan P., et al. (1994). A nursing rehabilitation program for women with breast cancer receiving adjuvant chemotherapy. *Oncol Nurs Forum 21*(5), 899–907; discussion 908.

Ofman, U.S. (1995). Preservation of function in genitourinary cancers: Psychosexual and psychosocial issues. *Cancer Invest 13*(1), 125–131.

Pickard-Holley, S. (1995). The symptom experience of alopecia. *Semin Oncol Nurs 11*(4), 235–238.

Rhodes, V.A., McDaniel, R.W., & Johnson, M.H. (1995). Patient education: Self-care guides. *Semin Oncol Nurs 11*(4), 298–304.

Schover, L.R., Yetman, R.J., Tuason, L.J., et al. (1995). Partial mastectomy and breast reconstruction. *Cancer 75*(1): 54–64.

4

Cultural Issues

Joanne K. Itano, RN, PhD, OCN

Theory

   I. Demographics of the United States (U.S.) population have shifted dramatically with marked increases in the number of cultural minorities and elderly and economically disadvantaged persons experiencing cancer.
      A. Until recently, the cultural diversity of the U.S. was largely limited to Caucasian immigrants from Europe who made up the majority of the population.
      B. In the 1950s, nine out of 10 Americans were of European descent.
      C. In the 1990s, one out of every four adults and one out of every three children was of African, Latin American, or Asian origin.
   II. Oncology nursing practice reflects respect for the unique cultural background of the client and family.
      A. Nurse must provide culturally competent care.
         1. Care provided with an awareness and appreciation of the cultural differences between the caregiver and client.
         2. Care given is individualized. Caregivers respect the client's cultural background.
   III. Culture refers to the learned, shared, and transmitted values, beliefs, norms, and life ways of a particular group that guides their thinking, decisions, and actions in patterned ways.
      A. Although basic human needs are the same for all people, the way a person seeks to meet those needs is influenced by culture.
      B. The way culture influences behaviors, attitudes, and values depends on many factors and may not be the same for individual members of a cultural group.
   IV. Health care beliefs and practices of many cultural groups may not be congruent with those of mainstream, Westernized medicine.
      A. Conflicts and nonadherence may result because health professionals are commonly ethnocentric—the tendency to view people unconsciously by using one's group and one's own customs as the standard for all judgments.
      B. Important to avoid stereotyping, assuming that all members of the cultural group are alike.
      C. Overgeneralization is often a concern and must be avoided because enormous differences exist across cultural groups and within cultural groups.
      D. Health care system is also a subculture with its own rules, customs, and language.

V. Epidemiology.
   A. In 1996 about 1,359,150 cancers will be diagnosed.
      1. 136,380 (10%) will be among African Americans.
      2. 38,000 (2.7%) among other minority Americans.
   B. Tables 4–1, 4–2, and 4–3 summarize the incidence, mortality, and 5-year
      survival rates among different cultural groups.
   C. Differences among cultural groups.
      1. African Americans include immigrants from African countries, the West
         Indies, the Dominican Republic, Haiti, and Jamaica.
         a. Constitute about 10% of the total U.S. population.
            (1) Represent about 1/3 of the population below the poverty line.
            (2) One fourth are unemployed.
            (3) Are disproportionately represented among the poor.
         b. Highest cancer incidence rate of all sites in comparison with other
            race and ethnic groups.
         c. Highest incidence rates of cancers of the esophagus, colon and rec-
            tum, pancreas, lung, and prostate.
         d. Highest mortality rates of cancers of the esophagus, colon and rec-
            tum, pancreas, uterus, cervix, oral cavity, and prostate.
         e. Second lowest 5-year survival rates due to later stage at diagnosis.
            (1) Often occurs at sites for which screening tests are available.
            (2) Early detection and timely treatment could increase survival
                rates.
      2. Hispanic is the umbrella term for persons of Mexican, Puerto Rican,
         Cuban, Caribbean, and Central and South American origin.
         a. Ranks in the middle for cancer incidence and mortality rates when
            compared with other race and ethnic groups.
         b. Has second highest incidence of gallbladder and pancreatic cancers
            and third highest rates for cervical, ovarian, prostate, and stomach
            cancers.
         c. Highest mortality rates for gallbladder cancer and second highest
            for pancreatic cancer.
      3. Asian and Pacific Islanders are the fastest growing cultural minority
         group in U.S., comprising those originating from 28 Asian countries
         and 25 identified Pacific Island cultures.
         a. Native Hawaiians have highest incidence rates for breast, stomach,
            uterine, and ovarian cancers.
         b. Japanese, Chinese, and Filipino Americans have overall lower cancer
            incidence and mortality rates.
         c. Japanese have high incidence rates for stomach and colorectal
            cancers.
         d. Chinese Americans have high incidence rates for oral cavity (naso-
            pharyngeal) and liver cancers.
         e. Filipino women have the highest incidence rates for thyroid cancer
            but have the lowest cancer mortality and incidence rates after Na-
            tive Americans.
      4. Native Americans, once called American Indians, include natives of
         the continental U.S., Aleuts, and Alaskan Eskimos.
         a. Lowest cancer incidence rates and second lowest cancer mortality
            rates.
            (1) Misleading because they have a shorter life expectancy.

TABLE 4-1. SEER Incidence Rates, 1988–1992, Selected Sites

Cancer Site	Alaska Native M	Alaska Native W	American Indian M	American Indian W	Black M	Black W	Chinese M	Chinese W	Filipino M	Filipino W	Hawaiian M	Hawaiian W	Japanese M	Japanese W	Korean M	Korean W	Vietnamese M	Vietnamese W	White M	White W	Hispanic (Total) M	Hispanic (Total) W
All sites	372	348	196	180	560	326	282	213	274	224	340	321	322	241	266	180	326	273	469	346	319	243
Brain and nervous system	*	*	*	*	4.5	3.4	3.1	2.1	3.6	2.8	*	*	2.1	*	*	*	*	*	7.8	5.4	5.2	3.8
Breast, invasive	*	78.9	*	31.6	1.2	95.4	*	55.0	*	73.1	*	105.6	*	82.3	*	28.5	*	37.5	0.9	111.8	0.6	69.8
Cervix uteri		15.8		9.9		13.2		7.3		9.6		9.3		5.8		15.2		43.0		8.7		16.2
Colon and rectum	79.7	67.4	18.6	15.3	60.7	45.5	44.8	33.6	35.4	20.9	42.4	30.5	64.1	39.5	31.7	21.9	30.5	27.1	56.3	38.3	38.3	24.7
Corpus uteri		*		10.7		14.4		11.6		12.1		23.9		14.5		3.8		8.4		22.3		13.7
Esophagus	*	*	*	*	15.0	4.4	5.3	*	2.9	*	9.4	*	5.6	*	*	*	*	*	5.4	1.7	4.4	0.9
Kidney and renal pelvis	*	*	15.6	*	12.8	6.0	4.6	2.3	5.8	2.8	9.8	*	7.3	2.3	6.3	*	*	*	11.9	5.9	10.0	5.5
Larynx	*	*	*	*	12.7	2.5	2.8	*	2.4	*	*	*	2.5	*	*	*	*	*	7.5	1.5	5.1	0.7
Leukemias	*	*	*	*	11.5	6.8	7.2	4.4	10.7	6.6	10.8	7.2	6.6	4.5	6.5	4.7	9.5	8.3	13.5	7.9	9.4	6.4
Liver and intrahepatic bile duct	*	*	*	*	6.9	2.4	20.8	5.3	10.5	3.4	*	*	6.3	3.9	24.8	10.0	41.8	*	3.7	1.5	6.7	2.6
Lung and bronchus	81.1	50.6	14.4	*	117.0	44.2	52.1	25.3	52.6	17.5	89.0	43.1	43.0	15.2	53.2	16.0	70.9	31.2	76.0	41.5	41.8	19.5

Site																				
Lymphomas: Non-Hodgkin's lymphoma	*	*	*	*	*	13.2	7.6	12.4	6.8	12.9	9.0	12.5	11.6	7.8	5.8	6.0	**15.8**	*	**18.7**	12.0	14.1	9.1
Lymphomas: Hodgkin's disease	*	*	*	2.3	2.0	*	*	*	*	*	*	*	*	*	*	*	*	*	3.3	2.6	2.5	1.6
Melanoma of the skin	*	*	*	1.0	0.7	*	1.8	*	*	2.6	*	*	1.6	*	*	*	*	*	14.5	10.1	2.7	3.2
Multiple myeloma	*	*	*	11.3	7.4	2.3	4.8	3.9	2.6	5.3	*	1.6	*	*	*	*	*	5.0	3.2	4.2	3.0
Nasopharynx	*	*	*	1.0	*	10.8	3.9	3.9	*	*	*	*	*	7.7	*	*	0.6	0.2	0.6	*
Oral cavity (excluding nasopharynx)	*	*	*	20.4	5.8	5.3	2.3	5.4	5.3	11.7	*	7.0	*	3.3	*	11.6	*	14.6	5.8	8.9	2.7
Ovary	—	17.5	—	10.2	—	9.3	—	10.2	11.8	—	11.8	10.1	—	7.0	—	13.8	9.8	15.8	15.8	8.0	11.4
Pancreas	*	*	*	14.0	11.5	8.0	4.9	6.5	6.0	**10.9**	**8.7**	8.7	7.3	**7.6**	*	*	9.8	7.4	8.0	6.9
Prostate	46.1	52.5	—	180.6	46.0	69.8	57.2	88.0	40.0	24.2	134.7	89.0	89.0	8.0
Stomach	27.2	*	*	17.9	7.6	15.7	8.3	8.5	5.3	20.5	13.0	15.3	48.9	25.8	19.1	**30.5**	10.2	4.4	15.3	8.0
Testis	*	*	—	0.8	*	1.7	1.3	*	*	2.3	*	5.4	*	2.6	5.0	2.9
Thyroid	*	*	*	1.4	3.3	2.1	6.5	4.1	**14.6**	*	**9.1**	1.6	5.4	7.8	10.5	2.6	6.5	2.0	6.2
Urinary bladder	*	*	*	15.2	5.8	13.0	3.7	8.3	2.1	*	13.7	4.1	10.4	*	**31.7**	7.8	15.8	4.3

Note: Rates are ''average annual'' per 100,000 population, age-adjusted to 1970 U.S. standard; N/A = information not available. **Numbers in bold face = Top three rates, as applicable.**

* = rate not calculated when fewer than 25 cases.

† These figures are for **general comparison** only as this group may overlap the other ethnic populations in this table.

From Miller, B.A., Kolonel, L.N., Bernstein L., et al. (eds.). (1996). *Racial/Ethnic Patterns of Cancer in the United States 1988–1992*. Bethesda, MD: National Cancer Institute. NIH Pub. No. 96-4104.

TABLE 4–2. United States Cancer Mortality Rates, 1988–1992

Cancer Site	Alaska Native M	Alaska Native W	American Indian M	American Indian W	Black M	Black W	Chinese M	Chinese W	Filipino M	Filipino W	Hawaiian M	Hawaiian W	Japanese M	Japanese W	White M	White W	Hispanic[†] (Total) M	Hispanic[†] (Total) W
All sites	225	179	123	99	319	168	139	86	105	63	239	168	133	88	213	140	129	85
Brain and nervous system	*	*	*	*	3.1	2.1	2.1	1.4	1.6	1.4	*	*	1.3	1.1	5.4	3.7	3.0	2.0
Breast, invasive	*	*	*	*	0.4	31.4	*	11.2	*	11.9	*	25.0	*	12.5	0.2	27.0	0.1	15.0
Cervix uteri	—	*	—	*		6.7		2.6		2.4	*	*		1.5		2.5		3.4
Colon and rectum	27.2	24.0	*	*	28.2	20.4	15.7	10.5	11.4	5.8	23.7	11.4	20.5	12.3	22.9	15.3	12.8	8.3
Corpus uteri	—	*	—	*		6.0		2.2		1.3	—	8.4		1.9		3.2		2.3
Esophagus	*	*	*	*	14.8	3.7	4.2	*	2.2	*	*	*	4.8	0.9	5.3	1.2	3.4	0.7
Kidney and renal pelvis	*	*	*	*	5.1	2.2	1.3	0.9	1.9	*	*	*	2.4	0.8	5.0	2.3	3.7	1.7
Larynx	*	*	*	*	5.6	0.9	0.9	*	*	*	*	*	*	*	2.3	0.5	1.9	0.2
Leukemias	*	*	*	*	8.0	4.6	3.6	2.4	5.7	2.9	7.8	*	4.4	2.2	8.5	5.0	5.1	3.4
Liver and intrahepatic bile duct	*	*	*	*	6.6	2.7	17.7	4.6	7.8	2.3	9.2	*	6.2	4.0	3.8	1.8	5.9	2.8
Lung and bronchus	69.4	45.3	*	*	105.6	31.5	40.1	18.5	29.8	10.0	88.9	44.1	32.4	12.9	72.6	31.9	32.4	10.8

Site																		
Lymphomas: Non-Hodgkin's lymphoma	*	*	*	**5.8**	3.4	5.2	2.3	5.0	3.0	**8.8**	*	7.3	*	4.8	**3.9**	**8.1**	**5.3**	5.3
Lymphomas: Hodgkin's disease	*	*	*	**0.7**	**0.4**	*	*	*	*	*	*	*	*	*		**0.7**	**0.4**	0.6
Melanoma of the skin	*	*	*	0.5	0.4	*	*	*	*	*	*	*	*	*		**3.4**	**1.7**	0.8
Multiple myeloma	*	*	*	7.3	5.0	1.2	1.3	2.2	1.0	*	*	*	*	*		3.4	2.2	2.7
Nasopharynx	*	*	*	0.6	0.2	**4.6**	**1.2**	1.7	*	*	*	*	*	2.1		0.3	0.1	0.3
Oral cavity (excluding nasopharynx)	*	*	*	**8.7**	2.1	1.6	0.7	1.2	**1.3**	*	*	*	2.1	0.8	**3.8**	**1.5**	**2.7**	2.7
Ovary	—	*	*	**6.6**	—	4.0	—	3.4	7.3	—	—	5.0		—	**8.1**	—		
Pancreas	*	*	*	**14.4**	10.4	6.7	5.1	4.5	3.5	**12.8**	**9.1**	8.5	6.7	**9.7**	**6.9**	7.1	5.2	
Prostate	*	16.2	—	**53.7**	6.6	13.5	**19.9**	—	11.7	**24.1**	15.3	5.2						
Stomach	*	*	*	**13.6**	**5.6**	10.5	4.8	3.6	2.5	**12.8**	14.4	17.4	**9.3**	6.1	2.8	8.4	4.2	
Testis	*	*	*	0.1	*	*	*	*	*	*	*	*		0.3	0.2			
Thyroid	*	*	*	0.3	0.4	*	*	1.1	*	*	*	*	0.3	0.3	0.2	0.5		
Urinary bladder	*	*	*	**4.8**	2.4	2.0	1.0	1.2	1.0	*	2.0	1.2	**5.8**	**1.7**	**2.8**	0.9		

Note: Rates are "average annual" per 100,000 population, age-adjusted to 1970 U.S. standard; N/A = information not available. **Numbers in bold face = Top three rates, as applicable.**
* = rate not calculated when fewer than 25 cases. No mortality data available for Korean and Vietnamese groups.
† These figures are for **general comparison** only as this group may overlap the other ethnic populations in this table.
From Miller, B.A., Kolonel, L.N., Bernstein, L., et al. (eds.). (1996.) *Racial/Ethnic Patterns of Cancer in the United States 1988–1992.* Bethesda, MD: National Cancer Institute. NIH Pub. No. 96-4104.

TABLE 4–3. Five-Year Relative Survival Rates (%) by Race/Ethnic Group, 1975–1984

Cancer Site	White	Black	Chinese	Japanese	Filipino	American Indian	Mexican American	Native Hawaiian
All sites	51.9	39.6	47.5	53.1	46.1	35.4	48.4	43.2
Oral cavity	54.0	33.0	55.7	44.4	46.6	38.6	60.7	42.8
Esophagus	6.5	4.2	11.5	5.8	3.4	—	0.0	0.0
Stomach	15.3	17.5	21.6	29.8	18.8	8.9	17.8	12.9
Colon and rectum	53.2	46.7	53.1	61.7	44.8	39.7	45.0	58.4
Liver	3.8	3.1	2.0	1.5	6.7	0.0	0.0	6.6
Gallbladder	9.2	8.9	—	16.2	—	2.8	8.5	26.2
Pancreas	2.7	3.2	0.0	2.6	5.2	0.0	1.2	0.0
Lung	13.2	11.7	15.1	14.3	13.2	0.0	10.8	13.0
Melanoma (skin)	81.2	57.5	—	81.0	—	—	82.1	—
Breast	76.1	63.2	80.8	85.4	73.7	46.2	70.6	68.0
Cervix uteri	68.2	61.6	74.6	70.2	73.0	63.5	70.5	67.7
Corpus uteri	86.0	54.9	86.1	84.1	79.9	82.7	77.0	74.6
Ovary	37.6	40.9	43.3	43.5	44.7	42.9	38.7	46.8
Prostate	72.6	63.4	72.5	80.5	71.7	54.2	72.4	72.0
Urinary bladder	76.6	53.4	78.5	80.8	58.4	—	64.6	51.4
Kidney	51.9	56.3	60.7	63.1	47.0	49.7	51.4	59.0
Brain and CNS	23.3	28.5	35.9	40.6	29.6	37.6	32.2	38.9
Hodgkin's disease	74.7	71.0	—	—	43.5	—	69.0	74.1
Non-Hodgkin's lymphoma	50.2	47.9	50.3	41.1	33.8	31.1	41.1	40.2
Leukemia	35.5	28.0	19.8	26.0	22.3	21.4	25.7	21.1

From American Cancer Society (1991). *Cancer Facts and Figures for Minority Americans 1991*. Atlanta: American Cancer Society.

        (2) Often do not live long enough to develop cancer.

        (3) Have high rates of obesity and diseases associated with alcohol and tobacco use, which are risk factors for many cancers

    b. Stomach, gallbladder, and cervix are high incidence sites for cancer.

    c. Lowest 5-year survival rates.

VI. Six cultural phenomena that vary among cultural groups.

  A. Communication.

    1. Means by which culture is transmitted and preserved.

    2. Consists of verbal, nonverbal, and written words.

    3. Most obvious cultural difference is language.

      a. Most important factor in culturally competent care because it affects all stages of the nursing process.

      b. If the client does not speak the nurse's language, a translator may be needed.

      c. More likely, the client speaks nurse's language with limited ability and uses language with denotative or connotative meanings different from nurse's meanings.

    4. Common nurse responses to client's loss of ability to communicate verbally.

      a. Avoid clients.

      b. Shout the same words louder.

      c. Focus on tasks rather than the clients.

      d. Stop talking with clients.

        (1) Start doing things for them instead of with them.

        (2) May be interpreted as implying client inferiority.

      e. Result is isolation of clients who do not speak the dominant language with possible reactions of withdrawal, hostility or belligerence, or uncooperativeness.

    5. Nonverbal communication includes use of touch, facial expressions, eye movement, body language, and silence.

      a. Need to know the meaning of nonspecific nonverbal behaviors in the client's culture.

  B. Space.

    1. Includes the individual, body, surrounding environment, and objects within that environment.

    2. Relationship among the above is learned and influenced by one's culture.

    3. People are by nature territorial.

      a. For territoriality needs to be met, the person must be in control of some space, must establish some rules for the space, and must be able to defend it against invasion or misuse by others.

      b. The nurse often invades this personal space.

  C. Social organization.

    1. Patterns of cultural behavior are learned through enculturation; involves acquiring knowledge and internalizing values.

    2. These patterns are important to the nurse because they provide explanations for behavior related to life events.

    3. Includes knowledge of family structure and organization, religious values and beliefs that dictate culturally accepted role behaviors of different members of the group and rules for behavior.

    4. Behaviors are prescribed for significant life events such as birth, death, childbearing, child rearing, role and care of the elderly, and illness.

    5. Social barriers to health care.
       a. Poverty is a major social barrier that affects entry into health care system.
       b. Poverty, not race, accounts for 10 to 15% lower survival rate from cancer in many cultural groups.
       c. Impact of poverty on cancer is felt in ethnic minorities because a disproportionate number of cultural minorities comprise the poor of America.
       d. "Culture of poverty" includes unemployment; unskilled occupations; no savings; no health insurance; frequent daily food purchases in small amounts; crowded living quarters; women as single parents; low education level; critical attitudes toward the dominant class; feelings of helplessness, inferiority, fatalism, and dependency; or a present time orientation with inability to defer gratification.
       e. Contributes to increased cancer incidence and mortality through risk factors of chronic malnutrition, occupational exposure through unskilled jobs, early initiation into sex and multiple partners, smoking, and alcoholism.
       f. Secondary prevention may be absent because of present orientation wherein survival needs take precedence over screening and early detection.
       g. Critical attitudes toward middle class and sense of fatalism may decrease participation in screening programs.
       h. Delayed tertiary prevention due to lack of insurance, inability to pay fee-for-service, or limited health care access.
       i. Emergency rooms used inappropriately and referral to clinics may result in fragmented care, impersonal service, long waiting hours, and transportation and child care problems.
  D. Time.
    1. Meaning and influence of time from a cultural perspective.
    2. May be present, past, or future.
    3. In present orientation, time is flexible and events begin when the client arrives, which may result in client arriving late for appointments.
    4. Past orientation emphasizes influence of past events and ancestors on present events.
    5. Future orientation emphasizes planning and schedules, which is often the value perspective of the health professional.
    6. Most cultures combine all three time orientations but one is more likely to dominate.
    7. When time orientation differs between nurse and client, long-term planning is affected.
       a. If present oriented, for example, emphasize short-term problems rather than only long-term problems when teaching about the potential effects of medications.
  E. Environment control.
    1. Ability of members of a particular cultural group to plan activities that control nature or direct environmental factors.
    2. Beliefs about causes of illness, health behaviors, and actions taken when illness or disease occurs are influenced by the individual perception of the environment, which is influenced by the individual's culture.

   3. Types of health beliefs:
       a. Magico-religious health belief view in which health and illness are controlled by supernatural forces.
           (1) Illness is the result of being bad or opposing God's will.
           (2) Use of charms, holy words, and holy actions to prevent and cure illnesses.
       b. Scientific or biomedical health belief.
           (1) Life and life processes are controlled by physical and biochemical processes that can be manipulated by humans.
           (2) Illness is caused by microorganisms or breakdown of the body.
           (3) Client expects medication, a treatment, or surgery to cure the health problem.
       c. Holistic health view.
           (1) Forces of nature must be maintained in balance or harmony.
           (2) If the natural balance is disturbed, illness results.
           (3) Use of natural environment and use of herbs, plants, minerals, and animal substances to prevent and treat illnesses.
   4. Folk medicine.
       a. Beliefs and practices relating to health, illness, and prevention that come from cultural traditions.
       b. Consistent with holistic health view.
           (1) Healing is viewed as restoration of a person to a state of harmony between body, mind, and spirit.
       c. Often involves a healer who prepares a treatment and involves some ritual practice.
       d. Healer understands the problem within a cultural context, speaks the same language, and shares a similar world view as the client.
       e. Healer often is consulted first by client because the healer is heritage-consistent.
       f. Consultation occurs within the community.
   F. Biologic variations.
       1. Differences in skin, eye or hair color, facial characteristics, amount of body hair, body size, and body shape.
       2. Enzymatic and genetic variations causing differences in metabolism of drugs and alcohol.
       3. Increased susceptibility to certain diseases.
       4. Dietary practices.
VII. Table 4–4 summarizes specific information on five major ethnic minority groups using the six cultural phenomena described above.
   A. This information should be used as guidelines for practice.
   B. Nursing interventions that consider the cultural background of a client and family must be based on sound assessment and validation of the role that culture plays in the life of the client and family.
   C. Many subgroups that vary in beliefs and practices exist within any ethnic group.
   D. Clients vary in the degree to which they identify with their dominant and traditional culture.
       1. Values and beliefs of the children of immigrants to the U.S. may be less traditional than their parents.
       2. Need to assess health beliefs determining people's ties to traditional beliefs and their stage of acculturation.
       3. Table 4–5 outlines this heritage continuum.

TABLE 4–4. Cross-cultural Examples of Cultural Phenomena Impacting on Nursing Care

Regions of Origin	Communication	Space	Time Orientation	Social Organization	Environmental Control	Biological Variations*
Asian China Hawaii Philippines Korea Japan Southeast Asia (Laos, Cambodia, Vietnam)	National language preference Dialects, written characters Use of silence Nonverbal and contextual cuing	Noncontact people	Present	Family: hierarchical structure, loyalty Devotion to tradition Many religions, including Taoism, Buddhism, Islam, and Christianity Community social organizations	Traditional health and illness beliefs Use of traditional medicines Traditional practitioners: Chinese doctors and herbalists	Liver cancer Stomach cancer Coccidioidomycosis Hypertension Lactose intolerance
African West Coast (as slaves) Many African countries West Indian Islands Dominican Republic Haiti Jamaica	National languages Dialect: Pidgin, Creole, Spanish, and French	Close personal space	Present over future	Family: many female, single parent Large, extended family networks Strong church affiliation within community Community social organizations	Traditional health and illness beliefs Folk medicine tradition Traditional healer: root-worker	Sickle cell anemia Hypertension Cancer of the esophagus Stomach cancer Coccidioidomycosis Lactose intolerance
Europe Germany England Italy Ireland Other European countries	National languages Many learn English immediately	Noncontact people Aloof Distant Southern countries: closer contact and touch	Future over present	Nuclear families Extended families Judeo-Christian religions Community social organizations	Primary reliance on modern health care system Traditional health and illness beliefs Some remaining folk medicine traditions	Breast cancer Heart disease Diabetes mellitus Thalassemia
Native American 170 Native American tribes Aleuts Eskimos	Tribal languages Use of silence and body language	Space very important and has no boundaries	Present	Extremely family oriented Biological and extended families Children taught to respect traditions Community social organizations	Traditional health and illness beliefs Folk medicine tradition Traditional healer: medicine man	Accidents Heart disease Cirrhosis of the liver Diabetes mellitus
Hispanic countries Spain Cuba Mexico Central and South America	Spanish or Portuguese primary language	Tactile relationships Touch Handshakes Embracing Value physical presence	Present	Nuclear family Extended families *Compadrazzo:* godparents Community social organizations	Traditional health and illness beliefs Folk medicine tradition Traditional healers: *Curandero, Espiritista, Partera, Senora*	Diabetes mellitus Parasites Coccidioidomycosis Lactose intolerance

Modified from Spector, R.E. (1993). Culture, ethnicity, and nursing. In P.A. Potter, A.G. Perry (eds.). *Fundamentals of Nursing: Concepts, Process, and Practice* (3rd ed.). St. Louis: Mosby-Year Book. p. 101.

TABLE 4–5. **Heritage Continuum**

Heritage Consistency Factors	Heritage Inconsistency Factors
Childhood development occurred in the individual's country of origin or in a U.S. neighborhood of like ethnic group.	Childhood development did not occur in the individual's country of origin or in an immigrant neighborhood of like ethnic group.
Extended family members encouraged participation in traditional religious or cultural activities.	Extended family members did not encourage participation in traditional religious or cultural activities.
Individual engaged in frequent visits home to the country of origin or to the "old neighborhood" in the United States.	Individual does not engage in visits home to the country of origin or the "old neighborhood" in the United States.
Family homes are within the ethnic community.	Family was not in the ethnic community.
Individual participates in ethnic cultural events such as religious festivals, "national holidays," singing, dancing, and costumes.	Individual does not participate in ethnic cultural events.
Individual was raised in an extended family setting.	Individual was not raised in an extended family setting.
Individual maintains regular contact with the extended family.	Individual does not maintain contact with the extended family.
Individual's name has not been Americanized.	Individual's name has been Americanized.
Individual was educated in a parochial (nonpublic) school with a religious or ethnic philosophy similar to personal background.	Individual was educated in public schools.
Individual engages primarily in social activities with others of the same ethnic background.	Individual does not engage primarily in social activities with others of the same ethnic background.
Individual has knowledge about the ethnic culture and language.	Individual does not have knowledge about ethnic culture and language.
Individual possesses elements of personal pride about the national and ethnic origin.	Individual does not possess elements of personal pride about the national and ethnic origin.
Individual incorporates elements of historical beliefs and practices into personal philosophies.	Individual does not incorporate elements of historical beliefs and practices into personal philosophies.

From Spector, R.E. (1991). *Cultural Diversity in Health and Illness* (3rd ed.). Stamford, CT: Appleton & Lange.

Assessment

I. Accurately assessing a client's culture must start with the nurse and the influence of one's own culture on the nurse.
   A. Who is the nurse from a cultural perspective?
   B. What is the nurse's culture?
   C. What are the health traditions of the nurse's culture?
   D. What are the nurse's attitudes and emotions toward providing care to clients from diverse cultural backgrounds?

II. Assessing the client's culture.
   A. Culture.
      1. Does the client identify with a particular ethnic or racial or cultural group?
      2. Where was the client born?
      3. How long has the client lived in this country?
   B. Communication.
      1. What language is spoken?
      2. Can the client communicate in English?
         a. Both spoken and written?
         b. To what extent is English spoken?
      3. Does the client speak for self or defer to another?
      4. What nonverbal communication behaviors are observed (e.g., touching, eye contact)?
         a. What significance do these behaviors have for the nurse-client interaction?
   C. Space.
      1. Observe the client's proximity to other people and objects within the environment.
      2. How does the client react to the nurse's movement toward the client?
      3. Assess the client's physical environment (especially important in home health care, community nursing, and long-term care nursing).
      4. What cultural objects within the environment have importance for health promotion and health maintenance?
   D. Social organization.
      1. What are the client's roles?
      2. Is the client the primary decision maker for health care behaviors?
      3. Must the client consult another to make health decisions?
         a. If so, who?
      4. What other family members are important to the client's decision making?
      5. Are there cultural or religious leaders that are important in the client's health decision making?
      6. Is there a religious affiliation linked with the cultural affiliation?
   E. Time.
      1. What is the client's time orientation: past, present, or future?
      2. What is the significance of time for the client?
      3. Does the client talk about time in specifics, such as dates or times, or in generalities such as "a long time" or a "short time."
   F. Environmental control.
      1. How is health defined by the culture?
      2. What does the client believe to be the cause of the cancer?
      3. Has the client used the services of a cultural healer?
      4. What healing practices has the client used?
      5. Have folk healing behaviors been used?
      6. Is the client wearing or carrying any amulets or artifacts that are believed to have healing properties?
   G. Biologic variations.
      1. Are there normal variations in anatomic characteristics (e.g., body structure or size, skin color, facial characteristics)?
      2. What are the dietary preferences of the client?
         a. Are the dietary preferences related to the client's ethnicity?
      3. Is the client at risk for nutritional deficiencies because of ethnicity (e.g., pernicious anemia, lactose intolerance)?

4. Are there variations in physiologic functioning related to the client's race (e.g., drug metabolism, alcohol metabolism)?
5. Are there illnesses or diseases for which the client is at risk because of ethnicity or race (e.g., hypertension, diabetes mellitus, sickle-cell anemia, specific cancers)?

Nursing Diagnoses

I. Impaired verbal communication.
II. Anxiety.
III. Fear.
IV. Altered health maintenance.
V. Ineffective individual coping.
VI. Altered family processes.
VII. Decisional conflict.
VIII. Spiritual distress.
IX. Altered role performance.
X. Impaired social interaction.
XI. Sleep pattern disturbance.
XII. Body image disturbance.

Outcome Identification

I. Nurse ensures that the plan of care reflects sensitivity and respect for the cultural and ethnic practices of the client.
II. Client is able to effectively communicate needs.
III. Client and family are able to modify cultural and health practices to achieve an optimal level of health.
IV. Client maintains cultural practices, as appropriate.
   A. Client selects foods consistent with cultural heritage.
   B. Client is able to practice cultural and religious rituals.

Planning and Implementation

I. Interventions related to the nurse.
   A. Recognize that cultural diversity exists.
   B. Assess personal beliefs surrounding persons from different cultures.
      1. Review personal beliefs, past experiences, biases, prejudices, and stereotypes.
      2. Set aside any values, biases, ideas, and attitudes that are judgmental and may negatively affect care.
   C. Respect the unfamiliar.
   D. Analyze own communication (e.g., facial expressions and body language) and how they may be interpreted.
   E. Recognize that the client's definitions of health and illness and practices to promote health and cure illness may differ from own.
      1. Identify sources of discrepancy between the client and own concepts of health and illness.
   F. Be sensitive to the uniqueness of the client.
II. Interventions related to interacting with clients of different cultures.
   A. Increase knowledge about the different beliefs and values of the major ethnic or cultural groups with whom one is likely to have contact.

B. Use the client and family as sources of information whenever possible.

C. Recognize that cultural symbols and practices can often bring a client comfort.

D. Appreciate that each person's cultural values are ingrained and therefore very difficult to change.

E. Do not expect all members of one cultural group to behave in exactly the same way.

F. Remember that the color of a client's skin does not always determine the client's culture.

G. During illness clients may return to their preferred cultural practices.
   1. A client who has learned English as a second language may revert to the primary language.

H. Be willing to modify health care delivery in keeping with the client's cultural background.

I. Support the client's practices and incorporate them into nursing practice whenever possible and when they are not contraindicated for health reasons.
   1. Do not impose a cultural practice on a client without knowing whether it is acceptable.

J. Recognize differences in the ways clients communicate and do not assume the meaning of a specific behavior (e.g., lack of eye contact) without validating its meaning.

K. Understand that respect for the client and communicated needs is central to the therapeutic relationship.
   1. Communicate respect by using a kind and attentive approach.
   2. Learn how listening is communicated in the client's culture.
   3. Use appropriate active listening techniques.
   4. Adopt an attitude of flexibility, respect, and interest to help bridge barriers imposed by culture.

L. Be considerate of reluctance to talk when the subject involves sexual matters.
   1. Sexual matters are not freely discussed with members of the opposite sex in some cultures.

III. Interventions related to communication.

A. Relate to the client in an unhurried manner that takes into account the social and cultural amenities.
   1. Give time for the client to answer.
   2. Engage in appropriate social conversation before discussing more intimate personal details.

B. Use validating techniques in communication.
   1. Be alert for feedback that the client is not understanding.
   2. Note that big smiles and frequent head nodding or lack of questions may indicate that the client is trying to please, not necessarily that the client understands.

C. Be aware that in some groups discussion concerning the client with others may be offensive and may impede the nursing process.

D. Use interpreters to improve communication.
   1. Be sure that the language the client speaks at home is known.
   2. Avoid interpreters from a rival tribe, state, region, or nation.
   3. Be aware of sex, gender, and relationship differences between the interpreter and client.
      a. Same-gender interpreters are preferred.

       b. Caution is needed because the client may be hesitant to reveal personal information if the interpreter is a child or a friend.

    4. Be aware of age differences between the interpreter and client.

       a. Older, more mature interpreter is preferred.

  E. Adopt special approaches when there is no interpreter.

    1. Use a caring tone of voice and appropriate facial expressions to help alleviate client fears.

       a. Proceed in an unhurried manner.

       b. Pay attention to any effort by the client and family to communicate.

    2. Speak slowly and distinctly but not loudly.

       a. Be polite.

    3. Greet the person using the last or complete name.

    4. Use gestures, pictures, and play acting to help the client understand.

    5. Use any words known in the client's language.

    6. Ask who among the client's family and friends could serve as an interpreter.

    7. Try a third language.

       a. Some Indo-Chinese speak French.

       b. Many Koreans speak Japanese.

    8. Keep the message simple and repeat frequently.

       a. Avoid medical jargon.

    9. Learn key phrases in the language of the client.

    10. Validate whether the client understands by having him or her repeat instructions, demonstrate procedure, or act out meaning.

IV. Interventions to enhance access to health care.

  A. Involve trusted and respected members of cultural groups in the planning and delivery of health care services to their communities.

  B. Develop culturally sensitive client education materials.

  C. Use the navigator concept to assist individuals in overcoming health care access barriers.

    1. Use of a navigator, often an individual of similar cultural background, who can guide the client around and through the labyrinth of the health care system.

    2. Navigator also provides education and support to the client.

Evaluation

The oncology nurse systematically and regularly evaluates the client's and/or family's responses to interventions to determine progress toward the achievement of expected outcomes. Relevant data is collected and actual findings are compared with expected findings. Nursing diagnoses, outcomes, and plans of care are reviewed and revised as necessary.

BIBLIOGRAPHY

American Cancer Society. (1996). *Cancer Facts and Figures*. Atlanta: American Cancer Society.

American Cancer Society. (1989). A summary of the American Cancer Society report to the nation: Cancer in the poor. *CA Cancer J Clin 39*, 263–265.

American Cancer Society. (1989). *Cancer in the Economically Disadvantaged: A Special Report*. Atlanta: American Cancer Society.

American Cancer Society. (1991). *Cancer Facts and Figures for Minority Americans 1991*. Atlanta: American Cancer Society.

Black, B.L., & Ades, T.B. (1994). American Cancer Society urban demonstration projects: Models for successful intervention. *Semin Oncol Nurs 10*, 96–103.

Black, B.L., Schweitzer, R., & Dezelsky, T. (1993). Report on the American Cancer Society workshop on community cancer detection, education, and prevention demonstration projects for underserved populations. *CA Cancer J Clin 43,* 226–233.

Bralwey, O.W. (1995). Minority accrual and clinical trials. *Oncology Issues 10,* 22–24.

Day, J C. (1993). *Population Projections of the United States, by Age, Sex, Race, and Hispanic origin: 1993 to 2050* (U.S. Bureau of the Census, Current Populations Reports, P25–1104). Washington, D.C.: U.S. Government Printing Office.

Frank-Stromborg, M., & Olsen, S.J. (eds.). (1993). *Cancer Prevention in Minority Populations: Cultural Implications for Health Care Professionals.* St. Louis: Mosby-Year Book.

Giger, J.N., Davidhizar, R.E. (eds.). (1995). *Transcultural Nursing: Assessment and Intervention* (2nd ed.). St. Louis: Mosby-Year Book.

Kagawa-Singer, M. (1995). Socioeconomic and cultural influences on cancer care of women. *Semin Oncol Nurs 11,* 109–119.

Kozier, B., Erb, G., Blais, K., & Wilkinson, J.M. (1995). *Fundamentals of Nursing: Concepts, Processes and Practice* (5th ed.). Redwood City, CA: Addison-Wesley.

Lewin, M., & Rice, B. (eds.). (1994). *Balancing the Scales of Opportunity: Ensuring Racial and Ethnic Diversity in the Health Professions.* Committee on Increasing Minority Participation in the Health Professions, Institute of Medicine. Washington, D.C.: National Academy Press.

McCabe, M.S., Varricchio, C.G., & Padberg, R.M. (1994). Efforts to recruit the economically disadvantaged to national clinical trials. *Semin Oncol Nurs 10,* 123–129.

Mack, E., McGrath, T., Pendleton, D., et al. (1993). Reaching poor populations with cancer prevention and early detection programs. *Cancer Pract 1,* 35–39.

Miller, B.A., Kolonel, L.N., Bernstein, L., et al. (eds.). (1996). *Racial/ethnic Patterns of Cancer in the United States 1988–1992* (NIH Publication No. 96-4104). Bethesda, MD: National Cancer Institute.

Palos, G. (1994). Cultural heritage: Cancer screening and early detection. *Semin Oncol Nurs 10,* 104–113.

Potter, P.A., & Perry, A.G. (1995). *Basic Nursing: Theory and Practice* (3rd ed.). St. Louis: C.V. Mosby.

Spector, R.E. (1991). *Cultural Diversity in Health and Illness* (3rd ed.). Stamford, CT: Appleton & Lange.

Spector, R.E. (1993). Culture, ethnicity, and nursing. In P.A. Potter, & A.G. Perry (eds.). *Concepts, Process, and Practice* (3rd ed.). St. Louis: Mosby-Year Book, pp. 94–119.

Varricchio, C. (1987). Cultural and ethnic dimensions of cancer nursing care. *Oncol Nurs Forum 14*(3), 57–73.

Wilkes, G., Freeman, H., & Prout, M. (1994). Cancer and poverty: Breaking the cycle. *Semin Oncol Nurs 10,* 79–88.

Coping: Survivorship Issues and Financial Concerns

Susan Leigh, RN, BSN

Theory

I. Definition.
   A. When cancer was considered an incurable disease, the family members or significant others who lost a loved one to cancer were the original cancer *survivors.*
   B. As potentially curative therapies became available, clinicians and researchers used a 5-year landmark to define cancer survivors—free of disease 5 years from diagnosis or from the completion of therapy.
   C. Many health care providers today differentiate between *clients* who are receiving therapy and *survivors* who have completed treatment.
   D. A broader, more encompassing definition of cancer survivor (*"from the time of its discovery and for the balance of life, an individual diagnosed with cancer is a survivor"*) has been proposed by the National Coalition for Cancer Survivorship (NCCS).
      1. Implications of the NCCS definition for health care providers and the public:
         a. Cancer survival begins at the moment of diagnosis and proceeds along a continuum through and beyond treatment to remissions, recurrences, cure, and the final stages of life.
         b. Survivorship can be seen as a dynamic, evolutionary process rather than a predetermined stage of survival. It is living with, through, or beyond a diagnosis of cancer, regardless of outcome.
      2. Survivorship issues also affect persons other than the diagnosed client—family members, significant others, friends, coworkers, health care professionals, and social support networks.
II. "Seasons of Survival" (Mullan)—a dynamic model of life after a cancer diagnosis consists of three *stages*—the acute, extended, and permanent stages of survival.
   A. Acute stage.
      1. Begins at the moment of diagnosis and extends through the initial treatments.
      2. Individuals may be dealing with:
         a. Acute or potential losses.
         b. Fear of dying or impending death.
         c. Acute side effects from treatment.
         d. Disruption in family and social roles.

B. Extended stage.
 1. Follows the completion of the initial treatment.
 2. Individuals may be in remission or on maintenance therapy, or their condition may be terminal.
 3. Individuals may be dealing with:
  a. Severing of treatment-based support systems.
  b. Feeling ambiguous about the joy of being alive and feeling fear of recurrence or fear of death.
  c. Adjusting to physical or psychosocial compromise.
  d. Reintegrating and reorganizing individual and family concerns.
  e. Isolating the individual because of external or self-imposed forces.
  f. Seeking community-based support systems.
C. Permanent stage.
 1. Gradual evolution to a time of diminished probability for disease recurrence.
 2. If cancer is arrested permanently, some survivors may be considered "cured."
 3. Individuals may be dealing with:
  a. Discrimination in the workplace.
  b. Procurement or maintenance of adequate insurance coverage.
  c. Adaptation to the physical and psychosocial changes resulting from disease.
  d. Treatment for long-term or late effects of disease and therapy (Tables 5–1 and 5–2).
   (1) Long-term effects are chronic sequelae that may develop during or result from treatment and may persist for months to years

TABLE 5–1. **Examples of Common Chemotherapy Agents and Possible Long-Term or Late Effects**

Agent	Effect
Actinomycin D	Hepatic fibrosis, cirrhosis
Adriamycin	Cardiomyopathy
BCNU	Pulmonary fibrosis, ovarian failure, azoospermia
Bleomycin	Pulmonary fibrosis, hyperpigmentation, digital cutaneous ulcerations
Chlorambucil	Progressive germinal aplasia, azoospermia
Cisplatin	Hearing loss, peripheral neuropathy
Cyclophosphamide	Progressive germinal aplasia, azoospermia, ovarian failure, chronic hemorrhagic cystitis
5-fluorouracil	Irreversible tear-duct fibrosis
Ifosfamide	Reduced bladder capacity, tubular dysfunction, chronic hemorrhagic cystitis, ovarian failure
Methotrexate	Hepatic fibrosis, cirrhosis, leukoencephalopathy, renal failure
Nitrogen mustard	Azoospermia, oligospermia
Procarbazine	Azoospermia, oligospermia, ovarian failure
Steroids	Cataracts, osteonecrosis, avascular necrosis
Vincristine	Peripheral neuropathy
VP-16	Testosterone deficiency, peripheral neuropathy

BCNU = bis-chloroethyl-nitrosourea

TABLE 5–2. **Examples of Radiation Sites
and Possible Long-Term or Late Effects**

Site	Effect
Abdomen/intestines	Adhesions, fibrosis
Bladder	Fibrosis, hypoplasia
Central nervous system	Stroke, blindness, myelitis, focal necrosis, peripheral neuropathy, leukoencephalopathy, neurocognitive deficits
Chest	Breast cancer, soft tissue sarcomas, difficulty swallowing, pulmonary fibrosis
Head and neck	Hypothyroidism, hyperthyroidism, osteonecrosis of mandible, increased dental caries, alopecia, chronic otitis, hearing loss, xerostomia, hoarseness
Heart	Pericarditis, coronary artery disease, cardiomyopathy, pericardial effusion, myocardial infarction
Liver	Fibrosis, cirrhosis
Ovaries	Ovarian failure, premature menopause
Skeletal system	Late fractures, osteonecrosis
Skin	Fibrosis, necrosis, basal cell carcinoma, hyperpigmentation
Testicles	Oligospermia, azoospermia, testosterone deficiency
Urinary tract	Fibrosis, strictures
Vagina	Fibrosis, decreased vaginal secretions

after the cancer is eradicated and treatment is complete (amputations, hair loss, neuropathies, scarring).
   (2) Late effects are clinically obvious or clinically subtle or are subclinical sequelae that may become apparent months to years after completion of treatment (pulmonary fibrosis, infertility, second malignancies, disease recurrence).
   e. Maintenance of adequate follow-up care.
III. Impact of survival.
   A. The impact of cancer survival may be long-term or delayed.
   B. Multiple factors determine the occurrence, frequency, and severity of actual or potential effects.
      1. Type of cancer.
      2. Location of disease.
      3. Size and extent of the primary tumor.
      4. Type and aggressiveness of therapy.
      5. Age of the individual at diagnosis.
      6. State of general physical and mental health of the individual at diagnosis.
      7. Quantity and quality of psychosocial support available.
      8. Individual coping strategies.
   C. Effects can be categorized as physiologic, psychological, social, or spiritual.
      1. Physiologic effects.
         a. Recurrence of disease.
         b. Second malignancies.
            (1) Overall risk is low but remains a serious problem for those affected.

        (2) Risk of second malignancies does not contraindicate therapy for first malignancy.
    c. Physical changes or losses such as amputations or scars.
    d. Decreased physical stamina.
    e. System-related effects.
        (1) Neurologic—neuropathies, delayed radiation necrosis, and neuralgias.
        (2) Cardiovascular—cardiomyopathy, pericardial effusion, and arterial and venous obstruction or occlusion.
        (3) Pulmonary—fibrosis, pleural effusions, and spontaneous pneumothorax.
        (4) Urologic—nephritis, tubular atrophy, cystitis, and urinary diversions.
        (5) Gastrointestinal—transient liver enzyme elevations, bowel diversions, adhesions, obstruction, and hepatic venoocclusive disease.
        (6) Sexual/reproductive—sterility, impotence, testicular atrophy, premature menopause, and changes in sexual response times.
        (7) Musculoskeletal—late fractures, muscle atrophy.
2. Psychological effects.
    a. Fear of recurrence (Damocles syndrome).
    b. Heightened sense of vulnerability.
    c. Recurrent episodes of anxiety during routine health care follow-up or cancer-related anniversaries.
    d. Ambivalence about health care follow-up, ranging from hypochondriacal obsession to complete avoidance.
    e. Changes in body image or self-concept that result in less-than-satisfactory expression of self and sexuality.
    f. Continued need for psychosocial support after therapy.
3. Social effects.
    a. Social stigma associated with external sources (shunning by others) or internal sources (isolation).
    b. Difficulties with transition from sick role to previous roles or to the development of new roles and responsibilities.
    c. Inconsistent perceptions of the state of health of the survivor among individual, family, and social acquaintances.
    d. Employment-related problems may include avoidance by coworkers; demotion or lack of promotion; job-lock for fear of losing benefits; and dismissal from the job.
        (1) Legal protection is provided through the Federal Rehabilitation Act of 1973 that prohibits discrimination against the handicapped or those perceived as handicapped by employers who receive federal funding (federal agencies, hospitals, and universities).
        (2) Additional protection is provided for workers not protected by the Federal Rehabilitation Act under the Americans With Disabilities Act (ADA) of 1990.
        (3) Federal and state laws specifically prohibit cancer-related employment discrimination; contain information on how to file a complaint and with whom; prohibit employers from requiring preemployment examinations; and allow medical questions only after one is offered the job and only if the questions are related specifically to the job.

e. Insurance-related problems may include refusal of new applications, waiver or exclusion of preexisting conditions, extended waiting periods, an increase in premiums and reduction of benefits for the employee and employer, or cancellation of health and life insurance policies.

    (1) Legal protection includes Consolidated Omnibus Budget Reconciliation Act (COBRA) of 1986, which mandates that employers of more than 20 workers offer group medical coverage to employees (18 months) and their dependents (36 months) if they lose a job or need to work fewer hours.

    (2) Other protection includes high-risk insurance pools in some states for the medically uninsurable—insurers share both the risks and expenses with the high-risk population.

    (3) Social Security Disability Insurance Program is available to individuals who have paid into the program previously; eligibility begins 6 months after being declared medically or mentally impaired.

    (4) Portability of insurance and deletion of preexisting conditions for insurability through recent legislation will be modest improvements in insuring people with histories of cancer.

4. Spiritual and existential issues.

    a. Changes in life priorities and values after critical evaluation and a search for meaning.

    b. Deepening sense of spirituality, which may or may not include organized religion.

    c. Expressed concerns about the quality of one's life.

    d. Increased self-love or self-acceptance.

    e. An increased passion or zest for life.

    f. Ambivalent feelings about occasional periods of depression.

    g. Survivor's guilt, especially experienced during follow-up examinations when confronted with others who are not doing well, who are more debilitated, or whose condition is terminal.

Assessment

I. Identification of stage of survival.

    A. Acute—diagnosis and treatment.

    B. Extended—at completion of treatment or on maintenance therapy.

    C. Permanent—long-term survival, "cured."

II. Evaluation of cancer history.

    A. Individual diagnosis and treatment plan.

        1. Chemotherapy drugs and doses.

        2. Radiation fields and doses.

        3. Surgeries.

    B. Risk or probability for:

        1. Recurrence of original disease.

        2. Long-term (chronic) effects or symptoms.

        3. Late (delayed) effects or symptoms.

III. Psychosocial interview.

    A. Client.

        1. Psychological issues.

        2. Social issues.

        3. Financial issues.

B. Family and significant others.
   1. Psychological issues.
   2. Social issues.
   3. Financial issues.

Nursing Diagnoses

  I. Disturbance in self-esteem.
  II. Spiritual distress.
 III. Ineffective individual or family coping.
 IV. Sexual dysfunction.
  V. Anxiety.
 VI. Post-trauma response.
VII. Fatigue.

Outcome Identification

   I. Client and family receive appropriate information and referrals to optimize acute and long-term treatment plans.
  II. Nurse discusses measures to identify, treat, decrease, or eliminate physiologic sequelae.
 III. Nurse identifies institution and community-based resources to help client deal with psychosocial issues.
 IV. Client understands need for continued long-term medical follow-up.

Planning and Implementation

  I. Planning and interventions are guided by two beliefs and values.
    A. From diagnosis to death, all people with histories of cancer are survivors.
    B. Cancer survivors are entitled to certain rights (Figure 5–1):
      1. Assurance of lifelong medical care, as needed.
      2. Pursuit of happiness.
      3. Equal job opportunities.
      4. Assurance of adequate public or private health insurance.
 II. Acute-stage interventions.
    A. Begin to incorporate rehabilitation models of care at the time of diagnosis; for example, referring to local support groups, encouraging appropriate exercise and nutrition plans, and assisting with information gathering.
    B. Encourage client and family involvement in treatment decisions and planning for transitions in the level of care and services.
    C. Introduce survivorship potential and support with factual information and available resources.
    D. Assess changes in individual and family coping demands and resources throughout the seasons of survivorship.
    E. Establish exit interviews as clients complete initial treatment to assist in the transition to the extended stage.
III. Extended-stage interventions.
    A. Encourage periodic follow-up examinations and continued access to health care.

THE CANCER SURVIVORS' BILL OF RIGHTS

The American Cancer Society presents this Survivors' Bill of Rights to call public attention to survivor needs, to enhance cancer care, and to bring greater satisfaction to cancer survivors, as well as to their physicians, employers, families and friends:

1. **Survivors have the right to assurance of lifelong medical care, as needed. The physicians and other professionals involved in their care should continue their constant efforts to be:**
   - Sensitive to the cancer survivors' lifestyle choices and their need for self-esteem and dignity;
   - Careful, no matter how long they have survived, to have symptoms taken seriously, and not have aches and pains dismissed, for fear of recurrence is a normal part of survivorship;
   - Informative and open, providing survivors with as much or as little candid medical information as they wish, and encouraging their informed participation in their own care;
   - Knowledgeable about counseling resources, and willing to refer survivors and their families as appropriate for emotional support and therapy that will improve the quality of individual lives.

2. **In their personal lives, survivors, like other Americans, have the right to the pursuit of happiness. This means they have the right:**
   - To talk with their families and friends about their cancer experience if they wish, but to refuse to discuss it if that is their choice and not to be expected to be more upbeat or less blue than anyone else;
   - To be free of the stigma of cancer as a "dread disease" in all social relations;
   - To be free of blame for having gotten the disease and of guilt for having survived it.

3. **In the workplace, survivors have the right to equal job opportunities. This means they have the right:**
   - To aspire to jobs worthy of their skills, and for which they are trained and experienced, and thus not to have to accept jobs they would not have considered before the cancer experience.
   - To be hired, promoted, and accepted on return to work, according to their individual abilities and qualifications, and not according to "cancer" or "disability" stereotypes;
   - To privacy about their medical histories.

4. **Since health insurance coverage is an overriding survivorship concern, every effort should be made to ensure all survivors adequate health insurance, whether public or private. This means:**
   - For employers, that survivors have the right to be included in group health coverage, which is usually less expensive, provides better benefits, and covers the employee regardless of health history;
   - For physicians, counselors, and other professionals concerned, that they keep themselves and their survivor-clients informed and up-to-date on available group or individual health policy options, noting, for example, what major expenses like hospital costs and medical tests outside the hospital are covered and what amount must be paid before coverage (deductibles);
   - For social policymakers, both in government and in the private sector, that they seek to broaden insurance programs like Medicare to include diagnostic procedures and treatment, which help prevent recurrence and ease survivor anxiety and pain.

Figure 5–1. The Cancer Survivors' Bill of Rights. (Adapted from Spingarn ND. *The Cancer Survivors' Bill of Rights.* Atlanta: American Cancer Society.)

B. Make referrals to appropriate supportive services within the treatment center and the community such as the American Cancer Society, Leukemia Society, United Ostomy Association, community-based resource and support centers, and vocational rehabilitation programs (see Chapter 8).

C. Give client, family, and children updated information and keep them informed of changes in the status of the client.

IV. Permanent stage interventions.

A. Encourage the development of systematic follow-up programs for long-term survivors for both pediatric and adult oncology.

B. Encourage participation in activities related to changes in public and private policies affecting cancer survivors.

C. Assist in the development of guidelines for continued care that transfers to other care providers; for example, algorithms for specific disease follow-up to primary care physicians.

Evaluation

The oncology nurse systematically and regularly evaluates the client's and/or family's responses to interventions to determine progress toward the achievement of expected outcomes. Relevant data are collected and actual findings are compared with expected findings. Nursing diagnoses, outcomes, and plans of care are reviewed and revised as necessary.

BIBLIOGRAPHY

Baez, S.B., Dodd, M.J., & DiJuleo, J.E. (1991). Nursing management of persons treated for cure: Prototype-Hodgkin's disease. In S.B. Baird, R. McCorkle, & M. Grant (eds.). *Cancer Nursing: A Comprehensive Textbook.* Philadelphia: W.B. Saunders, pp. 673–688.

Card, I. (1994). *What Cancer Survivors Need to Know About Health Insurance.* A publication of the National Coalition for Cancer Survivorship (NCCS), Silver Spring, MD.

Carter, B.J. (1989). Cancer survivorship: A topic for nursing research. *Oncol Nurs Forum 16*(3), 435–437.

Ferrell, B.R., Hassey Dow, K., Leigh, S., et al. (1995). Quality of life in long-term cancer survivors. *Oncol Nurs Forum 22*(6), 915–922.

Haberman, M. (1996). Suffering and survivorship. In B.R. Ferrell (ed.). *Suffering.* Sudbury, MA: Jones & Bartlett, pp. 121–140.

Hancock, S., Tucker, M., & Hoppe, R. (1993). Breast cancer after treatment of Hodgkin's Disease. *J Natl Cancer Institute 85*(1), 25–31.

Harpham, W.S. (1994). *After Cancer: A Guide to Your New Life.* New York: W.W. Norton & Company.

Hoffman, B. (1993). *Working It Out: Your Employment Rights as a Cancer Survivor.* A publication of the National Coalition for Cancer Survivorship (NCCS), Silver Spring, MD.

Leigh, S. (1994). Cancer survivorship: A consumer movement. *Semin Oncol 21*, 783–786.

Loescher, L.J., Welch-McCaffrey, D., Leigh, S.A., et al. (1989). Surviving adult cancer. Part 1: Physiologic effects. *Ann Intern Med 3*, 411–432.

Mayer, D.K. (1992). The healthcare implications of cancer rehabilitation in the twenty-first century. *Oncol Nurs Forum 19*, 23–27.

Mullan, F. Seasons of survival: Reflections of a physician with cancer. *N Engl J Med 313*, 270–273.

Quigley, K.M. (1989). The adult cancer survivor: Psychosocial consequences of cure. *Semin Oncol Nurs 5*, 63–69.

Rose, M.A. (1989). Health promotion and risk prevention: Applications for cancer survivors. *Oncol Nurs Forum 16*, 335–340.

Schwartz, C.L., Hobbie, W.L., Constine, L.S., & Ruccione, K.S. (1994). *Survivors of Childhood Cancer: Assessment and Management.* St. Louis: C.V. Mosby.

Welch-McCaffrey, D., Hoffman, B., Leigh, S.A., et al. (1989). Surviving adult cancer. Part II: Psychosocial implications. *Ann Intern Med 3*, 411–432.

Sexuality

Patricia W. Nishimoto, MPH, DNS

Theory

I. Including sexuality in holistic nursing care of oncology patients is important because:
   A. Of improved treatment and outcome.
      1. Clients are living longer.
         a. Client's sexual dysfunction can increase risk of emotional morbidity.
         b. Increased comfort of clients to ask questions about sexuality.
      2. Focus on quality of life (QOL).
         a. QOL includes sexual functioning.
         b. To optimize clients' QOL, nurses need to be able to:
            (1) Conduct nursing assessment of sexual health.
            (2) Inform clients of possible changes in function due to treatment.
            (3) Educate clients and partners.
            (4) Provide suggestions for adapting to changes.
            (5) Know resources available and refer when needed.
   B. World Health Organization.
      1. Recognizes sexuality as an important aspect of health care.
      2. Definition of sexual health integrates the somatic, emotional, intellectual, and social aspects of a sexual being.
   C. Nurses often do not incorporate sexuality into holistic care (Table 6–1).
II. Multiple theories have been used to explore the phenomenon of sexuality.
   A. Each has strengths and weaknesses, with no one theory being perfect.
   B. One theory with the ability to provide direction for appropriate nursing intervention is Johnson's Behavioral Model (JBM).
      1. Person seen as behavioral system, not simple biologic system.
      2. Biologic, psychological, and sociologic factors considered.
      3. Consists of seven subsystems—interrelated, yet open.
         a. Attachment/affiliative.
         b. Dependency.
         c. Ingestive.
         d. Eliminative.

The views expressed in this chapter are those of the author and do not reflect the official policy or position of the Department of the Army, Department of Defense, or the United States Government.

TABLE 6–1. **Staff Beliefs That Prevent Intervention With Client Sexuality**

Someone else will do it	They are not worried about it
They never bring up the subject	They are too (young, old, sick)
I do not know how to help	It will offend them if I ask
I do not have time	There is no privacy
Only perverts have questions	I am not married
I do not believe in sex for single people	I do not have the specialized education
They should be grateful to be alive	

  e. Sexual.
  f. Aggressive.
  g. Achievement.
 4. Disturbance in one subsystem affects other subsystems (e.g., when eliminative subsystem is disrupted owing to incontinence after radical prostatectomy, it affects sexual subsystem).
C. Symbolic interaction theory combines with JBM to include how the individual interpretation of a symbol can affect behavior.
 Example:
 1. When chemotherapy stops menses, one woman may interpret this as she is "no longer a woman" and stops coitus.
 2. Another woman may have the same side effect but may interpret it as "no more mess" and increase sexual activity based on her interpretation.
III. "PLISSIT" Model for Intervention.
 A. Useful model for levels of nursing intervention based on the nurse's comfort with subject of sexuality.
 B. Ability to intervene at an appropriate level based on nurse's expertise.
 C. Nurse may refer to another provider at any level of intervention.
  1. "P" = Permission.
   a. First level of intervention.
    (1) All nurses are able to provide this level of intervention.
    (2) Sexuality is part of human functioning.
    (3) Addressing sexual concerns is part of nursing care.
    (4) Nurses initiate discussion to convey acceptability of the topic.
   b. Nurses need to know basic information about sexuality.
    (1) Anatomy and physiology.
    (2) How disease affects sexual functioning.
    (3) How treatment affects sexual functioning.
    (4) Sexual response cycle.
   c. Example: Many women after mastectomy have questions about if or when to let their partner see the incision.
  2. "LI" = Limited Information.
   a. Second level of intervention.
    (1) Most nurses are able to intervene at this level.
    (2) Addresses concerns, questions, myths, misconceptions.
   b. Nurses need to know facts about how diagnosis and treatment can affect sexuality.
   c. Example: Sometimes men have worried that if they have intercourse

with their wife after treatment of cervical cancer with a radiation implant, their penis will "glow in the dark."
3. "SS" = Specific Suggestions.
   a. Third level of intervention.
      (1) Many experienced or advanced practice nurses are able to intervene at this level.
      (2) Suggestions need to be appropriate for:
         (a) Cultural beliefs.
         (b) Client's value system.
         (c) Partner's value system.
   b. Example: Hormonal therapy can sometimes decrease vaginal lubrication. (LI level) Water-soluble lubrication can decrease the risk of vaginal tears or dyspareunia.
4. "IT" = Intensive Therapy.
   a. Requires in-depth knowledge level about sexuality and counseling.
   b. Usually needed for long-standing or severe concerns.
   c. Example: If treatment brings up issues of childhood abuse, intensive therapy is needed.

Assessment, Planning, and Implementation

I. Reproductive issues.
   A. Three components—pregnancy prevention, treatment, fertility.
      1. Prevention of pregnancy.
         a. Risk factors.
            (1) Risk of birth defects, miscarriages.
               (a) Radiation from diagnostic workups and radiation therapy.
               (b) Mutagenic, teratogenic effects of chemotherapy.
               (c) Spontaneous abortion following surgical procedure.
            (2) May use unreliable birth control because of:
               (a) Cultural beliefs.
               (b) Lack of access to birth control.
               (c) Partner may not accept birth control.
               (d) Denial they have cancer.
               (e) Desire to get "accidentally" pregnant.
                  (i) Yearning for "return to normal."
                  (ii) Opportunity for adolescent to rebel.
                  (iii) May worry treatment will cause infertility, so seen as "last chance."
         b. Prevention.
            (1) Need to assess above risks.
               (a) Work with client to choose appropriate intervention for prevention of pregnancy based on belief system, religious belief, culture, other reasons.
               (b) Assess "meaning" of pregnancy to client.
               (c) Explain to clients the rationale for no conception during workup, treatment, and minimum of 1 year posttreatment.
            (2) Limited information level of intervention needed.
               (a) Intrauterine device (IUD)—risk of infection if client is neutropenic.
               (b) Diaphragm—need for refitting if weight change; risk of infection if client is neutropenic.

(c) Hormonal birth control—not appropriate for hormone-dependant tumors; can affect vaginal lubrication and increase risk of dyspareunia.

(d) Condoms—allow prevention of sexually transmitted diseases (STD).

c. Management

(1) Ensure referrals for birth control counseling.

(2) Use PLISSIT model for intervention management.

(3) Discuss importance of not becoming pregnant after treatment (specific time based on type of treatment given and follow-up needed, e.g., scans that have radiation risk).

2. Treatment issues during pregnancy.

a. Risk factors (depend on trimester).

(1) Diagnostic tests.

(a) May be risk to the fetus.

(b) Diagnosis of cancer itself may be more difficult because of pregnancy changes.

(i) Example: 1 to 4% of women with breast cancer are pregnant at the time of diagnosis.

(ii) Diagnosis of breast cancer may be delayed owing to vascular, lymphatic, and density changes in the breast consequent to pregnancy.

(iii) Diagnostic tests may be delayed owing to pregnancy, which may affect survival of client.

(2) Chemotherapy agents.

(a) Type of agent affects risk to fetus.

(i) Avoid antimetabolites (especially methotrexate), alkylating agents, and folic acid antagonists in the first trimester.

(ii) Teratogenic potential affected by drug dosage, ability of drug to enter fetal circulation, route of administration.

(b) First trimester is greatest time of risk.

(i) National Cancer Institute (NCI) set up database in 1985 to examine pregnancy outcomes after use of chemotherapy.

(ii) 29 babies born to the first 210 registered mothers had abnormal outcomes.

(iii) Most data available based on a single agent, not the combination regimens that are now used.

(3) Radiation therapy.

(a) Usually delayed until after delivery.

(b) Risk depends on field, amount of Gy.

b. Prevention of complications during treatment while pregnant.

(1) Diagnostic tests considerations.

(a) May adjust workup to reduce risk to fetus.

(i) May order ultrasound instead of radiologic test if possible.

(ii) Magnetic resonance imaging instead of computed tomography (CT) scan so no radiation exposure to fetus.

(iii) If early stage disease, may omit late stage workup, e.g., bone scan.

(b) May be able to modify diagnostic test procedure, e.g., shield fetus.

(c) Consult with obstetrician when making diagnostic decisions.

  (2) Chemotherapy agents.

   (a) Usually safer to give chemotherapy during the second or third trimester.

   (b) May increase risk to fetus of:

    (i) Low birth weight.

    (ii) Mutagenesis.

    (iii) Teratogenic effects.

   (c) Weigh risks/benefits of various regimens.

   (d) Consider delay of treatment initiation if possible.

   (e) Address issue of pregnancy termination but keep in mind cultural and religious beliefs.

  (3) Radiation therapy.

   (a) Shield fetus if possible.

   (b) Delay therapy until after delivery if possible.

  (4) Surgery.

   (a) Timing of surgery (trimester of pregnancy).

   (b) Type of surgery.

   (c) Anesthetic agent used:

    (i) Relatively safe.

    (ii) Compensate for pregnancy-induced physiologic and anatomic changes.

   (d) Length of surgery.

 c. Management of pregnant client during oncologic treatment.

  (1) Review choices concerning continuation of pregnancy.

  (2) If the client remains pregnant, provide high-risk prenatal care.

   (a) Risk of thrombocytopenia.

   (b) Risk of disseminated intravascular coagulation.

   (c) Risk of premature delivery due to physical stress of illness, treatment, or side effects.

  (3) Evaluate treatment options with client and discuss one with lowest risk to fetus.

  (4) Initiate discussion about which life is a priority if an emergency occurs.

  (5) Carefully evaluate each drug for safety.

   (a) Assess if crosses placental barrier.

   (b) Example: Lorazepam increases risk of floppy baby syndrome.

   (c) After delivery, need to counsel mother about risk to baby if she breastfeeds while on chemotherapy.

    (i) Potential for immune suppression/neutropenia.

    (ii) Unknown effect on growth.

    (iii) Possible risk of carcinogenesis.

3. Fertility.

 a. Risk factors.

  (1) Type and amount of chemotherapy.

   (a) Lomustine, doxorubicin, melphalan can suppress gonadal function.

   (b) Cyclophosphamide, cytarabine, fluorouracil usually have reversible germ cell toxicity.

   (c) Age of patient (e.g., puberty or perimenopausal) affects risk to fertility.

   (2) Single versus combination chemotherapy affects risk.
       (a) 80% of men who receive mechlorethamine, vincristine (On-
           covin), procarbazine, and prednisone (MOPP) combination
           therapy have fertility affected.
       (b) Fertility affected in 35% of men treated with Adriamycin, bleo-
           mycin, vinblastine, dacarbazine (ABVD) combination therapy;
           fertility is usually recovered.
       (c) Fertility may reverse as late as 4 years after treatment, so serial
           measurements of serum follicle-stimulating hormone (FSH)
           sperm counts need to be done.
   (3) Amount of radiation therapy.
       (a) For males receiving pelvic radiation.
            (i) Age of male does not affect risk of sterility.
           (ii) Less than 4 Gy results in temporary sterility.
          (iii) Greater than 5 Gy results in permanent sterility.
       (b) For females:
            (i) Age and amount of radiation dosage affect risk of sterility.
           (ii) 95% women under the age of 40 receiving 20 Gy fraction-
                ated over 5 to 6 weeks will have sterility.
          (iii) Over age 40, a dose of only 6 Gy affects sterility.
   (4) Field of radiation therapy, i.e., abdomen or pelvis.
   (5) Type of surgery.
       (a) Bilateral orchiectomy.
       (b) Total penectomy.
       (c) If affects prostatic nerve plexus or presacral sympathetic nerves.
       (d) Complete removal of prostate and seminal vesicles.
       (e) Hysterectomy.
   (6) Age of client at time of treatment.
   (7) Type of malignancy.
       (a) Diagnosis itself may affect fertility.
       (b) Examples: Many men when diagnosed with Hodgkin's disease
           or testicular cancer have low sperm count.
 b. Prevention.
   (1) Choose treatment with least risk to fertility.
   (2) Sperm banking if the client meets criteria.
   (3) Use of oophoropexy reduces ovarian exposure by as much as 50%.
   (4) No direct radiation treatment to gonads.
   (5) Methods to preserve fertility (Table 6–2).

TABLE 6–2. **Preservation of Fertility**

Sperm banking
Egg retrieval (experimental)
Zone drilling of egg (experimental)
Careful selection of chemotherapy agents
Shielding of gonads during radiation therapy
Retrieval of sperm from retrograde ejaculation
Oophoropexy

    c. Management.
       (1) Grief counseling for loss of fertility.
       (2) Treatment for retrograde ejaculation may restore fertility.
           (a) Certain drugs can temporarily close sphincter so the man can ejaculate sperm.
           (b) Example: sympathomimetic phenylpropanolamine.
  B. Sexuality dysfunction.
    1. Risk factors.
       a. Hormonal.
          (1) Hormonal therapy in men.
              (a) Gynecomastia.
              (b) Feminization.
              (c) Erection dysfunction.
              (d) Decreased fertility.
              (e) Penile/testicular atrophy.
              (f) Decrease or loss of libido.
          (2) Hormonal therapy in women.
              (a) Decreased vaginal lubrication.
              (b) Change in libido.
              (c) Masculinization.
       b. Radiation therapy.
          (1) Amount of radiation (Gy).
          (2) Type of radiation.
              (a) External can cause fibrosis to blood vessels.
              (b) Internal can cause vaginal stenosis.
          (3) Area of radiation field.
              (a) Temporary or permanent erectile dysfunction or decreased vaginal lubrication from vascular or nerve damage to pelvis.
              (b) See Table 6–3 for sexual dysfunction after pelvic radiation in women.
       c. Chemotherapy.
          (1) Decrease or loss of libido.
          (2) Retarded ejaculation.
          (3) Erectile dysfunction or loss of vaginal lubrication.
          (4) Neuropathies.
              (a) If pain in fingers, affects ability to touch partner.
              (b) If pain in jaw, affects ability to kiss partner.
          (5) Antimetabolites and antitumor antibiotics as single agents do not directly cause sexual dysfunction but may potentiate dysfunction when given with alkylating agents.
          (6) Chemotherapy side effects of oral or vaginal stomatitis, nausea, fatigue, and others affect sexual functioning.

TABLE 6–3. **Sexual Dysfunction After Pelvic Radiation Therapy (Female)**

Decreased vaginal lubrication	Change in usual sexual expression
Dyspareunia	Shortening of vaginal vault
Change in vaginal sensation	Decreased elasticity of vagina
Risk of infection due to decreased vaginal lubrication	Increased vaginal irritation

d. Surgical intervention.
   (1) Prostatectomy.
       (a) Retrograde ejaculation.
       (b) Erectile dysfunction if there is damage to autonomic nerve plexus.
       (c) Occasionally, diminished orgasm intensity.
   (2) Orchiectomy.
       (a) No change if only one testicle is removed.
       (b) Risk of erectile dysfunction, decreased libido, premature ejaculation, decreased orgasm intensity if radical abdominal lymph node dissection is done.
       (c) Bilateral orchiectomy may decrease libido and cause atrophy of the penis.
   (3) Cystectomy.
       (a) Damages nerves.
       (b) Loss of vaginal lubrication in women or erection dysfunction in men.
       (c) Change in vaginal diameter and length.
       (d) Retrograde ejaculation.
   (4) Head and neck surgery.
       (a) Appearance affects body image and the way in which others view client.
       (b) Change in speech and ability to whisper during lovemaking.
       (c) Removal of spinal accessory nerve affects ability to turn the head.
       (d) Change in smell and taste sensations.
       (e) Drooling or the sensation of respirations on the neck of partner may affect partner's sexual desire.
2. Prevention.
   a. Education and anticipatory guidance.
      (1) Explain physiology of sexual functioning and ways in which diagnosis and treatment may affect functioning.
          (a) See Table 6–4 for psychological factors that affect sexual functioning.
          (b) See Table 6–5 for physiologic factors that influence sexual functioning.
      (2) Do not assume that the client knows basic sexuality information.
      (3) Use models or drawings.
      (4) Dispel myths or misconceptions (e.g., fear that anal stimulation caused rectal cancer).

TABLE 6–4. **Psychological Factors That Affect Sexual Functioning**

Anxiety	Low self-esteem
Fear	Feelings of isolation
Depression	Change in body image
Change in affect/personality	Fear of transmitting cancer
Grief	Heightened sense of vulnerability
Guilt	Withdrawal

TABLE 6–5. **Physiologic Factors That Affect Sexuality**

Fatigue	Lymphedema
Pain	Change in skin texture/pigmentation
Sleep deprivation	Decreased vaginal lubrication
Constipation/diarrhea	Weight fluctuations/muscle atrophy
Respiratory compromise	Menopausal symptoms
Alopecia	Decreased complete blood counts
Fistulas/draining wounds	Severity of cancer
Neuropathy	Comorbidity of chronic diseases
Shingles	Phantom uterine contractions after hysterectomy
Availability of partner	

    b. Encourage the couple's intercommunications.
        (1) Serve as a role model for couple by speaking openly when discussing sexual functioning.
        (2) Use a nonjudgmental approach as they discuss their fears or feelings.
        (3) Allow them to conduct role playing in a safe environment demonstrating how they may begin conversation with a partner about changes in sexual functioning.
    c. Be a client advocate.
        (1) Be aware of medications that affect sexual functioning (e.g., narcotics, hormones, sedatives).
        (2) Suggest medications with fewer side effects.
  3. Management.
    a. Conduct a sexual history.
        (1) Use PLISSIT model to intervene.
        (2) Incorporate client's value system and cultural beliefs into intervention.
    b. Help client expand sexual options to accommodate changes in sexual functioning.
        (1) Massage, fantasy, change in positions, use of sexy lingerie to cover incision site or ostomy, use of lubricants, penile stuffing.
        (2) Facilitate referrals for medical intervention for penile implants, penile injections, vacuum devices, vaginal reconstruction.
    c. Provide strategies to enlarge clients' knowledge base.
        (1) Encourage attendance at support groups.
        (2) Inform them of written resources on sexuality and cancer.
        (3) Write a short article on sexuality and cancer for the local support group newsletter or offer to present a class to them.

Nursing Diagnoses

  I. Nursing diagnoses specific to sexuality.
    A. Body image disturbance.
    B. Situational low self-esteem.
    C. Sexual dysfunction.

    D. Altered sexuality patterns.

    E. Impaired social interaction.

II. In accordance with JBM, other nursing diagnoses (activity intolerance, anxiety, bowel incontinence, decreased cardiac output, caregiver role strain, self-care deficit) can affect sexual functioning.

    A. With a diagnosis of impaired gas exchange, client may become easily fatigued during sexual activity.

    B. Example of how to use PLISSIT model to intervene for this nursing diagnosis:

      1. "P" = bring up subject that shortness of breath (SOB) may affect sexuality.

      2. "LI" = inform couple how SOB can affect stamina.

      3. "SS" = help couple explore ways to conserve energy by a change in position.

      4. "IT" = refer to sex therapist if above three levels of intervention not effective.

Outcome Identification

I. Client identifies potential or actual alterations in sexuality due to disease or treatment (e.g., infertility, dry mucous membranes, decreased/lack of libido, erection dysfunction, and premature menopause).

II. Client expresses feelings about alterations (e.g., alopecia, body image changes, and altered sexual functioning). (Caution: these outcomes are specific to Western culture.)

III. Client engages in open communication with partner.

IV. Client describes strategies he/she can use in response to actual or potential sexual changes (e.g., change in position to decrease fatigue or penile implant if erection dysfunction is present).

V. Client identifies satisfactory alternative methods for expressing sexuality.

VI. Client identifies personal and community resources to assist with changes in body image and sexuality.

Evaluation

    The oncology nurse systematically and regularly evaluates the client's and/or the family's responses to interventions to determine progress toward the achievement of expected outcomes. Relevant data are collected and actual findings are compared with expected findings. Nursing diagnoses, outcomes, and plans of care are reviewed and revised as necessary.

BIBLIOGRAPHY

Bello, L.K., & McIntire, S. (1995). Body image disturbances in young adults with cancer: Implications for the oncology clinical nurse specialist. *Cancer Nurs 18*(2), 138–143.

Cartwright-Alcarese, F. (1995). Addressing sexual dysfunction following radiation therapy for a gynecologic malignancy. *Oncol Nurs Forum 22*(8), 1227–1232.

Filiberti, A., Audisio, R.A., Gangeri, L. (1994). Prevalence of sexual dysfunction in male cancer patients treated with rectal excision and coloanal anastomosis. *Eur J Surg Oncol 20*(1), 43–46.

Ghizzani, A., Pirtoli, L., & Bellezza, A. (1995). The evaluation of some factors influencing the sexual life of women affected by breast cancer. *J Sex Marital Ther 21*(1), 57–63.

Hughes, M.K. (1996). Sexuality changes in the cancer patient. *Nurs Interventions Oncol 8,* 15.

Hulter, B., & Lundberg, P.O. (1994). Sexual function in women with hypothalamo-pituitary disorders. *Arch Sex Behav 23*(2), 171–183.

Lamb, M.A. (1995). Effects of cancer on the sexuality and fertility of women. *Semin Oncol Nurs 11*(2), 120–127.

Nishimoto, P.W. (1995). Sex and sexuality in the cancer patient. *Nurs Pract Forum 6*(4), 221–227.

Ofman, U.S. (1995). Preservation of function in genitourinary cancers: Psychosexual and psychosocial issues. *Ca Invest 13*(1), 125–131.

Shell, J.A., & Smith, C.K. (1994). Sexuality and the older person with cancer. *Oncol Nurs Forum 21*(3), 553–558.

Smith, D.B. (1994). Sexuality and the patient with cancer: What nurses need to know. *Oncol Pt Care 4*, 1.

Zarcone, J., Smithline, L., Koopman, C., et al. (1995). Sexuality and spousal support among women with advanced breast cancer. *Breast J 1*(1), 52–57.

Symptom Management and Supportive Care: Dying and Death

Margaret J. Crowley, RN, MSEd, CRNH

PALLIATIVE CARE AND HOSPICE CARE

Theory

I. Palliative care is symptom management that is intended to relieve but not cure.
II. Hospice care is a system of care designed to provide for the needs of the client and family/significant others as they deal with the client's terminal illness.
  A. Care is provided by a team of hospice workers.
  B. The nurse is the coordinator of care.
  C. The client/family or significant others is the unit of care.
  D. Care is usually provided in the home.
III. Palliative or hospice care may be indicated in the following situations:
  A. Metastasis is documented.
  B. Disease is progressing with treatment.
  C. Disease recurs after remission.
  D. Poor prognosis at diagnosis and client not eligible for treatment.
  E. Poor prognosis at diagnosis and client elects no treatment.
  F. Prognosis is less than 6 months.

Assessment

I. Identify primary physician for palliative care.
II. Obtain medical history from physician.
III. Evaluate the client and family understanding of care goals.
IV. Determine that the client and family chose hospice/palliative care.

Nursing Diagnosis

I. Knowledge deficit related to care of the terminally ill.

Outcome Identification

I. Client and family receive care appropriate to the disease prognosis.
II. Client chooses a hospice/palliative care program.

Planning and Implementation

I. Provide client and family with palliative care/hospice options.

II. Inform client and family of appropriate agencies.

III. Complete referral to agency.

IV. Obtain informed consent from client for palliative care/hospice care

Evaluation

The oncology nurse systematically and regularly evaluates the client's and/or family's response to interventions to determine progress toward the achievement of expected outcomes. Relevant data are collected and actual findings are compared with expected findings. Nursing diagnoses, outcomes, and plans of care are reviewed and revised as necessary.

PAIN

Theory

I. 85% of cancer patients have pain that responds well to usual treatment.

II. 15% of patients have pain that requires specialized knowledge or techniques to control pain.

III. According to the American Pain Society, cancer pain may be acute, chronic, or intermittent, and it often has a definable etiology, which is usually related to tumor recurrence or treatment.

IV. Most pain in advanced cancer is related to the disease and is chronic and progressive.

    A. Acute pain can occur that may or may not be related to the cancer.

    B. Constant monitoring and adjustment of the pain control regimen is required.

V. Morphine sulfate is the drug of choice for severe pain.

VI. Adjuvant medications enhance pain control (see Chapter 10).

    A. Steroids.

    B. Tricyclics.

    C. Anticonvulsants.

    D. Nonsteroidal antiinflammatory drugs (NSAIDs).

VII. Physical and behavioral interventions may be used in addition to pharmacologic therapy.

    A. Cutaneous stimulation (e.g., heat and cold, massage).

    B. Behavioral interventions (e.g., relaxation technique).

VIII. Nonpharmacologic invasive interventions may be used for pain not responsive to pharmacologic and behavioral interventions.

    A. Radiation at either primary or metastatic sites.

    B. Radiopharmaceuticals (e.g., strontium 89).

    C. Surgical intervention to interfere with pain transmission (i.e., cordotomy).

    D. Nerve blocks to interfere with pain transmission.

IX. Intraspinal or epidural infusion may be considered.

    A. When pain not relieved with systemic opioids.

    B. If side effects of systemic opioids limit escalation.

X. Exercise is important for the treatment of chronic pain.
   A. Strengthens muscles.
   B. Mobilizes stiff joints.
   C. Restores coordination and balance.
XI. Barriers to adequate pain control include:
   A. Fear of addiction to narcotics.
   B. Concern regarding side effects of medications.
   C. Fear of what the pain represents.

Assessment

I. Obtain current pain rating on a scale of 0 to 10 with 0 equal to no pain and 10 equal to the worst pain the client can imagine.
II. Evaluate pain status via pain assessment tool (see Chapter 1).
III. Obtain history of drugs used for pain management.
IV. Obtain history of nonpharmacologic, noninvasive management techniques employed.
   A. Guided imagery.
   B. Relaxation technique.
   C. Distraction.
   D. Heat and cold applications.
V. Continuously evaluate pain control and pain status.
   A. Determine if pain is changing in location or quality.
   B. Determine if pain is not responding to current interventions.
VI. Determine client and family goals for pain control.
VII. Evaluate for side effects of narcotics.
   A. Constipation.
   B. Nausea and vomiting.
   C. Sedation.
VIII. Determine barriers to pain control.

Nursing Diagnoses

I. Acute or chronic pain.
II. Impaired physical mobility.
III. Altered role performance.
IV. Sleep pattern disturbance.
V. Management of therapeutic regimen, ineffective individual.
VI. Spiritual distress.
VII. Social isolation.

Outcome Identification

I. Client and family have adequate knowledge related to pain regimen.
II. Client and family goals for pain relief are met.

III. Client is independent in activities of daily living for as long as possible.
IV. Client is comfortable at the time of death.

Planning and Implementation

   I. Instruct the client and family on the pain control regimen.
      A. Round-the-clock dosing.
      B. Keeping a log of medication used and client's response to medication.
      C. Proper use of delivery system for intravenous, subcutaneous, or epidural administration of medication.
  II. Consult with physician regarding the appropriate titration of medications for pain relief.
 III. Assess the client's ability to take oral medications and use alternate route when necessary.
      A. Transdermal.
      B. Sublingual.
      C. Rectal suppositories.
      D. Subcutaneous, intermittent.
      E. Intravenous or subcutaneous, continuously.
      F. Intravenous or subcutaneous continuously and with patient-controlled bolus dosing as needed.
  IV. Consult with physician regarding the use of adjuvant medications for pain.
   V. Collaborate with physician regarding nonpharmacologic invasive interventions and ensure client understanding of modalities.
  VI. Collaborate with physician regarding nonresponsive pain and consider referral to pain team or clinic.
 VII. Teach and evaluate psychological interventions dependent upon the client's cognitive functions.
VIII. Consult with social worker and chaplain regarding psychosocial and spiritual components of pain.
  IX. Encourage activity and consult with physical therapists and occupational therapists.

Evaluation

The oncology nurse systematically and regularly evaluates the client's and/or family's response to interventions to determine progress toward the achievement of expected outcomes. Relevant data are collected and actual findings are compared with expected findings. Nursing diagnoses, outcomes, and plans of care are reviewed and revised as necessary.

ELIMINATION

Theory

  I. The most common cause of constipation in clients with cancer is opioid use without adequate doses of laxatives.
 II. Additional causes of constipation include low fiber diet, dehydration, reduced defecation, depression, and hypercalcemia.

III. Persons who are not eating continue to produce waste in the bowel.
IV. Causes of diarrhea include fecal impaction, malignant intestinal obstruction, laxative imbalance, and loss of sphincter control.
V. Urinary retention and/or urinary incontinence may result from spinal cord involvement by tumor, increased weakness and confusion, side effects of medication, urinary tract infection, and dehydration.

Assessment

I. Obtain history of the bowel problem including those laxatives that have been used.
II. Complete abdominal physical assessment.
   A. Examine abdomen for presence of fecal masses and tenderness.
   B. Palpate for full bladder.
   C. Perform rectal examination for presence of impacted feces, malignant stenosis, and empty balloon rectum (higher impaction).
   D. Assess bowel sounds.
III. Obtain history of usual elimination patterns.
IV. Obtain intake history and evaluate for dehydration.
V. Assess for urinary tract infection—frequency, burning on urination, and urgency.
VI. Assess signs of spinal cord involvement.
   A. Back pain.
   B. Lower extremity weakness.
   C. Loss of rectal sensation.

Nursing Diagnoses

I. Constipation.
II. Bowel incontinence.
III. Functional incontinence.
IV. Urinary retention.
V. Risk for impaired skin integrity.

Outcome Identification

I. Constipation is eliminated.
II. Diarrhea is controlled.
III. Urinary retention is relieved.
IV. Skin remains intact.
V. Family copes with client's needs.

Planning and Implementation

I. Teach use of laxatives (Table 7–1).
II. Remove impaction.

TABLE 7–1. **Constipation Management in Pharmacologic Management of Cancer Pain**

Start all patients on
   Senokot-S 2 tabs po hs
If no bowel movement in any 24-hour period:
   Senokot-S 2 to 4 tabs po bid–tid
If no bowel movement in any 48-hour period:
   Dulcolax 2 to 3 tabs po hs–tid
If no bowel movement in any 72-hour period:
   Nonimpacted
      Haley's MO 45–60 ml po
      Magnesium citrate 8 oz po
      Lactulose 45–60 ml po
      Dulcolax suppository 1 pr
      Fleet phosphasoda enema 1 pr
   Impacted
      Disimpact
      Enemas until clear
   Increase daily Senokot-S and Dulcolax

Abbreviations: tabs, tablets; po, orally; hs, at bedtime; bid, twice daily; tid, three times daily; pr, per rectum.

From Levy, M.H. (1994). Pharmacologic management of cancer pain. *Semin Oncol 21*(6), 730.

  III. Teach dietary interventions (see Chapter 14).

  IV. Teach use of protective skin barriers and adult incontinence pads.

   V. Teach use of antidiarrheal medications.

  VI. Obtain urine for culture if appropriate.

 VII. Insert Foley catheter for retention and teach the family the care of the catheter.

VIII. Encourage increased intake of fluids.

     A. Intravenous hydration is rarely used in the care of terminally ill patients.

     B. A short course of hydration may be considered if symptoms are temporary and are expected to be controlled.

  IX. Notify physician if spinal cord involvement is suspected.

Evaluation

The oncology nurse systematically and regularly evaluates the client's and/or family's response to interventions to determine progress toward the achievement of expected outcomes. Relevant data are collected and actual findings are compared with expected findings. Nursing diagnoses, outcomes, and plans of care are reviewed and revised as necessary.

DYSPNEA

Theory

   I. Some shortness of breath is reported in 40% of patients on admission to hospice.

     A. Dyspnea is a subjective symptom that can be undetected by an outside observer.

B. Dyspnea is accompanied by feelings of anxiety and frustration.
II. Causes of dyspnea in advanced cancer are multiple (Table 7–2).
III. Morphine sulfate is an effective drug for the treatment of dyspnea.
IV. The role of oxygen therapy in nonhypoxic, dyspneic cancer patients is uncertain, but it may increase comfort.

Assessment

I. Assess respiratory status.
   A. Auscultate breath sounds in all lung fields.
      1. Breath sounds present or absent?
      2. Crackles or wheezes present?
      3. Cough present?
      4. Secretions are present. What color?
   B. Evaluate respiratory pattern.
      1. Respiratory rate.
      2. Depth of respirations.
      3. Irregular breathing patterns.
   C. Obtain history.
      1. Onset: sudden, gradual.
      2. Impact on activity.
      3. Frequency and duration.
      4. Pulmonary metastases.

TABLE 7–2. **Causes of Dyspnea in Patients with Advanced Cancer**

Carcinoma of the lung
   Obstruction lesions with atelectasis and pneumonia
   Restrictive ventilatory defect
   Lymphangitic spread
   Metastases
   Impaired diaphragmatic function
   Pleural effusions
   Superior vena cava syndrome
   Bleeding
   Pneumothorax

Prior cancer therapy
   Postpneumonectomy
   Postradiation fibrosis
   Chemotherapy

Generalized debility

Thrombotic pulmonary embolism

Tumor pulmonary embolism

Aspiration pneumonia

Pneumonia due to infection

Underlying chronic obstructive pulmonary disease or congestive heart failure

Massive ascites

Anxiety

From Enck, R. (1994). *The Medical Care of Terminally Ill Patients*. Baltimore: Copyright The Johns Hopkins University Press, p. 42. Reprinted by permission of The Johns Hopkins University Press.

    D. Assess for anemia (see Chapter 15).

    E. Assess for congestive heart failure.

       1. Auscultate lungs for rales.

       2. Check for peripheral edema.

II. Evaluate subjective symptoms.

    A. Weakness.

    B. Suffocation.

    C. Tightness.

    D. Panic or anxiety.

Nursing Diagnoses

   I. Anxiety

  II. Activity intolerance.

 III. Impaired gas exchange.

 IV. Knowledge deficit related to dyspnea.

Outcome Identification

   I. Client is able to manage episodes of dyspnea.

  II. Client is relieved of the perception of breathlessness.

 III. Client's respiratory rate remains at a comfortable level.

Planning and Implementation

   I. Collaborate with the physician regarding pharmacologic management and teach the family and client proper use of medications.

    A. Bronchodilators.

    B. Anxiolytics.

    C. Steroids.

    D. Morphine by mouth, intravenously (IV), subcutaneously (SQ), or via nebulizer.

    E. Furosemide (Lasix) for congestive heart failure.

  II. Collaborate with physician regarding blood transfusions for anemia.

 III. Teach behavioral interventions.

    A. Positioning.

       1. Sitting up, using a table to support the arms and upper body.

       2. Elevate head of bed.

    B. Pacing of activities.

       1. Provide periods of rest between activities.

       2. Change times of activities.

       3. Transfer responsibilities to someone else.

       4. Shower while sitting.

    C. Pursed-lip breathing.

    D. Use of electric fan to create a stream of air against cheek.

 IV. Provide reassurance.

    A. Instruct family to remain with the client during acute attacks.

B. Instruct that dyspnea can be controlled and nurse is available 24 hours by telephone.

Evaluation

The oncology nurse systematically and regularly evaluates the client's and/or family's response to interventions to determine progress toward the achievement of expected outcomes. Relevant data are collected and actual findings are compared with expected findings. Nursing diagnoses, outcomes, and plans of care are reviewed and revised as necessary.

ANOREXIA

Theory

 I. Anorexia is related to the disease process.
 II. Anorexia causes a great deal of stress and anxiety between caregivers and clients.
 III. Enteral feedings are not suggested for patients with end-stage disease.
 IV. Parenteral feedings are not appropriate.

Assessment

 I. Explore the meaning of not eating with the client and family.
 II. Identify factors that discourage eating.
 III. Obtain dietary history.

Nursing Diagnosis

I. Altered nutrition, less than body requirements.

Outcome Identification

 I. Client and family accept the client's inability to eat.
 II. Client eats what he/she wishes.

Planning and Implementation

 I. Normalize the feelings of the caregiver and client.
    A. Caregiver may feel frustrated with preparation of foods that are not eaten.
    B. Client may feel unable to live up to caregiver expectations.
 II. Explain possible causes of anorexia.
 III. Inform the caregiver that the client is unable and not unwilling to eat.
 IV. Suggest small meals and liquid supplements.
 V. Consult with physician to determine if stimulants or steroids (e.g., megestrol) are appropriate.

Evaluation

The oncology nurse systematically and regularly evaluates the client's and/or family's response to interventions to determine progress toward the achievement

of expected outcomes. Relevant data are collected and actual findings are compared with expected findings. Nursing diagnoses, outcomes, and plans of care are reviewed and revised as necessary.

NAUSEA AND VOMITING

Theory

   I. Multiple causes of nausea and vomiting in terminal illness (Table 7–3).
      A. Attempt should be made to identify underlying etiologies, and corrective measures may be instituted.
      B. Client preferences and prognostic expectations must be weighed when considering therapeutic interventions.
  II. Palliative treatment most often consists of antiemetic medications, dietary manipulation, and behavioral interventions.
 III. Bowel obstructions may be treated conservatively with antiemetics, stool softeners, and soft or liquid diets.
      A. Initiation of intravenous fluids and antiemetics with the use of a nasogastric suction may be considered for severe obstruction and vomiting.

TABLE 7–3. **Common Causes of Nausea and Vomiting in Patients with Advanced Disease**

Fluid and electrolyte disturbances
  Hypercalcemia
  Volume depletion
  Water intoxication (syndrome of inappropriate antidiuretic hormone [SIADH] secretion)
  Adrenocortical insufficiency

Gastrointestinal causes
  Mouth: infections (*Candida albicans,* herpes simplex) and ulceration
  Taste: postchemotherapy and tumor effect
  Esophagus: fungal infections, obstruction, and postradiation therapy inflammation
  Stomach: irritation and stasis
  Obstruction of the small bowel
  Constipation

Pancreatic carcinoma—gastric stasis

Hepatic metastases

Peritonitis

Central nervous system metastases
  Brain
  Meninges

Renal failure with uremia

Local infections and septicemia

Tumor toxins

Drugs
  Opioid analgesics
  Other medications such as digoxin and nonsteroidal antiinflammatory drugs

Radiation therapy, especially treatment of the gastrointestinal tract

Syndrome of cardiovascular autonomic insufficiency

Behavioral/psychogenic problems

From Enck, R. (1994). *The Medical Care of Terminally Ill Patients.* Baltimore: Copyright The Johns Hopkins University Press, p. 13. Reprinted by permission of the Johns Hopkins University Press.

B. Nasogastric tubes are uncomfortable, and medical management without suction may be preferred.

Assessment

  I. Assess for possible causes of nausea and vomiting.
   A. Constipation.
   B. Opioid-induced.
   C. Hypercalcemia.
   D. Bowel obstruction.
   E. Increased intracranial pressure.
 II. Obtain history of occurrences of nausea and vomiting.

Nursing Diagnoses

  I. Altered nutrition, less than body requirements.
 II. Risk for fluid volume deficit.

Outcome Identification

  I. Nausea and vomiting are controlled.
 II. Adequate nutrition and hydration are maintained, as appropriate, to promote client comfort.

Planning and Implementation

    I. Report signs and symptoms of nausea and vomiting to physician.
   II. Treat causes of nausea and vomiting when possible; for example, relieve constipation.
  III. Collaborate with physician in selecting antiemetics.
   IV. Teach client and family use of medications.
    V. Suggest dietary changes.
       A. Cold foods or foods at room temperature (decrease odors).
       B. Clear liquid diet.
       C. Avoidance of sweet, fatty, highly salted, or spicy foods.
   VI. Limit sights, sounds, or smells that can induce vomiting.
  VII. Provide fresh air.
 VIII. Provide distraction and relaxation techniques.
   IX. Consult client, family, and physician if nasogastric suction is appropriate and initiate.

Evaluation

The oncology nurse systematically and regularly evaluates the client's and/or family's response to interventions to determine progress toward the achievement of expected outcomes. Relevant data are collected and actual findings are compared with expected findings. Nursing diagnoses, outcomes, and plans of care are reviewed and revised as necessary.

DEHYDRATION

Theory

I. Dehydration in terminally ill clients may be considered predictable and does not necessarily require an attempt to reverse the condition.

II. Major physical problem of dehydration is dry mouth.

III. Dehydration is an emotional issue for the family.

IV. Positive effects of dehydration include:

A. Decreased urine output with the effect of less incontinence and less need for catheterization.

B. Decreased gastric secretions and less vomiting.

C. Decreased pulmonary secretions and edema with quieter breathing and less need for suctioning.

D. Decreased ascites and peripheral edema.

Assessment

I. Assess client's intake and output.

II. Evaluate client and family wishes for intervention.

III. Assess condition of client's mouth.

Nursing Diagnoses

I. Fluid volume deficit.

II. Altered oral mucous membrane.

Outcome Identification

I. Family recognize dehydration as predictable event in the dying process.

II. Client is comfortable at the time of death.

III. Client and family are comfortable with the decision regarding hydration.

Planning and Implementation

I. Describe possible positive effects of dehydration.

II. Discuss disadvantages of hydration.

A. Invasive procedures.

B. Increased pulmonary and cardiac load.

C. Possible need for urinary catheterization.

D. May decrease patient comfort.

III. Recognize family needs and respect wishes if the family chose hydration.

IV. Consult with physician and initiate hydration if appropriate.

V. Teach oral care every 2 hours to moisten mouth and protect mucous membranes.

VI. Provide small amounts of fluids for comfort.

Evaluation

The oncology nurse systematically and regularly evaluates the client's and/or family's response to interventions to determine progress toward the achievement

of expected outcomes. Relevant data are collected and actual findings are compared with expected findings. Nursing diagnoses, outcomes, and plans of care are reviewed and revised as necessary.

RESTLESSNESS AND AGITATION

Theory

I. Causes of restlessness and agitation include:
   A. Unrelieved pain.
   B. Distended bladder or rectum.
   C. Hypercalcemia.
   D. Cerebral anoxia.
   E. Dyspnea.
   F. Inability to move.
II. Delirium may occur and is characterized by its acute onset and hallucinations, disorientation, and clouding of consciousness.

Assessment

I. Assess for reversible causes of agitation.
II. Review medications for drugs that may contribute to agitation, such as steroids or neuroleptics.
III. Note degree of agitation and the effects on the family.
   A. Caregivers unable to sleep at night.
   B. Disorganization in the home because of client demands.
IV. Assess for safety.
   A. Client not left alone.
   B. Bedrails provided.
   C. Room uncluttered.

Nursing Diagnoses

I. Confusion.
II. Altered thought processes.
III. Caregiver role strain.

Outcome Identification

I. Client is calm and suffers a minimal amount of agitation as death approaches.
II. Client is not injured.
III. Caregiver has support needed to allow death to occur at home.

Planning and Implementation

I. Treat reversible causes.
II. Collaborate with physician to discontinue medications or change doses.
III. Provide well-lit room and familiar objects.
IV. Minimize disturbance and keep environment calm.

V. Support family with additional help in the home.

VI. Provide respite in a community skilled nursing facility if the family needs relief from stress.

VII. Consult with physician if drugs, such as haloperidol (Haldol) or chlorpromazine (Thorazine), are needed to control symptoms.

Evaluation

The oncology nurse systematically and regularly evaluates the client's and/or family's response to interventions to determine progress toward the achievement of expected outcomes. Relevant data are collected and actual findings are compared with expected findings. Nursing diagnoses, outcomes, and plans of care are reviewed and revised as necessary.

IMMINENT DEATH

Theory

I. Dying due to chronic illness is rarely rapid and may last from a few hours to a few days.

II. Dying is a continuous process because the body is unable to cope with hypoxia, malnutrition, electrolyte imbalance, tumor burden, and toxins that are not cleared as hepatic and renal failure occur.

III. Emotion, cognition, thinking behavior, and autonomic function all slowly deteriorate, and coma usually occurs before death.

Assessment

I. Assess for signs of impending death.

A. Mental changes such as withdrawal from social interaction, dreaming or visualizing persons who have died, or talking about going away on a trip or going back home.

B. Decreased fluid and food intake.

C. Dysphagia.

D. Increased sleeping.

E. Decreased urine output.

F. Restlessness and agitation.

G. Changes in breathing pattern.

H. Noisy or moist breathing.

I. Decreased circulation with mottling of the skin.

J. Coma.

II. Assess caregiver recognition of impending death.

Nursing Diagnosis

I. Impending death.

Outcome Identification

I. Family is prepared for client's death.

II. Client dies with dignity.

Planning and Implementation

    I. Ensure that all comfort measures are provided.
       A. Continue pain medications.
       B. Provide mouth care.
       C. Provide preventive skin care.
       D. Ensure proper positioning of client.
    II. Consult with physician for medications, such as anticholinergics for moist breathing and benzodiazepines for restlessness.
   III. Instruct the family in the symptoms of impending death.
   IV. Plan with the family for the death event.
       A. Will there be adequate caregivers in the home?
       B. Does the family wish that the nurse, chaplain, or social worker visit at the time of death?
       C. Are funeral arrangements in place?
       D. Does the family understand the need to call the hospice nurse at the time of death?
       E. Is the family aware of the local requirements regarding pronouncement at the time of death?
    V. Encourage the family members to say good-bye and to give permission to the dying person to let go.

SOCIAL SUPPORT

Theory

    I. Psychosocial factors influence the client's level of comfort with the dying process.
       A. Major family reorganization may occur with the terminal diagnosis.
       B. Different family systems react differently to hospice/palliative care.
          1. Open family systems emphasize a flexible, adaptive approach to group operations.
             a. Realizes each individual's interests.
             b. Amenable to outside interventions
          2. Closed family systems are authoritarian in construct with clearly defined head of household.
             a. One individual may be responsible for all decision making.
             b. Clear guidelines within which each family member interacts.
             c. Resistant to outside intervention.
          3. Random family systems emphasize variety, individuality, and excitement.
             a. High regard for individual freedom.
             b. May be inviting to outside intervention but chaotic and unmanageable.
             c. Social support has significant influence on psychological adjustment for cancer patients.
          4. Social support is primarily the emotional assistance that one receives from significant others.
          5. The dying person has increased needs for affection and for relationships with others.
    II. Anticipatory grieving occurs in the expectation of future losses.
       A. Family members mourn the eventual loss of the individual family member.
       B. The individual mourns his/her own losses: independence, traditional role in the family and eventual death.

Assessment

I. Identify the type of family system.
II. Collaborate with the social worker to complete a family assessment.
III. Identify the primary caregiver.
IV. Identify the learning needs and abilities of the caregiver.

Nursing Diagnoses

I. Ineffective individual coping related to terminal diagnosis.
II. Ineffective family coping related to terminal diagnosis.
III. Knowledge deficit related to terminal care needs.

Outcome Identification

I. The family/significant other provides the comfort care that the client requires.
II. The client and family/significant other begin the work of anticipatory grief.
III. The client experiences a death with dignity.

Planning and Implementation

I. Interventions to strengthen the family.
  A. Encourage communication among family members.
    1. Listen to family members and client.
    2. Encourage the family and client to "tell their own stories."
    3. Address fears directly and provide information to allow the family to deal with fears.
  B. Respect the privacy of the family and accept the family's coping styles.
  C. Contact outside resources to provide additional social support.
    1. Offer volunteers from the hospice.
    2. Refer to community agencies.
    3. Provide homemaker support.
    4. Provide respite care in a community facility.
II. Interventions to teach caregiving skills to primary caregiver.
  A. Provide instruction regarding technical skills and comfort measures.
  B. Demonstrate appropriate skills.
  C. Provide 24-hour availability for emergency situations or caregiver questions and concerns.
III. Help the client redefine long-term goals and set more immediate goals such as seeing friends, listening to music, or completing unfinished business.

Evaluation

The oncology nurse systematically and regularly evaluates the client's and/or family's response to interventions to determine progress toward the achievement of expected outcomes. Relevant data are collected and actual findings are compared with expected findings. Nursing diagnoses, outcomes, and plans of care are reviewed and revised as necessary.

SPIRITUAL

Theory

I. Spiritual needs need to be considered in the care of the individual with terminal diagnosis.

II. Spiritual needs include:
  A. Finding meaning.
    1. Meaning of the illness.
    2. Meaning of life as it was lived.
    3. Meaning of the remaining days.
  B. Finding hope.
    1. Expectation of a good that is yet to come.
    2. Desire not to die alone.
    3. Exploration of belief in afterlife, resurrection, or rebirth.
  C. Defining relatedness.
    1. To God.
    2. To others.
  D. Finding forgiveness.
    1. Finding a means of dealing with mistakes or sins.
    2. Acceptance of life, mistakes, suffering.

Assessment

I. Assess for spiritual distress and determine spiritual needs.
  A. What does being in this situation mean to you?
  B. Are there things in your life about which you feel particularly proud? Regret?
  C. What is left undone in your life?
  D. What is your hope for yourself?
  E. What are your spiritual needs?
II. Identify religious practices that have meaning for the client.
  A. Religious affiliation.
  B. Degree of involvement with church, synagogue, or other institutions.
  C. Rituals or sacrament that are meaningful to the client.

Nursing Diagnoses

I. Spiritual distress.
II. Potential for enhancement of spiritual well-being.

Outcome Identification

I. The client and family/significant other are sustained during the dying process by their own spiritual values.

Planning and Implementation

I. Primary intervention is the nurse's willingness to stay in an active presence with the client.
  A. Listen to the client as he/she questions spiritual issues.
  B. Remain nonjudgmental as the client questions as well as finds answers.
  C. Encourage the family to remain present with the client.
II. Share normative information.
  A. Fears, guilt, doubts, and failure of faith are not uncommon.
  B. Virtually everyone involved in this work has similar struggles.
III. Activate the client's spiritual resources.
  A. Refer to clergyman or hospice chaplain.

B. Acquire reading material and read with client.

C. Pray with the client, if appropriate.

Evaluation

The oncology nurse systematically and regularly evaluates the client's and/or family's response to interventions to determine progress toward the achievement of expected outcomes. Relevant data are collected and actual findings are compared with expected findings. Nursing diagnoses, outcomes, and plans of care are reviewed and revised as necessary.

BEREAVEMENT

Theory

I. Bereavement care is part of a comprehensive palliative/hospice care program.

II. Bereavement is a normal human experience.

III. Tasks of bereavement include:

A. Accepting the reality of the loss.

B. Experiencing the pain of grief.

C. Adjusting to the new environment.

IV. Manifestations of grief associated with loss of loved one may include:

A. Social withdrawal.

B. Restlessness.

C. Loss of weight.

D. Inability to sleep.

E. Exhaustion.

F. Heart palpitations.

G. Anxiety.

H. Decreased interest, motivation, or initiative.

V. Complicated grief is manifested by an increased intensity of response and increased length of response.

VI. Risk factors for developing complicated grief include:

A. Reawakening of an old loss.

B. Multiple losses.

C. Guilt associated with relationship with deceased.

D. Angry or ambivalent relationship with deceased.

E. Social isolation.

F. Lack of financial support.

G. History of physical and/or mental illness.

Assessment

I. Assess family for risk factors associated with unresolved grief.

II. Evaluate family members for manifestations of grief.

III. Assess social support available to family.

Nursing Diagnoses

I. Potential for growth in family coping.

II. Ineffective family coping.

III. Knowledge deficit related to bereavement.

Outcome Identification

I. Family completes the tasks of bereavement.

Planning and Implementation

   I. Before death occurs, encourage family members and significant others to say good-bye to client.
  II. Provide time for family/significant others to relive the traumatic events of the death and "tell their stories."
 III. Add to the stability of the family's social world.
     A. Make bereavement visit.
     B. Attend or participate in funeral.
     C. Ensure bereavement follow-up.
        1. Refer to appropriate counseling.
        2. Collaborate with social worker and chaplain in completing referral.
 IV. Provide information regarding grief response.

Evaluation

The oncology nurse systematically and regularly evaluates the client's and/or family's response to interventions to determine progress toward the achievement of expected outcomes. Relevant data are collected and actual findings are compared with expected findings. Nursing diagnoses, outcomes, and plans of care are reviewed and revised as necessary.

BIBLIOGRAPHY

American Pain Society (1992). *Principles of Analgesic Use in the Treatment of Acute Pain and Cancer Pain* (3rd ed.). Skokie, IL: American Pain Society.
Coyne, P. (1995). Standard of care for pain management interventions. *Oncol Nurs Forum 22*(9), 1437–1438.
Dudgeon, D., & Rosenthal, S. (1996). Management of dyspnea and cough in patients with cancer. *Hematol Oncol Clin North Am 10*(1), 157–169.
Enck, R.E. (1994*). The Medical Care of Terminally Ill Patients.* Baltimore: The Johns Hopkins University Press.
Enck, Robert (1992). The last few days. *Am J Hosp Palliat Care 9*(4), 11–13.
Gulla, J.P. (1992). Family assessment and its relation to hospice care. *Am J Hosp Palliat Care 9*(4), 30–33.
Jacox, A., Carr, D.B., Payne, R., et al. (1994). *Management of Cancer Pain, Clinical Practice Guideline No. 9.* AHCPR Publication No. 94-0592. Rockville, MD. Agency for Health Care Policy and Research, U.S. Department of Health and Human Services, Public Health Service.
Kaye, P. (1993). *Symptom Control in Hospice and Palliative Care.* Essex, CT: Hospice Education Institute.
Kemp, C. (1994). Spiritual care in terminal illness. *Am J Hosp Palliat Care 1*(5), 31–36.
Kemp, C. (1995). *Terminal Illness: A Guide to Nursing Care.* Philadelphia: J.B. Lippincott Co.
Levy, M. (1993). Controlling cancer and its symptoms. *Am J Hosp Palliat Care 10*(1), 19–27.
Levy, M.H. (1994). Pharmacologic management of cancer pain. *Semin Oncol 21*(6), 718–739.
McCann, R.M., Hall, W.J., & Groth Juncker, A. (1994). Comfort care for terminally ill patients: the appropriate use of nutrition and hydration. *JAMA 272*(16), 1263–1266.
Meares, C.J. (1994). Terminal dehydration: A review. *Am J Hosp Palliat Care 11*(3), 10–14.
Morgan, A.E., Lindley, C.M., & Berry, J.I. (1994). Assessment of pain and patterns of analgesic use in hospice patients. *Am J Hosp Palliat Care 11*(1), 13–25.
Rousseau, P. (1995). Antiemetic therapy in adults with terminal disease: A brief review. *Am J Hosp Palliat Care 12*(1), 13–18.
Storey, P. (1994). *Primer of Palliative Care.* Gainesville, FL: The Academy of Hospice Physicians.
Worden, J.W. (1985). Bereavement. *Semin Oncol 12*(4), 472–475.
Zerwekh, J.V. (1995). A family caregiving model for hospice nursing. *Hospice J 10*(1), 27–43.

Symptom Management and Supportive Care: Rehabilitation and Resources

Doris Ahana, RN, MSN, OCN

Theory

I. Rationale for rehabilitation.
   A. Over 10 million Americans alive today have a history of cancer.
      1. Estimated 7 million are living 5 years or more after a cancer diagnosis.
   B. Increasing need for rehabilitation to improve the quality of life of cancer clients whose lives have been extended with advancement in technology and treatment.
II. Synopsis of *Rehabilitation of People with Cancer: An ONS Position Statement.*
   A. Definition—rehabilitation is the process by which individuals are assisted, within their environments, to achieve optimal functioning and wellness.
   B. Structure—rehabilitation services available to address the individual's physical, psychological, spiritual, social, vocational, and educational potential.
   C. Process—services provided according to the individual's preventive, restorative, supportive, or palliative needs.
   D. Outcome—individuals achieve optimal functioning and wellness.
III. Cancer rehabilitation concepts.
   A. The interdisciplinary team of health professionals, volunteers, and, most importantly, the client and family, contributes to the rehabilitation plan.
      1. Composition of team varies according to client need and resource availability.
         a. Health professionals involved may include: Oncology nurse—inpatient, outpatient, home care; physiatrist; social worker; physician; physical therapist; occupational therapist; dietitian; chaplain/minister; financial counselor; enterostomal therapist; pharmacist; recreational therapist; dentist; psychiatrist; speech language pathologist.
         b. Case manager or other specialist may serve as coordinator of the rehabilitation process.
   B. Continuity of cancer care requires coordinated and comprehensive system of care throughout the health care and community-based settings.
   C. Rehabilitation enhanced through the process of sharing and developing a common bond with others who have similar problems.
   D. Human needs that include the physiologic, psychosocial, and spiritual dimensions addressed through a holistic approach.

IV. Goals of rehabilitation.
   A. Goal-setting requires interaction between the client and family and health professionals.
      1. Validate strengths, limitations, and rehabilitation potential with client.
      2. Identify goals that are realistic and achievable within the context of the client and family situation.
   B. Goals for rehabilitation services.
      1. Preventive rehabilitation.
         a. Reduce impact and severity of disabilities.
         b. Focus is on clients with a disability that can be predicted.
      2. Restorative rehabilitation.
         a. Resume pre-illness level of functioning with minimal residual disability.
         b. Focus is on clients who are cured.
      3. Supportive rehabilitation.
         a. Reduce cancer-related disability in clients who are maintained on treatment for ongoing disease to control cancer.
      4. Palliative rehabilitation.
         a. Reduce and eliminate complications, increase autonomy, provide comfort and emotional support when there is increasing disability from progressive disease.
         b. Focus is on terminally ill clients.
V. Barriers to cancer rehabilitation.
   A. Cancer viewed as terminal rather than curable, as compared with other chronic diseases, by both the public and health professionals.
   B. Control of health care cost in a managed care environment further constrains rehabilitation.
      1. Lack of available and appropriate resources.
      2. Limitations in rehabilitation benefits from health plans.
   C. Fiscal crisis in the federal and state government affects community support and resources for continuity of comprehensive services to clients and families.
VI. Major trends that affect rehabilitation.
   A. Growing numbers of elderly, ethnic minorities, and poor who need assistance to:
      1. Enroll in and utilize appropriate hospital and community services.
      2. Meet their basic extramedical needs such as housing, food, and clothing.
      3. Become well informed to make sound decisions about their treatment.
   B. Increasing use of alternative healing to promote mental and physical fitness—diet, exercise, stress reduction.
   C. Increasing consumer awareness related to wellness, prevention, self-determination, and quality of life.
   D. Shift from in-client care to out-client care requires increased technologic skills and complex care in the community setting and produces increasing demands on the caregiver.

Assessment

I. Data collection.
   A. Use a comprehensive, reliable, and valid tool to assess rehabilitation needs.

B. Upon entry to a health care facility, obtain baseline assessment data.
   1. Trigger cues for further evaluation by appropriate health professionals (Figure 8–1).
C. Data should include:
   1. Demographic and medical information.
      a. Disease process—type and stage of disease, location of cancer, prognosis.
      b. Type and duration of treatment.
      c. Other comorbidities.
      d. Biographic data—age, occupation, socioeconomic status, religion, education, marital status, insurance.
   2. Psychosocial.
      a. Personal characteristics—attitudes toward cancer, coping abilities, problem-solving skills, self-concept, motivation to learn, recreational interest.
      b. Family characteristics—perception of cancer; reaction to stress, roles, and relationships.
      c. Support systems.
         (1) Identify available support—spouse or significant other, children, friends, peers, minister, chaplain or church member, school counselor, teacher, employer.
         (2) Assess type of support family member or significant other is able to provide—educational, emotional, instrumental (care and tasks).
   3. Physical assessment.
      a. Body system review for physiologic problems or symptoms that may affect rehabilitation potential.
      b. Functional health patterns—cognition, communication, mobility, activities of daily living, nutritional, bowel and bladder functioning, pain.
D. Continue assessment as needs change.

Sample of Admission Database

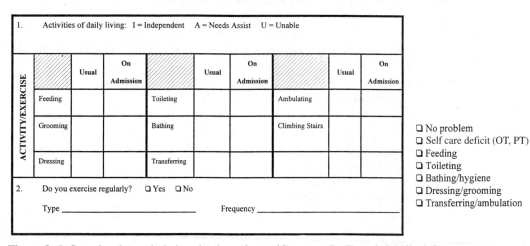

Figure 8–1. Sample of an admission database form. (Courtesy St. Francis Medical Center, Honolulu, HI, 1996.)

Nursing Diagnoses

    I. Ineffective individual coping.
   II. Ineffective family coping.
  III. Altered role performance.
  IV. Body image disturbance.
   V. Knowledge deficit.
  VI. Self-care deficit: feeding, bathing, hygiene, dressing, grooming, toileting.
 VII. Activity intolerance.
VIII. Impaired home maintenance management.

Outcome Identification

    I. Client participates in decision making and care.
   II. Client and family/significant other demonstrate measures to manage symptoms from disease process and treatment.
  III. Client achieves maximal level of activity.
  IV. Client demonstrates skills in self-care.
   V. Client and family/significant other use appropriate sources of support to cope with alterations in:
      A. Body image
      B. Roles
      C. Lifestyle
  VI. Client and family/significant other demonstrate knowledge of complications related to immobility.
 VII. Client and family/significant other identify available organizations that can provide assistance at home.

Planning and Implementation

   I. Interventions to promote client autonomy and independence.
     A. Encourage client to participate in decisions that affect his or her care.
     B. Provide and reinforce information on cancer, treatment plan, symptom management, and cancer resources in the community.
     C. Praise client for positive self-care behaviors to build self-confidence and facilitate mastery of technical skills.
     D. Work collaboratively with physician and other health professionals to identify and control or treat factors that interfere with self-care activities—electrolyte imbalance, hyponatremia, fatigue, cognitive changes, malnutrition, situational depression, uncontrolled pain, edema.
     E. Support family members in their role as coach to encourage the client to assume greater responsibility for self-care.
     F. Empower client through education—coping skills, self-care skills, symptom management, community resources.
     G. Explore the cultural expectations of client and family and adapt teaching to meet their needs.
  II. Interventions to help cancer clients and their families cope with cancer-associated treatment, losses, and lifestyle changes.

A. Support client in expression of feelings about changes in appearance, function, and lifestyle.
B. Encourage open communication between client and family to meet their individual and collective needs (e.g., reassignment of roles, social activities).
C. Refer client to the local office of the American Cancer Society for support groups, volunteer visitation programs, and educational programs.
D. Make referrals to mental health professionals and social services for individual and family counseling to resolve issues related to body image and role alterations.
E. Provide information about prosthetic devices, wigs, cosmetics, and reconstructive surgery to enhance self-esteem in clients facing mastectomy or lumpectomy, amputation, head and neck surgery, chemotherapy- or radiation-associated skin changes and hair loss.

TABLE 8–1. **Comprehensive Rehabilitation: Multidisciplinary Team Resources**

Rehabilitation Issues	Resources

Cancer education
  Disease
  Treatment
  Nutrition
  Community resources
  Levels of care
	Individual or group teaching:
	  Nurse, physician, dietitian,
	  social worker

Physical—functional status
  Self-care skills
  Technical skills
    Ostomy care
    Incontinence management
    Assistive devices
    Symptom management, e.g., pain, nausea and
      vomiting
	Physical therapist, occupational
	  therapist, nurse,
	  enterostomal therapist,
	  physical/occupational
	  therapist, pain specialist,
	  clinical pharmacist,
	  nutritionist

Communication/speech	Speech/language pathologist

Psychological support
  Coping skills
  Lifestyle changes
	Social worker, psychiatric nurse
	  specialist, psychiatrist, sex
	  therapist

Spiritual support, beliefs and practices	Minister, priest

Economic issues
  Financial resources
  Insurance—life and medical
  Disability benefits
  Vocational—employment discrimination
	Social worker, financial
	  counselor

Legal and ethical issues
  Client rights
  Advanced directives: wills, power of attorney
	Nurse, client advocate, social
	  worker, attorney

School-related issues
  School re-entry and academic performance
	Social worker, nurse, school
	  counselor or teacher

Housing	Social worker

Personal care: grooming, bathing, dressing, toileting,
  mobility, meal preparation, shopping, household
  chores, child care, transportation, equipment
	Home care nurse, physical
	  therapist, occupational
	  therapist, home health aides

III. Interventions to rehabilitate cancer clients with functional status limitations.
  A. Consult with an occupational therapist, physical therapist, nutritionist, social service worker, and members of other appropriate disciplines to assist with the identification of resources, special equipment, devices, and environmental modification necessary to permit maximal functioning.
  B. Encourage progressive mobility from active range of motion exercises to functional activities.
  C. Coordinate treatment and activities to minimize fatigue.
  D. Provide positive reinforcement for activities out of bed. Avoid immobilization or long confinement in bed.
  E. Maintain normal range of motion and exercises to increase endurance and strength.
IV. Interventions to provide comprehensive care and continuity of services.
  A. Conduct a client and family meeting with physicians and other appropriate health professionals before treatment (surgery, chemotherapy, and radiation) to:
    1. Clarify myths and misconceptions.
    2. Identify potential and actual problems.
    3. Identify resource availability in the acute care setting and at home.
  B. Initiate site- or treatment-specific client and family education using educational materials appropriate to their level of understanding. Utilize a language interpreter for non-English–speaking client and family.
  C. Recognize the developmental needs of the young and the elderly cancer clients when planning the rehabilitation goals, interventions, and outcome.
  D. Support family in their role of caregiver by encouraging use of self-help groups and volunteers to supplement care.
  E. Refer client to cancer rehabilitation team members to assist with the physical, psychosocial, spiritual, vocational/economic, legal/ethical, and home care/personal care issues (Table 8–1).
  F. Assist client and family to contact and use:
    1. Local agencies for non-medical needs.
      a. Agencies on aging.
      b. Legal Aid Society.
      c. Social Security Administration.
      d. Veterans Affairs Center.
  G. Refer to local, regional, national, and international organizations for information and support services (Table 8–2).

TABLE 8–2. **National Cancer Resources**

American Brain Tumor Association 2720 River Road, Suite 146 Des Plaines, IL 60018 (800) 886-2282 (client line) (708) 827-9910	Provides: • Educational publications about brain tumors and related treatment to clients and families. • List of brain tumor support groups, referrals to support organizations and a pen-pal program.
American Cancer Society (L) 1599 Clifton Road, NE Atlanta, Ga 30329-4251 (404) 320-3333 (General Nursing)	Operates through 157 divisions and 3000 local units throughout the United States. Provides: • Printed and audiovisual materials for clients.

TABLE 8–2. **National Cancer Resources** (*Continued*)

(404) 329-7616
(Dept. of Nursing)
	• Educational programs for nurses and other health professionals.
	• Site-specific support programs, including visitations by trained volunteers:
	  1. Reach to Recovery (Breast)
	  2. International Association of Laryngectomies (Larynx)
	  3. Local Ostomy Association (Colorectal, Urostomy, Ileostomy)
	• Resources and educational programs:
	  1. I CAN COPE—Series of classes to assist clients and families cope with the diagnosis of cancer.
	  2. Community Connection: Resources, Information and Guidance (RIG). Provides current information about community and American Cancer Society resources for cancer clients and families.
	  3. Can Surmount: One-to-one visitation.

American Foundation for Urologic Disease 300 West Pratt Street Suite 401 Baltimore, MD 21201-2463 (410) 727-2908	Offers a prostate cancer support group network that facilitates intergroup communications, program development, and leadership development for prostate cancer survivor support groups.
Candlelighters Childhood Cancer Foundation 7910 Woodmont Avenue, Suite 406 Bethesda, MD 20814 (301) 657-8401 (800) 366-2223 *or* (800) 366-CCCF	International organization of parents whose children have or had cancer. • Provides information, support, referral, and access to survivors of childhood cancer to parents of children with cancer.
Cancer Care, Inc. (L) 1180 Avenue of the Americas New York, NY 10036 (800) 813-HOPE 4673 (212) 302-2400	A voluntary social service agency that offers: • Free professional social work counseling and guidance to help clients and families cope with cancer. • Financial assistance to eligible families to help with home care, child care, transportation, pain medication. • Toll-free counseling line to provide information and referral to local community resources, counseling support, and education.
Cancer Information Service (CIS) (I) (800) 4-CANCER (R)	National Cancer Institute program that provides: • Information about cancer causes, prevention, diagnosis, treatment, rehabilitation, and research. • Information about resources in local area. • PDQ data to public and healthcare professionals.
COPE 2019 North Carothers Franklin, TN 37064 (615) 790-2400	Publishes journal for America's oncologists and oncology nurses. Provides information to empower clients and professionals to cope with the many issues confronting their daily lives. Assists health professionals to establish comprehensive breast cancer rehabilitation services.

Table continued on following page

TABLE 8–2. **National Cancer Resources** (*Continued*)

Encore Plus (L) YWCA of USA Office of Women's Health Initiative 624 9th Street, NW 3rd Floor Washington, DC 20001 (202) 628-3636 FAX: (202) 783-7123	Offers postdiagnostic support that includes a specially designed exercise regimen and peer group or individual support session.
Johanna's On Call to Mend Esteem Cancer Rehabilitation Nurse Consultants 199 New Scotland Avenue Albany, NY 12208 (518) 482-4178	Offers private client consultation for pre– and post–breast surgery. Provides information on exercise, arm and hand care, positive self-image, and support organizations.
Leukemia Society of America, Inc. (L) 600 Third Avenue New York, NY 10016 (212) 573-8484 (800) 955-4LSA	Provides information, support groups, financial assistance for outclient chemotherapy drugs and therapy, transportation, and transfusions to persons with leukemia, lymphoma, and multiple myeloma.
Lymphedema Foundation P.O. Box 834 San Diego, CA 92014-0834 (800) LYMPH-DX *or* (800) 596-7439	Provides information and resources to persons with lymphedema and to health professionals who treat it.
Make Today Count (L) (I) 101 1/2 South Union Street Alexandria, Va 22314-3323	Provides support groups, informational materials, and educational programs to persons and families with cancer or other life-threatening illness.
National Association for Continence P.O. Box 8306 for Consumers P.O. Box 8310 Spartanburg, SC 29305 (800) BLADDER (803) 579-7900 FAX: (864) 579-7902	Provides information on the management of incontinence and resources on incontinence devices and absorbent products. Publishes and disseminates educational materials about diagnosis, treatment, and management of incontinence. Continent referral service.
National Brain Tumor Foundation 785 Market Street, Suite 1600 San Francisco, CA 94103 (800) 934-2873 or (415) 284-0208 FAX: (415) 284-0209	Provides: • "The Support Line," composed of a network of nurses, clients, and their families who offer one-to-one support by phone. • Brain Tumor guide and directory for brain tumor clients and family members.
National Cancer Institute Office of Cancer Communications Public Inquiries Bethesda, MD 20892 (301) 496-5583	Offers education programs and up-to-date information about cancer to clients, the public, and health professionals.
National Coalition for Cancer Survivorship 1010 Wayne Avenue Silver Spring, MD 20910 (301) 650-8868	Coalition of key organizations in the cancer community working together to: • Advocate the interests of cancer survivors. • Serve as a clearinghouse for information, materials, and programs on survivorship.
National Hospice Organization 1901 North Moore Street, Suite 901 Arlington, VA 22209 (793) 243-5900 (800) 658-8898 (Hospice Helpline)	Provides educational materials and information about hospice care to clients and their families.

TABLE 8–2. **National Cancer Resources** (*Continued*)

National Lymphedema Network 2211 Post Street, Suite 404 San Francisco, CA 94115 (800) 541-3259	Provides information on the prevention and management of primary and secondary lymphedema.
Prostate Cancer Support Network (L) 300 West Prutt Street, Suite 401 Baltimore, MD 21201 (410) 727-2908	Provides education and advocacy for prostate cancer issues through a network of prostate cancer survivors and support groups.
The Oley Foundation 214 Hun Memorial A23 Albany, NY 12208 (518) 262-5079 (800) 776-OLEY	Provides free information and emotional support to clients requiring home nutritional support that includes enteral and parenteral nutrition.
United Ostomy Association, Inc. (L) (I) 36 Executive Park, Suite 120 Irvine, CA 92714 (714) 660-8624	Offers support, mutual aid, and information to persons with colostomy, ileostomy, or urostomy. Volunteer visitations by trained ostomates.
The Wellness Community 2200 Colorado Avenue Santa Monica, CA 94040-3506 FAX: (310) 453-2300	Provides psychosocial support to cancer clients and their families.
The Women's Cancer Network 2413 West River Road Grand Island, NY 14072	Provides information and referral system to help women with cancer meet their physical and psychosocial needs and understand the health care system. Offers support group and telephone access for women confined at home.
Y-ME National Organization for Breast Cancer Information and Support 18220 Harwood Avenue Homewood, IL 60430-2104 (708) 799-8228	Offers counseling, educational programs, and self-help support groups for breast cancer clients and their families and friends.

(L) = local resource; PDQ = physician data query; (I) = international resource
From ONS Education Committee. (1995). Cancer resources in the United States. *Oncol Nurs Forum* 22(9), 1265-1272.

BIBLIOGRAPHY

American Cancer Society. (1996). Cancer Facts and Figures. Atlanta: American Cancer Society.

Baker, C. (1995). A functional status scale for measuring quality of life outcomes in head and neck cancer clients. *Cancer Nurs 18,* 452–457.

Bedder, S.M., & Aikin, J.L. (1994). Continuity of care: A challenge for ambulatory oncology nursing. *Semin Oncol 10,* 254–263.

Frymark, S. (1992). Rehabilitation resources within the team and community. *Semin Oncol Nurs 8,* 212–218.

Groenwald, S.L., Frogge, J.H., Goodman, M., & Yarbro, C.H. (eds.). (1995). *A Clinical Guide to Cancer Nursing: A Companion to Cancer Nursing.* Boston: Jones & Bartlett.

Leigh, S. (1994). Cancer survivorship: A consumer movement. *Semin Oncol 21,* 783–786.

Mayer, D.K., & O'Conner-Kelleher, L. (1993). Rehabilitation of People with Cancer: ONS Position Statement.

Mellette, S.F., & Blunk, K. (1994). Cancer rehabilitation. *Semin Oncol 21,* 779–782.

Mock, V., Burke, B.B., Sheehan, P., et al. (1994). A Nursing rehabilitation program for women with breast cancer receiving adjuvant chemotherapy. *Oncol Nurs Forum 21,* 899–906.

Oncology Nursing Society Education Committee (1995). Cancer resources in the United States. *Oncol Nurs Forum 20,* 1265–1272.

9

Symptom Management and Supportive Care: Therapies and Procedures

Jan Petree, RN, MS, FNP

Special thanks to Lynn Erdman, RN, MN, OCN, and Marcia Rostad, RN, MS, OCN, NS for work on the previous edition of these chapters, with material used from those previous chapters.

VASCULAR ACCESS: GENERAL CONSIDERATIONS FOR VENOUS, ARTERIAL, AND PERITONEAL DEVICES

Theory

I. Vascular access devices are essential in the care of clients with cancer because of:
   A. Increased use of combination intravenous therapy (antineoplastics, biologic response modifiers, immunotherapy) in the treatment of cancer.
   B. Increased use of supportive therapy (nutritional support, antibiotics, and blood component therapy) in cancer care.
   C. Increased laboratory monitoring required with aggressive therapy.
II. Types of venous catheters.
   A. Short-term or intermediate-term catheters.
      1. Description—single-lumen or multilumen catheters inserted peripherally or centrally.
         a. Inserted in forearm or antecubital fossa into the cephalic, basilic, or median cubital veins.
         b. In the neck or chest inserted into jugular (external or internal) or subclavian veins.
         c. Made out of silicone elastomer, polyurethane, or elastomeric hydrogel.
      2. Types.
         a. Catheter-over-needle or butterflies, inserted into peripheral veins.
         b. Midline catheters 6 to 8 inches long, use for therapy 2 to 6 weeks or longer, considered an intermediate-term device.
         c. Short-term central venous pressure (CVP) lines used for 7 to 10 days.
   B. Long-term venous catheters.
      1. Description—single-lumen or multilumen catheters inserted into jugular, subclavian, femoral veins.
      2. Tunneled.
         a. Description—single-lumen or multilumen catheters tunneled subcutaneously into jugular, subclavian, basilic, cephalic, and femoral veins.

    b. Tip of catheter, which is open or closed, is inserted to the distal superior vena cava and sometimes in the right atrium (for monitoring purposes).

    c. A Dacron cuff along the length of the catheter becomes embedded into the subcutaneous tissue, which:

      (1) Stabilizes the catheter.

      (2) Minimizes the risk of ascending infections up the tunnel.

    d. Silver-ion embedded cuff, in a biodegradable collagen matrix, at the exit site to prevent ascending microbes; or chlorhexidine and silver sulfadiazine embedded into polyurethane catheters.

    e. Materials are polyurethane or elastomeric silicone, or Silastic (cheaper grade material).

  2. Nontunneled.

    a. Description—catheters placed directly into jugular, femoral, or subclavian veins

    b. Long- or short-term catheters depending on catheter materials (silicone, Silastic, polyurethane).

    c. Catheter tip placement in jugular vein, subclavian vein, superior vena cava, inferior vena cava, or right atrium (depending on entry site).

C. Implanted ports.

  1. Description—single or double unit implanted surgically.

    a. Port (reservoir with self-sealing septum or reservoir) is sutured into a subcutaneous pocket near the vessel in which the catheter is inserted.

    b. Size of reservoir and gauge of the catheter vary.

    c. Entry to the port may be parallel or perpendicular to the skin (i.e., side or top entry).

    d. Port is reached with a straight or angled noncoring needle or noncoring catheter-over-needle (needle removed and catheter left in port).

  2. Types.

    a. Vascular—venous and arterial (direct administration of chemotherapy into tumor, low systemic toxicity) ports.

    b. Peripheral ports—placed in basilic, cephalic, or median cubital veins with port above or below antecubital fossa.

    c. Epidural or intraspinal ports—for administration of anesthetics, narcotics, or both for pain management.

    d. Intraperitoneal—temporary or permanent placement in abdominal cavity for peritoneal chemotherapy, surgically or percutaneously placed; either a port or catheter.

  3. Catheter materials—elastomeric silicone, Silastic, or polyurethane.

  4. Size—various French sizes according to needs of client.

D. Peripherally inserted central catheters (PICC) (Fig. 9–1).

  1. Description—central catheters placed in antecubital fossa in cephalic, basilic, or median cubital veins for short- or intermediate-term therapy.

  2. Inexpensive access device with low thoracic complications; major complications are malposition, bleeding at access site, thrombophlebitis.

  3. Advantages—decreased risk of infection; decreased risk of insertion complications; decreased costs; increased satisfaction with lack of multiple intravenous sticks; decreased air embolism, pneumothorax, thrombosis (due to small catheter size).

  4. Types—open or closed ends, single- or double-lumen (staggered ends), made out of silicone, Silastic, or polyurethane materials.

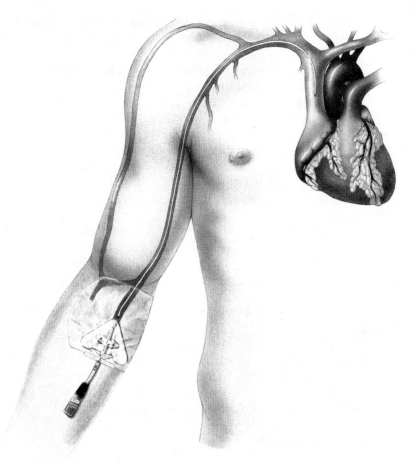

Figure 9–1. Peripherally inserted central catheter. (Courtesy of HDC Corporation, San Jose, CA.)

III. Solving problems with catheter occlusions.
   A. Catheter withdrawal occlusions.
      1. Occlusion by medications or lipids.
         a. Lipids dissolved with ethyl alcohol, 70%, via a 22 μg filter, with dwell (time it takes to dissolve precipitate) time of 1 to 2 hours.
         b. Other drugs can be dissolved with sodium bicarbonate (NaHCO$_3$) (1 mEq/mL) or with hydrochloric acid (HCl) 0.1 N, depending on whether the solution is acidic or basic, as advised by the pharmacist. Ask the pharmacist: will the change in pH dissolve the precipitate? If yes: fill catheter with volume of device, dwell time 5 minutes to 1 to 2 hours.
         c. For precipitate—increase the pH with NaHCO$_3$ or decrease pH with HCl.
      2. Use of thrombolytic agents for clotted catheters.
         a. Urokinase, 5000 IU/mL, a fibrinolytic and thrombolytic drug; allow dwell time of 30 to 60 minutes.

      b. If vein patency restored, withdraw urokinase, waste 5 to 6 mL of blood, flush with normal saline and heparin, or restore intravenous infusion.

   3. Mechanical withdrawal occlusions.

      a. Pinch-off syndrome, wherein catheter becomes pinched between the clavicle and the first rib.

      b. Secondary collapse of catheter lumen due to negative pressure.

      c. Catheter is abutted against a vein wall, such that attempts to aspirate will cause an occlusion (Valsalva maneuver, cough, deep breathe, raising arms, change position, lie in Trendelenburg position).

      d. A fibrin sheath can form at the lumen of the catheter causing a one-way valve effect, allowing infusion of IV fluids into the client but causing withdrawal occlusion.

IV. Noninfectious complications.

   A. Fibrin sheath.

   B. Catheter migration.

   C. Catheter constriction by a suture.

   D. Contrast extravasation.

   E. Malpositioned catheter tips.

   F. Catheter leak.

   G. Catheter fracture.

   H. Vascular access device maximal pressure recommendations are exceeded, which may lead to catheter rupture, catheter separation, or septum rupture; usually occurs when positive or negative force is used to clear an occlusion.

      1. Ports—usually maximal pounds per square inch (psi) are 40, with most manufacturers recommending that a smaller than 10-mL syringe not be used for flushing.

      2. Groshong catheters—maximal psi 40, with a 10- to 20-mL syringe for flushing.

      3. Pressure exerted by 3-pound weight force (your hand can exert more pressure) on an empty 3-mL syringe is 25 psi; same force with 10-mL syringe will exert 10 psi. A fluid-filled syringe of under 10 mL volume can generate 40 psi.

      4. An empty 1-mL tuberculin syringe with a 12-pound weight can force 120 to 150 psi. If fluid-filled, force may exceed 300 psi.

Assessment

  I. Identification of potential candidates for venous, arterial, and intraperitoneal access devices (Table 9–1).

 II. Physical examination.

   A. Evaluate site of potential insertion.

   B. Evaluate condition of skin over potential insertion site.

III. Psychosocial examination.

   A. Ability of client/family to care for the catheter or port.

   B. Knowledge of procedures for use of device for therapy.

   C. Concerns expressed about implications of insertion of device.

Nursing Diagnoses

  I. Risk for infection.

 II. Pain.

TABLE 9–1. **Criteria and Indications for Vascular Access Devices**

Type of Device	**Clinical Indications**	**Client Selection Criteria**
Short-term venous catheters	Infusions of chemotherapy, antibiotics, TPN, PPN, blood components, and analgesics Infusions of vesicant or irritating agents that may damage peripheral veins Urgent venous access needed	Limited venous access available Frequent venous access required Peripheral lines and midlines: need to consider osmolality of solution infused through vein (dextrose 12.5% or less)
Long-term venous catheters	Infusions of chemotherapy, antibiotics, TPN, blood components, analgesics Collection of blood samples	Limited venous access available, frequent venous access needed for prolonged period of time Long-term catheterization desired by client, ability to take care of device is necessary
Implanted ports	Infusions of all above agents Collection of blood samples	Limited venous access available for continuous or intermittent therapy anticipated, client/family unable to take care of device (infections are feared)
Peripherally inserted central catheters (PICCs)	All above therapies Blood collection samples	Client does not desire device in chest, intermediate-term therapy for 4–6 weeks or longer
Arterial catheters and implanted ports	Delivery of high concentrations of chemotherapy directly into tumor	Tumor with direct vascular access Tumor sensitive to antineoplastic agents
Intraperitoneal catheters or implanted ports	Delivery of high concentrations of chemotherapy to disease in peritoneal cavity	Metastatic cancer into the abdomen and peritoneum. Diagnosis of cancers of the ovary or colon; mesothelioma; or malignant ascites

TPN = total parenteral nutrition; PPN = peripheral parenteral nutrition

III. Risk for body image disturbance.
IV. Knowledge deficit.
V. Risk for injury.

Outcome Identification

I. Client describes the rationale, benefits, and risks of venous, arterial, or peritoneal catheters or ports.
II. Client and family/significant other participate in strategies to decrease the risks of complications of venous, arterial, or peritoneal catheters or ports.
III. Client and family/significant other list the signs and symptoms of complications of venous, arterial, or peritoneal catheters or ports to report to a member of the health care team.
IV. Client and family/significant other identify community resources for obtaining supplies for care of device.

TABLE 9–2. **Interventions for Complications of Venous, Arterial, and Peritoneal Devices**

Complication	Prevention	Restoration
Loss of blood return	Maintain flushing routine, flush with push-stop method causing swirling action in device	Change client position, roll right or left side, sit up, lie flat Change intrathoracic pressures: have client inhale fully and hold breath, or exhale fully and hold breath. Attempt push-pull method using normal saline-filled syringe (avoid using high force or high pressure) or a thrombolytic agent
Occlusion	Maintain flushing routines, flush with push-stop method causing swirling, prevent clotting. Always flush with normal saline before and after drug administration. Avoid incompatible drugs	If occlusion the result of clotted blood, urokinase may be instilled with a physician order If drug precipitate, determine type drug, check with pharmacist for drug to dissolve precipitate *Lipids* dissolve with ethyl alcohol 70% for 1–2 hours via 22 μg filter. Drugs dissolve with *sodium bicarbonate (1 mEq/mL) or hydrochloric acid (0.1 N)*
Pinch-off syndrome	Proper placement by surgeon	Put client in Trendelenburg position, with arms raised, and attempt to redraw blood
Infection	Wash hands thoroughly Follow strict aseptic techniques when using device	Administer antibiotics as ordered by the physician. Remove device as ordered by the physician, if allowed by institutional policy
Dislodgement	Avoid pulling on the catheter Tape catheters to body Teach client to avoid manipulation of catheter or port, and prevent from trauma to catheter	Refer to physician for resuturing if tip of the catheter remains in the vessel Remove device if cannot be used safely
Catheter migration	Protect device from trauma Anchor device appropriately with sutures	Refer to physician for repositioning catheter under fluoroscopy Remove device if cannot be used safely
Catheter pinholes, tracks, cuts	Avoid use of scissors or sharp objects near the catheter Clamp properly, moving device up and down length of clamping area	Repair using appropriate repair kit Move up and down to prevent areas from being worn with clamp
Erosion of port through subcutaneous tissue	Maintain adequate nutrition status. Avoid placing port at sites of actual or potential tissue damage (in radiation field) Avoid trauma or pressure over port	Refer to physician to remove the device

(Table continued on following page)

TABLE 9–2. **Interventions for Complications of Venous, Arterial, and Peritoneal Devices** (*Continued*)

Complication	Prevention	Restoration
Port-catheter separation	Avoid trauma and high-pressure infusions, or flushing with 1 mL or 3 mL syringes when clogged	Refer to physician for removal of device Use devices that are preconnected by manufacturer, instead of attaching in OR
Dislodgement of port access needle	Tape needle securely in place. Avoid tension on the needle or tubing. Place clear dressing over needle, securely fastening	Remove needle and reaccess the port using a sterile noncoring needle

V. Client and family/significant other demonstrate appropriate care of vascular access devices.

Planning and Implementation

I. Interventions to maximize safety for the client.
  A. Maintain aseptic technique when entering or manipulating the system.
  B. Teach client and family emergency procedures if the catheter is severed.
  C. Await radiographic confirmation of catheter or port placement before using device (except for midlines, radiographic examination not necessary).
II. Interventions to minimize risks for complications of venous, arterial, or peritoneal devices (Table 9–2).
III. Interventions to monitor for complications of venous or peritoneal devices.
  A. Occlusion—inability to infuse fluids with minimal pressure or inability to withdraw samples of blood or peritoneal fluid.
  B. Air embolism—presence of sudden-onset pallor or cyanosis, shortness of breath, cough, or tachycardia.
  C. Pneumothorax—presence of shortness of breath, chest pain, or tachycardia.
  D. Infection—presence of redness, pain, swelling, warmth, or drainage.
  E. Dislodgement—increase in the length of the external catheter, pain during infusion of fluids, or swelling along the catheter tract or insertion site.
  F. Migration—regional discomfort, pain, swelling, or difficulty in using device.
IV. Interventions to manage complications of venous, arterial, or peritoneal catheters or ports (see Table 9–2).

Evaluation

The oncology nurse systematically and regularly evaluates the client's and/or family's responses to interventions to determine progress toward the achievement of expected outcomes. Relevant data are collected and actual findings are compared with expected findings. Nursing diagnoses, outcomes, and plans of care are reviewed and revised as necessary.

INFUSION SYSTEMS

Theory

 I. Infusion systems have become critical in the care of clients with cancer because of:
  A. Increased emphasis on timing of antineoplastic therapy.
  B. Increased number of intravenous therapies.
  C. Need to minimize entry into the infusion system to minimize risk of infection.
 II. Infusion systems are used for:
  A. Controlling the rate of infusions.
  B. Providing positive pressure for infusions.
  C. Providing alarms; if there is a problem with the infusion, an alarm sounds.
III. Types of infusion systems.
  A. Large-volume.
   1. Examples—controllers (computer-controlled infusion pumps), volumetric pumps (mechanical pumps), variable flow systems (systems that allow large flow volumes), and multiinfusion devices or pumps.
   2. Used to administer blood components, antibiotics, parenteral nutrition, and intravenous fluids (including chemotherapy).
  B. Small-volume.
   1. Examples—intermittent syringe devices, continuous and intermittent peristaltic devices (fluid released by pressure, from a spring-like device), elastomeric (release of fluid by pressure-filled balloon-like device), and programmable portable single or multiinfusion devices (used in home, office, or hospital).
   2. Used to administer products similar to those in large-volume systems except in smaller volumes.
  C. Patient-controlled.
   1. Systems controlled by the client—deliver infusions at continuous, variable, intermittent, and basal rates.
   2. Used to administer antibiotics, antiemetics, and analgesics.
 IV. Potential complications associated with infusion systems.
  A. Occlusion.
  B. Severed or leaking infusion tubing.
  C. Mechanical errors—power failure, error in programming, insufficient fluid volume, or error in setting up the system.
  D. Infection.

Assessment

 I. Identification of potential candidates for infusion systems.
  A. Requires long-term or short-term, controlled-rate intravenous therapy.
  B. Has peripheral or central venous access established.
 II. Physical examination.
  A. Site of venous access—color, temperature, contour, drainage of entry site, exit site, or tunnel of catheter.
  B. Patency of venous access device.
III. Psychological examination.
  A. Ability of client and family to care for infusion device if intended for home use.
  B. Concerns expressed about infusion device use.

Nursing Diagnoses

I. Risk of infection.
II. Risk of injury.
III. Anxiety.
IV. Knowledge deficit.

Outcome Identification

I. Client and family/significant other participate in procedures to minimize risks of infection when manipulating the system.
II. Client and family/significant other participate in strategies to limit electrical hazards from system use.
III. Client and family/significant other participate in routine assessments to monitor for system malfunction.
IV. Client and family/significant other report signs of potential complications to appropriate health personnel.

Planning and Implementation

I. Interventions to maximize safety for the client.
   A. Maintain aseptic technique when entering or manipulating the system.
   B. Teach client and family emergency procedures to use if the system is disengaged.
   C. Maintain electrical safety—check all wiring, plugs, and accessory power packs; keep electrical equipment away from water hazards; and do not overload electrical outlets.
II. Interventions to minimize risks of complication of infusion system.
   A. Check patency of system with each system component change.
   B. Assess intactness of system, rate of infusion, remaining volume to be infused, and site of infusion at regular intervals.
   C. Use accessory components designed for the specific system.
   D. Operate infusion systems only for their intended use.
   E. Replace equipment and accessory components at intervals recommended by the manufacturer or institutional policy.
III. Interventions to monitor for complications of infusion system.
   A. Assess for redness, pain, swelling, and pus at infusion site.
   B. Assess client response to fluids being infused.
   C. Assess the system when any alarm sounds.

Evaluation

The oncology nurse systematically and regularly evaluates the client's and/or family's responses to interventions to determine progress toward the achievement of expected outcomes. Relevant data are collected and actual findings are compared with expected findings. Nursing diagnoses, outcomes, and plans of care are reviewed and revised as necessary.

BLOOD COMPONENT THERAPY

Theory

I. Use of blood component therapy in cancer care has increased with:
   A. Advancement of surgical oncology techniques.
   B. Use of more aggressive single and multimodality cancer therapy and resulting marrow suppression.

    C. Development of donor programs, hemapheresis technology, advent of peripheral stem cell programs and bone marrow transplantation.

  II. Types of blood component therapy (Table 9–3).

 III. Sources of blood components.

    A. Homologous blood—blood collected from donors for transfusion to another individual.

    B. Autologous blood—blood collected from the intended recipient.
      1. Self-donation usually made before elective surgery.
      2. Red blood cell salvage during surgery by use of automated "cell saver" device or manual suction equipment.

    C. Directly donated blood—blood collected from a donor designated by the intended recipient.

 IV. Potential complications of blood component therapy.

    A. Allergic reactions.

    B. Febrile reactions.

    C. Hemolytic reactions.

    D. Bacterial contamination.

    E. Volume overload.

    F. Hypothermia.

    G. Air emboli.

    H. Transmission of viruses.

Assessment

    I. All clients with a diagnosis of cancer may need some form of blood component therapy during the course of their illness.

  II. Factors that increase the likelihood that blood component therapy will be needed.

    A. Cancer treatment—surgery, radiation therapy, and chemotherapy.

    B. Cancer that has invaded the bone marrow.

    C. Drugs that suppress bone marrow production such as chloramphenicol, cimetidine, and ganciclovir (DHPG).

    D. Chronic infection.

    E. Chronic or acute virus infection.

    F. Aging.

    G. Malnutrition.

    H. Stress.

    I. Chronic immune deficiency.

 III. Physical assessment (see Chapter 12 and Chapter 15).

 IV. Evaluation of laboratory data.

    A. ABO type.

    B. Hemoglobin: less than 9 g/dL.

    C. Platelet count.
      1. Less than $10,000/mm^3$, with or without bleeding.
      2. Less than $20,000/mm^3$, with active bleeding.
      3. Less than $50,000/mm^3$ and scheduled for surgical procedure.

    D. Neutrophils—less than $500/mm^3$, with an infection unresponsive to antibiotic therapy.

Nursing Diagnoses

  I. Fluid volume excess.

 II. Altered body temperature.

TABLE 9–3. **Types of Blood Component Therapy**

Blood Component	Indication	Consideration
Whole blood	Replacement of blood volume Replacement of RBCs	Rarely used, except in extreme loss of volume
Red blood cells (packed)	Anemia, for replacement of RBCs	Volume overload
Leukocyte-poor packed red blood cells	Prior febrile reactions to packed RBCs May delay alloimmunizations	May use a leukocyte filter to further reduce risk of reaction
Washed or plasma-poor red blood cells.	Prior urticarial reaction, IgA deficiency, need to avoid complement transfusion	Increased viscosity of blood, thin with normal saline before transfusion
Frozen packed red blood cells	Rare blood types, autologous donations; a separation process removes plasma and leukocytes.	Used for severe RBC reactions
Platelets, random	Control or prevent bleeding; platelet count <10,000–20,000/mm^3 or client is bleeding or preoperative	Few red cells present, ABO compatibility not required
Single-donor platelets	May delay alloimmunization, lower risk of infection, exposure to one donor	
Leukocyte poor platelets	Prior febrile reactions to red cells of platelets	
HLA-matched platelets	Poor response to prior platelets transfusion due to alloimmunization	
Granulocytes	Documented infection to bacteria or fungus not responsive to therapy, with severe neutropenia, not expected to recover for several days to 1 week	Long-term therapeutic effect questionable
Fresh frozen plasma	Increase the level of clotting factors in client with documented deficiency	Plasma compatibility preferred; when thawed must transfuse within 24 hours. Watch for fluid overload
Cryoprecipitate	Increase levels of factors VIII and XIII, fibrinogen, and von Willebrand factor	Plasma compatibility preferred. If thawed, transfuse within 6 hours, if pooled within 4 hours
Factor VIII	Hemophilia A, or low ATIII levels	Clients with volume overload problems, plasma cannot be used
Factor IX	Hemophilia B deficiency	
Colloid solutions	Expand blood volume	ABO compatibility not required
Plasma substitutes	Chiefly 5% and 25% albumin and plasma protein fraction (PPF)	Provide volume expansion and colloid replacement without risk of hepatitis or HIV
Serum immune globulins	Provide passive immunity protection (i.e., against cytomegalovirus) or treat hypogammaglobulinemia	Avoid transfusion for client with allergic reactions to plasma

HLA = human leukocyte antigen; HIV = human immunodeficiency virus

III. Knowledge deficit.
IV. Risk of injury.

Outcome Identification

 I. Client describes personal risk factors for blood component therapy.
 II. Client discusses the rationale for blood component therapy.
III. Client lists signs and symptoms of reactions to blood component therapy that should be reported to the health care team.

Planning and Implementation

 I. Interventions to maximize client safety.
   A. Obtain blood components according to the institutional protocol.
   B. Check blood component type with physician order.
   C. Check blood component type and identification numbers with another registered nurse or physician.
   D. Compare blood component identification information with client identification information before administration.
   E. Examine blood product for clots, bubbles, and discoloration.
   F. Never add medications to blood products.
 II. Interventions to decrease incidence and severity of side effects.
   A. Premedicate client with antipyretics and antihistamines as ordered by physician.
   B. Attach appropriate filter and/or blood component set to the blood product.
   C. Use 20-gauge or larger needle for infusion, preferably a needle-free system.
   D. Infuse component over time, according to institutional guidelines.
      1. Packed red blood cells—infuse slowly over initial 15 minutes then remainder over 1 to 2 hours per unit.
      2. Platelets—infuse 8 units of random donor platelets over 30 to 60 minutes, and single donor platelets over 30 to 60 minutes or according to volume.
      3. Granulocytes—infuse slowly over 2 to 4 hours, premedicate with acetaminophen (Tylenol) and diphenhydramine (Benadryl).
      4. Fresh frozen plasma—administer each unit slowly or as tolerated by fluid volume.
      5. Cryoprecipitate—infuse rapidly.
      6. Concentrated factor VIII, or factor IX, infuse rapidly.
   E. Observe for signs and symptoms of transfusion reaction (fever, chills, shortness of breath, hives, kidney or back pain, blood in urine, hypotension, tachycardia, chest pain, headache).
      1. If a reaction occurs:
         a. Stop infusion and keep intravenous line open with normal saline solution.
         b. Report reaction to the physician and the transfusion service or blood bank.
         c. Check identifying tags and numbers on the blood component at the bedside.
         d. Treat symptoms noted, as ordered by the physician.
            (1) Benadryl—administer (25 to 50 mg IV)
            (2) Hydrocortisone—have available, (50 to 100 mg)
            (3) Oxygen.

(4) Meperidine (Demerol) (25 to 50 mg IV), to treat uncontrolled rigors or shaking.

(5) Tylenol (650 to 1000 mg)

(6) In the future, client should be premedicated with acetaminophen (Tylenol) and diphenhydramine (Benadryl).

    e. Monitor vital signs.

    f. Send blood bag and attached administration set and labels to the transfusion service or blood bank.

    g. Collect blood and urine samples and send to the laboratory.

2. Document transfusion reaction.

    a. Date and time noted.

    b. Signs and symptoms observed.

    c. Actions taken.

    d. Response of client after transfusion discontinued.

III. Interventions to monitor for complications of blood component therapy.

    A. Assess for general signs and symptoms—fever, chills, muscle aches and pain, back pain, chest pain, headache, and heat at site of infusion or along vessel.

    B. Assess for respiratory signs and symptoms—shortness of breath, tachypnea, apnea, cough, wheezing, rales, and/or air embolism.

    C. Assess for cardiovascular signs and symptoms—bradycardia or tachycardia, hypotension or hypertension, facial flushing, cyanosis of extremities, cool clammy skin, distended neck veins, and edema.

    D. Assess for integumentary signs and symptoms—rash, hives, swelling, urticaria, posttransfusion purpura, and diaphoresis.

    E. Assess for gastrointestinal signs and symptoms—nausea, vomiting, abdominal cramping and pain, and diarrhea.

    F. Assess for renal signs and symptoms—dark, concentrated, red- to brown-colored urine.

    G. Assess for other delayed complications—delayed hemolytic transfusion reaction, graft-versus-host disease (from nonirradiated blood), iron overload, alloimmunization, and infections: hepatitis, human immunodeficiency virus (HIV), cytomegalovirus (CMV), bacterial contamination, and parasites.

    H. Assess for changes in laboratory values such as hypocalcemia and hyperkalemia, resulting from anticoagulants in blood products combining with electrolytes.

IV. Interventions to incorporate client and family into care.

    A. Teach the purpose of the transfusion.

    B. Teach the signs and symptoms of transfusion reaction to report to the health care team.

V. Interventions to monitor for response to blood component therapy.

    A. Assess changes in laboratory values.

    B. Monitor changes in subjective responses of clients to blood component therapy.

Evaluation

The oncology nurse systematically and regularly evaluates the client's and/or family's responses to interventions to determine progress toward the achievement of expected outcomes. Relevant data are collected and actual findings are compared with expected findings. Nursing diagnoses, outcomes, and plans of care are reviewed and revised as necessary.

NUTRITION SUPPORT THERAPY

Theory

I. Nutritional complications are a common consequence in clients with a diagnosis of cancer or its treatment.

   A. Effects of malignant tumors.

      1. Cancer cells compete with normal cells for nutrients needed for cellular division and growth.

      2. Exact demands of the tumor on the host are unknown; the following metabolic changes are proposed:

         a. Altered carbohydrate metabolism—glucose is mobilized for energy and results in glucose intolerance in selected clients, and causing:

            (1) Anaerobic glycolysis—produces 2 adenosine triphosphate (ATP) molecules where complete oxidation of glucose yields 36 ATP molecules, thus anaerobic glycolysis is less efficient. Tumors use anaerobic glycolysis.

            (2) Increased rate of gluconeogenesis—estimated a 10% increase in energy expenditure for an individual with cancer.

            (3) Glucose intolerance—evidenced by a delayed clearing of intravenous or oral glucose, which could be due to lack of tissue response to insulin or defect of insulin response to hyperglycemia.

         b. Altered protein metabolism—muscle tissue is mobilized to meet increased metabolic demands and results in muscle wasting, especially in those clients with cachexia (a severe syndrome of malnutrition).

            (1) Serum albumin is often used to measure protein status.

            (2) Hypoalbuminemia is common with clients with cancer.

               (a) Normal albumin level is 4.0 g/dL.

               (b) In a client with cancer, average albumin level is 2.9 g/dL.

            (3) Increased uptake of amino acids by tumor.

            (4) Decreased protein synthesis.

            (5) Increased protein degradation; muscle protein breakdown is accelerated.

            (6) Protein loss by abnormal leakage or exertion leads to depletion of protein stores and decreased muscle mass.

            (7) Use of protein for energy needs.

               (a) For healthy individuals fat is used first.

               (b) In cancer cachexia, protein is wasted despite intake of protein.

               (c) Fat is mobilized as an energy source and results in depletion of fat stores, because glucose stores are exhausted.

         c. Fluid and electrolyte disturbances (see Chapter 13).

            (1) Hypercalcemia—high calcium levels in blood caused by certain tumors.

            (2) Hyperuricemia—along with hyperphosphatemia and hyperkalemia are a result of chemotherapy breakdown of cells in some leukemias and lymphomas, leading to tumor lysis syndrome.

            (3) Hyponatremia—common presentation with bronchogenic and oat cell carcinoma causing syndrome of inappropriate antidiuretic hormone secretion (SIADH) and causing persistent loss of sodium and excessive retention of water by the kidneys.

            (4) Hypokalemia—low potassium level caused by secretion of aldosterone, resulting in hypokalemic alkalosis. Polyuria and nocturia

are symptoms. Hypokalemia may be due to treatment by chemotherapy or antifungal therapy.

2. Cancer cells also produce biochemical substances that affect the desire for food, altering taste, causing anorexia (by central mechanisms or neurotransmitters).

3. Malignant tumors may invade or compress structures and organs vital to the ingestion, digestion, and elimination of food and fluids or may increase metabolic demands.
   a. Fistula formation.
   b. Obstruction.
   c. Decubiti.
   d. Ulcerations.

B. Effects of cancer treatment.
   1. Structural changes in the gastrointestinal system may result from surgery and result in:
      a. Inability to feed oneself.
      b. Inability to masticate or swallow.
      c. Inability to move food through the stomach and bowel.
      d. Bowel diversion.
   2. Functional changes may occur as a result of surgery, radiation therapy, or chemotherapy, and may result in:
      a. Malabsorption of fat.
      b. Gastric hypersecretion of acid.
      c. Water and electrolyte loss.
      d. Dumping syndrome.
      e. Xerostomia.
      f. Constipation.
      g. Changes in taste and smell.
   3. Metabolic changes many occur as a result of treatment or side effects of treatment such as increased energy demands that result from fever, stress, diarrhea, vomiting, and cell division or destruction.

II. Nutritional assessment.
   A. Nutritional screening—should be performed before therapy or shortly after starting therapy.
      1. Extensive nutrition history and dietary habits taken.
      2. Anthropometric measurements—height, weight, midarm circumference, skinfold thickness, calculation of ideal body weight, and body surface area.
      3. Biochemical measurements of protein status—serum albumin (half-life 20 days), transferrin (half-life 8 days), prealbumin (half-life 2 days); assessing long-term, intermediate-term, and short-term protein status.

III. Principles of medical management.
   A. Controversies exist in nutritional support for long-term management in clients with cancer.
      1. Nourishing a client with cancer may enhance tumor growth by improving its nutrient supply.
      2. Beneficial effects of nutritional support are temporary.
   B. Goals of nutritional therapy should be established.
      1. Increase client's weight.
      2. Maintain weight.
      3. Maintain fluid and electrolyte balance.

4. Improved sense of well-being.
5. Prolonged life.
6. Establishment of calories needed and calculation of basal metabolic rate (BMR).

C. Selection of type of nutritional therapy (enteral or parenteral) depends on:
1. Function of gastrointestinal tract.
2. Severity of nutritional problem.
3. Ability of client to masticate and swallow.
4. Length of proposed therapy and prognosis.
5. Community resources for management at home.
6. Cost.

D. Type of nutritional support (only after inadequate oral intake).
1. Enteral therapy—provision of nutritional replacement through the gastrointestinal tract through an entry other than the mouth such as a gastrostomy (button), jejunostomy, or nasogastric (temporary) feeding tube.
   a. Indicated if the need for nutritional support is anticipated for more than 1 month and attempts at oral intake have been unsuccessful; clients need at least 30 cm of functioning small bowel.
   b. May require percutaneous endoscopic feeding tube placement.
   c. Potential complications of enteral tube placement and feedings are included in (Table 9–4).
   d. Selection of appropriate formula is essential and many may need to be tried.
2. Parenteral therapy—provision of feeding through an intravenous route when the gastrointestinal tract cannot be used for nutritional replacement. It is a mixture of amino acids, glucose, fluid, vitamins, minerals, electrolytes, and trace elements. Lipid emulsions can be added to increase calories with smaller volume.
   a. Requires placement of a central venous line (or PICC line), although peripheral parenteral nutrition (PPN) can be given with lower glucose percentages.
   b. Potential mechanical, metabolic, and infectious complications of parenteral therapy are presented in (Table 9–5).

Assessment

I. Nutritional assessment includes an evaluation of the desire and ability of the client to ingest and process nutritional products.
A. Ingestion.
1. Desire to eat.
2. Patterns of dietary intake.
3. Ability of client to prepare food and feed self.
4. Food allergies and preferences.
5. Dentition.
6. Ability of client to moisten, chew, and swallow nutrients.
B. Digestion.
1. Ability to digest food in stomach and small intestine.
2. Ability to move digested stomach contents through bowel.
C. Metabolism.
1. Presence of abnormal carbohydrate, fat, or protein metabolism.
2. Presence of vitamin and mineral deficiencies.

TABLE 9–4. **Potential Complications of Enteral Tube Placement and Feedings**

Complication	Nursing Intervention
Nasogastric	

Malpositioned tube	Verify proper placement via chest x-ray examination
	Check placement each time before using tube by:
	    Aspirating gastric contents
	    Observing for air bubbles by placing distal end of tube in
	       water
	    Injecting air and listening with stethoscope over stomach
	Tape tube securely to nose

Aspiration	Give bolus feeding rather than continuous feeding
	Administer no more than 350–400 mL over 20 minutes every
	    3–4 hours while client is awake
	Administer initial volume of 240 mL
	Keep head of bed elevated 30 degrees during and 1 hour
	    after infusion

Contaminated equipment, clogged tube	Change feeding bag and tube daily
	Flush nasogastric tube with 30 mL of water or cranberry
	    juice after each feeding
	If tube is clogged, flush with 30 mL cranberry juice and 1/4
	    teaspoon meat tenderizer

Abdominal distention, vomiting, cramping, diarrhea	Regulate infusion accurately over 20 minutes
	Give formula at room temperature, may need to decrease
	    volume of formula given. Diarrhea may be due to formula,
	    lactose intolerance, bacterial contamination, osmolality,
	    antibiotics, *Clostridium difficile*

Nasoduodenal	

Aspiration	Decreased risk of occurrence because tube is in the small
	    bowel
	Give continuous rather than bolus feeding
	Small bowel is sensitive to osmolarity; therefore, administer
	    at initial rate of 30–50 mL/hr for isotonic formula and
	    increase by 25 mL/hr every 12 hours until desired volume
	    is reached

Contaminated equipment	Do not allow amount of formula in bag to exceed that which
	    can be administered in 4 hours
	Change entire administration set every 24 hours, and rinse
	    out with hot water every 8 hours

    D. Excretion.
        1. Bowel elimination patterns.
        2. Urinary elimination patterns.
        3. Characteristics of urine and stool.
  II. Nutritional assessment includes evaluation of the effects of dietary intake on
    the person.
    A. Physical assessment.
        1. Skin turgor.
        2. Weight in comparison to ideal body weight.
        3. Muscle mass as measured by the midarm circumference.
        4. Fat stores as measured by triceps skinfold thickness.
    B. Evaluation of laboratory data.
        1. Serum albumin, total protein, and serum transferrin to assess protein
           stores.

TABLE 9–5. **Potential Complications of Parenteral Therapy**

Complication	Nursing Intervention
Technical or Mechanical	
Pneumothorax	May occur during insertion of subclavian catheter
	Observe client during insertion for chest pain, dyspnea, cyanosis
	Obtain chest x-ray examination after insertion to verify placement
	Verify blood return before connecting intravenous (IV) tubing to catheter
Arterial puncture	May occur during insertion
	Observe for bright red blood, pulsating from catheter
	Client may complain of pain at site
	Apply pressure to site for 15 minutes; may need to apply a sandbag after this
Malpositioned catheter	Monitor catheter for migration from the superior vena cava to another vein. Note client complaint of neck and shoulder pain, swelling in the surrounding area
Clotted catheter	NOTE: if unable to infuse solution through catheter and unable to obtain blood return. "Declot" according to institutional policy (see recommendations, Vascular Access Devices, withdrawal occlusions, p. 126). Infuse 10% dextrose in water solution peripherally or through other lumen of catheter, at the same rate as TPN to prevent hypoglycemia
Fluid overload	Regulate infusion on a volumetric pump for accuracy
	Place a time tape on infusion, checking volume infused over each hour
	Obtain daily weights
Air emboli	Secure all IV tubing connections with tape to prevent disconnection
	If air emboli are suspected, clamp tubing immediately and place client on left side in Trendelenburg position
Metabolic	
Hyperglycemia	Increase rate of infusion gradually
	Check urine for sugar and acetone every 6 hours
	Monitor serum glucose levels daily
Hypoglycemia	Observe for signs and symptoms of hypoglycemia
	Monitor serum glucose levels.
	If sudden cessation of TPN occurs, infuse 10% dextrose in water solution peripherally at same rate as TPN
	Per physician's order, administer 50 mL of 50% dextrose IV
Infections	
Contaminated solution	Do not leave solution unrefrigerated for longer than 4 hours
	Check each bottle before and during infusion for color and clarity of solution
Contaminated equipment	Change all IV tubing per institutional/agency procedure, using aseptic technique
	Do not interrupt TPN for other infusions or blood collecting
Local site infection	Change dressing, using aseptic technique, and following institutional procedure
	Observe site for redness, tenderness, swelling, and exudate
Fever	Monitor vital signs every 4 hours
	Obtain both peripheral and central line blood cultures to identify source of infection

2. Nitrogen balance to assess energy balance.
3. Creatinine height index to assess protein stores.
4. Hemoglobin and hematocrit index.
5. Electrolyte levels.

Nursing Diagnoses

   I. Alteration in nutrition: less than body requirements.
  II. Fluid volume deficit.
 III. Impaired swallowing.
  IV. Self-care deficit: feeding.
   V. Anxiety.

Outcome Identification

   I. Client describes personal risk factors for malnutrition and the ability to assess her/his nutritional status.
  II. Client describes measures that enhance oral intake of food and fluids to enhance nutritional status.
 III. Client lists signs and symptoms of complications of nutritional support to report to the health care team.
  IV. Client describes interventions to relieve symptoms such as nausea, vomiting, and stomatitis that interfere with nutritional intake.
   V. Client identifies nutritional goals such as a low-fat, high-fiber diet, or ability to maintain weight.

Planning and Implementation

   I. Interventions to maximize client safety.
      A. Administer nutritional therapy according to institutional protocol.
      B. Examine nutritional supplement for abnormalities in color or clarity.
      C. Check expiration date on nutritional supplement.
      D. Confirm placement of feeding tube or catheter before administering nutritional supplement.
  II. Interventions to decrease the incidence and severity of complications of nutritional therapy (see Table 9–5).
 III. Interventions to monitor for complications of nutritional therapy.
      A. Infection—fever and redness, swelling, pus, or pain along feeding tube, catheter tract, or exit site.
      B. Respiratory complications—chest pain, dyspnea, cough, or cyanosis.
      C. Fluid overload—weight gain, edema, shortness of breath, and distended neck veins.
      D. Hyperglycemia—glucose monitoring every 6 hours and pattern of urinary elimination.
      E. Gastrointestinal—character of stool, bloating, and pattern of bowel elimination.
      F. Electrolyte abnormalities—changes in mental status, weakness, fatigue, and changes in neurologic examination (restlessness and agitation).
  IV. Interventions to incorporate client and family into care.
      A. Teach client and family self-care procedures needed to manage the feeding tube or catheter.
      B. Teach client and family signs and symptoms of complications of nutritional therapy.

C. Encourage participation of client and family in decision-making about nutritional therapy.

Evaluation

The oncology nurse systematically and regularly evaluates the client's and/or family's responses to interventions to determine progress toward the achievement of expected outcomes. Relevant data are collected and actual findings are compared with expected findings. Nursing diagnoses, outcomes, and plans of care are reviewed and revised as necessary.

BIBLIOGRAPHY

Alexander, H.R. (1993). Vascular access and other specialized techniques of drug delivery. In V.T. DeVita, Jr., S. Hellman, & S.A. Rosenberg (eds.). *Cancer: Principles and Practice of Oncology* (4th ed.). Philadelphia: J.B. Lippincott Co., pp. 556–563.

Borlase, B.C., Bell, S.J., Blackburn, G.L, et al. (1995). *Enteral Nutrition.* New York: Chapman and Hall.

Conn, C. (1993). The importance of syringe size when using implanted vascular access devices. *J Vasc Access Network 3*(1), 11–18.

Cunningham, R.S., & Bonam-Crawford, D. (1993). The role of fibrinolytic agents in the management of thrombotic complications associated with vascular access devices. *Nurs Clin North Am 28*(4), 899–909.

D'Amelio, L.F., & Greco, R.S. (1996). Biologic properties of venous access devices. In S.E. Wilson (ed.). *Vascular Access: Principles and Practice* (3rd ed.). St. Louis: C.V. Mosby Co., pp. 42–53.

Doane, L.S. (1993). Administering intraperitoneal chemotherapy using a peritoneal port. *Nurs Clin North Am 28*(4), 885–897.

Fischer, J.E. (1991). *Total Parenteral Nutrition* (2nd ed.). Boston: Little, Brown.

Freedman, S.E., & Bosserman, G. (1993). Tunneled catheters: Technologic advances and nursing care issues. *Nurs Clin North Am 28*(4), 851–858.

Gullo, S.M. (1993). Implanted ports: Technologic advances and nursing care issues. *Nurs Clin North Am 28*(4), 859–871.

Jassak, P.F., & Goodwin, J. (1991). Blood Component Therapy. In R. McCorkle & M. Grant (eds.). *Cancer Nursing.* Philadelphia: W.B. Saunders Co., pp. 370–378.

Johnson, G.B. (1993). Nursing care of patients with implanted pumps. *Nurs Clin North Am 28*(4), pp. 873–883.

Herbst, S.F. (1993). Accumulation of blood products and drug precipitates in VAD's: A setup for trouble. *J Vasc Access Network 3*(3), 9–13.

Merrick, H.W. (1995). Vascular access, infusion, and perfusion. In R.T. Skeel (ed.). *Handbook of Cancer Chemotherapy* (4th ed.). Boston: Little, Brown, pp. 680–688.

Myers, J.S., & Kylem K.S. (1993). Intermediate term intravenous therapy: A pilot study. *J Post Anesth Nurs 8*(1), 21–25.

Orr, M.E. (1993). Issues in the management of percutaneous central venous catheters: Single and multiple lumens. *Nurs Clin North Am 28*(4), 911–919.

Paice, J.A. (1993). Intraspinal devices for pain management. *Nurs Clin North Am 28*(4), 921–935.

Reymann, P.E. (1993). Chemotherapy: Principles of administration. In S.L. Groenwald (ed.). A Clinical Guide to Cancer Nursing. Boston: Jones & Bartlett, pp. 293–330.

Ryder, M.A. (1993). Peripherally inserted central venous catheters. *Nurs Clin North Am 28*(4), pp. 937–971.

Tenenbaum, L., & Scelsi, D.B. (1994). Central venous access devices. In Tenenbaum, L. (ed.). *Cancer Chemotherapy and Biotherapy: A Reference Guide* (2nd ed.). Philadelphia: W.B. Saunders Co., pp. 411–428.

Tominaga, G., & Jakowatz, J.G. (1996). Placement of indwelling venous access systems. In S.E. Wilson (ed.). *Vascular Access: Principles and Practice* (3rd ed.). St. Louis: C.V. Mosby Co., pp. 56–66.

Turgeon, M.L. (1995). *Fundamentals of Immunohematology: Theory and Technique* (2nd ed.). Baltimore: Williams & Wilkins.

Walker, R.H. (1990). *Technical Manual.* Arlington, VA: American Association of Blood Banks.

Wile, A. (1996). Indications and devices for chronic venous access. In S.E. Wilson (ed.). *Vascular Access: Principles and Practice* (3rd ed.). St. Louis: C.V. Mosby Co., pp. 54–58.

Yeslin, A.E., Hood, D.B., & Weaver, F.A. (1996). Axillosubclavian vein thrombosis. In S.E. Wilson (ed.). *Vascular Access: Principles and Practice* (3rd ed.). St. Louis: C.V. Mosby Co., pp. 104–109.

10

Symptom Management and Supportive Care: Pharmacologic Interventions

Carolyn S. J. Ma, PharmD
Karen N. Taoka, RN, MN, AOCN

ANTIMICROBIALS

Theory

   I. Infections are a major complication of cancer and cancer therapy.
      A. Infections are the most common cause of death in persons with cancer.
      B. As a result of changes in immune functions, many of the usual signs and symptoms of infection are absent in the client diagnosed with cancer or receiving cancer treatment.
  II. Types of antimicrobial therapy (Table 10–1).
 III. Principles of medical management.
      A. At the first sign of temperature greater than 100.4°F, a fever workup is initiated.
          1. Physical examination.
          2. Blood cultures—peripheral and central.
          3. Central venous catheter or port cultures.
          4. Urine culture.
          5. Chest x-ray examination.
          6. Other cultures from wound and drainage, if applicable.
      B. Initiation of empiric antimicrobial therapy.
          1. Selection of antibiotics based on:
             a. Coverage for common infectious organisms among persons with cancer.
             b. Prevalence rates for microorganisms and the patterns of resistance within the institution.
          2. Most regimens include an antipseudomonal penicillin, an aminoglycoside, and/or a first- or third-generation cephalosporin.
          3. Intravenous doses and schedules are designed to provide bactericidal serum levels for as long as possible between each dose interval.
          4. Duration of treatment is sufficient for the resolution of the fever without exposure to unnecessary side effects of the agents.
             a. Negative culture results—if no organisms were isolated, treatment continues for a minimum of 7 days.

       b. Afebrile for 3 days.

       c. Neutrophil count greater than 500 cells/mm^3.

    5. If fever is unresponsive to initial antibiotic therapy, the risk of nonbacterial cause, infectious organisms resistant to antimicrobial therapy (e.g., methicillin-resistant *Staphylococcus aureus,* vancomycin-resistant *Enterococcus*), inadequate serum and tissue levels of antimicrobials, or drug fever should be considered.

       a. Continue current antimicrobials if clinical condition is unchanged and evaluation reveals no new information.

       b. Change antimicrobial program if evidence of progressive infection is present.

       c. Add amphotericin B to the antimicrobial program.

          (1) One third of febrile neutropenic clients who do not respond to 1 week of antimicrobial therapy have a systemic fungal infection.

          (2) Most common organisms include *Candida* or *Aspergillus.*

    6. Antiviral therapy should be considered if client has a past history of positive titers (e.g., herpes zoster).

IV. Potential complications of antimicrobial therapy.

  A. Suprainfection.

  B. Renal toxicity—acute renal tubular necrosis, nephritis, and electrolyte imbalances.

  C. Hematologic—bleeding, neutropenia, and anemia.

  D. Hepatotoxicity—elevated liver function tests.

  E. Cardiovascular—phlebitis, hypotension, and arrhythmias.

  F. Gastrointestinal—nausea, vomiting, anorexia, and colitis.

  G. Neurotoxicity—seizures, dizziness, ototoxicity.

  H. Dermatologic—rash, Stevens-Johnson syndrome, thrush, esophagitis, vaginitis.

  I. Fluid and electrolyte imbalances—hypokalemia, hypernatremia, dehydration, fluid volume overload.

  J. Hypersensitivity reactions.

Assessment

  I. Identification of clients at risk for infection.

    A. Disruption of primary barriers to organisms.

      1. Surgical disruption of skin.

      2. Invasive procedures (e.g., insertion of central vascular access catheters, indwelling urinary catheters).

      3. Extravasation of vesicant antineoplastic agents.

      4. Stomatitis/mucositis.

      5. Rectal fissures.

      6. Burns.

    B. Alteration in phagocytic defenses.

      1. Neutropenia with granulocyte count less than 1000/mm^3.

      2. Length of time client has been neutropenic.

      3. Steroid use.

      4. Previous antibiotic therapy.

    C. Concurrent disease states.

      1. Diabetes.

      2. Renal disease.

(*Text continued on page 155*)

TABLE 10–1. Types of Antimicrobial Therapy

Antimicrobial Agent	Indications	Potential Side Effects of Group	Nursing Implications
Penicillins			
Penicillin G	*Streptococcus pneumoniae, S. pyogenes, S. viridans, S. bovis, Neisseria,* and most anaerobes (except *B. fragilis*)	Skin rash—hypersensitivity up to 0.05% 5–10% fatal Dizziness, neuromuscular hyperirritability, seizures, decreased sense of taste and smell, stomatitis, flatulence, diarrhea, pancytopenia, hypokalemia, and changes in liver and kidney function studies	Monitor for skin rash Monitor for neurologic changes at regular intervals. Provide safety measures for clients with dizziness. Evaluate the effects of changes in taste and smell, nausea, and stomatitis on nutritional intake. Implement strategies to control flatulence and diarrhea Evaluate the effect of diarrhea on perineal skin and rectum
Methicillin sodium Nafcillin sodium Oxacillin sodium	*Staphylococcus aureus* and streptococci		
Ampicillin	*Streptococcus fecalis, Listeria monocytogenes, Haemophilus, Escherichia coli, Salmonella,* and *Proteus*	Nausea and vomiting Hypokalemia	Evaluate laboratory studies as ordered by physician Monitor volume, patterns, and character of urinary output Administer potassium supplement, as ordered Assess for signs of low potassium: paralytic ileus, muscle weakness, dysrhythmias
Ampicillin sulbactam	Coverage same as ampicillin but with more reliable gram-negative activity and broader anaerobic coverage. Active against ampicillin-resistant bacteria—*S. aureus, Bacteroides fragilis* and β lactamase–producing Enterobacteriaceae		
Carbenicillin disodium	*Pseudomonas aeruginosa, Enterobacter, Proteus, Serratia* seraha, *Acinetobacter,* and *Providencia*		
Ticarcillin disodium	Anaerobes		

Drug	Activity/Description	Adverse Effects	Nursing Considerations
Ticarcillin disodium and clavulanate potassium (Timentin)	Improves activity against *Haemophilus influenzae*, *Klebsiella* spp. and anaerobes, but not against *Pseudomonas aeruginosa* and *Enterobacter cloacae*		
Mezlocillin sodium	*P. aeruginosa*, *Enterobacter*, *Proteus*, *Serratia seraha*, *Acinetobacter*, *Providencia*, *Klebsiella* spp.		
Piperacillin sodium	Plus increased activity against *P. aeruginosa*	Prolonged bleeding	Monitor sites of invasive procedures for bleeding Assess client for signs and symptoms of internal or external bleeding Evaluate coagulation laboratory studies as ordered by physician
Azlocillin	Same as piperacillin		
Piperacillin Tazobactam (Zosyn)	Increased activity over piperacillin alone against gram-negative rods and anaerobes. Better β lactamase inhibitor.		
Cephalosporins *First Generation*			
Cephalothin sodium	*E. coli*, *Klebsiella*, *Proteus*, *Haemophilus*, *S. aureus*, *Staphylococcus epidermidis*, streptococci	Cross sensitivity of 5–15% in clients with history of penicillin allergy Skin rash without fever and eosinophilia—13% Seizures in high doses with renal failure	Monitor for skin rash Monitor for neurologic changes at regular intervals. Provide safety measures for client experiencing dizziness and vertigo
Cefazolin sodium	Similar to cephalothin but more active against *Klebsiella* and *E. coli*	Dizziness, vertigo, headache, nausea, vomiting, diarrhea, anorexia, abdominal cramping, pancytopenia, changes in SGOT, changes in SGPT, changes in alkaline phosphatase, changes in BUN and creatinine clearance, oliguria Hypersensitivity	Evaluate laboratory studies as ordered by physician Monitor food and fluid intake and output Evaluate effect of diarrhea on perineal skin and rectum Monitor urinary output
Second Generation			
Cefamandole	Most active against *Haemophilus*, *Klebsiella*, *E. coli*, *Enterobacter* spp., *Proteus*, and less active against gram-positive cocci		

(Table continued on following page)

147

TABLE 10–1. **Types of Antimicrobial Therapy** (*Continued*)

Antimicrobial Agent	Indications	Potential Side Effects of Group	Nursing Implications
Cefoxitin sodium	Same as cephalothin plus *Proteus* spp. and anaerobes	→	Implement strategies to control pain, nausea, and diarrhea See Chapter 12, discussion on thrombocytopenia, leukopenia, and anemia Monitor for signs and symptoms of hypersensitivity reactions—respiratory status, itching, hives, fever, pain, changes in pulse rate, decrease in blood pressure, decrease in urinary output
Third Generation			
Cefotaxime sodium	Same as cephalothin plus *Enterobacter* spp., *Proteus*, *H. influenzae*, *Citrobacter* spp., *Serratia* spp., and some *P. aeruginosa* and *Bacteroides* spp.	Hypersensitivity Transient leukopenia and thrombocytopenia Phlebitis	Assess local reactions at site of infusion—pain, swelling, and redness
Moxalactam disodium	Same as cefotaxime but better anaerobe coverage	Bleeding reactions	
Ceftriaxone	Similar to cefotaxime but with better coverage of *Streptococcus pneumoniae* and *pyogenes*, *S. aureus*. Maintain high activity against *E. coli*, *Klebsiella* spp. *Proteus mirabilis*, *Providencia*, and *Serratia*		
Cefoperazone	Better *P. aeruginosa* coverage		
Ceftizoxime	Same as cefotaxime		
Ceftazidime	Same as cefoperazone but with less anaerobic activity. Most active against *P. aeruginosa*		

Drug	Antimicrobial Activity	Side Effects / Nursing Considerations
Fourth Generation		
Cefepime	*E. coli, Klebsiella pneumoniae, P. mirabilis, Pseudomonas,* Methicillin-resistant *S. aureus, S. pyogenes*	
Miscellaneous β Lactams		
Aztreonam	Similar to third-generation cephalosporins. Gram-negative bacteria including *Pseudomonas* and Enterobacteriaceae	Hypersensitivity, diarrhea, nausea, vomiting, eosinophilia, slight prolongation of PT, PTT; transient increases in liver function test (LFT) values
Imipenem/cilastatin (Primaxin)	Broad-spectrum gram-negative aerobic including *Pseudomonas,* Enterobacteriaceae, *Klebsiella* spp. Anaerobic gram-positive and gram-negative anaerobes including *B. fragilis* and some mycobacteria Gram-positive cocci including *S. aureus* and *epidermidis, S. pneumoniae* and *pyogenes,* and *Enterococcus*	
Fluoroquinolones		
Ciprofloxacin	Gram-negative rods, Enterobacteriaceae; most active against *P. aeruginosa, Haemophilus, Chlamydia,* some *Mycoplasma legionella.* Less active against gram-positive organisms, especially *Streptococcus* and *Staphylococcus* spp.	GI irritation, nausea, vomiting, diarrhea Decreased oral absorption with aluminum, calcium, and magnesium antacids. Administer 1–2 hr before or after these antacids are given
Norfloxacin	No pseudomonal activity. Used in gastrointestinal (GI) and urinary tract infections	
Ofloxacin	Most active against *Chlamydia*	Changes in blood sugar—hyper or hypo Monitor blood sugars; assess for signs and symptoms of hypo- or hyperglycemia

(Table continued on following page)

TABLE 10–1. **Types of Antimicrobial Therapy** (*Continued*)

Antimicrobial Agent	Indications	Potential Side Effects of Group	Nursing Implications
Aminoglycosides Gentamicin sulfate	*P. aeruginosa*, Enterobacteriaceae, and *Enterococcus*. Synergistic use with penicillin/vancomycin for gram-positive cocci, e.g., streptococci	Vestibular toxicity. Hearing loss, loss of balance, high-frequency deafness, peripheral neuritis, numbness, tingling of skin Granulocytopenia, anemia, thrombocytopenia purpura Proteinuria, changes in BUN, oliguria, nephrotoxicity	Evaluate neurologic status before initiation of therapy. Assess hearing status before therapy or prolonged treatment See Chapter 12 for granulocytopenia and thrombocytopenia, and Chapter 15 for anemia Monitor urinary output Evaluate laboratory studies as ordered by physicians Evaluate serum peak/trough or serial troughs with prolonged use
Tobramycin sulfate	Similar to gentamicin except not as active against *Enterococcus*	Changes in SGOT, SGPT, and LDH; pancytopenia, nausea, vomiting, headache, fever, lethargy	Implement measures to increase comfort Monitor amount and type of fluid and food intake Monitor amount and character of emesis output Assist with activities of daily living as needed Monitor for signs and symptoms of bleeding or infection
Amikacin sulfate	*Serratia, Proteus, Pseudomonas,* Enterobacteriaceae, and *Providencia*	Drowsiness, headache, unsteady gait, paresthesias, tremors Hypotension, tachycardia Oliguria, hematuria, thirst	Provide assistance with activities of daily living and ambulation as needed Teach client and family about use of assistive aids for ambulation Monitor blood pressure and pulse rate at regular intervals Monitor amount and character of urinary output

Drug	Spectrum/Uses	Adverse Effects	Nursing Implications
		Ringing or buzzing in ears, high-frequency hearing loss Bleeding reactions	Assess levels of hearing before and periodically during treatment Monitor for signs and symptoms of bleeding
Antifungals			
Amphotericin B	*Candida, Aspergillus, Zygomycetes, Torulopsis, Cryptococcus,* and *Histoplasma*	Fever, headache, sedation, weakness, paresthesia, flushing, arrhythmias, hypotension/hypertension, tinnitus, hearing loss, vertigo, nausea, vomiting, diarrhea, coagulation deficits, electrolyte imbalances (decreased potassium, magnesium, sodium), pancytopenia, and hepatic dysfunction Increased serum creatinine, renal failure	Monitor temperature, blood pressure, and pulse at regular intervals Evaluate changes in sensory perception over time Assess effect of vertigo, nausea, diarrhea, and neurologic changes on ability to accomplish activities of daily living Monitor changes in laboratory study results as ordered by physician Assess client for symptoms of electrolyte changes See Chapters 12 and 15, discussion on thrombocytopenia, leukopenia, and anemia
Liposomal amphotericin	Patients intolerant or hypersensitive to amphotericin B. Patients with compromised renal function		
Flucytosine	*Cryptococcus, Candida, Torulopsis,* chromomycosis		
Clotrimazole	*Candida* spp., dermatophytes	Erythema, stinging, blistering, peeling, edema, and pruritus with topical application	Evaluate condition of skin before initiation of treatment Implement strategies to minimize symptoms of local skin reactions (see Chapter 11)
Miconazole nitrate	*Candida* spp., *Aspergillus* spp., Zygomycetes, *Torulopsis, Cryptococcus, Petiellidium, Blastomyces, Histoplasma, Coccidioides,* Paracoccidioides, *Sporothrix*		
Ketoconazole	Similar to miconazole	Gynecomastia and adrenal insufficiency	Monitor for signs of adrenal insufficiency—weakness, fever, abdominal pain, nausea, vomiting, diarrhea, decreased blood pressure, headache, and confusion Assess changes in volume of breast tissue

(Table continued on following page)

TABLE 10–1. Types of Antimicrobial Therapy (*Continued*)

Antimicrobial Agent	Indications	Potential Side Effects of Group	Nursing Implications
Fluconazole	*Candida*, cryptococcal meningitis	Nausea, vomiting, diarrhea, abdominal pain, rash, CNS (headache, dizziness, somnolence), decreased libido. Hypertension, hypokalemia, increased LFT values, increased triglycerides	
Itraconazole	Aspergillosis: refractory to amphotericin B or intolerant Plastomycosis—pulmonary and extra-pulmonary Histoplasmosis—pulmonary, disseminated nonmeningeal		
Antivirals			
Adenosine	Herpes simplex virus and varicella zoster virus	Anorexia, nausea, vomiting, diarrhea, myelosuppression, hallucinations, confusion, psychosis, dizziness, and metabolic encephalopathy	Assess nutritional intake Monitor fluid intake and output Evaluate effect of diarrhea on perineal skin and rectum Provide safety measures for clients with neurologic changes Evaluate laboratory study results as ordered by physician
Acyclovir	Herpes simplex virus and varicella zoster virus	Renal toxicity and neurotoxicity Arthralgias	Monitor flow rate for infusion and maintain hydration Monitor blood pressure, pulse rate, and respiratory rate
Ganciclovir	Cytomegalovirus retinitis, pneumonia, colitis CMV pneumonia with IVIG in BMT	Hematologic: granulocytopenia, thrombocytopenia; fever, rash, increase in liver function test values	
Foscavir	Cytomegalovirus (CMV) retinitis, ganciclovir resistance or intolerance, acyclovir-resistant CMV	Headache, fatigue nausea, fever, electrolyte disturbances, seizures, increase in serum creatinine, neuropathy, decrease in white cell count	
Interferons (alpha, beta, and gamma)	Herpes simplex virus and varicella zoster virus	Local pain, fever, alopecia, fatigue, anorexia, and myelosuppression	Assess local reactions at site of infusion Evaluate effect of fatigue on activities of daily living

Miscellaneous

Drug	Organisms	Side/Adverse Effects	Nursing Implications
Chloramphenicol	*Haemophilus, B. fragilis, S. pneumoniae, Neisseria, Salmonella, Klebsiella, Rickettsia,* and most anaerobes	Headache, depression, confusion Nausea, vomiting, diarrhea, perianal irritation, stomatitis, xerostomia, abdominal distention, blotching skin, cyanosis, hypothermia, and bone marrow depression	Monitor for neurologic changes at regular intervals. Provide safety measures if confusion is present Encourage consultation with psychiatrist for evaluation of depression Monitor food and fluid intake and output Evaluate pulmonary status at least each shift—respiratory rate, effort Assess rectal area for irritation Teach perianal hygiene and protective measures Monitor for signs and symptoms of bleeding or infection
Erythromycin	*Legionella* and *Mycoplasma*	Transient deafness, decreased liver or renal function Abdominal cramping and distention, diarrhea, and phlebitis	Assess volume and character of stool Encourage client to exercise in hallway, room, or bed
Clindamycin	*B. fragilis, Clostridia, S. pneumoniae, S. viridans, S. pyogenes,* and *S. aureus*	Diarrhea, abdominal pain, bloating, nausea, vomiting, decreased taste, neutropenia, thrombophlebitis, jaundice, and abnormal liver function study results	Assess skin every day for changes in integrity, color or texture Evaluate liver function study results as ordered by physician
Metronidazole	All anaerobes including *B. fragilis Clostridium difficile* toxin—po or IV	Metallic taste in mouth, darkened stools, dizziness, vertigo, and paresthesias. Peripheral neuropathy can occur with high doses and prolonged treatment	
Vancomycin	*C. difficile, S. aureus, S. epidermidis, S. fecalis,* corynebacteria, and *S. bovis.* Methicillin-resistant *S. aureus.* Oral form: *C. difficile* toxin	Anaphylaxis, vertigo, dizziness, phlebitis, tinnitus, ototoxicity, increased BUN and creatinine levels, suprainfection	Provide for environmental safety with dizziness Monitor client responses to change in hearing Evaluate renal function studies as ordered by physician

(Table continued on following page)

TABLE 10–1. **Types of Antimicrobial Therapy** (*Continued*)

Antimicrobial Agent	Indications	Potential Side Effects of Group	Nursing Implications
Trimethoprim-sulfamethoxazole	*P. carinii, S. aureus, S. pneumoniae, S. pyogenes, Salmonella, Listeria, E. coli, Proteus, Serratia, Haemophilus,* and *Neisseria*	Myelosuppression	Monitor signs and symptoms of infection or bleeding
Rifampin	Mycobacteria, most gram-positive and gram-negative bacteria, *Neisseria* meningitis. Used mainly to enhance bactericidal activity of other anti-staphylococcal agents in refractory or chronic infections. Develops resistance quickly if used singly		

SGOT = serum glutamic-oxaloacetic transaminase; SGPT = serum glutamate pyruvate transaminase; BUN = blood urea nitrogen; PT = prothrombin time; PTT = partial thromboplastin time; LDH = lactate dehydrogenase; CNS = central nervous system; IVIG = intravenous immune globulin; BMT = bone marrow transplant.
Adapted from Erdman, L. (1992). Nursing implications of supportive therapies in cancer care. In J.C. Clark & R.F. McGee (eds.). *Oncology Nursing Society Core Curriculum* (2nd ed.). Philadelphia: W.B. Saunders Co., pp. 378–383; and Pizzo, P.A., Meyers, J., Freifeld, A.G., & Walsh, T. (1993). Infections in the cancer patient. In V.T. DeVita, Jr., S. Hellman, & S. Rosenberg (eds.). *Cancer: Principles and Practice of Oncology* (4th ed.). Philadelphia: J.B. Lippincott Co., pp. 2300–2307.

   3. Liver disease.
   4. Gastrointestinal disease.
   5. Fistula, abscesses.
   6. Stress.
  D. Tumor necrosis and invasion.
  E. Previous cancer therapy.
  F. History of drug allergies/drug reaction or intolerance.
 II. Physical examination.
  A. Integumentary—rash, ulceration, redness, swelling, and warmth.
  B. Vital signs—temperature, blood pressure, pulse, and respirations.
  C. Pulmonary—respiratory rate, rhythm, effort, presence of adventitious sounds, oxygen saturation.
  D. Renal—character of urine and urinary output.
  E. Neuromuscular—mental status.
III. Evaluation of laboratory data.
  A. Culture and sensitivity: blood, urine, sputum, throat.
  B. Chest x-ray examination.
  C. Complete blood count with differential.
  D. Other—computed tomography (CT), magnetic resonance imaging (MRI), ultrasound, esophagogastroduodenoscopy (EGD), bronchoscopy.

Nursing Diagnoses

  I. Knowledge deficit.
 II. Risk for altered body temperature.
III. Risk for infection.
IV. Risk for fluid volume deficit.

Outcome Identification

  I. Client and family describe personal risk factors for infection.
 II. Client and family discuss the rationale for immediate evaluation of fever.
III. Client and family list signs and symptoms of side effects of antimicrobial therapy to report to the health care team.

Planning and Implementation

  I. Implement strategies to educate client and family of risk factors for infection (see Assessment).
 II. Assess client's and family's cultural and ethnic background, particularly health care practices and values and beliefs related to pharmacotherapy.
  A. Assess understanding and compliance to Western/mainstream prescribed therapy.
  B. Determine if client and family are also consulting traditional healers and/or taking herbal preparations (potential drug interactions).
  C. Determine client's racial group because biologic variations among racial groups may affect drug metabolism rates, clinical drug responses, and side effects to drugs.
III. Implement interventions to decrease the incidence and severity of side effects of antimicrobial therapy (see Table 10–1).
IV. Implement strategies to monitor for complications of antimicrobial therapy (see Table 10–1).

V. Implement measures to monitor for response to antimicrobial therapy.
   A. Monitor temperature, pulse, respirations, and blood pressure.
   B. Discuss with the client and family rationale for immediate evaluation of fever.
   C. Assess changes in laboratory values/fluid volume status.

Evaluation

The oncology nurse systematically and regularly evaluates the client's and/or family's responses to interventions to determine progress toward the achievement of expected outcomes. Relevant data are collected and actual findings are compared with expected findings. Nursing diagnoses, outcomes, and plans of care are reviewed and revised as necessary.

ANTIINFLAMMATORY AGENTS

Theory

I. Although the inflammatory process is a protective mechanism, in certain situations it may cause harm and pain to the individual.
   A. The inflammatory process involves the production of prostaglandins by the action of the enzyme cyclooxygenase (also known as prostaglandin synthetase). Prostaglandins are particularly associated with the pain that accompanies inflammation.
   B. Inhibition of cyclooxygenase by antiinflammatory agents will inhibit production of prostaglandin. This break in the cascade suppresses the inflammatory response of white blood cell and macrophage migration to the site of injury and results in or contributes to symptom relief.
II. Types of antiinflammatory agents.
   A. Nonsteroidal antiinflammatory drugs (NSAIDs) (Table 10–2).
   B. Corticosteroids (Table 10–3).
III. Principles of medical management.
   A. To treat mild to moderate pain.
   B. Adjuvant pharmacologic pain management with opiates.
   C. Symptom management of tumor lysis fever, bony metastases, nausea and vomiting from chemotherapy.
IV. Potential complications. See Table 10–4 for adverse effects and nursing implications.

Assessment

I. Identification of clients at risk.
   A. For pain (see Chapter 1).
   B. For nausea/vomiting (see Chapter 13).
   C. Clients with cancers that commonly metastasize to bone (e.g., prostate, breast, lung).
   D. Clients with fever from tumor lysis.
II. Physical examination.
   A. Pain assessment (see Chapter 1).
   B. Temperature, vital signs.
   C. Nausea/vomiting (see Chapter 13).
III. Evaluation of laboratory data.
   A. Complete blood count.
   B. Hepatic and renal function.

TABLE 10–2. **Commonly Used Nonsteroidal Antiinflammatory (NSAID) Agents in Cancer**

Nonsteroidal Agent	Notable Drug Information
Propionic Acids	
Fenoprofen (Nalfon)	Possible fluid retention. May cause somnolence
Ibuprofen (Motrin, Advil)	Short half-life
Ketoprofen (Orudis)	Possible photosensitivity reactions
Naproxen (Naprosyn, Aleve)	Useful in bone metastases. Fluid retention
Acetic Acids	
Diclofenac (Voltaren)	Associated with increased hepatotoxicity
Etodolac (Lodine)	Possible photosensitivity reactions
Indomethacin (Indocin)	High incidence for central nervous system effects—drowsiness, dizziness, mental confusion, and frontal lobe headache
Ketorolac tromethamine (Toradol)	Available parenteral form
Sulindac (Clinoril)	Long half-life of metabolites
Tolmetin (Tolectin)	Higher frequency of anaphylactoid reaction
Oxicams	
Piroxicam (Feldene)	High incidence of gastrointestinal side effects Photosensitivity reactions
Salicylates	
Acetylsalicylic acid/aspirin (various brands)	May affect platelet aggregation and prolong bleeding time. Hearing impairment, visual disturbances, nausea, vomiting, gastric upset, and occult bleeding
Choline magnesium trisalicylate (Trilisate)	Has no antiplatelet effect. May administer to patients with aspirin sensitivity
Salsalate (Disalcid)	Similar to choline magnesium trisalicylate

TABLE 10–3. **Various Corticosteroids Used in Cancer Patients**

Corticosteroids	Notable Drug Information
Short-acting (8–12 hr)	
Cortisone (various)	Needs to be metabolized to active species
Hydrocortisone (various)	
Intermediate-acting (12–36 hr)	
Methylprednisolone (Medrol)	Minimal sodium-retaining activity
Prednisolone (various)	Same as above
Prednisone (various)	Metabolized to prednisolone
Long-acting	
Dexamethasone (Decadron)	No sodium-retaining activities with lower doses

TABLE 10–4. **Adverse Reactions of Nonsteroidal Antiinflammatory Drugs (NSAIDs) and Corticosteroids**

Adverse Effects	Nursing Implications
Nonsteroidals	
Gastrointestinal	
Ulceration, bleeding, gastritis, dyspepsia, abdominal pain, constipation, peptic ulcer disease (PUD). Risks increase with age, chronic use, concomitant corticosteroid use, history of PUD. Misoprostol (Cytotec) can be used to prevent NSAID-induced ulcers	Administer with food or milk. Guaiac stool. Assess for signs/symptoms of gastrointestinal (GI) bleeding.
Pancreas	
Pancreatitis reported with Sulindac	Monitor laboratory results. Monitor for signs/symptoms of pancreatitis, e.g., sudden and intense epigastric pain, vomiting
Hepatic	
Increase ALT, AST, bilirubin. Risks for hepatotoxicity include alcoholism, chronic active hepatitis, history of hepatitis, cirrhosis, CHF	Monitor laboratory results
Central Nervous System	
Dizziness, drowsiness, lightheadedness/vertigo. Malaise, fatigue, somnolence, mental confusion, headache	Neurologic examination for alertness and orientation. Advise clients/families to avoid driving or other hazardous activities that require mental alertness until CNS effects can be determined
Cardiovascular	
CHF, peripheral edema, fluid retention, and hypertension	Monitor fluid status, pitting edema, vital signs
Renal	
Acute renal failure, elevated BUN and serum creatinine levels, proteinuria. Risks include advanced age, chronic renal disease, and CHF	Monitor intake and output. Monitor renal function tests, blood pressure. Assess for edema
Hematologic	
Neutropenia, leukopenia, pancytopenia, thrombocytopenia, decreased hemoglobin/hematocrit levels	Monitor laboratory results, neutropenic precautions, bleeding precautions—exception: choline magnesium trisalicylate (Trilisate)
Platelet Aggregation	
Prolonged bleeding time	No IM shots; bleeding precautions
Special Senses	
Visual disturbance, blurred vision, photophobia, ocular cataracts, glaucoma, myopathy; ear pain, tinnitus	Clients should have regular eye examinations, hearing tests
Hypersensitivity	
Asthma, anaphylaxis, acute respiratory distress	NSAIDS contraindicated in clients with ASA allergy, nasal polyps, and bronchospastic disease
Respiratory	
Dyspnea, hemoptysis, bronchospasm, shortness of breath	Respiratory assessment; monitor breath sounds
Dermatologic and Skeletal	
Rash, erythema, urticaria, photosensitivity, osteoporosis, poor wound healing, skin thinning, growth arrest	Observe for rash. Advise clients to use sunblock, wear protective clothing, avoid prolonged exposure to sunlight

TABLE 10–4. **Adverse Reactions of Nonsteroidal Antiinflammatory Drugs (NSAIDs) and Corticosteroids** (*Continued*)

Adverse Effects	Nursing Implications
Electrolyte Imbalance Hyperglycemia with glycosuria, hypokalemia, hypernatremia. Disturbances can lead to hypertension and possible edema.	Monitor blood glucose and electrolytes. Monitor vital signs, presence of peripheral edema
Pituitary Adrenal insufficiency: due to prolonged use and rapid withdrawal	
Infectious Disease Immunosuppressive with increased risk of infections—fungal, viral. Activation of tuberculosis, spread of herpes conjunctivitis	Cultures, dermatologic examination. Be aware that signs/symptoms of infection may be masked by NSAIDs
Corticosteroids	
Cushing Syndrome with Long-Term Use Central obesity, moon face, buffalo hump, easy bruising, acne, hirsutism, striae	Assess client's body image concerns; fatigue, weakness
Electrolyte and Metabolic Imbalances Hyperglycemia, hypernatremia, hypokalemia, hypocalcemia. With resulting edema, hypertension, diabetes, and osteoporosis.	Monitor laboratory results (blood glucose, electrolytes, calcium), vital signs, body weight. Assess for edema.
Suppression of Pituitary-Adrenal Function With long-term use and sudden withdrawal may cause acute adrenal insufficiency and dependence. Fever, myalgia, arthralgia, and malaise. Unable to respond to stress	Monitor blood pressure for hypotension. Monitor electrolytes for hyponatremia. Assess for dehydration, fatigue, diarrhea, and anorexia
Psychiatric Disturbances Paranoia	Observe for and report any emotional status changes. Suicide precautions, if needed
Gastrointestinal Peptic ulcers, GI bleed.	Assess for epigastric pain 1–3 hr after meals; assess for nausea/vomiting, hematemesis; monitor CBC; guaiac stools/emesis.
Miscellaneous Poor wound healing, immunosuppression, menstrual irregularities, ocular cataracts, glaucoma, arrest of growth, myopathy	Monitor intraocular pressure. Monitor clients for signs and symptoms of infection; WBC count

ALT = alanine aminotransferase; AST = aspartate aminotransferase; CBC = complete blood count; CHF = congestive heart failure; CNS = central nervous system; BUN = blood urea nitrogen; IM = intramuscular; WBC = white blood cell.

Nursing Diagnoses

I. Knowledge deficit.

II. Risk for activity intolerance.

III. Risk for altered body temperature.

IV. Pain.

V. Risk for altered bowel elimination pattern (constipation or diarrhea).

VI. Risk for infection.
VII. Altered protection.
VIII. Body image disturbance.
IX. Risk for fluid volume deficit.
X. Risk for fluid volume excess.

Outcome Identification

I. Client and family discuss the rationale for the use of antiinflammatory agents.
II. Client and family describe personal risk factors for potential side effects of antiinflammatory agents.
III. Client and family list signs and symptoms of side effects of antiinflammatory agents to report to the health care team.
IV. Client experiences adequate symptom relief (e.g., of pain, nausea/vomiting).

Planning and Implementation

I. Assess client's and family's cultural and ethnic background, particularly health care practices and values and beliefs related to pharmacotherapy (see Antimicrobials, Planning and Implementation).
II. Implement interventions to decrease the incidence and severity of side effects of antiinflammatory agents (see Table 10–4).
   A. Establish client's allergies before administering NSAIDs. NSAIDs are contraindicated in clients with aspirin allergy or hypersensitivity to acetylsalicylic acid (ASA), nasal polyps, and bronchospastic disease.
   B. Review client's current medications for potential drug interactions; for example, NSAIDs can increase the effects of phenytoin (Dilantin), sulfonamide, and warfarin (Coumadin).
III. Implement strategies to monitor for complications of antiinflammatory agents (see Table 10–4).
IV. Implement measures to monitor for response to antiinflammatory agents.
   A. Assess client for adequate symptom relief (e.g., of pain, nausea and vomiting).
   B. Assess client for infection because the antipyretic and antiinflammatory actions of NSAIDs may mask signs and symptoms of infection.

Evaluation

The oncology nurse systematically and regularly evaluates the client's and/or family's responses to interventions to determine progress toward the achievement of expected outcomes. Relevant data are collected and actual findings are compared with expected findings. Nursing diagnoses, outcomes, and plans of care are reviewed and revised as necessary.

ANTIEMETIC THERAPY

Theory

I. Goal/indication.
   A. Goal—to prevent nausea and vomiting by pharmacologically inhibiting neurotransmitters that stimulate the reflex arc of nausea and vomiting.

   B. Indication.
     1. Chemotherapy with moderate to highly emetogenic potential (Table 10–5).
     2. Nausea and vomiting related to:
       a. Radiation therapy alone or in combination with antineoplastic chemotherapy.
       b. Tumor-related problems such as intestinal obstruction or head and neck metastases.
       c. Concomitant pharmacologic therapy (e.g., opiates, antibiotics).
       d. Concomitant medical complications.
         (1) Fluid and electrolyte disturbances (e.g., hypercalcemia, volume depletion, water intoxication, hypoadrenalism).
         (2) Infection (e.g., septicemia, central nervous system infection [meningitis]).
         (3) Constipation and bowel obstruction.
II. Classifications of nausea and vomiting.
   A. Anticipatory.
     1. Arises from the cortex and limbic region of the brain.
     2. Classic Pavlovian conditioned response in clients with prior episodes of poorly controlled nausea and vomiting.
     3. Nonthreatening cues (auditory, visual, or sensory) may trigger reaction.
     4. Provoked by anxiety.
   B. During and after chemotherapy.
     1. Nausea, mediated through the autonomic nervous system.
     2. Acute vomiting phase.
       a. Occurs within 24 hours of antineoplastic administration.
       b. Stimulation of reflex arc that includes the intestinal tract and release of various neurotransmitters, the chemoreceptor trigger zone (CTZ) located in the area postrema of the brainstem and the vomiting center (VC) located in the medulla oblongata.
     3. Delayed vomiting phase.
       a. Delayed emesis may persist for more than 24 hours after chemotherapy.
       b. This phase is common after cisplatin administration. Vomiting may last up to 7 days, peaking at 48 to 72 hours.
       c. With administration of carboplatin, symptoms may persist up to 5 days.
   C. Refractory.
     1. Resistant or nonresponsive to antiemetic therapy.
III. Principles of medical management.
   A. Selection of appropriate antiemetics (Table 10–6) for phase or indication and appropriate timing of antiemetic.
     1. Administer antiemetics prophylactically to cover onset, peak, and duration period of each antineoplastic agent.
IV. Potential complications.
   A. Uncontrolled nausea and vomiting.
     1. Fluid and electrolyte imbalance.
     2. Anorexia and weight loss.
     3. Esophageal tear or hemorrhage.
     4. Loss of quality of life.
     5. Potential noncompliance with therapeutic regimen.

TABLE 10–5. **Emetogenic Potential, Onset, and Duration of Action of Select Chemotherapeutic Agents**

Incidence	Agent	Onset (Hours) Nausea/Vomiting	Duration (Hours) Nausea/Vomiting
Very high (>90%)	Cisplatin*	1–6	24–72+
	Dacarbazine	1–3	1–12
	Mechlorethamine	0.5–2	8–24
	Melphalan (high-dose)	3–6	6–12
	Dactinomycin D	1–2	4–20
High (60–90%)	Carmustine*	2–4	4–24
	Cyclophosphamide#	4–12	12–24
	Procarbazine	24–27	Variable
	Etoposide#	4–6	24+
	Methotrexate*	1–12	24–72
	Cisplatin*	1–6	24–72+
Moderate (30–60%)	Doxorubicin	4–6	6+
	Mitoxantrone	4–6	6+
	5-Fluorouracil*	3–6	24+
	Mitomycin-C*	1–4	48–72
	Carboplatin*	4–6	12–24
	Ifosfamide	3–6	24–72
	Cytarabine*	6–12	3–12
	Idarubicin	2 (p.o.)/15′–30′ IV	———
	Pentostatin	———	———
	DaunoXome	———	———
	Gemcitabine	———	———
	Irinotecan	———	———
	Topotecan	———	———
Low (10–30%)	Bleomycin	3–6	———
	Daunorubicin*	1–2	———
	Etoposide#	3–8	———
	Melphalan*	6–12	———
	6-Mercaptopurine	4–8	———
	Methotrexate*	4–12	3–12
	Mitomycin-C*	1–4	48–72
	Vinblastine	4–8	———
	Lomustine*	2–6	2–24
	Altretamine	———	———
	Asparaginase	———	———
	Vinorelbine	———	———
	Vindesine	———	———
Very low (<10%)	Vincristine	4–8	———
	Chlorambucil	48–72	———
	Paclitaxel	4–8	———
	Aldesleukin	———	———
	Flutamide	———	———
	Fludarabine	———	———
	Tretinoin	———	———
	Goserelin	———	———
	Bacillus Calmette-Guérin (BCG)	———	———

*Dose-related, potential increases with higher doses.
#Route- and dose-related.
Adapted from Cleri, L.B. (1995). Serotonin antagonists: State of the art management of chemotherapy-induced emesis. *Oncology Nursing: Patient Treatment and Support 2*(1), 4; and Craig, J.B. & Powell, B.L. (1987). The management of nausea and vomiting in clinical oncology. *Am J Med Sci 293*, 39–44.

   B. Complications of drug therapy.
      1. Adverse effects (see Table 10–6).
      2. Administration difficulties.
         a. Erratic absorption due to client variables (e.g., gastric resection).
         b. Special needs for compounding alternative drug formulations (e.g., suppositories, suspensions).

Assessment

   I. Identification of clients at risk for nausea and vomiting.
      A. Type of chemotherapy agent, dose, and schedule.
      B. Client-related factors.
         1. Age less than 50 years old—may have more anticipatory vomiting.
         2. Heavy ethanol intake—may have lower incidence.
         3. Women more than men.
         4. Positive history of prenatal nausea and vomiting.
  II. Physical examination and/or clinical information.
      A. Number and volume of emetic episodes.
      B. Retching.
      C. Lack of oral intake.
      D. Fluid balance, signs and symptoms of dehydration—poor skin turgor, concentrated urine, low urine output, orthostatic hypotension.
      E. Presence of blood in vomitus.
      F. Vital signs—orthostatic hypotension.
      G. History of present health problems (e.g., clients with glaucoma should avoid many of the antiemetics).
 III. Evaluation of laboratory data.
      A. Electrolytes.
      B. Intake and output/fluid balance.

Nursing Diagnoses

   I. Knowledge deficit.
  II. Altered nutrition, less than body requirements.
 III. Risk for fluid volume deficit.
  IV. Altered thought processes.
   V. Anxiety.

Outcome Identification

   I. Client and family describe personal risk factors for nausea and vomiting.
  II. Client and family discuss the rationale for the use of antiemetics and their schedule of administration.
 III. Client and family list signs and symptoms of side effects of antiemetic therapy to report to the health care team.
  IV. Client obtains adequate control of nausea and vomiting, remains euvolemic, and maintains body weight.
   V. Client and family verbalize concerns regarding antiemetic therapy.

Planning and Implementation

   I. Assess client's and family's cultural and ethnic background, particularly health

(*Text continued on page 168*)

TABLE 10–6. Antiemetic Therapy: Select Pharmacologic Agents for the Control of Chemotherapy-Induced Nausea and Vomiting, Acute

Classification	Generic Name	Trade Name(s)	Route	Dose/Schedule	Adverse Effects of Class	Nursing Implications
Serotonin antagonist	Ondansetron	Zofran	IV	0.15 mg/kg, Q8H × 3 doses or 32 mg, or 20–24 mg or 10–12 mg × 30 min prechemo × 1, *OR*	Headache, diarrhea, constipation, fever, transient increases in serum AST/SGPT	Give higher doses over at least 30 min to prevent dizziness, headache, hypotension. Administer acetaminophen for headache; stool softeners and stimulants to prevent constipation. Monitor liver function test results
			PO	8 mg TID or BID		
	Granisetron	Kytril	IV	10 µg/kg over 5 min, within 30 min of chemo	Headache, asthenia, somnolence, diarrhea, constipation, fever	→
			PO	1–2 mg QD before chemotherapy		
Substituted benzamide	Metoclopramide	Reglan	IV	2.0 mg/kg Q2H × 4	Sedation; extrapyramidal reactions (EPS), e.g., akathisia, acute dystonic reactions (increased incidence in clients <40 yrs); diarrhea (high doses), dry mouth, anticholinergic side effects	Monitor for diarrhea. Do not administer to clients with prior hypersensitivity to procaine or procainamide; epilepsy or pheochromocytoma or where stimulation of gastrointestinal (GI) motility is contraindicated (e.g., mechanical obstruction, GI bleeding)
			PO	0.5–2.0 mg/kg Q3–4H		

Class	Generic	Trade	Route	Dose	Side Effects	Nursing Considerations
Phenothiazines	Prochlorperazine	Compazine	IM IV PO Spansule PR	10 mg Q4–6H 10–40 mg Q4–6H 10 mg Q4–6H 15–30 mg Q12H 25 mg Q4–6H	Sedation, akathisia, EPS, dry mouth, orthostatic hypotension, blurred vision. Anticholinergic crisis with overuse	Monitor vital signs (VS) for orthostatic hypotension; dizziness. Concurrent administration of diphenhydramine to alleviate EPS, anxiety or agitation
	Chlorpromazine	Thorazine	IM IV PR	12.5–50 mg Q4–6H 12.5–50 mg Q4–6H 12.5–50 mg Q4–6H	Sedation, hypotension, dizziness, akathisia, EPS, dry mouth	Monitor level of consciousness for sedation; monitor VS for orthostatic hypotension; monitor for and be prepared to treat EPS
	Perphenazine	Trilafon	PO IM IV	4 mg Q4–6H 5 mg Q4H 5 mg intravenous bolus (IVB) followed by an infusion at 1 mg/hr for 24 hr: max dose 30 mg (inpatients) and 15 mg (outpatients) in 24 hr	Sedation, constipation, EPS, dry mouth, rash. Contraindicated in clients with blood dyscrasias. Seizure threshold may be lowered	⟶
	Thiethylperazine maleate	Torecan Norzine	IM PO PR	10 mg QD–TID 10 mg QD–TID 10 mg QD–TID	Drowsiness, extrapyramidal side effects (dystonia, torticollis, akathisia, gait disturbances), hypotension	Do not give IV—causes hypotension. Torecan injection contraindicated in patients allergic to sulfites

(Table continued on following page)

TABLE 10–6. **Antimetic Therapy: Select Pharmacologic Agents for the Control of Chemotherapy-Induced Nausea and Vomiting, Acute** (*Continued*)

Classification	Generic Name	Trade Name(s)	Route	Dose/Schedule	Adverse Effects of Class	Nursing Implications
Corticosteroids	Dexamethasone	Decadron	IV	4–20 mg (10–20 mg given × 1, otherwise Q4–6H	Dyspepsia, hiccoughs, increased appetite, euphoria, insomnia, fluid retention, hyperglycemia, hypokalemia, adrenal gland suppression	Slow IV infusion to prevent perineal itching/burning. Monitor blood glucose and potassium levels. See Table 10–4
		Hexadrol	PO	4–8 mg Q6H × 4 doses		
	Prednisolone	Deltasone	PO	2.5–15 mg Q4–12H	Dyspepsia, hiccoughs, increased appetite, euphoria, insomnia, fluid retention, hyperglycemia	See Table 10–4
Butyrophenones	Haloperidol	Haldol	IM	2–5 mg Q2H × 3–4 doses/24 hr	Sedation, akathisia, EPS, orthostatic hypotension	Assess baseline level of consciousness and monitor for oversedation
			PO	2–5 mg Q2H × 3–4 doses/24 hr		
			IV	2 mg × 1		
	Droperidol	Inapsine	IM	2–5 mg Q4–6H	Sedation, akathisia, EPS, hypotension	→
			IV	2–5 mg Q4–6H or drip		
Cannabinoids	Dronabinol	Marinol	PO	2.5–10 mg 1–3 hr before chemotherapy, then Q2H × 4–6 doses/day	Sedation, dry mouth, euphoria or dysphoria, dizziness, orthostatic hypotension	Central nervous system (CNS) adverse reactions more common in the elderly
Drugs used to augment antiemetics	Diphenhydramine	Benadryl	PO	25–50 mg Q4H PRN	Sedation, dizziness, blurred vision/diplopia, dry mouth	Assess client's level of consciousness and risk for oversedation
			IM	25–50 mg Q4H PRN		
			IV	25–50 mg Q4H PRN		

		Route	Dose	Side effects	Nursing considerations
Hydroxyzine	Vistaril	IM	25 mg Q 4–6H PRN	Drowsiness, dry mouth	Never give IV. Client/family teaching to avoid concurrent ethyl alcohol (ETOH) ingestion and hazardous activities that require mental alertness. Assess and monitor for excessive sedation. When administering IM, may cause marked discomfort at injection site; Z-track method is preferred, deep into large muscle mass
Lorazepam	Ativan	IV PO SL	0.5–2 mg 0.5–2 mg 0.5–2 mg	Sedation, anterograde amnesia, dizziness, weakness, unsteadiness, disorientation, hypotension	Assess client's level of consciousness and risk for sedation. Monitor VS. Fall precautions
Diazepam	Valium	PO IV	2–4 mg Q4–6H 2–5 mg Q4–6H	Drowsiness, confusion, anterograde amnesia, impaired physical coordination. Phlebitis, pain at injection site. Hypotension, bradycardia, cardiovascular collapse, respiratory depression	Baseline assessment of level of consciousness, mental status. Client/family teaching to avoid concurrent ETOH ingestion, avoid driving, operating machinery, and other hazardous activities that require mental alertness
Miscellaneous					
Promethazine	Phenergan	PO IV, IM	25 mg Q4H PRN 12.5–25 mg Q4H PRN	Phenothiazine derivative. Sedation, lower seizure threshold	Assess baseline level of consciousness and monitor elderly clients for confusion, sedation. Monitor VS especially during IV administration because hypotension may occur

Adapted from Cleri, L.B. (1995). Serotonin antagonists: State of the art management of chemotherapy-induced emesis. *Oncology Nursing: Patient Treatment and Support* 2(1), 6–7.

care practices and values and beliefs related to pharmacotherapy (see Antimicrobials, Planning and Implementation).
II. Implement strategies to maximize client safety.
  A. Assess for mental status changes, dizziness, sedation and implement safety measures (e.g., fall precautions) as needed.
III. Implement interventions to decrease the incidence and severity of side effects of antiemetic therapy and monitor for complications of antiemetic therapy (see Table 10–6).
IV. Implement measures to monitor for response to antiemetic therapy.
  A. Follow recommended schedules for administration (e.g., administer oral antiemetics 30–40 minutes before treatment, intravenous bolus approximately 10–30 minutes before treatment).
  B. Monitor intake and output.
  C. Monitor number of vomiting events.
  D. Monitor client's complaints of nausea.

Evaluation

The oncology nurse systematically and regularly evaluates the client's and/or family's responses to interventions to determine progress toward the achievement of expected outcomes. Relevant data are collected and actual findings are compared with expected findings. Nursing diagnoses, outcomes, and plans of care are reviewed and revised as necessary.

ANALGESICS

Theory

  I. Rationale/indication.
    A. The use of pharmacologic interventions to reduce the effect of noxious stimuli caused by heat, cold, or mechanical injury that elicit a response known as pain.
    B. To intervene with the pain transmission initiated by the pain receptors, primary afferent neuronal fibers, the spinothalamic tract, collateral fibers and higher brain centers.
    C. Indications—include musculoskeletal, visceral, neuronal pain.
  II. Types of analgesics.
    A. Opiate agonist compounds.
      1. Morphine sulfate.
      2. Hydromorphone hydrochloride (Dilaudid).
      3. Codeine sulfate and codeine phosphate.
      4. Hydrocodone bitartrate.
      5. Oxycodone hydrochloride.
      6. Oxymorphone hydrochloride (Numorphan).
      7. Levorphanol tartrate (Levodromoran).
      8. Fentanyl citrate (Fentanyl).
      9. Sufentanyl citrate (Sufenta).
      10. Methadone hydrochloride (Dolophine).
      11. Meperidine hydrochloride (Demerol).
      12. Propoxyphene napsylate (Darvon compounds).
      13. Alfentanyl citrate (Alfenta).
    B. Agonist-antagonist compounds.
      1. Buprenorphine hydrochloride (Buprenex).
      2. Butorphanol tartrate (Stadol).

3. Nalbuphine hydrochloride (Nubain).
4. Pentazocine (Talwin)
C. Nonopioid analgesics (see NSAIDs section).
D. Miscellaneous.
1. Acetaminophen.
2. Tramodol
E. Adjuvant agents (see Psychotropics and NSAIDs sections).
III. Principles of medical management.
A. Assessment of type of pain—description, etiology, classification, degree of pain.
B. History of past and current analgesia regimens and their effectiveness.
1. Time to onset of pain relief.
2. Duration of time of pain relief.
3. Quality or rating of decrease of pain.
C. Assessment of side effects from previous regimens.
1. Description of side effects.
2. Onset and duration of side effects.
3. Pharmacologic and/or other interventions to control or alleviate side effects.
4. Severity of side effects.
D. Physical examination; review of systems; laboratory indices (e.g., electrolytes, renal and liver function tests).
E. Selection of appropriate analgesia based on pharmacokinetic factors and client's physical needs, age, history of analgesia usage, and organ function (Table 10–7).
F. Reassessment of effectiveness and side effect profile (see also section on pain in Chapter 1).

TABLE 10–7. **Pharmacokinetic Factors of Opiates and Nonopiates**

Drug (Oral)	Onset of Effect (Minutes)	Peak Effect (Minutes)	Duration of Effect (Hours)	Plasma Half-life (Hours)
Morphine	30	30–90	3–7	2–3
Codeine	30	45–90	4–6	3–4
Fentanyl	10	20–30	1–2	3–4
Hydromorphone	30	30–90	4–5	2–4
Levorphanol	30	60–90	4–8	10–12
Meperidine	15	30–60	2–4	3–4*
Methadone	15	60–120	4–6	22–55**
Oxycodone	15	45–60	4–6	———
Oxymorphone	10	30–90	3–6	———
Propoxyphene	60	60–90	4–6	6–12
Sufentanil	1–3	5	avg. 40 min	2
Buprenorphine	15	45–60	4–6	2–3
Butorphanol	10	30–60	3–4	2–4
Nalbuphine	15	45–60	3–6	4–6
Pentazocine	15	30–60	2–3	2–3
Acetaminophen	15	30–60	4–6	1.25–3

*Active metabolite normeperidine 14–24 hours in normal renal function.
**Half-life extends with chronic dosing.

IV. Potential complications.
    A. Side effect profile of opioid analgesics (Table 10–8).
    B. Tolerance and dependence.
    C. Opioid withdrawal.
    D. Drug interactions with multidrug regimens (Table 10–9).
        1. Other sedative hypnotic drugs—potentiate sedative properties of opiates and combination opiate substances.

TABLE 10–8. **Side Effect Profile of Opioid Analgesics**

Side Effect	Nursing Implications
Gastrointestinal	
Nausea, vomiting, constipation, narcotized bowel	Concomitant antiemetic therapy Stool softeners and/or stimulant cathartics Assist client in ambulation as needed; increase fluid and dietary fiber intake; monitor bowel sounds and bowel regularity
Cardiovascular	
Arteriolar vasodilation and reduced peripheral resistance. Decrease in blood pressure. Tachycardia, bradycardia	Monitor VS, blood pressure for orthostatic hypotension
Respiratory	
Depressant effect on brainstem reduces respiratory rate, minute volume, and tidal exchange. Irregular and periodic breathing. Respiratory arrest	Monitor level of sedation; respiratory rate, depth; arterial blood gases, vital signs, O_2 saturations. Have available narcotic antagonist and measures for respiratory assistance
Decreased cough reflex	Monitor coughing ability postoperatively Aspiration precautions
Central Nervous System	
Drowsiness, alteration in mood, mental clouding. Visual and auditory hallucinations, euphoria, dizziness, disorientation, paranoia. Lethargy, inability to concentrate, apathy. Seizure, uncontrollable twitching, myoclonus	Monitor mental status changes, institute fall precautions Monitor for preseizure activity especially in patients on meperidine. Monitor for twitching Level of sedation may indicate degree of respiratory depression
Pupil	
Miosis	Monitor pupil size, contraction
Smooth Muscle	
Contraction of gallbladder, bile duct, and sphincter of Oddi	
Genitourinary	
Urinary retention	Monitor urine output, catheterization (straight or indwelling) as needed
Dermatologic	
Skin rash, cutaneous vasodilation	Monitor skin integrity. Administer antihistamines for allergic reactions

VS = vital signs

TABLE 10–9. Common Drug Interactions of Analgesics

Drug	Effect
Acetaminophen (APAP) plus (+)	
Barbiturates	Reduced APAP effect, increased toxicity of APAP overdose
Ethanol (ETOH)	Chronic ETOH causes increased toxicity of APAP overdose
Food	Delayed APAP absorption
Phenytoin	Increased hepatic metabolism of APAP
Metoclopramide	Increased APAP absorption
Diazepam	Decreased diazepam bioavailability
Methadone +	
Phenytoin	Reduced methadone plasma levels
Opioid Analgesics +	
Barbiturates	Enhanced central nervous system (CNS) depressant effects
Cimetidine	Enhanced opioid effects
Chlorpromazine	Enhanced CNS depression and hypotension
Ethanol	Enhanced CNS depressant effects
Neuromuscular blockers	Additive respiratory depression
Rifampin	Decreased opioid plasma levels
Pentazocine +	
Smoking	Increased metabolism of pentazocine
Meperidine +	
Monoamine oxidase inhibitors	Increased adverse reactions (excitation, sweating, rigidity, and hypertension)
Phenytoin	Reduced meperidine plasma levels
NSAID +	
ACE inhibitors	Reduced antihypertensive effect
β-adrenergic receptor blockers	Reduced antihypertensive effect
Corticosteroids	Increased incidence of gastrointestinal ulceration
Hydralazine	Reduced antihypertensive effect
Prazosin	Reduced antihypertensive effect
Potassium-sparing diuretics	Decreased renal function
Salicylates +	
Warfarin	Increased risk of bleeding
Acetazolamide	May enhance renal salicylate excretion and increase salicylate penetration into the brain causing CNS salicylate toxicity
ETOH	Increased risk of gastrointestinal blood loss
Heparin	Increased risk of bleeding
Methotrexate	Increased risk of methotrexate toxicity
Probenecid	Inhibit uricosuric effects of probenecid
Sulfinpyrazone	Inhibits uricosuric effects of sulfinpyrazone
Antacids	Reduce salicylate levels. Increased renal elimination of salicylates
Antidiabetic agents	Increased response of sulfonylureas Chlorpropamide most likely affected

NSAIDs = nonsteroidal antiinflammatory drugs

2. Drugs that lower seizure threshold—increase potential for seizure disorder.
3. Concomitant drugs that alter mental status equilibrium.
4. Other drugs that alter hepatic metabolism, renal excretion.
5. Other drugs that alter bioavailability, absorption, or pharmacokinetics of the administered drug. Abnormalities in absorption caused by:
    a. Gastrointestinal.
        (1) Surgical resections including gastrectomy, jejunectomy, duodenectomy; may increase transit time and/or decrease absorption.
        (2) Feeding tubes inserted at various points in the gastrointestinal tract may not be appropriate point of absorption of individual drug. Tube feedings or fluids administered through tubes may increase transit time and decrease absorption.
        (3) Pharmacologically induced changes in gut motility (e.g., laxatives, muscarinics, metoclopramide prokinetic agents—cisapride, antidiarrheal drugs, narcotics).
    b. Topical absorption.
        (1) Skin integrity—moisture content, friability, fat-to-lean body ratio, homogeneous epidermis without ulcerations.
        (2) Occlusive dressings increase absorption.
        (3) Location of application—areas of high vascularity may have higher absorption.
E. Potential adverse effects due to compromised organ systems.
    1. Renal insufficiency—may slow rate of elimination of drug and/or metabolites leading to increased potential for toxicities.
    2. Hepatic insufficiency—may increase amount of drug available to body due to decreased first pass effect, altered enzyme pathways, or other metabolic pathways.
    3. Central nervous system (CNS)—brain metastases, underlying seizure disorders may predispose to CNS toxicity.
    4. Urinary—benign prostatic hypertrophy may contribute to urinary retention.
    5. Respiratory—underlying lung disorders including emphysema, lung metastases, asthma; acute pulmonary distress syndromes may additionally compromise respiratory drive.
    6. Gastrointestinal—history of nausea and vomiting, impaired cough reflex.
    7. Cardiovascular—coronary artery disease, congestive heart failure.

Assessment

I. Identification of clients at risk for pain (see Chapter 1).
II. Physical examination.
    A. Review of systems.
    B. Examination of area of pain and/or originating site of pain—redness, temperature changes, atrophy, tenderness (see Chapter 1).
III. Evaluation of laboratory data.
    A. Renal indices—serum creatinine and blood urea nitrogen (BUN), intake and output.

B. Hepatic indices—aspartate aminotransferase (AST), serum glutamic-pyruvic transaminase (SGPT), bilirubin, transaminase.
C. Electrocardiogram (ECG), EEG if available.
D. X-ray examination, bone scan, MRI, ultrasound.

Nursing Diagnoses

I. Knowledge deficit.
II. Risk for activity intolerance.
III. Pain.
IV. Risk for altered bowel elimination pattern.
V. Impaired gas exchange.
VI. Altered thought processes.

Outcome Identification

I. Client and family discuss the rationale for the use of analgesics including the schedule of administration, if applicable.
II. Client and family describe personal risk factors for potential side effects of analgesic agents.
III. Client and family list signs and symptoms of side effects of analgesics to report to the health care team.
IV. Client experiences adequate/acceptable pain relief with minimal side effects or with satisfactory management of his/her side effects.
V. Client and family discuss that the risk of addiction is extremely rare.

Planning and Implementation

I. Assess client's and family's cultural and ethnic background, particularly health care practices and values and beliefs related to pharmacotherapy (see Antimicrobials, Planning and Implementation).
II. Implement strategies to decrease the incidence and severity of side effects of analgesics.
   A. Assess baseline data (e.g., vital signs, CNS—orientation, alertness, affect; respiratory effort, rate, and depth).
   B. Review client's medical history for existing or previous conditions such as acute alcoholism, impaired hepatic or renal function, advanced age, increased intracranial pressure.
   C. Review client's medications for possible drug interactions.
III. Implement strategies to monitor for complications of analgesic agents (see Table 10–8).
IV. Implement measures to monitor for response to analgesia.
   A. Assess client's pain experience.
   B. Assess for adverse effects, toxicity, and drug interactions.

Evaluation

The oncology nurse systematically and regularly evaluates the client's and/or family's responses to interventions to determine progress toward the achievement of expected outcomes. Relevant data are collected and actual findings are compared with expected findings. Nursing diagnoses, outcomes, and plans of care are reviewed and revised as necessary.

PSYCHOTROPIC DRUGS

Sedative/Hypnotic and Antianxietal Agents

Theory

    I. Rationale/indication.

        A. Anxiety is a commonly identified response to the uncertainty, loss of control, and hopelessness frequently experienced by cancer patients and families. This anxiety can be further exacerbated by preexisting psychological disorders.

            1. Antianxietal agents are used to reduce behavioral and physiologic abnormalities caused by anxiety disorders.

            2. Antianxietal agents are also used to control anxiety induced by other medical conditions, psychiatric disorders, or pharmacologic disorders.

        B. Sedative/hypnotic and antianxietal agents are also used as adjuvant pharmacologic management for pain associated with marked anxiety or manic-like symptoms.

        C. Sedative/hypnotic agents used for sleep disorders, e.g., insomnia.

        D. Alcohol or narcotic withdrawal.

    II. Types of sedative/hypnotic and antianxietal agents.

        A. Barbiturates (Table 10–10).

        B. Benzodiazepines (Table 10–10).

        C. Neuroleptics (Table 10–11).

   III. Principles of medical management.

        A. Identify signs and symptoms of anxiety (see Chapter 2).

        B. Selection of therapy.

            1. Psychotherapy.

            2. Pharmacologic (see Tables 10–10 and 10–11).

                a. Half-life.

                b. Sedative properties.

                c. Psychomotor and memory impairment.

                d. Dose-response profiles.

                e. Cost.

                f. Duration of therapy.

                g. Dosage conversion.

                h. Routes of administration.

                i. Compromised organ function.

                j. Elderly.

        C. Potential complications.

            1. Dependence and withdrawal.

            2. Drug interactions.

            3. Respiratory depression.

            4. Combative behavior.

            5. Noncompliance.

Assessment

    I. Identify clients at risk for anxiety disorders (see Chapter 2).

    II. Signs and symptoms (see Chapter 2).

   III. Evaluation of laboratory data.

        A. Electrolyte abnormalities and blood glucose levels.

        B. Drug level abnormalities.

Nursing Diagnoses

    I. Knowledge deficit.

II. Anxiety.

III. Ineffective individual coping.

IV. Altered thought processes.

Outcome Identification

I. Client and family discuss the rationale for the use of sedative/hypnotic and/or antianxietal agents.

II. Client and family describe personal risk factors for potential side effects of sedative/hypnotic and/or antianxietal agents.

III. Client and family list signs and symptoms of side effects of sedative/hypnotic and/or antianxietal agents to report to the health care team.

IV. Client experiences adequate symptom control or management with minimal side effects.

Planning and Implementation

I. Assess client's and family's cultural and ethnic background, particularly health care practices and values and beliefs related to pharmacotherapy (see Antimicrobials, Planning and Implementation).

   A. Determine client's racial group because biologic variations among racial groups may affect drug metabolism rates, clinical drug responses, and drug side effects. For example, Asians may require lower doses of neuroleptics; Chinese may require lower doses of benzodiazepines and may be more sensitive to the sedative effects of this class of drugs.

II. Implement strategies to decrease the incidence and severity of side effects of sedative/hypnotics and antianxietal agents (see Tables 10–10 and 10–11).

   A. Assess baseline data (e.g., vital signs, CNS—orientation, alertness, affect; respiratory effort, rate, and depth).

   B. Review client's medical history for existing or previous conditions.

   C. Review client's medications for potential drug interactions.

III. Implement strategies to monitor for complications of sedative/hypnotics and/or antianxietal agents (see Tables 10–10 and 10–11).

IV. Implement measures to monitor for response to sedative/hypnotics and/or antianxietal agents.

   A. Psychiatric/psychological consult as needed.

   B. Assess for adverse effects, toxicity, and drug interactions.

Evaluation

The oncology nurse systematically and regularly evaluates the client's and/or family's responses to interventions to determine progress toward the achievement of expected outcomes. Relevant data are collected and actual findings are compared with expected findings. Nursing diagnoses, outcomes, and plans of care are reviewed and revised as necessary.

Antidepressants

Theory

I. Rationale/indications.

   A. Depression is a commonly identified response of cancer patients to the cancer experience. Depression can range from minor mood changes to major emotional responses of suicidal ideation.

     1. Antidepressants are used to treat clinical unipolar or bipolar depression.

   B. Used in depression associated with chronic pain.

   C. Used as adjuvant pharmacologic pain management in pain conditions in-

(*Text continued on page 182*)

TABLE 10–10. **Common Sedative/Hypnotic and Antianxietal Agents**

Drug	Indications and Notable Pharmacologic Facts	Potential Adverse Effects of Class	Nursing Implications
Sedative/Hypnotic Agents			
Barbiturates		Lethargy, drowsiness; rash → Stevens-Johnson syndrome; apnea; barbiturate toxicity (e.g., hypotension; cold, clammy skin; insomnia; nausea; vomiting; delirium; weakness)	Monitor Hgb/Hct, RBCs, LFTs; assess mental status (e.g., affect, mood); monitor respiratory status; safety measures (e.g., assist with ambulation). Give on empty stomach for best absorption. Physical dependency may occur if long-term use. Do not discontinue drug abruptly, taper off over 1–2 weeks
Short-acting Secobarbital	Insomnia, basal hypnosis for anesthesia, emergency control of convulsions. Incompatible with several medications (e.g., codeine, cimetidine, diphenhydramine, hydrocortisone, insulin, meperidine, methadone, vancomycin); decreased effect of oral anticoagulants, corticosteroids	Tolerance builds quickly to hypnotic effect after approximately 2 weeks	Aqueous solutions must be prepared with sterile water for injection. Use solution within 30 min due to instability. Aqueous polyethylene glycol vehicles should be given slowly intravenously (IV) and client monitored closely with emergency equipment available
Intermediate Amobarbital (Amytal)	Use as sedative, hypnotic, preanesthetic, anticonvulsant. Used in management of catatonic or manic reactions	Effects of class may be increased by central nervous system (CNS) depressants, monoamine oxidase inhibitors. Other sedative hypnotic, alcohol, narcotics, phenothiazines, general anesthetics, antihistamine, centrally acting muscle relaxants	Use injection within 30 min after opening vial. Inject deep IM or slow IV (100 mg/min maximum IV rate)

Drug	Use	Side Effects	Nursing Considerations
Long-acting Phenobarbital	Sedation, grand mal and focal seizures alone or in combination with other antiepileptic drugs. IV in acute convulsive states	Loss of concentration, mental dulling, depression of affect. Skin rashes. Folate deficiency can occur. May increase metabolic activity of liver enzymes and decrease effects of drugs biotransformed by these enzymes	Assess convulsive activity; monitor drug levels; respiratory assessment. Use injection within 30 min after opening vial. Long half-life and too frequent dosing can lead to accumulation toxicity
Benzodiazepines *Long-acting* Flurazepam (Dalmane)	Insomnia. Sedation. Active metabolite	Drowsiness, dizziness, headache, ataxia, lightheadedness common in elderly. Adverse effects may include lethargy, disorientation, slurred speech, faintness, confusion, anorexia, nervousness, apprehension, weakness, irritability, palpitation, short-term memory impairment, depression	Longest acting benzodiazepine hypnotic. Daytime carryover effects are common (e.g., decreased alertness, impaired coordination, confusion, and personality changes). Safety measures (e.g., fall precautions, assist with ambulation), mental status checks. Side effects may persist for days after discontinuation of drug. Use with caution in the elderly
Intermediate Temazepam (Restoril)	Insomnia. Sedation. No accumulation of metabolites	Lethargy, drowsiness, daytime sedation, nausea, vomiting, constipation, diarrhea	Monitor labs (Hgb/Hct, LFTs); assess mental status; safety measures. Minimal hangover effect. May take two nights before beneficial effects felt. Sleep disturbances can occur for several nights after discontinuance
Short-acting Triazolam (Halcion)	Insomnia. Sedation. Inactive metabolites	Anterograde amnesia may occur. Headache, lethargy, drowsiness	Monitor labs (Hgb/Hct, LFTs); assess mental status; safety measures. Minimal daytime hangover effect. May take two nights before beneficial effects felt. Increased wakefulness during the last third of the night

(Table continued on following page)

TABLE 10–10. **Common Sedative/Hypnotic and Antianxietal Agents** (*Continued*)

Drug	Indications and Notable Pharmacologic Facts	Potential Adverse Effects of Class	Nursing Implications
Antianxietal Agents **_Benzodiazepines_** *Short-acting*			
Alprazolam (Xanax)	Anxiety	Antidepressant activity at higher doses. Drowsiness and lightheadedness are common during early stages of therapy. Orthostatic hypotension, blurred vision	Monitor VS. Assess for orthostatic hypotension—if systolic BP drops 20 mm Hg, hold drug, notify prescriber. Monitor laboratory results. Assess mental status, monitor affect, drowsiness, suicidal tendencies. Safety measures (e.g., assist with ambulation)
Chlordiazepoxide (Librium)	Used in anxiety and for ETOH withdrawal. Less potent than diazepam and less anticonvulsive activity. Excreted slowly by kidneys	Dizziness, drowsiness, orthostatic hypotension, blurred vision	Monitor VS. Assess for orthostatic hypotension—if systolic BP drops 20 mm Hg, hold drug, notify prescriber. Monitor laboratory test results. Assess mental status, monitor affect, drowsiness, suicidal tendencies. Safety measures (e.g., assist with ambulation) IM solution prepared immediately before administration. IM solution not to be given IV due to air bubbles from solution. Inject IM slowly and deeply. IV solution to be reconstituted with sterile water or saline. Give IV over 1 min. Do not give IV preparation IM because of pain on injection. Do not add IV dose to IV solution because of instability and quick deterioration

Drug	Use	Adverse effects	Nursing considerations
Diazepam (Valium)	Used in anxiety, acute seizure control, operating procedures	Dizziness, drowsiness, orthostatic hypotension, blurred vision	Monitor VS. Assess for orthostatic hypotension—if systolic BP drops 20 mm Hg, hold drug, notify prescriber. Monitor laboratory test results. Assess mental status; monitor affect, drowsiness, suicidal tendencies. Safety measures (e.g., assist with ambulation) Can be given IM or IV. Do not add to IV fluids. When administering IV: use large vein, inject slowly, maximum rate no greater than 5 mg/min. Assess site for phlebitis. Be prepared to provide respiratory assistance
Lorazepam (Ativan)	Acute anxiety, preoperative sedation, insomnia. Shortest acting drug used for anxiety and preanesthetic. No active metabolite formed, so less danger of accumulation	Dizziness, drowsiness, orthostatic hypotension, blurred vision. May impair short-term memory	Monitor VS. Assess for orthostatic hypotension—if systolic BP drops 20 mm Hg, hold drug, notify prescriber. Monitor laboratory test results. Assess mental status; monitor affect, drowsiness, suicidal tendencies. Safety measures (e.g., assist with ambulation)

Hgb = hemoglobin; Hct = hematocrit; RBCs = red blood cells; LFTs = liver function tests; VS = vital signs; BP = blood pressure; ETOH = ethanol; IM = intramuscular; IV = intravenous

TABLE 10–11. Neuroleptics for Anxiety

Drug and Indications	Side Effect Frequency				Nursing Implications
	Sedation	Anticholinergic	Extrapyramidal	Orthostatic Hypotension	
Phenothiazines					
Used in pain management with behavioral problems such as anxiety or psychoses					
Chlorpromazine (Thorazine)	High	Moderate	Moderate	High	Monitor VS; assess BP, pulse lying and standing/sitting. Assess mental status: level of consciousness, affect, oversedation. Prevent constipation (e.g., stool softeners/stimulants, increase bulk/fluids, increase ambulation). Safety measures (e.g., fall precautions, assist with ambulation). Dilute IV solution to 1 mg/mL in saline and administer at 1 mg/min.
Fluphenazine (Prolixin, Permitil)	Low	Low	Very high	Low	Assess and be prepared to treat extrapyramidal symptoms (EPS). Monitor liver/renal function and CBC. Monitor VS; assess BP, pulse lying and standing/sitting. Assess mental status: level of consciousness, affect, oversedation. Prevent constipation (e.g., stool softeners/stimulants, increase bulk/fluids, increase ambulation). Safety measures (e.g., fall precautions, assist with ambulation). Protect solution from light. Moisture may cloud solution so use dry syringe and needle for injection. Due to impaired GI absorption, avoid antacids with oral forms. Effects can be prolonged; teach client/family to report side effects immediately. Instruct client/family that urine may turn pink to reddish brown.

Drug					Nursing Implications
Perphenazine (Trilafon)	Low	Low	High	Low	Assess and be prepared to treat extrapyramidal symptoms (EPS). Monitor liver/renal function and CBC. Monitor VS; assess BP, pulse lying and standing/sitting. Assess mental status: level of consciousness, affect, oversedation. Prevent constipation (e.g., stool softeners/stimulants, increase bulk/fluids, increase ambulation). Safety measures (e.g., fall precautions, assist with ambulation). Monitor BP/pulse when administering IV because hypotension can occur. Oral concentrate: dilute (60 mL diluent/5 mL concentrate) in water, fruit juices except apple; no caffeinated beverages.
Thioridazine (Mellaril)	High	High	Low	Low	Assess level of consciousness, affect, mental status. Monitor patient for excessive sedation. Monitor cardiac status. Monitor VS; assess BP, pulse lying, and standing/sitting. Prevent constipation (e.g., stool softeners/stimulants, increase bulk/fluids, increase ambulation). Safety measures (e.g., fall precautions, assist with ambulation). Monitor urine output. Monitor CBC, liver function tests. Male patients: potential impotence. Oral concentrate: dilute immediately before use with fruit juice or water. After IM injection: instruct client to remain lying for 30 min
Butyrophenones Haloperidol (Haldol)	Very low	Very low	Very high	Very low	Assess for and be prepared to treat extrapyramidal symptoms (EPS). May lower seizure threshold—use cautiously in individuals with epilepsy. Assess mental status (e.g., affect, level of consciousness). Monitor CBC and liver function tests. Monitor VS; assess BP, pulse lying, and standing/sitting. Prevent constipation (e.g., stool softeners/stimulants, increase bulk/fluids, increase ambulation). Safety measures (e.g., fall precautions, assist with ambulation). Monitor urine output. Dose reduction in the elderly. IM injection into deep muscle mass; patient to remain lying for 30 minutes after injection. Do not mix oral concentrate in coffee or tea

BP = blood pressure; CBC = complete blood count; GI = gastrointestinal; IM = intramuscular; VS = vital signs

cluding postherpetic neuralgia, migraine and chronic tension headaches, sundowner syndrome.
    D. Insomnia.
  II. Types of antidepressants (Table 10–12).
    A. Tricyclic antidepressants.
    B. Selective serotonin reuptake inhibitors (SSRI).
 III. Principles of medical management.
    A. Identify signs and symptoms of depression (see Chapter 2).
    B. Types of depression.
      1. Bipolar—with manic phase.
      2. Major depression—unipolar only.
      3. Situational depression.
      4. Drug- or food-induced depression.
    C. Selection of therapy.
      1. Psychotherapy.
      2. Pharmacologic therapy (see Table 10–12).
    D. Potential complications (see Table 10–12).
      1. Drug interactions.
      2. Dietary restrictions.

Assessment
  I. Identification of clients at risk.
    A. Age—younger more than older persons.
    B. Health conditions (e.g., advanced stage of disease), negative body image.
    C. Mental health history—family or individual history of depression or substance abuse.
    D. Disease recurrence, treatment failure.
    E. Unrelieved symptoms, especially pain.
    F. Pharmacologically induced risk factor.
      1. Antihypertensive and cardiovascular drugs: guanethidine, methyldopa, reserpine, propranolol, metoprolol, prazosin, clonidine, digitalis.
      2. Sedative-hypnotic agents: alcohol, chloral hydrate, benzodiazepines, barbiturates, meprobamate.
      3. Anti-inflammatory agents and analgesics: indomethacin, phenylbutazone, opiates, pentazocine.
      4. Steroids: corticosteroids, oral contraceptives, estrogen withdrawal.
      5. Miscellaneous: antiparkinsonian drugs, antineoplastic agents (interferon), ethambutol, neuroleptics, stimulant withdrawal.
    G. Concomitant medical diseases.
      1. Endocrine disorders: hypothyroidism, hyperthyroidism, diabetes mellitus, hyperparathyroidism, Cushing's disease, Addison's disease.
      2. Central nervous system disorders: brain tumors, Parkinson's disease, multiple sclerosis, Alzheimer's disease, Huntington's disease.
      3. Cardiovascular disorders: myocardial infarction (MI), cerebral vascular accident (CVA), congestive heart failure (CHF).
      4. Miscellaneous disorders: rheumatoid arthritis, pancreatic disease, carcinoma, systemic lupus erythematosus, infectious disease, metabolic abnormalities, pernicious anemia, malnutrition.
  II. Signs and symptoms (see Chapter 2).
 III. Evaluation of laboratory data.
    A. Electrolyte disorders.
    B. Fluid imbalances.

Nursing Diagnoses
I. Knowledge deficit.
II. Ineffective individual coping.
III. Dysfunctional grieving.
IV. Risk for injury.
V. Pain.
VI. Disturbance in self-esteem (situational low).
VII. Hopelessness.
VIII. Altered thought processes.

Outcome Identification
I. Client and family discuss the rationale for the use of antidepressants.
II. Client and family describe personal risk factors for potential side effects of antidepressants.
III. Client and family list signs and symptoms of side effects of antidepressants to report to the health care team.
IV. Client experiences adequate management of his/her depression with minimal side effects.

Planning and Implementation
I. Assess client's and family's cultural and ethnic background, particularly health care practices and values and beliefs related to pharmacotherapy (see Antimicrobials, Planning and Implementation).
II. Implement strategies to decrease the incidence and severity of side effects of antidepressants (see Table 10–12).
   A. Assess baseline data including vital signs; orthostatic blood pressures; laboratory test results (complete blood count, hepatic profile); CNS (orientation, alertness, affect, suicidal tendencies); respiratory effort, rate, and depth.
   B. Review client's medical history for existing or previous conditions.
   C. Review client's medications for potential drug interactions.
III. Implement strategies to monitor for complications of antidepressants (see Table 10–12).
IV. Implement measures to monitor for response to antidepressants.
   A. Monitor patient for emotional changes, suicidal ideation.
   B. Obtain psychiatric/psychological consultation as needed.
   C. Assess for adverse effects, toxicity, and drug interactions.

Evaluation
The oncology nurse systematically and regularly evaluates the client's and/or family's responses to interventions to determine progress toward the achievement of expected outcomes. Relevant data are collected and actual findings are compared with expected findings. Nursing diagnoses, outcomes, and plans of care are reviewed and revised as necessary.

ANTICONVULSANTS

Theory
I. Rationale/indications.
   A. For prophylaxis and treatment of seizure activity prompted by underlying medical condition or pharmacologic etiology.
   B. As adjuvant pharmacologic therapy for pain with neurologic etiology (trigeminal neuralgia, phantom limb pain, thalamic syndrome or lightning tabetic pain).

TABLE 10–12. **Common Antidepressants**

| Drug and Indications | Side Effect Frequency | | | Nursing Implications |
	Sedation	Anticholinergic	Orthostatic Hypotension	
Tricyclic Antidepressants				
Amitriptyline (Elavil, Endep) Used in endogenous depressions accompanied with anxiety. Adjuvant treatment for pain control	High	High	High	Assess mental status (e.g., excessive sedation, affect, suicidal tendencies). Give at bedtime to minimize daytime drowsiness. Monitor VS. Assess for orthostatic hypotension—if systolic BP drops 20 mm Hg, hold drug, notify practitioner. Institute safety precautions; teach patient to avoid rapid position changes. Monitor CBC, liver function tests; urinary output
Imipramine (Tofranil) Used in endogenous depression and in reducing enuresis in children	Moderate	Moderate	Moderate	Assess BP (lying/standing); if systolic BP drops 20 mm Hg, hold drug and notify practitioner. Take VS Q4H for clients with CV disease. Monitor cardiac status, CBC, liver function tests. Assess mental status: affect, suicidal tendencies. Interventions to prevent constipation: stool softeners/stimulants, increase bulk/fluid in diet, ambulation. If client consumes alcohol, hold dose
Desipramine (Norpramin) Active metabolite of imipramine with same uses	Low	Low	Moderate	Assess BP (lying/standing); if systolic BP drops 20 mm Hg, hold drug and notify practitioner. Take VS Q4H for clients with CV disease. Monitor CBC, liver function tests. Assess mental status: affect, suicidal tendencies. Monitor urinary output. If client consumes alcohol, hold dose. Teach client to avoid rapid position changes
Triazolopyridines				
Trazodone (Desyrel)	High	Very low	Moderate	Assess BP (lying/standing); if systolic BP drops 20 mm Hg, hold drug and notify practitioner. Take VS Q4H for clients with CV disease.

184

Drug				Nursing Implications
				Monitor CBC, liver function tests. Assess mental status: affect, suicidal tendencies. Monitor client for excessive sedation. Monitor urinary output. If client consumes alcohol, hold dose. Institute safety measures; teach client to avoid rapid position changes
Specific Serotonin Reuptake Inhibitors				
Fluoxetine (Prozac)	None	Very low	None	Assess mental status: affect, anxiety, suicidal tendencies; assess for insomnia. Assess BP (lying/standing); if systolic BP drops 20 mm Hg, hold drug and notify practitioner. Take VS Q4H for clients with CV disease. Monitor CBC, liver function tests. Monitor weights because anorexia is a potential side effect. Assess for urinary retention. Prevent constipation (e.g., stool softeners/stimulants, increase bulk/fluid in diet, ambulate). If client consumes alcohol, hold dose. Institute safety measures
Sertraline (Zoloft)	None	None	None	Assess mental status: affect, suicidal tendencies. Assess BP (lying/standing); if systolic BP drops 20 mm Hg, hold drug and notify practitioner. Take VS Q4H for clients with CV disease. Interventions to prevent constipation: stool softeners/stimulants, increase bulk/fluid in diet, ambulate. Assess for urinary retention. If client consumes alcohol, hold dose
Venlafaxine (Effexor) Inhibits both serotonin and norepinephrine uptake	Low	Low to none	Low to moderate	Assess BP (lying/standing); if systolic BP drops 20 mm Hg, hold drug and notify practitioner. Take VS Q4H for clients with CV disease. Sustained hypertension may occur in clients receiving doses >350 mg. Monitor cardiac status, CBC, liver function tests. Assess mental status: affect, suicidal tendencies

CBC = complete blood count; CV = cardiovascular; BP = blood pressure; VS = vital signs

II. Types of anticonvulsants (Table 10–13).
III. Principles of medical management.
    A. Diagnosis of appropriate seizure activity.
    B. Diagnosis of appropriate pain syndrome.
    C. Selection of appropriate pharmacologic therapy (see Table 10–13).
IV. Potential complications (see Table 10–13).

Assessment

I. Identification of clients at risk for seizure activity.
    A. Underlying seizure disorder.
    B. Drugs that lower seizure threshold (e.g., phenobarbital, ethanol, benzodiazepines, amphetamines, and salicylate toxicity).
    C. Medical conditions that lower seizure threshold.
        1. Trauma.
        2. Febrile episodes.
        3. Tumor pressing on CNS.
II. Physical examination.
    A. Level of consciousness, sensory perceptions.
    B. Eye examinations (e.g., for blurred vision, diplopia).
III. Evaluation of laboratory data.
    A. Subtherapeutic anticonvulsant serum levels.
    B. Electrolyte disorders.
    C. EEG, CT scan, or MRI.

Nursing Diagnoses

I. Knowledge deficit.
II. Risk for injury.
III. Impaired gas exchange.
IV. Altered thought processes.
V. Sleep pattern disturbance.

Outcome Identification

I. Client and family discuss the rationale for the use of anticonvulsants.
II. Client and family describe personal risk factors for seizure activity.
III. Client and family list the signs and symptoms of side effects of anticonvulsants to report to the health care team.
IV. Client experiences adequate seizure control with minimal side effects.

Planning and Implementation

I. Assess client's and family's cultural and ethnic background, particularly health care practices and values and beliefs related to pharmacotherapy (see Antimicrobials, Planning and Implementation).
II. Implement strategies to decrease the incidence and severity of side effects of anticonvulsants.
    A. Assess baseline data (e.g., neurologic status).
    B. Review client's medical history for existing or previous conditions.
    C. Review client's medications for potential drug interactions.
    D. Conduct client/family teaching (e.g., good oral hygiene; avoiding driving or other potentially hazardous activity that requires mental alertness).

TABLE 10–13. Common Anticonvulsants

Drug	Indications and Notable Pharmacologic Facts	Potential Adverse Effects of Class	Nursing Implications
Phenytoin (Dilantin)	Grand mal seizures; also to control psychomotor epilepsy. ETOH withdrawal syndrome. Ventricular arrhythmias, trigeminal neuralgias	Drowsiness, dizziness, hypotension, ventricular fibrillation, hepatitis, nephritis, hematologic disorders, systemic lupus erythematosus, Stevens-Johnson syndrome	Monitor and assess drug level. Monitor CBC; mental status, renal function, and liver function. Administer IV slowly and monitor VS. Do not exceed rate of 50 mg/min; avoid continuous infusion. Dilantin suspension: erratic absorption
Ethosuximide (Zarontin)	Petit mal seizures. Long half-life that can lead to cumulative toxicity	Drowsiness, dizziness, ataxia, headache, hiccoughs, gastrointestinal distress with too rapid dosing titration (e.g., nausea, cramping, diarrhea), rashes	Teach client that urine may turn pink to reddish brown from drug. Administer drug with meals to decrease GI upset. Assess mental status; ability to ambulate safely
Carbamazepine (Tegretol)	Spectrum of action similar to that of phenytoin. Also for treatment of trigeminal neuralgia and neuropathic pain in cancer patients	Blood dyscrasias (e.g., aplastic anemia, leukopenia, thrombocytopenia, eosinophilia, leukocytosis). Hyponatremia, drowsiness, dizziness, ataxia, nausea, blurred vision, diplopia with too rapid titration of dose	Monitor CBC, mental status. Administer drug with meals to decrease GI upset
Valproate/valproic acid (Depakene, Depakote)	Simple and complex absence seizures. Adjunct in treatment of multiple seizure types	Nausea, vomiting; diarrhea and abdominal cramps at initiation of therapy. Sedation, ataxia, tremor, behavioral disturbances more predominant if taken with other anticonvulsants. Elevated serum transaminase. Hepatic failure.	Monitor liver function tests. Administer antiemetics as needed. Assess mental status for excessive sedation. Administer with meals to decrease stomach upset. Do not break or crush the tablet or capsule; can cause irritation of mouth and throat
Phenobarbital	Sedation, grand mal and focal seizures alone or in combination with other antiepileptic drugs. IV in acute convulsive states	Loss of concentration, mental dulling, depression of affect. Skin rashes. Folate deficiency can occur. May increase metabolic activity of liver enzymes and decrease effects of drugs biotransformed by these enzymes	Assess mental status. Monitor drug levels; respiratory assessment. Use injection within 30 min of opening vials. Long half-life and too-frequent dosing can lead to accumulation toxicity
Gabapentin	Refractory partial (complex) seizures. Generalized seizures	Drowsiness, dizziness, fatigue, weight gain, skin rash, nausea, vomiting, blurred vision, tremor, slurred speech	Assess mental status, ability to ambulate safely. Monitor CBC. Discontinue drug gradually

III. Implement strategies to monitor for complications of anticonvulsants (see Table 10–13).
IV. Implement measures to monitor for response to anticonvulsants.
   A. Assess neurologic status.
   B. Assess for adverse effects, toxicity, and drug interactions.

Evaluation

The oncology nurse systematically and regularly evaluates the client's and/or family's responses to interventions to determine progress toward the achievement of expected outcomes. Relevant data are collected and actual findings are compared with expected findings. Nursing diagnoses, outcomes, and plans of care are reviewed and revised as necessary.

HEMATOPOIETIC GROWTH FACTORS

Theory

I. Rationale/indications.
   A. Hematopoietic growth factors are glycoproteins that stimulate the proliferation of bone marrow progenitor cells and their maturation into fully differentiated circulating blood cells. These compounds provide initiation, modification, and/or restoration of the hematopoietic and immune system and its various cell lines by exerting:
      1. Direct antitumor activity via cytotoxic or antiproliferative mechanisms of action.
      2. Biologic effects such as enhancing differentiation or maturation of immunologic cell lines, thus decreasing neutropenia and risk of infection.
   B. Indications (Table 10–14).
      1. Primary treatment of cancer (e.g., of hairy cell leukemia, Kaposi's sarcoma, renal cell carcinoma) (see Chapter 36).
      2. Supportive treatment.
         a. Granulocyte colony stimulating factors (G-CSF). Direct correlation exists between the duration of antineoplastic-induced neutropenia and risk of infection (see Table 10–14). In addition, clinical trials to investigate drug efficacy include:
            (1) Decreasing risk of infectious complications in human immunodeficiency virus (HIV) infection including CMV retinitis, in neonatal infections, and in clients with burns.
            (2) Dose-intensive chemotherapy.
            (3) Shortening time to engraftment in peripheral blood progenitor cell transplantation.
            (4) Radiotherapy.
         b. Granulocyte-macrophage colony stimulating factors (GM-CSF) (see Table 10–14). In addition, for investigational use to study drug efficacy in HIV infections, fungal and parasitic infections, chronic hepatitis B, peripheral blood progenitor cell transplantation, dose intensification.
         c. Erythropoietin (see Table 10–14). In addition, for clinical trials in augmenting autologous blood donations, acute blood loss, surgery, myelodysplastic syndromes.
         d. Monocyte colony stimulating factor. For clinical trials investigating effectiveness in fungal infections in bone marrow transplantation, in

TABLE 10–14. Growth Factors

Drug	Indications	Side Effects	Nursing Implications
GM-CSF or sargramostim (Leukine)	Myeloid recovery after autologous bone marrow transplant BMT graft failure or engraftment delay Following induction chemotherapy for acute myelogenous leukemia. Use if bone marrow hypoplastic with <5% blasts on day 10	Low dose: bone pain, local skin reaction. Fever, flu-like symptoms, headache, arthralgias, myalgias High dose: pericardial effusions, capillary leak syndrome, third spacing	May cause phlebitis with peripheral administration Bone pain alleviated with acetaminophen Monitor blood counts SQ administration standard. IV administration may require albumin in IV carrier
Interleukin-3	(Investigational)	Constitutional symptoms, bone pain	Monitor temperature spikes unrelated to drug administration Acetaminophen for bone pain
PIXY321	(Investigational)	Injection site erythema, flu-like symptoms with low-grade fever, nausea, and vomiting	Rotate sites of injection Monitor temperature spikes Symptom management
G-CSF or filgrastim (Neupogen)	Antineoplastic chemotherapy-induced neutropenia	Bone pain	Monitor blood counts Symptom management Contraindicated in clients with known hypersensitivity to *Escherichia coli*–derived products. Do not shake vial vigorously if giving subcutaneous injection
Erythropoietin (Epogen, Procrit)	Zidovudine-treated HIV-infected patients. Chronic renal failure Cancer patients receiving chemotherapy	Hypertension, thrombotic events, seizures, headaches, skin rashes, urticaria. Transient rash at injection site	Monitor blood pressure Rotate injection sites Monitor blood counts
M-CSF (macrophage-monocyte CSF)	(Investigational)	Thrombocytopenia, fever chills, palpitations, headaches, ocular discomfort, malaise. Reported dose-dependent lowering in cholesterol and lipoproteins	Thrombocytopenia precautions Symptom management

BMT = bone marrow transplant; SQ = subcutaneous; IV = intravenous; HIV = human immunodeficiency virus; CSF = colony stimulating factor refractory malignancies and as treatment for neutropenia, and in HIV patients.

II. Types of growth factors.
  A. Single lineage factors.
    1. Granulocyte colony stimulating factors (G-CSF).
      a. Stimulates target cells that include a late precursor committed to the neutrophil lineage and the mature neutrophil.
      b. Increases phagocytic activity.
      c. Increases antimicrobial killing.
      d. Enhances antibody-dependent cell-mediated cytotoxicity.
    2. Erythropoietin (r-HuEPO).
      a. Naturally produced by the kidneys. Production in normal hosts is regulated by a feedback mechanism involving the perception of decreased oxygen tension in tissue.
      b. Interacts with specific receptors on erythroid burst forming units and erythroid colony forming units.
      c. Binding of the stimulating factor and these units leads to erythropoiesis and subsequent production and differentiation of erythrocytes or red blood cells.
    3. M-CSF (rHuM-CSF, CSF-1, monocyte CSF, human urinary CSF). Monocyte-macrophage colony stimulating factor.
      a. Stimulates the proliferation, differentiation, and function of mononuclear cells.
      b. Indirect route of action by secreting a variety of cytokines that will interact with target cells.
        (1) Cytokines include interleukin-1 and tumor necrosis factor (TNF). These possess antitumor effects.
      c. Supports the proliferation and differentiation of macrophages. Enhances cellular function of macrophages.
    4. Platelet growth factors.
      a. Isolation of hormone thrombopoietin (TPO) thought to regulate platelet production or megakaryocytopoiesis, a function similar to erythropoiesis.
      b. Megakaryocyte growth and development factor under study in vitro.
      c. Interleukin-11: isolation and study of this factor's supporting role in the growth of megakaryocyte colonies.
    5. Stem cell factor (SCF)—also known as mast cell factor, steel factor, and c-kit ligand.
      a. Mechanism of action—works on primitive and mature progenitor cells. Murine SCF enhances erythropoietin-dependent colony-forming unit—granulocyte, erythrocyte, megakaryocyte, and monocyte (CFU-GEMM) and burst forming unit erythrocyte colony formation.
  B. Multilineage factors.
    1. GM-CSF—receptors exist on myeloid cell lines.
      a. Major effect stimulates the proliferation and differentiation of the cells destined for the neutrophil and macrophage lines.
      b. Enhances functional activities of neutrophils and monocytes lending to enhanced activity in clearing bacterial and fungal organisms.
      c. Stimulates production of secondary cytokines such as TNF, IL-1 and M-CSF.

2. Interleukin-3 (IL-3, multi-CSF)—T cell derived.
   a. Promotes proliferation and development of multipotential hemato-poietic stem cells as well as the committed progenitor cell lines of the granulocyte, macrophage, erythroid, eosinophil, megakaryocyte, mast cell, and basophil.
   b. Promotes activity of monocytes, macrophages, and eosinophils.
   c. Stimulates myelopoiesis, erythropoiesis, and thrombopoiesis.
   d. Clinical trials investigating use in reducing myelosuppression caused by antineoplastic therapy and bone marrow failure.
3. PIXY321 (GM-CSF/IL-3 fusion protein)
   a. Biologic effects of both factors listed earlier with reported greater lineage activity than either colony stimulating factor alone.
III. Principles of medical management.
   A. History of antineoplastic use, radiation therapy, surgery, or biotherapy.
   B. History of other medication use known to cause immunosuppression, neu-tropenia, anemia, and/or thrombocytopenia.
      1. Immunosuppressants—corticosteroids.
      2. H_2 antagonists—cimetidine, ranitidine.
      3. Aspirin-containing products, nonsteroidal antiinflammatory agents.
   C. Assessment of concurrent disease state or chronic illnesses contributing to neutropenia or anemic state.
      1. HIV infection.
      2. Immunosuppressive disorders: systemic lupus erythematosus.
   D. Assessment of chronic illnesses that may be exacerbated by use of growth factors.
      1. Cardiac—congestive heart failure, pericardial effusion, hypertension.
      2. Endocrine—hyperthyroid, diabetes.
      3. Neurologic or psychiatric disorders—seizure disorder or depressive dis-orders.
   E. Appropriate time from chemotherapy and nadir recovery. Colony stimulat-ing factor (CSF) to start no sooner than 24 hours after chemotherapy.
   F. Appropriate supportive therapy.
      1. Blood product support.
      2. Antiinfective therapy.
      3. Side effect management—nutrition, pain management, electrolyte and fluid balance, dermatologic and mucosal support.
IV. Potential complications.
   A. Side effects (see Table 10–14).

Assessment

I. Identification of clients at risk.
   A. Neutropenia—absolute neutrophil count less than 500 mm^3.
   B. Anemia—hemoglobin level less than 10 mg/dL.
   C. Risk for infection.(See antimicrobials section in this chapter.)
II. Physical examination (see Chapter 36).
III. Evaluation of laboratory data (see Chapter 36).

Nursing Diagnoses

I. Pain.
II. Risk for altered body temperature.

III. Knowledge deficit.

IV. Risk for infection.

Outcome Identification

I. Client and family identify the type of and describe the rationale for treatment with hematopoietic growth factors (HGF).

II. Client and family describe personal risk factors for potential side effects of HGF.

III. Client and family list signs and symptoms of side effects of HGF and those that need to be reported to the health care team.

IV. Client and family describe self-care measures to decrease the incidence and severity of side effects associated with HGF.

V. Client and family demonstrate self-care skills required to administer HGF, as applicable (e.g., subcutaneous injections).

Planning and Implementation

I. Assess client's and family's cultural and ethnic background, particularly health care practices and values and beliefs related to pharmacotherapy (see Antimicrobials, Planning and Implementation).

II. Implement strategies to decrease the incidence and severity of side effects of HGF.

A. Assess baseline data (e.g., vital signs, neurologic status).

B. Review client's medical history for existing or previous conditions.

C. Review client's medications for potential drug interactions.

D. Conduct client/family teaching (e.g., on side effects and self-management; medication administration).

III. Implement strategies to monitor for complications of HGFs (see Table 10–14).

IV. Implement measures to monitor for response to HGFs.

A. Monitor laboratory results (e.g., CBC).

B. Assess for adverse effects, toxicity, and drug interactions.

Evaluation

The oncology nurse systematically and regularly evaluates the client's and/or family's responses to interventions to determine progress toward the achievement of expected outcomes. Relevant data are collected and actual findings are compared with expected findings. Nursing diagnoses, outcomes, and plans of care are reviewed and revised as necessary.

BIBLIOGRAPHY

Bociek, R.G., & Armitage, J.O. (1996). Hematopoietic growth factors. *CA Cancer J Clin 46*(3), 165–184.

Brophy, L., & Rieger, P.T. (1992). Implications of biological response modifier therapy for nursing. In J.C. Clark & R.F. McGee (eds.). *Oncology Nursing Society Core Curriculum* (2nd ed.) Philadelphia: W.B. Saunders, pp. 346–358.

Cleri, L.B. (1995). Serotonin antagonists: State of the art management of chemotherapy-induced emesis. *Oncology Nursing: Patient Treatment and Support* 2(1), 1–20.

Craig, J.B., & Powell, B.L. (1987). The management of nausea and vomiting in clinical oncology. *Am J Med Sci 293*, 34–44.

DiGregorio, G.J., Barbieri, E.J., Sterling, G.H., et al. (1994). *Handbook of pain management* (4th ed.). West Chester, PA: Medical Surveillance.

Dorr, R.T., Van Horn, D. (1994). *Cancer Chemotherapy Handbook* (2nd ed.). Norwalk, CT: Appleton & Lange.

Erdman, L. (1992). Nursing implications of supportive therapies in cancer care. In J.C. Clark & R.F. McGee (eds.). *Oncology Nursing Society Core Curriculum* (2nd ed.). Philadelphia: W.B. Saunders, pp. 377–385.

Gralla, R. (1993). Antiemetic therapy. In V.T. DeVita, Jr., S. Hellman, & S. Rosenberg (eds.). *Cancer: Principles and Practice of Oncology* (4th ed.). Philadelphia: J.B. Lippincott, pp. 2338–2348.

Groenwald, S.L., Frogge, M.H., Goodman, M., & Yarbro, C.H. (eds.). (1996). *Cancer Symptom Management*. Boston: Jones & Bartlett.

Keltner, N.L., & Folks, D.G. (1992). Culture as a variable in drug therapy. *Perspect Psychiatr Care 28*(1), 33.

Knoben, J.E., & Anderson, P.O. (1993). *Handbook of Clinical Drug Data* (7th ed.). Hamilton, IL: Drug Intelligence Publications, Inc.

McEvoy, G.K. (ed.). (1996). *American Hospital Formulary Service Drug Information.* Bethesda, MD: American Society of Health-System Pharmacists.

McKenry, L.M., & Salerno, E. (1995). *Mosby's Pharmacology in Nursing* (19th ed.). St. Louis: Mosby-Year Book.

Malseed, R.T., Goldstein, F.J., & Balkon, N. (1995). *Pharmacology: Drug Therapy and Nursing Considerations* (4th ed.). Philadelphia: J.B. Lippincott.

Pitler, L.R. (1996). Hematopoietic growth factors in clinical practice. *Semin Oncol Nurs 12*(2), 115–129.

Pizzo, P.A., Meyers, J., Freifeld, A.G., & Walsh, T. (1993). Infections in the cancer patient. In V.T. DeVita, Jr., S. Hellman, & S. Rosenberg (eds.). *Cancer: Principles and Practice of Oncology* (4th ed.). Philadelphia: J.B. Lippincott, pp. 2293–2337.

Rhodes, V.A., Johnson, M.H., & McDaniel, R.W. (1995). Nausea, vomiting, and retching: The management of the symptom experience. *Semin Oncol Nurs 11*(4), 256–265.

Sanford, J.P., Gilbert, D.N., & Sande, M.A. (1995). *Guide to antimicrobial therapy.* Dallas: Antimicrobial Therapy, Inc.

Skidmore-Roth, L. (1996). *Mosby's Nursing Drug Reference.* St. Louis: Mosby-Year Book.

Wilkes, G.M., Ingwersen, K., & Burke, M.B. (1994). *Oncology Nursing Drug Reference.* Boston: Jones & Bartlett.

Williams, B.R. & Baer, C.L. (1994). Essentials of clinical pharmacology in nursing (2nd ed.). Springhouse, PA: Springhouse Corporation.

PART TWO

Protective Mechanisms

Alterations in Mobility, Skin Integrity, and Neurologic Status

Jennifer Douglas Pearce, RN, MSN, OCN

ALTERATIONS IN MOBILITY

Theory

I. Definition.
  A. State in which the client experiences limitation of independent physical movement.
  B. Voluntary motor function is primarily controlled by the corticospinal and corticobulbar tracts. These tracts originate in the posterior frontal lobe of the brain and descend through the brainstem to the point of discussion. Thus, voluntary motor function on one side of the body is controlled by the opposite side of the brain.
  C. The cerebellum controls much of the coordination of the extrapyramidal system.
  D. Motor impairment (spasticity, muscle weakness, paralysis, hemiparesis, ataxia) may occur in primary cancer (brain tumors), or as secondary effects in metastatic disease (spinal cord compression), infections, and cancer therapy.

II. Risk factors.
  A. Disease-related.
    1. Primary or metastatic tumors to the skeletal system.
    2. Primary and metastatic tumors of the brain and spinal cord.
    3. Obstruction in lymphatic or systemic circulation.
    4. Bone pain.
    5. Physical response to disease: pain, stiffness, fatigue.
    6. Spinal cord compression.
    7. Sensory-perceptual alterations.
  B. Treatment-related.
    1. Side effects of corticosteroid therapy.
    2. Side effects of radiation therapy.
    3. Side effects of chemotherapy.
    4. Residual effects of surgical intervention: nerve and muscle damage.
  C. Lifestyle-related.
    1. Changes in physical activity level.
    2. High or low stress level.
    3. Independent versus dependent personality.

Assessment

   I. History.
      A. Presence of risk factors.
      B. Recent treatment and anticipated side effects.
      C. Decreased activity level.
      D. Presence of pain, muscle weakness, fatigue.
      E. Current therapy.
  II. Physical examination.
      A. Changes in muscle tone and strength and muscle mass.
      B. Weight loss.
      C. Strength and motor function.
      D. Mobility function.
      E. Range of joints motion.
      F. Positive Babinski sign.
 III. Psychosocial examination.
      A. Depression.
      B. Anxiety.
      C. Lack of motivation.
 IV. Laboratory data.
      A. Hypercalcemia.
      B. Electrolyte abnormalities.
      C. Lumbar puncture results.

Nursing Diagnoses

   I. Impaired physical mobility.
  II. Self-care deficit.
 III. Risk for injury.
 IV. Risk for impaired skin integrity.
  V. Pain.

Outcome Identification

   I. Client increases mobility to maintain activities of daily living.
  II. Client states improvement in pain and an increase in daily activities.
 III. Client uses safety measures to minimize risk for injury.
 IV. Client demonstrates appropriate use of adaptive devices to increase mobility.

Planning and Implementation

   I. Interventions to maintain musculoskeletal function.
      A. Consult with rehabilitation services for physical and occupational therapy.
      B. Obtain appropriate assistive devices (e.g., splints, walker, cane, overhead trapeze).
      C. Perform active range of motion exercises (AROM) on unaffected limbs at least three to four times a day and passive range of motion (PROM) on affected limbs.
      D. Maintain the client's body alignment while in bed.
      E. Change the client's position every 2 to 4 hours.
      F. Monitor progress from AROM to functional activities.

II. Interventions to encourage involvement with activities of daily living.
   A. Establish a routine for activities of daily living.
   B. Provide adaptive devices as needed.
   C. Observe the client's ability to obtain supplies unassisted.
   D. Provide assistance and supervision as needed.
   E. Place call light within reach if the client is alone.
III. Interventions to maximize safety for the client.
   A. Protect areas of decreased sensation from extremes of heat and cold.
   B. Teach the client with decreased perception of lower extremities to check where the limb is placed when changing positions.
   C. Place the bed in low position and the siderails up.
   D. Clear pathways in room and hallways.
   E. Provide assistance as needed for activities of daily living.
IV. Interventions to enhance adaptation and rehabilitation.
   A. Positive reinforcement for behaviors that contribute to outcomes.
   B. Have the client and family be responsible for aspects of care.
   C. Initiate and follow up with referrals to rehabilitation services.
V. Interventions to incorporate client and family in care.
   A. Instruct client and family about signs and symptoms to report to health team.
   B. Discuss risk factors for impaired mobility.

Evaluation

The oncology nurse systematically and regularly evaluates the client's and/or family's responses to interventions to determine progress toward the achievement of expected outcomes. Relevant data are collected and actual findings are compared with expected findings. Nursing diagnoses, outcomes, and plans of care are reviewed and revised as necessary.

ALTERATIONS IN SKIN INTEGRITY

Theory

I. Definition.
   A. State in which a person's skin is adversely altered.
   B. The skin is the largest organ of the body.
   C. Intact skin provides protection from environmental assaults such as bacteria, heat, cold, physical trauma, and radiation.
   D. The skin is composed of three layers:
      1. The epidermis, the outer layer, serves as a barrier to prevent water loss; it renews itself continuously through cell division.
      2. The dermis, the inner connective tissue layer, is well supplied with blood, lymphatics, and afferent sensory nerve receptors; it provides nutritional support to the avascular epidermal layer.
      3. Derivatives of the integument, which include the cutaneous glands, hair, nails, and teeth.
   E. Mucous membranes line the alimentary canal from the lips to the anus, participating in digestion, absorption of food and fluids, and elimination of waste products.
   F. Mucous membranes also serve as a protective barrier to maintain the integrity of organs.

G. The mucosal lining consists of layers of epithelial cells and various structures that correlate with the function of different organs or parts of an organ.

H. Mucosal cells have a 10- to 14-day lifespan.

II. Risk factors.

A. Disease-related.

1. Thrombocytopenia.

2. Cutaneous metastases (late manifestation in the course of the illness for solid tumors of the breast and lung, squamous cell carcinoma of the head and neck, malignant melanoma, lymphoma, and Kaposi's sarcoma).

3. Primary malignant skin cancer (melanoma, basal cell carcinoma, squamous cell carcinoma, and Kaposi's sarcoma).

4. Mycosis fungoides (slow progressive cutaneous T-cell lymphoma).

5. Premalignant lesions (actinic keratosis, leukoplakia, dysplastic nevus syndrome).

B. Treatment-related.

1. Desquamative skin reaction (recall reactions) related to radiation therapy.

2. Fragile skin from steroid therapy.

3. Erythema multiforme (widespread, scattered, cutaneous vesicles) from penicillin therapy.

4. Erythema nodosum (tender, subcutaneous, anterior leg nodules) hypersensitivity reaction to penicillin or sulfonamides.

5. Graft-versus-host disease (skin reactions related to bone marrow transplantation).

6. Side effects of biologic response modifiers.

7. Extravasation of chemotherapy.

8. Breaks in skin integrity from intravenous (IV) lines, catheters, others.

9. Other effects—alopecia; decubitus ulcers; edema; pruritus; jaundice; incontinence; infection.

Assessment

I. History.

A. Presence of risk factors.

B. Client's age.

C. Exposure to infection.

D. Recent treatment and anticipated side effects.

E. Past and current skin conditions.

F. Review of personal and oral hygiene practices.

G. Dietary intake.

H. Incontinence of bowel or bladder.

II. Physical examination.

A. Presence of erythema, dry desquamation, moist desquamation.

B. Local inflammation at injection site (erythema, induration, blisters).

C. Ulcerations of mouth; dry, cracked mucous membranes and lips.

D. Presence of alopecia.

E. Presence of stomatitis.

F. Presence of pruritus.

G. Presence of redness, petechiae, purpura, ecchymosis, jaundice.

H. Integrity of tube sites, perirectal tissue, perineal tissue.

I. Presence of decubitus ulcers.

III. Psychosocial examination.
   A. Social isolation.
   B. Anxiety.
   C. Depression.
IV. Laboratory data.
   A. Complete blood count (CBC).
   B. Blood chemistries.
   C. Platelet count.

Nursing Diagnoses

  I. Impaired skin integrity.
 II. Risk for body image disturbance.
III. Alteration in nutrition, less than body requirement.
IV. Altered oral mucous membranes.
 V. Impaired physical mobility.

Outcome Identification

  I. Client manages mucosal and skin care.
 II. Client discusses effects of skin alterations on self-concept and body image.
III. Client increases and/or maintains adequate dietary and fluid intake.
IV. Client describes and demonstrates the proper techniques for oral care.
 V. Client contacts the appropriate health team member when initial signs and symptoms of mucosal trauma and skin breakdown occur.

Planning and Implementation

  I. Assess knowledge of risk factors and side effects of therapy.
 II. Interventions to increase or maintain dietary and fluid intake.
   A. Offer small frequent meals.
   B. Moisten foods with liquids, sauces, and gravy.
   C. Increase fluid intake to 3 L a day.
   D. Rinse the oral cavity before and after meals.
III. Interventions to teach self-care techniques and prevent complications.
   A. Teach the client and family to assess the skin every 2 to 4 hours.
   B. Assist with turning and positioning every 2 hours.
   C. Massage uninjured areas gently.
   D. Use a therapeutic mattress, specialty bed, or a water mattress for high-risk persons.
   E. Use dry, clean, wrinkle-free linens and devices such as sheepskin and an eggcrate mattress.
IV. Interventions to protect skin integrity.
   A. Discuss the effects of treatments on skin.
   B. Teach use of protective film, skin barriers, or collection devices around drains and tubes with copious drainage.
   C. Teach use of sterile technique for invasive procedures such as insertion of tubes.
   D. Teach handwashing.
   E. Teach reportable signs and symptoms of infection.
 V. Interventions for oral, perineal, and general hygiene practices.
   A. Use soft toothbrush or oral sponges.
   B. Apply moisturizers to oral mucosa.

     C. Cleanse the perineal area with mild soap, rinsing thoroughly, patting the area dry, and applying a skin barrier after each bowel movement.

     D. Gently clean the skin with mild soap, tepid water; pat dry with soft cloth, avoid washing radiation sites.

     E. Add emollients to bath water; skin lubricants to skin other than to irradiated sites.

  VI. Interventions to minimize hair loss (see Chapter 3).

 VII. Interventions to care for acute and chronic skin reactions to radiation therapy (see Chapter 35).

Evaluation

The oncology nurse systematically and regularly evaluates the client's and/or family's responses to interventions to determine progress toward the achievement of expected outcomes. Relevant data are collected and actual findings are compared with expected findings. Nursing diagnoses, outcomes, and plans of care are reviewed and revised as necessary.

NEUROPATHIES

Theory

  I. Definition.
     A. Neuropathies describe any functional disturbances and/or pathologic changes in the peripheral nervous system (PNS).
     B. The PNS consists of cranial, sensory, and motor nerves, and portions of the autonomic nervous system.
     C. Neuropathies with involvement of the central nervous system are seizures, encephalopathy, cerebellar dysfunction, opthalmologic and ototoxicities, mental status changes, and peripheral neuropathies with sensory and motor dysfunction.
     D. The incidence and severity of neuropathies may vary and may depend on the administration of immunosuppressive therapies.
     E. Toxicities may be dose-related and reversible upon discontinuation of therapy.
  II. Risk factors.
     A. Disease-related.
       1. Effects of cancer.
       2. Presence of infiltrative emergencies (i.e., spinal cord compression).
       3. Other diseases (i.e., history of hepatic or neurologic dysfunction).
     B. Treatment-related.
       1. Side effects of chemotherapy (e.g., cerebellar dysfunction, "stroke-like reaction," generalized weakness, gait disturbance, numbness of feet, loss of proprioception).
       2. Side effects of radiation therapy (e.g., ataxia, dysarthria, or nystagmus, radicular pain).

Assessment

  I. History.
     A. Presence of risk factors.
     B. Recent chemotherapy treatment and anticipated side effects.
     C. Presence of weakness.

    D. Presence of paresthesia of hands and feet, constipation, loss of deep tendon reflex.

    E. Presence of cerebellar involvement (e.g., tremors, loss of balance and fine motor movement).

    F. Inability to perform activities of daily living.

    G. Performance of occupational and recreational activities.

    H. Current medication therapy.

    I. Activity level.

 II. Physical examination.

    A. Vital signs.

    B. Baseline sensory, mobility, and motor function.

    C. Baseline autonomic function.

    D. Baseline cranial nerve assessment.

    E. Baseline cerebellar function.

    F. Speech or language ability.

    G. Sight-related changes (i.e., blurred vision, impaired color perception).

III. Laboratory data.

    A. Electromyogram, nerve conduction studies.

    B. Muscle or nerve biopsy.

Nursing Diagnoses

   I. Sensory perceptual alterations: kinesthetic, tactile.

 II. Risk for impaired skin integrity.

III. Risk for injury.

IV. Impaired physical mobility.

 V. Constipation.

VI. Pain

Outcome Identification

   I. Client verbalizes measures to maximize safety and manage self-care.

 II. Client demonstrates measures to maximize adaptation and rehabilitation.

III. Client maintains regular bowel and bladder function.

IV. Client maintains or increases mobility.

Planning and Implementation

   I. Interventions to increase participation in care.

    A. Assess knowledge of early signs and symptoms of peripheral and other neuropathies.

    B. Teach side effects of chemotherapy.

    C. Teach hand and foot care (use of massage and lotions).

    D. Refer to occupational and rehabilitation services.

 II. Interventions to maximize safety for the client.

    (See Alterations in Mobility: Planning and Implementation.)

III. Interventions to promote stool softening.

    A. Monitor and record stools.

    B. Use stool softeners.

    C. Increase fluid intake to 3000 mL/day.

    D. Offer small frequent meals.

    E. Modify diet to include gradual increase of high-fiber foods.

IV. Interventions to minimize diminished sensations.
   A. Protect hand and feet from cold through use of gloves.
   B. Avoid excess stimulation of skin; avoid tight clothing.
   C. Wear gloves for gardening activities.
   D. Teach inspection of affected areas for burns, cuts, abrasions.
V. Interventions to promote self-care and decrease mobility impairment.
   A. Collaborate with physical and occupational rehabilitation services.
   B. Develop an exercise and muscle strengthening program.
   C. Use assistive devices.
   D. Assist in performance of activities of daily living.
VI. Interventions to manage sexual dysfunction (see Chapter 6).

Evaluation

The oncology nurse systematically and regularly evaluates the client's and/or family's responses to interventions to determine progress toward the achievement of expected outcomes. Relevant data are collected and actual findings are compared to expected findings. Nursing diagnoses, outcomes, and plans of care are reviewed and revised as necessary.

ALTERATIONS IN MENTAL STATUS

Theory

I. Definition.
   A. Alterations in mental status are often diffuse and vague.
   B. There are changes in cognition, changes in behavior/personality, and changes in self-care skills.
   C. Cognition is a process that involves perception, memory, and thinking.
   D. Components of behavior/personality involve a person's presence or consciousness noted in thoughts, emotions, and actions.
   E. An alteration in mental status can also result in a loss of the ability to carry out activities of daily living and meet self-care needs.
II. Risk factors.
   A. Disease-related.
      1. Central nervous system neoplasm, primary or metastatic disease.
      2. Metabolic emergencies (e.g., hypercalcemia, hyperuricemia).
      3. Head injury.
      4. Depression.
      5. Human immunodeficiency virus (HIV)–related dementia.
      6. Opportunistic infections (e.g., toxoplasmosis encephalitis, cryptococcal meningitis).
      7. Liver disease.
   B. Treatment-related.
      1. Side effects of chemotherapy (e.g., sleep disturbance, headache, hyperkinesis).
      2. Side effect of biologic response modifier therapy (e.g., lethargy, somnolence, disturbance in recent memory).
      3. Side effect of steroid therapy (e.g., depression, psychotic reactions).
      4. Analgesics.
      5. Dehydration.
      6. Electrolyte imbalance (e.g., hyperuricemia, hyponatremia, hypokalemia).

    C. Situation-related.
       1. Emotionally traumatic situations.
       2. Significant loss.
       3. Rejection and abandonment.
       4. Hopelessness.
       5. Powerlessness.

Assessment

  I. History.
    A. Presence of risk factors.
    B. Analgesics.
    C. Recent head injury, trauma, falls.
    D. Medication history.
    E. Reported confusion at night.
 II. Physical examination.
    A. Neurologic examination results.
    B. Impaired memory, recent and remote.
    C. Impaired problem solving.
    D. Impaired communication and language.
III. Psychosocial examination.
    A. Changes in emotional and behavioral affect.
    B. Mood swings.
    C. Impaired judgment.
IV. Laboratory data.
    A. CBC.
    B. Serum electrolyte levels.
    C. Thyroid and liver function.

Nursing Diagnoses

  I. Altered thought processes.
 II. Self-care deficit.
III. Risk for injury.
IV. Sensory-perceptual alterations.

Outcome Identification

  I. Client demonstrates improvement or adjustment to altered thought processes.
 II. Client remains free from injury related to cognitive impairment.
III. Client regains ability to make decisions.
IV. Client participates in activities of daily living.

Planning and Implementation

  I. Interventions to maintain or regain client's cognitive functions.
    A. Assess degrees of altered attention and concentration.
    B. Reorient the client to time, place, and reason for hospitalization.
    C. Provide clear, concise information, using simple terms, with face-to-face interaction with the client.
    D. Provide a structured, organized environment.
    E. Provide cues for orientation: clock, calender, personal items.
    F. Maintain a quiet environment, approach the client in a slow, unhurried manner.

    G. Provide structure in routine activities: specific time for breakfast, hygiene, medications, lunch, visitors.

    H. Clarify distortion in feelings and thoughts.

    I. Allow time for response to questions and decisions.

II. Interventions to involve client and family in self-care activities.

    A. Assess the family's understanding and educate them about potential cognitive dysfunction.

    B. Provide opportunities for family members to ask questions and obtain information.

    C. Teach the family to monitor changes in cognitive status.

    D. Reinforce information that the health care provider discussed during visits.

    E. Teach avoidance of alcohol and unessential medications.

III. Interventions to ensure a safety environment.

    A. Maintain the bed in the lowest position; keep the call light within reach; have the bed locked and belt in place when the client is in bed.

    B. Assess limitations in and assist with activities of daily living.

    C. Assess for the presence of pharmacologic agents that can alter cognitive function.

    D. Assess the person's thoughts and feelings toward staff and the need for hospitalization.

    E. Discuss the client's fears and concerns.

Evaluation

The oncology nurse systematically and regularly evaluates the client's and/or family's responses to interventions to determine progress toward the achievement of expected outcomes. Relevant data are collected and actual findings are compared with expected findings. Nursing diagnoses, outcomes, and plans of care are reviewed and revised as necessary.

BIBLIOGRAPHY

Bender, C. (1994). Cognitive dysfunction associated with biological response modifier therapy. *Oncol Nurs Forum 21*(3), 515–523.

Brogden, M.J., & Nevidjon, B. (1995). Vinorelbine tartrate (Navelbine) drug profile and nursing implications of a new vinca alkaloid. *Oncol Nurs Forum 22*(4), 635–646.

Cain, J., & Bender, C. (1995). Ifosfamide-induced neurotoxicity: Associated symptoms and nursing implications. *Oncol Nurs Forum 22*(4), 659–668.

Carpenito, J.L. (1995). *Nursing Care Plans and Documentation: Nursing Diagnosis and Collaborative Problems* (2nd ed.). Philadelphia: J.B. Lippincott.

Clark, J., McGee, R., & Preston, R. (1992). Nursing management of responses to the cancer experience. In J.C. Clark & R.F. McGee (eds.). *Core Curriculum for Oncology Nursing* (3rd ed.). Philadelphia: W.B. Saunders, pp. 67–155.

Furlong, G.T. (1993). Neurologic complications of immunosuppressive cancer therapy. *Oncol Nurs Forum 20*(9), 1337–1354.

Groenwald, S., Frogge, M.H., Goodman, M., & Yarbro, C.H. (eds.). (1997). *Cancer Nursing: Principles and Practice* (4th ed.). Boston: Jones & Bartlett.

Haeuber, D., & Spross, J. (1994). Protective mechanisms. In J. Gross & B.L. Johnson (eds.). *Handbook of Oncology Nursing* (2nd ed). Boston: Jones & Bartlett, pp. 373–463.

Hausman, K.A. (1995). Interventions for clients with problems of the central nervous system: The brain. In D.D. Ignatavicius, L. Workman, & M. Mishler (eds.). *Medical-Surgical Nursing: A Nursing Process Approach* (2nd ed). Philadelphia: W.B. Saunders, pp. 1121–1168.

Lundquist, D., & Holmes, W. (1993). Documentation of neurotoxicity resulting from high-dose cytosine arabinoside. *Oncol Nurs Forum 20*(9), 1409–1412.

McCorkle, R., Grant, M., Frank-Stromberg, M., & Baird, S.B. (eds.). (1996). *Cancer nursing: A Comprehensive Textbook.* (2nd ed.) Philadelphia: W.B. Saunders.

McCorkle, R., & Grant, M. (eds.). (1994). *Pocket Companion for Cancer Nursing.* Philadelphia: W.B. Saunders.

NANDA Nursing Diagnoses: Definitions and Classification 1995–1996. (1994). Philadelphia: North American Nursing Diagnosis Association.

Otto, S.E. (1995). *Pocket Guide to Oncology Nursing.* St. Louis: C.V. Mosby.

Myelosuppression

Dawn Camp-Sorrell, RN, MSN, FNP, AOCN

Theory

I. Myelosuppression is a reduction in bone marrow function that results in a reduced production of red blood cells, white blood cells, and platelets into the peripheral circulation.
   A. Decreased red blood cell production results in anemia (see Chapter 15) and problems of fatigue (see Chapter 1).
   B. Decreased white cell production results in neutropenia and risk for infection.
   C. Decreased platelets result in thrombocytopenia and risk for hemorrhage.

NEUTROPENIA

Theory

I. Definition—a decrease in number of circulating neutrophils in the blood evidenced by an absolute neutrophil count (ANC) less than 1000 per mm^3.
   A. Neutrophils are the first line of the body's defense against bacterial infection by localizing and neutralizing bacteria.
   B. Normal range of neutrophil counts is 2500 to 6000 cells/mm^3 accounting for 50 to 60% of the total number of white blood cells (WBCs).
II. Risk factors.
   A. Client-related.
      1. Older clients, who have more fat and less cellular marrow than younger counterparts.
      2. Tumor cell invasion into the bone marrow.
      3. Prior treatment with chemotherapy, radiation therapy, or multimodal therapy.
      4. High negative nitrogen balance compromising the marrow.
      5. Certain diseases, such as aplastic anemia, have a decreased production of neutrophils.
      6. Interruption of the integrity of normal barriers such as from open wounds, mucositis, or vascular access devices.
   B. Treatment-related.
      1. Chemotherapy—destruction of the rapidly dividing hematopoietic cells, which results in decreased production of neutrophil precursors as well as other WBCs with eventual destruction of the mature neutrophil cells.
      2. Radiation therapy—treatment fields that receive 20 Gy or more that involve the major bone marrow production sites of the ilia, vertebrae, ribs, skull, sternum, and metaphyses of the long bones.

3. Biotherapy—because these agents modulate the immune system, the potential for alteration exists.

4. Steroids—prevent migration of neutrophils to the bacteria and the process of phagocytosis.

III. Principles of medical management

A. Antibiotics, antifungal, antiviral medications for the organism isolated (see Chapter 10).

1. Antibiotics are continued for a minimum of 7 days.

2. Antibiotics are continued until results of blood cultures indicate the causative organism to be eradicated.

3. Antibiotics are usually continued until the absolute neutrophil count (ANC) is greater than 500/mm^3.

4. Antibiotic therapy initially consist of a broad-spectrum cephalosporin or penicillin, which may be given in combination with an aminoglycoside.

5. If fever continues after the client has been on antibiotics for 3 days without a known cause, an antifungal agent is initiated.

6. Antiviral drugs are recommended if mucosal lesions or viral disease is suspected.

B. Hemopoietic growth factors are glycoprotein hormones that act as a natural regulator of hematopoiesis to promote the proliferation and differentiation of hematopoietic progenitor cells along multiple pathways (see Chapter 10).

1. Used to shortened the duration of neutropenia.

2. Dramatically reduces the occurrence of morbidity and mortality associated with infections as a result of neutropenia.

a. Granulocyte colony stimulating factor (G-CSF) predominantly enhances the growth of granulocyte colonies by affecting the proliferation and differentiation of neutrophil progenitor and precursor cells.

b. Granulocyte-macrophage colony stimulating factor (GM-CSF) is a multilineage hemopoietic growth factor that stimulates neutrophils, macrophages, monocytes, and eosinophils.

3. Recommended dose for CSF is to be administered daily.

a. G-CSF dose is 5 μg/kg/day subcutaneous injection for up to 14 days or until the ANC is greater than 10,000 per mm^3. Once discontinued, a precipitous drop in ANC occurs.

b. GM-CSF dose may be given by subcutaneous injection or intravenously in doses of 250 μg/m^2/day for up to 21 days.

4. Growth factors are started if the client is at a high risk for febrile neutropenia such as after receiving high-dose chemotherapy or bone marrow transplant and in the following situations:

a. Previous febrile neutropenic episode with a course of cancer treatment.

b. If a dose reduction is not recommended to cure the cancer.

IV. Potential sequelae of prolonged neutropenia.

A. Infectious organism resistant to antibiotics.

B. Sepsis and septic shock.

1. Infections increase in frequency and severity as the ANC decreases.

2. When the nadir persists for more than 7 to 10 days, the risk for severe infection increases.

C. Death.

Assessment

I. History.
  A. Review of previous cancer therapy such as chemotherapy, radiation therapy, biotherapy, or multimodal therapy.
  B. Review of current antibiotic regimen such as sulfamethoxazole-trimethoprim (Bactrim) or amphotericin B that can decrease the neutrophil count.
  C. Review of current hematopoietic growth factor use.
II. Physical examination.
  A. Assess access device exit sites for drainage, erythema, or tenderness.
  B. Assess nutritional status—protein-calorie malnutrition causes lymphopenia, diminished levels of the complement system, and a decrease of certain immunoglobulins.
  C. Assess vital signs—fever may be the only response to an infection.
    1. A fever of 100.5°F is significant in a client with an ANC less than 500/mm^3.
    2. If the client's pulse is over 100 beats per minute and the blood pressure is dropping, the client may be developing sepsis.
  D. Assess for signs of infection, which may not be apparent with the inhibition of phagocytic cells; therefore, redness, inflammation, and drainage may be minimal or absent.
    1. Most commonly infected sites include the periodontium, pharynx, lower esophagus, lung, perineum, anus, skin, and venous access exit sites.
    2. Assess all indwelling catheter sites.
  E. Assess for abnormal breath sounds.
  F. Assess the oral cavity for thrush.
III. Laboratory data.
  A. Complete blood count (CBC) with differential.
  B. Calculate the ANC (Table 12–1).
  C. Culture and sensitivity testing of urine, blood, stool, sputum, wound, drainage tubes or bags.

TABLE 12–1. **Calculation of Absolute Neutrophil Count**

The absolute neutrophil count (ANC) is calculated as follows:

$$ANC = \frac{(\% \text{ neutrophils } + \% \text{ bands})}{100} \times \text{white blood cell (WBC) count}$$

The example shows how to calculate the ANC of a client with the following counts: neutrophils = 50%, bands = 8%, WBC = 4000.

$$ANC = \frac{(50\% + 8\%)}{100} \times 4000$$

$$ANC = (.50 + .08) \times 4000$$

$$ANC = 2320$$

Infection Risk

Not significant	ANC = 1500 to 2000
Minimal	ANC = 1000 to 1500
Moderate	ANC = 500 to 1000
Severe	ANC = <500

From Liebman, M.C., & Comp-Sorrell, D. (1996). Multimodal Therapy in Oncology Nursing. St. Louis: Mosby-Year Book, p. 377.

Nursing Diagnoses

I. Risk for altered body temperature.
II. Risk for infection.
III. Knowledge deficit of infection precautions.

Outcome Identification

I. Client's ANC is greater than 1000/mm³.
II. Client does not develop any major complications as a result of neutropenia.
III. Client accurately describes appropriate infection precautions.

Planning and Implementation

I. Interventions to minimize the occurrence of infection.
   A. Employ strict handwashing technique.
   B. Restrict fresh fruits and vegetables in the client's diet.
   C. Restrict fresh flowers or other sources of stagnant water.
   D. Encourage client to bathe daily with meticulous personal hygiene and peri-neal care.
   E. Limit visitors to those without communicable illness.
   F. Give meticulous care to all catheters such as venous access devices, urinary or feeding tubes.
   G. Use aseptic technique for all nursing interventions.
II. Interventions to monitor for complications.
   A. Monitor for nadir (the lowest point of the blood cell levels after cancer treatment).
      1. As immature cells in the marrow and mature cells in the bloodstream are destroyed, the nadir becomes apparent.
         a. Usually 7 to 14 days after chemotherapy, except for the nitrosoureas, in which nadir occurs in 3 to 4 weeks, and except for cases employing radiation to the large bones.
         b. Occasional occurrence after biotherapy.
         c. Usually after multimodal treatment, the nadir occurs sooner and more severely than from single modality therapy.
      2. Nadir resolves within 3 to 4 weeks when the cells in the bone marrow mature and are released into the peripheral blood. With the exception of cases involving the administration of nitrosoureas, the nadir resolves in 6 to 8 weeks.
      3. Cancer treatment is usually held for an ANC less than 1500/mm³.
   B. Obtain cultures from the blood, urine, stool, and wound drainage.
      1. Approximately 85% of infections arise from endogenous microbial flora from the gastrointestinal and respiratory tracts.
      2. Bacteremia is principally caused by aerobic gram-negative bacilli (*Escherichia coli, Klebsiella pneumoniae,* and *Pseudomonas aeruginosa*) and gram-positive cocci (coagulase-negative staphylococci, streptococci species, and *Staphylococcus aureus*).
      3. Fungal infections commonly occur from *Candida albicans.*
III. Report critical changes in client assessment parameters to physician.
   A. Signs and symptoms of infection.
   B. Temperature greater than 100.5°F.
IV. Interventions to incorporate client and family in care.
   A. Teach personal hygiene measures to minimize the occurrence of infection,

such as wiping from front to back of the perineal area after voiding, and daily bathing.

  B. Teach infection precautions and how to minimize the risk of infection, such as strict handwashing.

  C. Teach subcutaneous administration of hematopoietic growth factors.

  D. Teach the symptoms for which to call the physician or nurse such as temperature greater than 100.5°F, productive cough, painful urination, or sore throat.

Evaluation

The oncology nurse systematically and regularly evaluates the client's and/or family's responses to interventions to determine progress toward the achievement of expected outcomes. Relevant data are collected and actual findings are compared with expected findings. Nursing diagnoses, outcomes, and plans of care are reviewed and revised as necessary.

THROMBOCYTOPENIA

Theory

  I. Definition—decrease in the circulating platelets below 100,000/mm^3.
  A. Normal count is 150,000 to 400,000/mm^3.
  B. Lifespan of platelets is 8 to 10 days.
  C. Major function of platelets is to maintain vascular hemostasis through clotting mechanisms.
 II. Risk factors.
  A. Disease-related.
   1. Idiopathic thrombocytopenia purpura or thrombotic thrombocytopenia purpura increases the use of platelets.
   2. Hypocoagulation disorders such as liver disease or vitamin K deficiency alter the development of prothrombin and several clotting factors.
   3. Hypercoagulation disorders such as paraneoplastic syndromes, disseminated intravascular coagulation, and thrombosis increases the use of platelets.
   4. Invasion of tumor cells in the bone marrow.
   5. Cancers involving the bone marrow, such as multiple myeloma, lymphoma, and leukemia, affect platelet production.
  B. Treatment-related.
   1. Chemotherapy—destruction of the rapidly dividing hematopoietic cells, which results in a decrease of the production of platelet precursors with eventual destruction of mature platelets.
    a. Platelet count usually decreases in 7 to 14 days after administration or sooner with multimodal treatment.
    b. Platelet count usually decreases after the drop in WBCs.
    c. Recovery usually occurs within 2 to 6 weeks.
   2. Radiation therapy—treatment field that receives 20 Gy or more that involves the major bone marrow production sites of the ilia, vertebrae, ribs, skull, sternum, and metaphyses of the long bones.
   3. Endotoxins released from bacteria during an infection can damage platelets and alter platelet aggregation.
   4. Some medications can alter platelet development, such as aspirin, digi-

talis, digoxin, furosemide, heparin, phenytoin, quinidine, sulfonamides, and tetracycline.

III. Principles of medical management.
   A. Administer platelets to increase the peripheral blood level approximately 10,000 to 12,000 cells/mm^3 per unit.
      1. Single donor platelets are taken from one donor.
      2. Random donor platelets are harvested from whole blood from several different donors. The client is exposed to multiple donor antigens.
      3. Human leukocyte antigen (HLA)-matched platelets are indicated if the client's platelet count fails to increase after repeated transfusion from non-HLA-matched products.
      4. Leukocyte-depleted filters may be used to eliminate WBCs from the product, which prevents alloimmunization.
   B. Platelet growth factors are investigational agents that promote maturation of the megakaryocyte; examples are thrombopoietin, interleukin-3, interleukin-6, and interleukin-11.
      1. Thrombopoietin is thought to be the hormone responsible for the production and maturation of megakaryocytes.
      2. No other biotherapeutic agent acts specifically on the megakaryocyte.
   C. Administer plasma to replenish clotting factors when client is actively bleeding and becomes refractory to platelets.
   D. Progestational agents may be prescribed to decrease menstrual bleeding.

IV. Potential sequelae of prolonged thrombocytopenia.
   A. Refractory to platelet transfusion.
   B. Internal bleeding such as intracranial, gastrointestinal, or respiratory tract bleeding.
   C. Death.

Assessment

I. History.
   A. Previous cancer treatment such as chemotherapy, radiation therapy, or multimodal therapy.
   B. Current medications that could alter platelet production.
   C. Social history of alcohol intake and illicit drug use.

II. Physical examination.
   A. Assess for bleeding such as from rectum, nose, ears, oral cavity.
      1. Platelet levels between 40,000 to 60,000/mm^3 are associated with an increased risk of postsurgical and traumatic bleeding.
      2. Platelet level less than 20,000/mm^3 is a major risk for spontaneous bleeding not due to trauma.
      3. Platelet level lower than 10,000/mm^3 is associated with fatal central nervous system bleeding or massive gastrointestinal tract or respiratory tract hemorrhage.
   B. Assess for petechiae, which usually appear initially on the upper and lower extremities, then on pressure points, elbows, and the oral palate.
   C. Assess all stool, urine, and vomitus for blood.
   D. Assess the skin for ecchymosis, purpura, or oozing of puncture sites.
   E. Assess for conjunctiva hemorrhage and sclera injection.

III. Laboratory data.
   A. Platelet count.
   B. Coagulation values—fibrinogen, prothrombin time, partial thromboplastin time.

Nursing Diagnoses

  I. Knowledge deficit related to bleeding precautions.

  II. Risk for injury.

Outcome Identification

  I. Client has resolution of thrombocytopenia.

  II. Client does not develop any complications as a result of thrombocytopenia.

  III. Client accurately describes appropriate bleeding precautions.

Planning and Implementation

  I. Interventions to minimize the occurrence of bleeding.
- A. Avoid using a blood pressure cuff or tourniquet when the platelet count is less than 20,000/mm^3.
- B. Avoid invasive procedures such as enemas, rectal temperatures, suppositories, bladder catheterizations, venipunctures, finger sticks, nasogastric tubes, subcutaneous or intramuscular injections.
- C. Prepare environment to avoid trauma, for example, pad siderails, arrange furniture to eliminate sharp corners, clear walkways.
- D. Apply firm direct pressure to venipuncture site for 5 minutes.
- E. Encourage client to wear shoes during ambulation to maintain skin integrity.
- F. Encourage client to avoid sharp objects, such as a straight-edge razor.
- G. If bleeding is not controlled, absorbable gelatin sponges or liquid thrombin can be applied.
  1. For nosebleeds, the client should be placed in a high Fowler position and pressure applied to the nose.
  2. Ice packs may help to decrease the bleeding.
- H. Implement a bowel regimen to prevent constipation.
- I. Use soft toothbrushes to avoid gingival trauma.
- J. Avoid physical activity that may lead to trauma.
- K. Monitor for menstrual bleeding and count sanitary napkins used.
- L. Monitor for changes that indicate intracranial bleeding such as changes in level of consciousness, restlessness, headache, seizures, pupil changes, ataxia.

  II. Monitor platelet levels.
- A. Cancer treatment is usually held for platelet count less than 100,000/mm^3.
- B. Platelets are usually administered if the count is 10,000 to 20,000/mm^3 or if the client is actively bleeding.

  III. Implement strategies to incorporate client and family in care.
- A. Teach the family and client bleeding precautions.
- B. Teach the family and client signs of bleeding that should be called to attention of the physician or nurse.
- C. Teach safety measures to decrease the occurrence of bleeding when performing activities of daily living.

Evaluation

The oncology nurse systematically and regularly evaluates the client's and/or family's responses to interventions to determine progress toward the achievement of expected outcomes. Relevant data are collected and actual findings are compared with expected findings. Nursing diagnoses, outcomes, and plans of care are reviewed and revised as necessary.

INFECTION

Theory

I. When the body or a part of the body is invaded by a microorganism or virus an infection develops, depending on three factors.
   A. Source of infectious organism.
      1. Endogenous organisms are within the body's normal flora and help to prevent colonization of microorganisms.
      2. Exogenous organisms are found in the environment.
   B. Methods of transmission include direct contact, indirect contact, and air-borne.
   C. Susceptible host, which refers to the ability to prevent or fight infection.
      1. Intact mechanical barriers such as the skin and mucous membranes.
      2. Chemical barriers such as the pH of the tissues.
      3. Intact inflammatory and immune responses.
II. Risk factors.
   A. Disease-related.
      1. Hematologic/lymphoid malignancy.
      2. Altered skin and mucosal barriers.
      3. Recent exposure to an infectious organism.
      4. Human immunodeficiency virus.
   B. Treatment-related.
      1. Myelosuppression induced from cancer treatment.
      2. Prolonged use of antibiotics or steroids.
      3. Multimodal cancer treatment.
III. Principles of medical management.
   A. Administer antibiotics according to organism isolated.
   B. Employ meticulous wound care.
IV. Potential sequelae of prolonged infection.
   A. Septic shock.
   B. Resistance to antibiotics or superinfection.
   C. Death.

Assessment

I. History.
      1. Review previous cancer therapy such as chemotherapy, radiation therapy, biotherapy or multimodal therapy.
      2. Review known allergies to medications, especially antibiotics.
      3. Review immunosuppressive therapy.
II. Physical examination.
   A. Comprehensive assessment every 4 to 8 hours or more often as indicated with special attention to access device sites, lungs, integument, oral cavity, and perineum for drainage, open wounds, erythema.
   B. Assess vital signs every 4 to 8 hours or more often as indicated for trends of deviations from the normal.
   C. Assess the character of the urine for sediment, color, odor, blood.
   D. Assess the mental status for orientation, confusion, memory recall, alertness.
III. Laboratory data.
   A. Complete blood count with differential.
   B. Culture and sensitivity testing of the urine, stool, blood, sputum, wounds, drainage bags or tubes.

Nursing Diagnoses

I. Risk for altered body temperature.
II. Risk for infection.
III. Knowledge deficit of infection precautions.
IV. Risk for impaired skin integrity.
V. Altered oral mucous membrane.

Outcome Identification

I. Client accurately describes appropriate infection precautions.
II. Client does not develop any major complications from the infectious process.

Planning and Implementation

I. Interventions to minimize infections.
   A. Employ strict handwashing before and after all contact with client.
   B. Promote and encourage daily meticulous personal hygiene, oral hygiene, and perineal care.
   C. Avoid unnecessary invasive procedures such as enemas, rectal temperatures, bladder catheterization, venipunctures.
   D. Administer vaccinations such as a flu shot to prevent communicable infections.
   E. Use aseptic technique when performing nursing interventions.
II. Interventions to locate source of infection by obtaining appropriate cultures such as blood, sputum, stool, urine, and wounds as indicated.
III. Educate the client/family about signs and symptoms of infection and when to call the physician or nurse.

Evaluation

The oncology nurse systematically and regularly evaluates the client's and/or family's responses to interventions to determine progress toward the achievement of expected outcomes. Relevant data are collected and actual findings are compared with expected findings. Nursing diagnoses, outcomes, and plans of care are reviewed and revised as necessary.

HEMORRHAGE

Theory

I. Definition—the occurrence of abnormal internal or external discharge of blood.
II. Risk factors.
   A. Disease-related.
      1. Cerebral hemorrhage can occur with severe thrombocytopenia or with brain metastases.
      2. Myeloproliferative disorders such as polycythemia vera, myelofibrosis, and thrombocythemia can cause hemorrhage phenomena.
      3. Disseminated intravascular coagulation from prostate cancer or acute promyelocytic leukemia.
      4. Paraneoplastic syndromes can stimulate bleeding.
   B. Treatment-related.
      1. Bone marrow transplantation can cause a diffuse alveolar hemorrhage clinically characterized by cough, dyspnea, and hypoxemia.

2. Disseminated intravascular coagulation as a result of cancer treatment.
3. High-dose chemotherapy such as cyclophosphamide can cause hemorrhagic cystitis or myocardial hemorrhage.
4. All types of surgical procedures have the risk for hemorrhage especially if the tumor is embedded within arteries or veins.

III. Principles of medical management.
   A. Administer appropriate blood products.
   B. Administer oxygen.
   C. Give vasopressin drugs, which may control severe bleeding.
   D. Lavage iced saline through a nasogastric tube, which may control gastric bleeding.

IV. Potential sequelae of prolonged hemorrhage.
   A. Hepatitis B from numerous blood transfusions.
   B. Shock.
   C. Death.

Assessment

I. History.
   A. Review previous cancer therapy such as chemotherapy, radiation therapy, or multimodal treatment.
   B. Ascertain recent traumatic events.
   C. Review the cancer disease.
      1. Evidence of metastasis to the brain or bone marrow.
      2. Leukemia, especially nonlymphocytic leukemia, can cause hemorrhage as a result of a paraneoplastic process.
   D. Review past medical history for the occurrence of peptic/gastric ulcer disease or esophageal varices.

II. Physical examination.
   A. Assess for signs of hemorrhage complications such as weak pulse, irregular pulse, pale skin, cold and moist skin.
   B. Assess all urine, stool, vomitus, and sputum for blood.
   C. Assess vital signs.
   D. Assess for neurologic deficits, such as reduced level of alertness or orientation.

III. Laboratory data.
   A. Complete blood count.
   B. Coagulation factors.
   C. Occult stool test.

Nursing Diagnoses

I. Decreased cardiac output.
II. Risk for fluid volume deficit.
III. Altered tissue perfusion.

Outcome Identification

I. Client does not develop complications as a result from hemorrhage.
II. Client does not have compromise of the tissue as a result of hemorrhage.
III. Client has resolution of hemorrhage.

Planning and Implementation

 I. Interventions to minimize the bleeding.
   A. Apply occlusive dressings to open bleeding wounds after cleansing the area.
   B. If applicable, elevate the body part above the heart level and apply firm pressure over the area.
 II. Interventions to monitor for complications.
   A. Hemodynamic measurements—decrease in cardiac output and decrease in blood pressure.
   B. Strict intake and output records to detect negative fluid balance.
 III. Report critical changes in the client's assessment parameters to the physician such as change in mental status, decrease in blood pressure, increase in bleeding.

Evaluation

The oncology nurse systematically and regularly evaluates the client's and/or family's responses to interventions to determine progress toward the achievement of expected outcomes. Relevant data are collected and actual findings are compared with expected findings. Nursing diagnoses, outcomes, and plans of care are reviewed and revised as necessary.

FEVER AND CHILLS

Theory

 I. Definition—elevation of body temperature above 98.6°F orally.
   A. Chills (shivering) occur as a body's response to heat loss when the body's temperature abruptly increases such as with fever.
     1. During shivering the body produces involuntary contractions of the skeletal muscles.
     2. The internal body temperature is maintained by shivering, which is a thermoregulatory mechanism.
     3. A subjective feeling of cold.
   B. Fever is initiated by the release of endogenous pyrogens from phagocytic WBCs.
     1. Vasodilation and sweating are the physiologic mechanisms used to increase heat loss.
     2. Vasoconstriction and shivering are the body's mechanisms for conserving or producing heat.
     3. Production of fever occurs as a response to the elevation of the set point in the temperature-regulating center in the hypothalamus.
     4. Results in an increase in metabolic activity and oxygen consumption brought about by an increase in muscle tone and shivering.
     5. Skin temperature drops because of vasoconstriction, which decreases heat loss.
 II. Risk factors.
   A. Disease-related.
     1. Tumor involving the hypothalamus where the temperature control for the body is located.
     2. Paraneoplastic syndrome.
       a. Pyrogens are released by the tumor cells producing a fever, especially in the presence of uncontrolled tumor growth.
       b. Most common tumors associated with tumor-induced fever include

Hodgkin's disease, osteogenic sarcoma, lymphoma, and liver metastasis.
  B. Treatment-related.
    1. Neutropenia following cancer treatment.
    2. Chemotherapy side effect from bleomycin, daunorubicin, thiotepa, methotrexate, dacarbazine, mithramycin.
    3. Blood transfusion reaction.
    4. Biotherapy side effect from interferon or interleukin-2.
    5. Steroid-induced adrenal insufficiency.
    6. Drug-induced such as vancomycin or amphotericin B.
III. Principles of medical management.
  A. Administer acetaminophen alternated with aspirin every 2 hours to decrease fever and drug toxicity. Use with caution in clients with thrombocytopenia.
  B. Administer nonsteroidal antiinflammatory drugs for tumor-induced fever. Use with caution in clients with thrombocytopenia.
  C. Administer meperidine to relieve chills.
IV. Potential sequelae of prolonged fever and chills.
  A. Increase in fatigue, muscle weakness, and myalgia.

Assessment

  I. History.
    A. Previous cancer treatments.
    B. Previous exposure to infections.
    C. Type of cancer.
    D. Previous blood transfusions.
    E. Current medications.
 II. Physical examination.
    A. Assess vital signs frequently.
    B. Perform a complete physical examination to ascertain the source of fever.
III. Laboratory data.
    A. Complete blood count.
    B. Appropriate cultures and sensitivities.

Nursing Diagnoses

  I. Altered body temperature.
 II. Risk for fluid volume deficit.
III. Risk for infection.
IV. Ineffective thermoregulation.

Outcome Identification

  I. Client's fever and chills resolve.
 II. Client does not develop complications as a result of fever and chills.

Planning and Implementation

  I. Interventions to locate the source of infection.
    A. Obtain cultures from the blood, throat, urine, stool, sputum, and wounds when an infection is suspected.
    B. Obtain cultures from all access devices.

II. Interventions to provide comfort.
   A. Promote slow cooling of the skin and mucous membranes.
      1. Tepid sponge baths.
      2. Reduced amount of client clothing.
      3. Mechanical cooling blankets.
      4. Reduction of the environmental temperature.
   B. Avoid rapid reduction in body temperature that can cause chilling by providing warm blankets or heating pads at the first sign of chilling.
   C. Change damp clothing immediately to prevent chilling.
   D. Administer acetaminophen to reduce fever every 4 hours not to exceed 4000 mg in a 24-hour period, which can be alternated with aspirin and nonsteroidal antiinflammatory drugs. Use with caution in clients with thrombocytopenia.
   E. Increase fluid intake to prevent dehydration.
III. Interventions to minimize the occurrence of infection in common sites.
   A. Encourage coughing and deep breathing every 4 to 8 hours while awake.
   B. Encourage oral hygiene every 4 hours while awake.
   C. Encourage client to void frequently.
   D. Avoid the use of douches or tampons.
   E. Encourage the client to eat well-balanced meals and increase fluid intake.

Evaluation

The oncology nurse systematically and regularly evaluates the client's and/or family's responses to interventions to determine progress toward the achievement of expected outcomes. Relevant data are collected and actual findings are compared with expected findings. Nursing diagnoses, outcomes, and plans of care are reviewed and revised as necessary.

BIBLIOGRAPHY

Bick, R.L. (1994). Platelet function defects associated with hemorrhage or thrombosis. *Med Clin North Am 78*, 511–543.
Camp-Sorrell, D. (1996). Hematologic toxicities. In M. Liebman & D. Camp-Sorrell (eds.). *Multimodal Therapy in Oncology Nursing.* St. Louis: Mosby-Year Book, pp. 367–385.
Carter, L.W. (1993). Influences of nutrition and stress on people at risk for neutropenia: Nursing implications. *Oncol Nurs Forum 20*, 1241–1250.
Finkbine, K.L., & Ernst, T.F. (1993). Drug therapy management of the febrile neutropenic cancer patient. *Cancer Pract 1*, 295–304.
Friedberg, R.C. (1994). Issues in transfusion therapy in the patient with malignancy. *Hematol Oncol Clin North Am 8*(6), 1223–1253.
Giamarellou, H. (1995) Empiric therapy for infections in the febrile, neutropenic, compromised host. *Med Clin North Am 79*(3), 559–580.
Holtzclaw, B.J. (1990). Shivering: A clinical nursing problem. *Nurs Clin North Am 25*(4), 977–986.
Miller, L.L., Anderson, J.R., Anderson, P.N., et al. (1994). American Society of Clinical Oncology recommendations for the use of hematopoietic colony-stimulating factors: Evidence-based clinical practice guidelines. *J Clin Oncol 12*, 2471–1508.
Pizzo, P.A. (1993). Management of fever in patients with cancer and treatment-induced neutropenia. *N Engl J Med 328*, 1323–1331.
Rutherford, C.J. & Frenkel, E.P. (1994). Thrombocytopenia: Issues in diagnosis and therapy. *Med Clin North Am 78*, 555–575.
Shuey, K.M. (1996) Platelet-associated bleeding disorders. *Semin Oncol Nurs 12*(1), 15–27.
von der Mass, H. (1994). Complications of combined radiotherapy and chemotherapy. *Semin Radiation Oncol 4*(2), 81–94.
Wujcik, D. (1993). Infection control in oncology patients. *Nurs Clin North Am 28*, 639–650.
Wujcik, D. (1993). An odyssey into biologic therapy. *Oncol Nurs Forum 20*, 879–887.

PART THREE

Gastrointestinal and Urinary Function

13

Alterations in Nutrition

Marilynn C. Berendt, RN, BSN, EdM, OCN

ANOREXIA

Theory

I. Definition—loss of appetite. May be insidious and may not be accompanied by obvious manifestations of disease other than progressive weight loss.

II. Etiology of anorexia.
   A. May be primary—cancer cachexia.
   B. May be secondary.
      1. Social causes—presentation and type of food, environment, and cultural influences.
      2. Physical causes.
         a. Local—dry/sore mouth, dysphagia, nausea and vomiting, abdominal mass or obstruction, ascites, early satiety, malodorous tumor, structural changes related to surgery, and/or dental involvement.
         b. General causes.
            (1) Concurrent physical or psychological responses to disease—pain, fatigue, anxiety, constipation, immobility, fear, depression.
            (2) Metabolic—hypercalcemia, hypokalemia, uremia, hyponatremia (tumor lysis syndrome).
            (3) Hepatic failure.
            (4) Medication side effects—narcotics, antibiotics, iron.
            (5) Treatment-related effects—chemotherapy, radiotherapy, surgery, and biotherapy.

III. Principles of medical management.
   A. Correct underlying cause.
   B. Support with nutritional supplementation or replacement.
   C. Employ nursing interventions to minimize occurrence and severity.

IV. Sequelae of prolonged anorexia.
   A. Contributes to decreased calorie and protein intake with subsequent weight loss, weakness.
   B. Weight loss can lead to cachexia, which can affect prognosis (weight loss >10% is a negative prognostic sign).
   C. Results in abnormalities of carbohydrate, protein, and fat metabolism.
   D. Visceral and lean body mass depletion—muscle atrophy, visceral organ atrophy, and hypoalbuminemia.
   E. Leads to compromised humoral and cellular immune function—decreased macrophage mobilization, depressed lymphocyte function, and impaired phagocytosis.

F. Protein/calorie malnutrition interferes with the delivery of oncologic therapy and enhances the severity of side effects of treatment.

Assessment

I. History.
   A. Previous dietary patterns, food preferences, eating habits, and history of anorexia with client/family.
   B. Patterns of anorexia.
      1. Onset, frequency, severity.
      2. Associated symptoms—food intolerances, taste abnormalities, mouth/throat pain, dysphagia.
      3. Other factors—precipitating, aggravating, alleviating factors.
   C. Previous self-care strategies.
      1. Ability to implement interventions to relieve anorexia.
      2. Use of food, nutritional supplements, and other remedies.
   D. Current or recent treatment for cancer and anticipated side effects.
II. Physical examination.
   A. Determine present weight and amount of total weight loss.
   B. Assess for presence of dehydration and/or electrolyte imbalances—dry mouth, poor skin turgor, and decreased urinary output.
   C. Assess client for associated ethnic, socioeconomic, emotional, and motivational factors that may affect the loss of weight or decreased oral intake.
   D. Assess psychosocial responses.
      1. Psychological responses—fear, anxiety, and depression.
      2. Response to noxious stimuli in environment.

Nursing Diagnoses

   I. Altered nutrition, less than body requirements.
  II. Risk for fluid volume deficit.
 III. Risk for impaired skin integrity.
  IV. Fatigue.

Outcome Identification

   I. Client states the goals of interventions related to anorexia.
  II. Client states the personal risk for complications related to loss of appetite and ways in which various cancer therapies may adversely affect nutritional reserves.
 III. Client and family participate in measures to minimize risk of occurrence, severity, and complications of anorexia.
  IV. Client's nutritional intake increases to 2000 calories/day.
   V. Client states the changes in condition that require professional assistance and/or intervention.
      A. Weight loss of more than 1 to 2 pounds per day.
      B. Dehydration and/or inability to eat or drink.
      C. Changes in skin integrity and wound healing.
      D. Any other area of concern for client's well-being related to lack of food intake.
  VI. Client and family state awareness of resources in the community to assist with nutrition.

Planning and Implementation

I. Interventions to increase calorie and nutritional value of oral intake—teach client/family to attempt the following:
   A. Consume nutritionally dense foods, such as cottage cheese, puddings, oatmeal, frequently, in small portions throughout the day.
   B. Maximize food intake during periods of greatest strength and appetite, usually early in the day.
   C. Increase the kilocalorie (kcal), protein content of foods by adding instant nonfat dry milk powder or instant breakfast powders to gravies, puddings, other foods.
   D. Maximize food preferences and access to favorite foods within dietary restrictions.
   E. Use high-protein, high-calorie supplements between meals.
   F. Try only cold or room temperature foods to improve intake.
   G. Avoid gas-forming foods.
   H. Limit liquids at mealtime because they may cause early satiety and nausea.
II. Interventions to promote maximal comfort and ease while eating. Teach client/family to:
   A. Administer pain medications, if needed, 30 to 60 minutes before meals.
   B. Assist with oral care, as needed, before and after meals.
   C. Plan activities according to client's activity level.
      1. Adequate rest period before meals.
      2. Encourage a short walk and fresh air before a meal to stimulate appetite.
   D. Minimize noxious stimuli in the environment.
III. Interventions to monitor complications related to anorexia. Stress the importance of:
   A. Maintaining a daily dietary intake record and weighing daily.
   B. Assessing for signs and symptoms of electrolyte imbalances and dehydration.
   C. Assessing overall skin and nail condition for adverse effects of poor nutrition or intake—skin breakdown, dehiscence, or poor wound healing.
IV. Interventions to incorporate client/family in care.
   A. Encourage family to provide foods within dietary restrictions.
   B. Teach family methods to enhance calorie/protein content of foods and methods to enhance food intake.
      1. Provide a list of high calorie/high protein foods.
      2. Offer suggestions for supplementing nutritional value by adding powders and supplements.
      3. Use medications as ordered by physician—pain medications, vitamin supplements, and Megace that may stimulate appetite.
      4. Plan mealtimes that are relaxed, unhurried, and pleasant.
      5. Utilize a variety of foods to avoid taste fatigue.
      6. Avoid fixating on intake to the point that it may become counterproductive.
   C. Teach client/family signs and symptoms of dehydration (dry skin and mucous membranes, poor skin turgor, decreased urinary output), delayed wound healing, malnutrition (wasting of skeletal mass, body fat decrease, weight loss, sepsis and decreased energy) and when to report critical symptoms to the physician.
   D. Develop a nurse/client contract for increasing the intake of calories and protein each day.

  V. Interventions to enhance adaptation and rehabilitation.
    A. Provide written and/or audiovisual materials on nutrition at the client's level of education and understanding.
    B. Initiate early referral to a dietitian for nutritional assessment and intervention, as indicated.

Evaluation

The oncology nurse systematically and regularly evaluates the client's and/or family's responses to the interventions to determine progress toward the achievement of expected outcomes. Relevant data are collected and actual findings are compared with expected findings. Nursing diagnoses, outcomes, and plans of care are reviewed and revised as necessary.

DYSPHAGIA

Theory

  I. Definition—difficulty in swallowing, usually accompanied by a sensation of material lodging in the esophagus.
 II. Etiology and risk factors.
    A. Neurologic impairment.
        1. Loss of innervation (i.e., of cranial nerves V, VII, IX, X, XI, and/or XII, thus loss of swallow reflex).
        2. Loss of vocal cord sphincter control.
    B. Tumor infiltration and impingement of the esophagus and mouth by tumor and/or treatment-related effects.
        1. Major surgery that impairs the ability to hold food in mouth, lateralize, masticate, form a bolus, and move a bolus through the oropharynx and esophagus.
        2. Radiation therapy (RT) causing fibrosis or stenosis.
        3. Mucositis.
        4. Aphthous ulceration.
        5. Candidiasis.
        6. Chemotherapy effects (e.g., of 5-fluorouracil [5-FU]) on the oral cavity and esophagus.
        7. Changes in character of oral secretions as a result of RT and chemotherapy.
    C. Iatrogenic factors.
        1. Psychotropic medications that impair gag reflex and swallowing.
        2. Anticholinergic drugs.
    D. Lifestyle-related effects (i.e., emotional responses to disease and treatment).
III. Progression of dysphagia.
    A. Usually insidious and slowly progressive.
    B. Usually manifested as difficulty swallowing solids progressing to difficulty swallowing liquids, including saliva, causing fluids and foods to flow into the lungs, increasing the risk for aspiration and/or pneumonia.
    C. Usually associated with weight loss, anorexia, nausea, dehydration, protein/calorie malnutrition, cachexia, muscle wasting, and negative nitrogen wasting.
    D. Elderly at increased risk, as well as clients with certain cancer types—head and neck cancer, esophageal and lung carcinomas with lymph node involvement.

IV. Principles of medical treatment.
  A. Treatment for underlying disease—nodal radiation, laser surgery, antifungal and antibiotic medications.
  B. Endoscopic laser therapy.
  C. Alternate method for feedings.
  D. Use of thickening agents (e.g., Thick-It, Nutra-Thik, and Thick'N Easy) to lessen the risk for flow of liquids into the airway causing choking and aspiration.
  E. Medications—steroids, expectorants, bronchodilators, pain and anxiety medications to relieve symptoms related to dysphagia.
  F. Swallowing therapy and/or direct swallowing exercises.

Assessment

  I. History.
    A. Previous treatments for cancer.
    B. Presence of underlying systemic disease—infection, cardiac, or stroke.
    C. Patterns of dysphagia—incidence, pattern, alleviating, aggravating, and precipitating factors.
    D. Impact on lifestyle, comfort, activities of daily living, and quality of life.
 II. Physical examination.
    A. Observe for presence of facial droop, drooling, oral retention, choking, coughing after swallowing, and gurgling voice quality.
    B. Determine ability to masticate, hold food in mouth and propel food to oropharynx with tongue.
    C. Elicit client's subjective report on pain or discomfort; weakness of lips, tongue, or jaw; and "lump in the throat."
    D. Assess lungs.

Nursing Diagnoses

  I. Altered nutrition, less than body requirements.
 II. Fear.
III. Risk for impaired skin integrity.
IV. Impaired swallowing.
 V. High risk for aspiration.

Outcome Identification

  I. Client states goals for therapy and rehabilitation for dysphagia.
 II. Client participates in measures to minimize the risk of occurrence, severity, and complications of dysphagia.
III. Client and family state signs and symptoms of dysphagia and techniques for minimizing these signs and symptoms.
IV. Client and family demonstrate competence in emergency techniques related to aspiration, regurgitation, and airway obstruction related to dysphagia.
 V. Client and family identify resources in the community to assist with rehabilitation.
VI. Client and family list symptoms or changes that require professional assistance and management.
    A. Aspiration.
    B. Airway obstruction.

C. Weight loss greater than 10%.

D. Dehydration.

E. Any change that constitutes a concern for client safety or well-being.

Planning and Implementation

I. Interventions that minimize the risk of occurrence or complications of dysphagia.

A. Manage the underlying cause of dysphagia.

B. Consult with speech or occupation therapy to perform a swallow test to determine extent of problem.

C. Perform and teach client/family methods to facilitate the effectiveness and ease of swallowing.

D. Provide appropriate assist devices—straws, plunger spoon, Asepto syringe, and/or pastry tube.

E. Maintain adequate food and calorie intake with high calorie/protein foods and/or enteral feedings, throughout the day—8 small feedings.

F. Institute and teach client/family other measures to decrease pain with swallowing—ice chips, soft or pureed foods, semisolid foods, avoidance of hot and spicy foods, and use of local anesthetics.

II. Interventions to maximize safety.

A. Prevent aspiration by mechanical techniques.

1. Elevate head of bed 45 to 90 degrees, with head slightly forward while eating and maintain position for 45 to 60 minutes after intake.

2. Assist with moving food from front of tongue to posterior area using a long-handled spoon or a syringe as needed.

B. Minimize swallowing difficulty by avoiding milk and milk products, alternating solids with liquids, and encouraging chewing thoroughly using the strongest side of the mouth.

C. Explain all procedures before occurrence to decrease fear or anxiety associated with attempts to swallow and stay with client during feedings.

D. Avoid small pieces of solids that can become lost in the mouth.

E. Consult with dietitian to provide thickening agents to minimize aspiration.

F. Utilize a variety of foods served in an appetizing way, in a progressive manner—pureed to ground to soft-textured to all textures.

III. Interventions to monitor complications related to dysphagia.

A. Maintain daily food record.

B. Weigh daily or at least every other day if daily weights upset client.

C. Assess for signs and symptoms—dehydration, aspiration, and increased/decreased secretions.

D. Explore the need for alternative methods for providing nutrition such as enteral feedings or total parenteral nutrition (TPN) if oral intake is not possible via oral route.

E. Elicit client's subjective reports of changes in patterns of dysphagia and measures that enhance or aggravate swallowing—room temperature foods versus cold or hot foods, consistency.

IV. Interventions to involve client/family in care.

A. Determine willingness of significant other to assist with care with meals and other aspects of overall care.

B. Teach client/family all aspects of care including emergency measures, pulmonary hygiene, oral hygiene, and appropriate time to report complications to a member of the health care team.

V. Interventions to enhance adaptation.
  A. Provide ongoing support to client in a situation that may potentially cause fear, anxiety, and inability to cope.
  B. Provide detailed written and/or audiovisual materials.
  C. Initiate early referral to speech therapist and dietitian for nutritional advice and suggestions.

Evaluation

The oncology nurse systematically and regularly evaluates the client's and/or family's responses to the interventions to determine progress toward the achievement of expected outcomes. Relevant data are collected and actual findings are compared with expected findings. Nursing diagnoses, outcomes, and plans of care are reviewed and revised as necessary.

XEROSTOMIA

Theory

  I. Definition—abnormal or excessive dryness of the mouth characterized by a decrease in the quality and quantity of saliva.
 II. Risk factors and etiology.
  A. Disease-related.
    1. Primary tumor involvement of the salivary/parotid glands.
    2. Metastatic tumor involvement of salivary glands.
    3. Other diseases or conditions—diabetes, infection, candidiasis, Sjögren's syndrome, obsessive-compulsive and anxiety states.
  B. Treatment-related.
    1. Surgical removal of salivary glands.
    2. Pharmacologic therapy for symptom management such as anti-histamines, decongestants, anticholinergics, diuretics, antidepressants, opioids, and phenothiazines, which can contribute to the problem.
    3. Radiation therapy effects.
      a. Can be transient or prolonged, leading to dental caries, taste dysfunction, mucosal lesions, pain, and *Candida* or other fungal infections.
      b. Symptoms develop within first week of therapy causing the mouth to become dry with thick, ropey saliva, which is directly proportional to the amount of radiation dose (Gy) given. As dose and percentage of tissue irradiated increases, damage to tissues increases.
        (1) 10 to 20 Gy results in a 50% decrease in saliva.
        (2) More than 30 Gy results in a 75% decrease in saliva.
        (3) More than 40 Gy may result in permanent, progressive inflammation and degeneration of acinar and ductal cells, replaced by fibrinous connective tissues.
  C. Lifestyle-related—alcohol, caffeine, and nicotine ingestion.
III. Principles of medical treatment.
  A. Artificial saliva/lubricants.
  B. Surgical interventions—salivary reservoirs and reconstruction with a mandibular denture.
  C. Dental prophylaxis with frequent cleaning and fluoride treatments before, during, and after radiation treatments.
  D. Prophylactic oral antimicrobial therapy.

Assessment

I. History.
    A. Previous therapy for cancer.
    B. Prescription and nonprescription medications.
    C. Pattern of xerostomia—incidence, frequency, alleviating and aggravating factors.
    D. Impact of xerostomia on food taste, intake, swallowing, digestion, and communication as well as psychosocial response to condition.
II. Physical examination.
    A. Dry, shiny mucous membranes of oral cavity.
    B. Thick, ropey, and/or scant saliva.
    C. Difficulty swallowing, chewing, and communicating.
III. Laboratory findings—decreased pH of oral secretions.
IV. Psychosocial examination—presence of fear and/or anxiety.

Nursing Diagnoses

I. Altered oral mucous membrane.
II. Altered protection.
III. Impaired swallowing.
IV. Impaired social interaction.

Outcome Identification

I. Client describes personal risk factors for development of xerostomia.
II. Client states signs, symptoms, and complications of xerostomia and participates in interventions that may prevent or alter severity of symptoms/complications.
III. Client and family list changes that require professional assistance in management—infection, lesions or ulcerations of the oral cavity, dental caries, and weight loss over 10 pounds.

Planning and Implementation

I. Interventions to minimize the risk of occurrence and severity of xerostomia.
    A. Measures to increase salivary flow by stimulating residual parenchyma.
        1. Offer sialagogues (agents that affect salivary glands).
            a. Tart sugar-free lemon candies and gum.
            b. Pilocarpine, a systemic parasympathomimetic that has been studied and used to reduce the severity of xerostomia and salivary dysfunction by stimulating remaining salivary gland function.
        2. Apply physical techniques tailored to client preference such as neck massage and/or pressure on the sternal notch.
    B. Measures to provide moisture to the oral mucosa.
        1. Moisten foods with liquids, milk, or gravies.
        2. Sip liquids with and between meals at frequent intervals.
        3. Increase intake to 8 glasses of liquid per day unless contraindicated.
        4. Use artificial saliva, ice chips, and popsicles.
        5. Use room humidifier and/or humidified face mask at night.
        6. Utilize protective enzymes present in some foods.
            a. Papain, which is found in papaya juice.
            b. Amylase present in pineapples (use frozen to minimize stinging).

c. Meat tenderizer, which helps dissolve and break up thick saliva (swab mouth before meals).

7. Lubricate mucosa with 1/8 teaspoon of butter or vegetable or corn oil before meals—starting 2 to 3 weeks after radiation is complete.

8. Use lip balm.

C. Measures to decrease risk of complications of xerostomia.

1. Make frequent assessments because early detection and prevention are key.

2. Encourage meticulous oral hygiene with mechanical and chemical débridement of accumulated plaque and microorganisms at regular intervals at least before and after each meal—every 2 hours is ideal.

3. Avoid physical, chemical, and thermal irritants such as poorly fitting dental prosthetics, hydrogen peroxide, alcohol, tobacco, commercial mouthwashes, and food items such as dry, bulky, spicy, and acidic foods.

II. Interventions to monitor for complications related to xerostomia.

A. Examine oral cavity daily (Table 13–1).

B. Encourage periodic dental examinations.

C. Seek prompt and appropriate medical treatment if infection develops.

Evaluation

The oncology nurse systematically and regularly evaluates the client's and/or family's responses to the interventions to determine progress toward the achievement of expected outcomes. Relevant data are collected and actual findings are compared with expected findings. Nursing diagnoses, outcomes, and plans of care are reviewed and revised as necessary.

MUCOSITIS

Theory

I. Definition—a general term that describes the inflammatory response of mucosal epithelial cells that are present on all surfaces of the gastrointestinal (GI) tract from the mouth to the rectum. These cells readily renew when exposed to normal wear and tear but are unable to do so when toxicity (mucositis) results from cancer treatments.

A. *Stomatitis* is mucositis in the oral cavity.

B. *Esophagitis* is mucositis in the esophagus.

C. *Enteritis* is mucositis in the intestine.

II. Risk factors.

A. Disease-related.

1. Infiltration of mucosal membranes of the GI tract by primary or metastatic tumor.

2. Type and location of tumor—frequency of oral problems two to three times higher in hematologic malignancies than solid tumors.

B. Treatment-related.

1. Can be acute, manifested by mucosal inflammation, ulceration, infection, and mucosal hemorrhage.

2. Can be chronic, manifested by changes in the healthy tissues resulting from xerostomia, taste alterations, trismus (spasms and muscular fibrosis), and soft tissue and bone necrosis.

TABLE 13–1. Oral Assessment Guide (OAG)

Category	Tools for Assessment	Methods of Measurement	Numerical and Descriptive Ratings		
			1	2	3
Voice	Auditory	Converse with patient	Normal	Deeper or raspy	Difficulty talking or painful
Swallow	Observation	Ask patient to swallow. To test gag reflex, gently place blade on back of tongue and depress	Normal swallow	Some pain on swallow	Unable to swallow
Lips	Visual/palpatory	Observe and feel tissue	Smooth and pink and moist	Dry or cracked	Ulcerated or bleeding
Tongue	Visual/palpatory	Feel and observe appearance of tissue	Pink and moist and papillae present	Coated or loss of papillae with a shiny appearance with or without redness	Blistered or cracked
Saliva	Tongue blade	Insert blade into mouth, touching the center of the tongue and the floor of the mouth	Watery	Thick or ropy	Absent
Mucous membranes	Visual	Observe appearance of tissue	Pink and moist	Reddened or coated (increased whiteness) without ulcerations	Ulcerations with or without bleeding
Gingiva	Tongue blade and visual	Gently press with tip of blade	Pink and stippled and firm	Edematous with or without redness	Spontaneous bleeding
Teeth or dentures (or denture-bearing area)	Visual	Observe appearance of teeth or denture-bearing area	Clean and no debris	Plaque or debris in localized areas (between teeth if present)	Plaque or debris generalized along gum line or denture-bearing area

From Goodman, M., Ladd, L.A., and Purl, S. (1993). Integumentary and mucous membrane alterations. In S.L. Groenwald, M.H. Frogge, M. Goodman, & C.H. Yarbro (eds.). *Cancer Nursing: Principles and Practice* (3rd ed.). Boston: Jones & Bartlet, pp. 762–781.

3. Drug administration—any drug known to cause neutropenia because the mouth has been identified as the source of infection in 25 to 54% of neutropenic patients.
   a. Antimicrobials.
   b. Steroids.
   c. Chemotherapy.
      (1) Mainly antimetabolites, antitumor antibiotics, and other miscellaneous drugs such as cyclophosphamide, nitrogen mustard, vinblastine, vincristine, hydroxyurea, and procarbazine, in which effects are dose-related and cumulative.
      (2) Depends on the method of infusion; for example, continuous infusion schedules have greater negative effect than short infusions.
   d. Radiation therapy—effects are greater when chest, abdomen, head and neck, and intestines are in the field, and are dose-related; that is, higher doses of radiation given to larger volumes over shorter periods increase the severity of mucositis.
   e. Oral graft versus host disease.
   f. Immunosuppression—cancer and cancer treatments decrease the body's immune system and alter protective barriers such as oral mucous membranes.
C. Lifestyle-related.
   1. Inadequate oral hygiene practiced, periodontal disease, and partially erupted third molars.
   2. Exposure to irritants—chemical (citrus, spicy, mouthwashes, tobacco, and alcohol) or physical (temperature extremes, poor-fitting prosthesis).
   3. Dehydration.
   4. Malnutrition.
   5. Age—frequency greater in younger than older age.
   6. Renal and hepatic dysfunction both alter drug metabolism.
III. Principles of medical treatment.
   A. Prophylactic antibacterial, antifungal, and antiviral drugs are controversial.
   B. Systemic therapy such as with acetaminophen or narcotics (for example, opioids) and/or topical analgesics and anesthetics (for example, Xylocaine solutions, dyclonine, Ulcerase, sucralfate, and vitamin E).
   C. Systemic and/or local antiinflammatory agents such as nonsteroidal antiinflammatory agents and/or antacids.
   D. Topical protective and coating agents such as Orabase, Hurricane, Oratect-gel, and Zilactin.
   E. Cryotherapy (ice).
   F. Dietary and vitamin supplements.
   G. Biologic response modifiers—prostaglandin E_2, interleukin, fibronectin, immunoglobin, beta carotene, and epidermal growth factors.
   H. Antidiarrheal medications, Tucks compresses, and sitz baths.
   I. Problem-specific approaches—xerostomia, taste changes, anorexia, and hemorrhage (thrombin-soaked collagen gauzes with ice and/or vasoconstricting agents).
IV. Potential sequelae of prolonged stomatitis, esophagitis, and mucositis.
   A. Impaired integrity of the mucous membranes.
   B. Infection, pain, and bleeding.
   C. Difficulty swallowing and speaking.

    D. Inadequate nutritional intake and/or absorption.

    E. Diarrhea.

    F. Bleeding/hemorrhage.

Assessment

I. History.
  - A. Previous therapy for cancer.
  - B. Medications.
  - C. Chemical and/or physical exposure.
  - D. Routine oral hygiene practices.
  - E. Patterns of mucositis—incidence; frequency; precipitating, alleviating, and aggravating factors.
  - F. Overall pattern of mucositis along the entire GI tract.
  - G. Impact of stomatitis, esophagitis, and/or mucositis on lifestyle, comfort, nutrition, activities of daily living, and quality of life.

II. Physical examination (see Table 13–1).
  - A. Utilize an assessment tool and grading scale on an ongoing basis so that changes can be consistently qualified as they occur and compared with the baseline assessment. Approach depends on severity. Grades of oral mucositis are:
    1. Grade 1—erythema of oral mucosa.
    2. Grade 2—isolated small white patches and ulcerations.
    3. Grade 3—confluent ulcerations covering less than 25% of oral mucosa
    4. Grade 4—hemorrhagic ulceration.
  - B. Be alert to timing of complications in relation to the chemotherapy and/or radiation treatments. For example, complaints of burning by client within 3 to 10 days of chemotherapy frequently precedes objective signs. May develop erythema and progress to erosion/ulceration over the next 3 to 5 days.
  - C. Examine and palpate the oral cavity and throat for redness, swelling, presence of white patches, shiny appearance, pain or burning, decreased or increased salivation, and presence of sensation changes.
  - D. Observe for inflammation of all mucous membranes—anal, stomal, and vaginal.

Nursing Diagnoses

    I. Body image disturbance.

   II. Altered oral mucous membrane.

  III. Altered protection.

  IV. Risk for infection.

   V. Altered nutrition, less than body requirements.

  VI. Risk for fluid volume deficit.

 VII. Diarrhea.

VIII. Altered sexual patterns.

  IX. Pain (acute).

   X. Impaired verbal communication.

Outcome Identification

  I. Client describes personal risk factors for mucositis.

 II. Client and family list signs, symptoms, and complications of mucositis to observe for and to report to the health care team.

III. Client discusses measures to minimize risk of occurrence, severity, and complications of mucositis.
IV. Client and family list situations that require professional assistance and intervention.
   A. Temperature elevations greater than 101°F.
   B. Significant decrease in oral intake.
   C. Poorly controlled pain or diarrhea, such as more than five stools a day.

Planning and Implementation

I. Interventions to minimize the risk of occurrence and severity of mucositis.
   A. Measures to decrease inflammation of mucous membranes.
      1. Encourage oral and perineal hygiene measures.
      2. Encourage fluid intake of greater than 3000 mL/day, if tolerated.
      3. Avoid exposures to chemical and physical irritants.
   B. Measures to increase comfort.
      1. Use topical protective agents.
      2. Increase frequency of oral hygiene, depending on grade of mucositis and use of appropriate cleansing devices according to extent of mucosal involvement and pain. Use rinses (normal saline, hydrogen peroxide [3% solution], and antimicrobial solutions [Peridex]).
      3. Give systemic or topical analgesics.
      4. Encourage sitz baths.
   C. Measures to decrease risk of complications of mucositis.
      1. Modify intake to bland, soft, liquid, high calorie/protein foods.
      2. Encourage oral assessment daily and a systematic oral care regimen consisting of cleansing, lubricating, and coating, because systematic performance (compliance) is of more value than the actual agents used.
      3. Discourage sexual intercourse and douching during the inflammatory stage of mucositis and encourage meticulous perineal care.
II. Interventions to monitor client response to symptom management.
   A. Monitor client's subjective reports of changes in the pattern of mucositis.
   B. Monitor changes in level of comfort.
   C. Monitor changes in integrity of the mucous membranes.
   D. Monitor compliance with measures to decrease severity of mucositis and to reduce the incidence of complications.
III. Interventions to incorporate client/family in care.
   A. Teach oral and perineal hygiene measures.
   B. Teach signs and symptoms of infection, impaired skin integrity, and complications to report to the health care team.
      1. Temperature elevations above 101°F.
      2. Significant changes in nutritional intake.
      3. Poorly controlled symptom management—diarrhea, discomfort.

Evaluation

The oncology nurse systematically and regularly evaluates the client's and/or family's responses to the interventions to determine progress toward the achievement of expected outcomes. Relevant data are collected and actual findings are compared with expected findings. Nursing diagnoses, outcomes, and plans of care are reviewed and revised as necessary.

TASTE ALTERATIONS

Theory

I. Definition—an actual or perceived change in taste sensation.
  A. Hypogeusesthesia—a decrease in the acuity of the taste sensation.
  B. Dysgeusia—an unusual taste perception, perceived as unpleasant.
  C. Ageusia—an absence of the taste sensation, "mouth blindness."

II. Etiology and risk factors.
  A. Disease-related.
     1. Excretion of amino acid–like substances from the tumor cells, which changes taste bud sensations (sweet, sour, bitter, and salty).
     2. Invasion of tumor into the oral cavity or salivary glands.
     3. Oral infections—candidiasis.
  B. Treatment-related.
     1. Specific surgical sites—oral cavity, tongue, salivary glands, pathway of the olfactory nerve, and tracheostomy.
     2. Radiation-induced—Changes in salivation usually precede mucositis.
        a. Destruction of the taste buds occurs at doses greater than 1 Gy at about day 10 to 14 and persists for 14 to 21 days.
        b. Saliva can become thick and tenacious early and membranes may become dry at about day 10 to 14, and the condition may continue for 2 to 4 months.
     3. Chemotherapy-induced.
        a. Certain drugs have greater effect on taste sensation than others. Examples are cisplatin, cyclophosphamide, dacarbazine, dactinomycin, mechlorethamine, methotrexate, vincristine, and 5-fluorouracil.
        b. Constant or intermittent metallic and bitter taste sensations.
        c. Increased or decreased threshold for the sweetness sensation, increased threshold for salty and sour tastes, usually decreased threshold for bitter taste.
        d. Aversion to meats.
  C. Lifestyle-related.
     1. Poor oral hygiene.
     2. Nutritional deficiencies—zinc, copper, nickel, niacin, and vitamin A.
  D. Developmental.
     1. Age-induced degeneration of the taste buds.
     2. Learned aversions.
        a. Taste changes or aversions that develop when a food is in association with unpleasant symptoms such as nausea and vomiting, pain.
        b. Seem to develop most rapidly to new or novel foods.

III. Principles of medical treatment.
  A. Nutritional replacement supplements.
  B. Experimentation with different combinations to mask or improve taste.

IV. Potential consequences to taste alterations.
  A. Anorexia—due mainly to decreased intake, decreased quality of foods consumed, decreased volume of saliva and gastric secretions, which are necessary for effective digestion to take place.
  B. Decreased intake due to food aversion that can persist up to 1 year after therapy.
  C. Altered or perverted sense of taste causing many to refuse meats, fish, poultry, eggs, tomatoes, and foods fried in light oil or fat, which can lead to protein/calorie malnutrition and weight loss.

Assessment

I. History.
   A. Presence of hypogeusesthesia, ageusia, or dysgeusia.
   B. History of risk factors including degree and duration of taste alterations.
   C. Subjective description of changes in taste and the impact of the taste alteration on the nutritional status and usual lifestyle patterns.
II. Physical examination.
   A. Oral assessment (see Table 13–1).
      1. Evaluate oral cavity and throat for presence of erythema, desquamation, dryness or excess saliva, and/or ulceration.
      2. Observe for signs and symptoms of secondary oral infection.
   B. Weight.
   C. Presence of other physical problems associated with altered intake.
III. Laboratory findings associated with compromised nutritional status.
   A. Decreased levels of albumin, transferrin, and total lymphocytes.
   B. Decreased levels of zinc, copper, and nickel.
   C. Decreased levels of niacin and vitamin A.

Nursing Diagnoses

I. Altered nutrition, less than body requirements.
II. Altered oral mucous membrane.
III. Sensory or perceptual, olfactory, gustatory alterations.

Outcome Identification

I. Client states the goal of interventions related to taste alteration.
II. Client describes the personal risk for changes in taste sensations.
III. Client reports signs and symptoms related to taste alteration to health care team.
IV. Client uses the appropriate interventions to achieve and maintain optimal nutrition.
V. Client uses interventions to minimize the degree and duration of taste alterations.

Planning and Implementation

I. Interventions to minimize risk of occurrence and severity of taste alterations.
   A. Institute measures to increase sensitivity of taste buds.
      1. Experiment with spices and flavorings to enhance taste.
      2. Use the aroma of foods to stimulate taste.
      3. Increase fluid intake with meals.
      4. Encourage oral hygiene before and after meals.
   B. Institute measures to decrease aversion to certain foods.
      1. Add increased sweeteners to foods.
      2. Marinate meats in sweet juices.
      3. Substitute other sources of protein for poorly tolerated foods.
      4. Avoid the sight and smell of foods causing unpleasantness.
      5. Consume candies such as lemon drops and gum to change taste before meals and before chemotherapy treatment to reduce metallic taste.
   C. Institute measures to increase salivation.
      1. Increase water or juices at frequent intervals—several times an hour.
      2. Spray water, saline, or artificial saliva on the mucous membranes.

      3. Have client suck on smooth flat tart candies or lozenges to stimulate saliva.

      4. Have client avoid alcohol, commercial mouthwashes, and smoking.

      5. Humidify the environmental air.

  II. Interventions to monitor for complications related to taste alterations.

    A. Weigh at regular intervals.

    B. Maintain a daily diet record.

    C. Teach clients the importance of diligent oral care and inspection and in which situations they should access the health care team.

  III. Interventions to incorporate client and family in care. (See Anorexia, Planning and Implementation.)

Evaluation

The oncology nurse systematically and regularly evaluates the client's and/or family's responses to the interventions to determine progress toward the achievement of expected outcomes. Relevant data are collected and actual findings are compared with expected findings. Nursing diagnoses, outcomes, and plans of care are reviewed and revised as necessary.

NAUSEA

Theory

  I. Definition—a subjective, unobservable phenomenon of an unpleasant sensation experienced in the back of the throat and the epigastrium that may or may not culminate in vomiting.

  II. Risk factors.

    A. Disease-related.

      1. Primary or metastatic tumor of the central nervous system (CNS) that includes the vomiting center (VC), or increased intracranial pressure.

      2. Obstruction of a portion of the GI tract.

      3. Food toxins, infection, or motion sickness.

      4. Metabolic abnormalities such as hyperglycemia, hyponatremia, hypercalcemia, and/or renal or hepatic dysfunction.

    B. Treatment-related.

      1. Stimulation of the receptors of the labyrinth in the inner ear.

      2. Obstruction, irritation, inflammation, and delayed gastric emptying stimulating the GI tract through vagal visceral afferent pathways.

      3. Stimulation of the true vomiting center (TVC) through the cellular by-products associated with cancer therapies.

      4. Stimulation of the TVC through afferent pathways from RT of the GI tract.

      5. Side effects of medications such as digitalis, morphine, antibiotics, iron, vitamins, and antineoplastic agents such as cisplatin, mechlorethamine, and dacarbazine.

      6. Side effects of concentrated nutritional supplements.

    C. Situational.

      1. Increased levels of tension, stress, emotions, and/or anxiety.

      2. Noxious odors or visual stimuli.

      3. Conditioned (anticipatory) responses to previous cancer and other stressful experiences.

        a. Occurs in 25% of chemotherapy patients.

        b. History of motion sickness, which increases risk.

III. Principles of medical treatment.
   A. Treatment of underlying disease.
   B. Antiemetic therapy (see Chapter 10).
   C. Behavioral interventions—relaxation training such as focused diaphragmatic breathing, guided imagery, hypnosis, and biofeedback.
IV. Potential sequelae of prolonged nausea.
   A. Vomiting.
   B. Anorexia with resultant weight loss, fluid and electrolyte imbalances, and dehydration.
   C. Noncompliance or refusal to complete treatment plan.
   D. Altered quality of life.

Assessment

I. History.
   A. Presence of risk factors for nausea.
   B. Presence of defining characteristics of nausea.
   C. Present symptoms, client's perception of possible correlation between occurrence of nausea and distress, and perceived meaning of nausea to the client and family, work, role responsibilities, and mood.
   D. Patterns of nausea—onset, frequency, associated symptoms, precipitating factors, aggravating factors, and alleviating factors.
II. Physical examination.
   A. Signs of sweating, tachycardia, dizziness, pallor, excessive salivation, and weakness.
   B. Laboratory reports to assess for other causes—serum electrolytes, liver and renal function tests.
   C. Weight.
III. Psychosocial assessment.
   A. Explore anxiety-producing events and coping abilities.
   B. Attempt to identify strengths of client/family.

Nursing Diagnoses

I. Altered nutrition, less than body requirements.
II. Risk for fluid volume deficit.
III. Ineffective coping, individual.

Outcome Identification

I. Client describes personal risk for nausea.
II. Client participates in measures to minimize the risk of occurrence of nausea.
III. Client demonstrates competence in self-care techniques for management of nausea.
IV. Client and family list changes in the condition of the client that require professional assistance in management.
   A. Presence of unrelieved nausea and/or inability to eat and drink.
   B. Weight loss greater than 10% of body weight.
   C. Presence of signs and symptoms of dehydration.

Planning and Implementation

I. Interventions to minimize the risk of occurrence, severity, or complications of nausea.

    A. Individualize drug regimen according to emetic potential of chemotherapy, expected duration of nausea and vomiting, and current pattern of symptoms.

    B. Modify the environment—cool, well ventilated, lowered lighting and noise levels, and absence of noxious sights and smells.

    C. Modify diet to include bland, chilled foods with liquids served separately.

    D. Avoid movement and reclining within 30 minutes after eating.

    E. Replace fluids with the use of popsicles, Gatorade, and fruit or yogurt bars.

    F. Administer antiemetics around the clock until cycle is broken.

    G. Encourage nonpharmacologic relaxation and distraction activities.

  II. Interventions to maximize safety.

    A. Position during vomiting episodes, if they occur, to reduce risk of aspiration.

    B. Anticipate needs due to weakness and/or sedative effects of antiemetics and provide assistance with ambulation, using raised siderails and emesis basin within reach.

 III. Interventions to monitor for complications of nausea.

    A. Observe for signs of dehydration, electrolyte imbalance, and profound loss of weight in a short time frame.

    B. Observe for side effects that may be associated with antiemetic therapy.

 IV. Interventions to incorporate client/family in care.

    A. Teach positioning techniques to decrease risk of aspiration.

    B. Teach home management techniques to avoid or minimize emetic events including use of medications around the clock, portable infusion devices, and medication combining for maximal effect.

    C. Encourage the use of self-care diaries and logs.

    D. Teach importance of reporting critical changes in client condition to the physician including presence of adverse or intensified pattern of vomiting; signs and symptoms of aspiration, dehydration, or other pathology.

Evaluation

The oncology nurse systematically and regularly evaluates the client's and/or family's responses to the interventions to determine progress toward the achievement of expected outcomes. Relevant data are collected and actual findings are compared with expected findings. Nursing diagnoses, outcomes, and plans of care are reviewed and revised as necessary.

VOMITING

Theory

    I. Definition—a somatic process performed by the respiratory muscles causing a forceful oral expulsion of gastric, duodenal, or jejunal contents through the mouth. Can be acute, 1 to 2 hours after chemotherapy, or delayed, 24 to 48 hours after chemotherapy.

   II. Etiology—the vomiting center (VC) located in the lateral reticular formation of the medulla is directly activated by the visceral and vagal afferent pathways from the GI tract, the chemoreceptor trigger zone (CTZ), vestibular apparatus, and the cerebral cortex. The damaged enterochromaffin cells in the GI tract release serotonin locally, resulting in activation of 5HT3 receptors on the visceral afferent fibers in the vagus nerve, which in turn induces impulses to the salivation, cardiac, and respiratory centers and then to the pharyngeal, GI, and abdominal muscles.

III. Risk factors.
   A. Disease-related.
      1. Primary or metastatic tumor of the CNS.
      2. Increased intracranial pressure from tumor or hemorrhage.
      3. GI or biliary obstruction.
      4. Metabolic abnormalities such as hypercalcemia, hyponatremia.
      5. Renal or hepatic dysfunction.
      6. Food toxins, infection, or motion sickness.
   B. Treatment-related (see Table 13–2).
      1. Stimulation of the VC and the CTZ by cancer therapies.
      2. Cellular damage to the enterochromaffin cells by chemotherapy and RT to the intradiaphragmatic area.
      3. Severity influenced by the emetic potential of the drugs.

TABLE 13–2. **Emetogenic Potential of Antineoplastic Agents**

Agent	% of Time Agent Induces Emesis	Onset of Emesis (h)	Duration of Emesis (h)
Cisplatin*	>90	1–6	24–120
Dacarbazine	>90	1–3	1–12
Mechlorethamine	>90	0.5–2	8–24
Carboplatin	60–90	1–6	4–24
Carmustine*	60–90	2–4	4–24
Cyclophosphamide*	60–90	4–12	4–24
Dactinomycin	60–90	2–6	12–24
Procarbazine	60–90	24–27	Varies
Cytarabine*	30–60	6–12	3–12
Daunorubicin	30–60	2–6	6–24
Doxorubicin	30–60	4–6	6–24
Ifosfamide	30–60	2–6	4–24
Mitoxantrone	30–60	2–6	6–24
Fluorouracil	30–60	3–6	2–24
Mitomycin	30–60	1–4	48–72
Bleomycin	10–30	3–6	1–4
Cytarabine*	10–30	6–12	3–5
Etoposide	10–30	3–8	1–4
Methotrexate*	10–30	4–12	3–12
Vinblastine	10–30	4–8	1–4
Vincristine	<10	4–8	1–4
Paclitaxel	<10	4–8	———

*Dose-related; potential for emesis increases with higher doses.
Data reprinted with permission from (1) Borison, H.L., & McCarthy, L.E. (1993). Neuropharmacology of chemotherapy-induced emesis. *Drugs* 25:8–17. [suppl 1] and (2) Dorr, R.T., & Fritz, W.L. *Cancer Chemotherapy Handbook*. Stamford, CT: Appleton & Lange, 1980, pp 143–150.
Reprinted from Rhodes, V.A., Johnson, M.H., & McDaniel, R.W. (1995). Nausea, vomiting and retching: The management of the symptom experience. *Semin Oncol Nurs 11*(4), 259–260.

4. Side effects of medications—digitalis, morphine, antibiotics, vitamins, iron, and narcotics.

5. Side effects of concentrated nutritional supplements.

C. Situational.

1. Increased levels of tension, stress, and/or anxiety.

2. Noxious odors or visual stimuli.

3. Conditioned (anticipatory) responses to poor previous emetic control (occurs in 25% of chemotherapy patients).

4. Being young.

5. History of motion sickness.

III. Principles of medical management (see Nausea, Theory).

IV. Potential sequelae of prolonged vomiting.

A. Fluid and electrolyte imbalances.

B. Anorexia with resultant weight loss.

C. Esophageal tears and/or aspiration.

D. Noncompliance or refusal to complete treatment plan.

E. Altered quality of life.

Assessment

I. History.

A. Presence of risk factors for vomiting or actual episodes of emesis.

B. Character of emesis.

C. Present symptoms, client's perception of possible correlation between occurrence of vomiting and stress, and the perceived meaning of vomiting to the client/family, work, role responsibilities, and mood.

D. Patterns of vomiting—onset, frequency, associated symptoms, precipitating factors, aggravating factors, and alleviating factors.

II. Physical examination.

A. Observe for sweating, tachycardia, dizziness, pallor, excessive salivation, weakness, increased blood pressure, and decreased muscle strength.

B. Monitor laboratory reports to assess other causes—serum electrolytes, liver and renal function tests.

C. Monitor weight.

III. Psychosocial assessment.

A. Explore anxiety-producing events and coping abilities.

B. Attempt to identify strengths of client and significant others.

Nursing Diagnoses

I. Altered nutrition, less than body requirements.

II. Fluid volume deficit (active loss)

III. Risk for aspiration.

IV. Fatigue.

V. Risk for injury.

VI. Ineffective individual coping.

Outcome Identification

I. Client describes personal risk for vomiting related to potential causes and timing of episodes related to chemotherapy and RT.

II. Client self-medicates with antiemetics to minimize the risk of occurrence, severity, and complications of vomiting.

III. Client performs safety measures to avoid injury related to the effects of vomiting.
IV. Client and family list changes in the condition of the client that require professional assistance in management.
   A. Presence of changes in amount or presence of blood or lack of relief from antiemetics.
   B. Weight loss greater than 10% of body weight.
   C. Presence of signs and symptoms of dehydration.
 V. Family/significant other involve themselves in distraction and relaxation techniques to assist client.

Planning and Implementation

I. See Nausea, Planning and Implementation.

Evaluation

The oncology nurse systematically and regularly evaluates the client's and/or family's responses to the interventions to determine progress toward the achievement of expected outcomes. Relevant data are collected and actual findings are compared with expected findings. Nursing diagnoses, outcomes, and plans of care are reviewed and revised as necessary.

WEIGHT CHANGES

Theory

 I. Effects of cancer and cancer treatments.
   A. Weight gain.
   B. Weight loss.
 II. Etiology of weight gain.
   A. Disease-related.
      1. Clients with breast cancer—often experience weight gain as a result of medications such as steroids and tamoxifen citrate.
      2. Effusions—pleural, pericardial, abdominal.
      3. Obstruction.
      4. Inactivity.
      5. Electrolyte imbalances.
      6. Biologic medications such as interleukin-2 (IL-2) (see Chapter 36).
   B. Treatment-related.
      1. Effects of hormonal drugs.
      2. Steroids.
      3. Electrolyte imbalances.
      4. Adjuvant chemotherapy for breast cancer patients.
III. Etiology of weight loss.
   A. May be primary—cancer cachexia.
   B. May be secondary—due to protein-calorie malnutrition, caused by the metabolic effects of the tumor.
      1. Altered carbohydrate metabolism.
         a. Anaerobic glycolysis.
         b. Increased rate of gluconeogenesis.
         c. Glucose intolerance.

2. Altered protein metabolism.
   a. Increased uptake of amino acids by the tumor.
   b. Decreased protein synthesis.
   c. Increased protein degradation.
   d. Protein loss.
   e. Use of protein for energy needs.
3. Altered lipid metabolism.
4. Fluid and electrolyte disturbances.
   a. Hypercalcemia.
   b. Hyperuricemia.
   c. Hyponatremia.
   d. Hypokalemia.
5. Increased energy expenditure.
6. Taste alterations.
7. Anorexia.
   a. Central mechanisms.
   b. Neurotransmitters.

C. Other causes.
1. Increased sweating, gastric suction, drains, fistulas, wounds.
2. Flu-like syndrome associated with biologic response modifiers.
3. Loss resulting from vomiting, malabsorption, surgery, infection, fatigue, diarrhea due to supplemental feedings, antibiotics, antacids, pain, stress/anxiety/depression, and infectious agents such as *Clostridium difficile.*

Assessment

I. History.
A. Previous dietary patterns, food preferences, eating habits, and history of weight changes with client/family.
B. Patterns of weight changes.
1. Type, onset, duration, severity.
2. Associated symptoms—food intolerances, taste abnormalities, mouth and throat pain, dysphagia.
3. Other factors—precipitating, aggravating, alleviating factors.
C. Previous self-care strategies.
1. Ability to carry out interventions to maintain weight.
2. Use of food, nutritional supplements, and other remedies.
D. Current or recent treatment for cancer and anticipated side effects.
II. Physical examination.
A. Determine present weight and amount of total weight loss or gain.
B. Assess for presence of dehydration and/or electrolyte imbalances.
C. Assess client for associated ethnic, socioeconomic, emotional, and motivational factors that may affect the loss of weight or weight gain.

Nursing Diagnoses

I. Altered nutrition, less than body requirements.
II. Altered nutrition, more than body requirements.
III. Risk for impaired skin integrity.
IV. Knowledge deficit.
V. Fatigue.

Outcome Identification

I. Client states the goals of interventions related to weight change.

II. Client states the personal risk for complications related to weight loss or gain and ways in which various cancer therapies may effect nutrition.

III. Client participates in measures to minimize risk of occurrence, severity, and complications of weight changes.

IV. Client states the changes in condition that require professional assistance and/or intervention.

    A. Weight loss or gain of more than 2 pounds per day.

    B. Dehydration, increased insensible losses, and edema.

    C. Changes in skin integrity, wound healing, respiratory or cardiovascular status, and presence of infection.

    D. Inability to eat or drink.

    E. Any area of concern for client's well-being related to intake or lack of intake.

V. Client and family state awareness of resources in the community to assist with nutrition.

Planning and Implementation

I. Interventions to minimize the risk of occurrence, severity, or complications of weight change.

    A. Measures to increase calorie and nutritional value of oral intake—teach client/family to:

        1. Consume frequent nutritionally dense meals in small portions throughout the day for weight loss.

        2. Maximize food intake during periods of greatest strength and appetite, usually early in the day.

        3. Maximize food preferences and access to favorite foods within dietary restrictions.

    B. Maximize measures to promote comfort and ease while eating—teach clients/family the importance of:

        1. Administering pain medications, if needed, 30 to 60 minutes before meals.

        2. Assisting with oral care, as needed, before and after meals.

        3. Planning activities according to client's activity level, such as rest periods and walking before meals to stimulate appetite.

        4. Minimizing noxious stimuli in the environment.

II. Interventions to monitor complications related to weight change—stress the importance of:

    A. Maintaining a daily dietary intake record and weighing daily.

    B. Assessing for signs and symptoms of dehydration or electrolyte imbalances.

    C. Assessing overall skin and nail condition for adverse effects of poor nutrition or intake—skin breakdown, dehiscence, or poor wound healing.

III. Interventions to incorporate client/family in care.

    A. Encourage family to provide foods within dietary restrictions.

    B. Teach family methods to enhance calorie/protein content of foods and methods to enhance food intake.

        1. List of high-calorie high-protein foods and/or low-residue foods.

        2. Suggestions for supplementing nutritional value by adding powders or supplements and vitamins.

        3. Use of medications as ordered by physician.

     4. Planning mealtimes that are relaxed, unhurried, and pleasant.

     5. Utilize a variety of foods to avoid taste fatigue.

     6. Employ proper quantities of foods from four food groups that provide a balanced, nutritious diet for weight control.

     7. Engage in regular excercise—may need consult with nutritionist.

  C. Teach signs and symptoms of dehydration, wound healing, third-spacing, and malnutrition.

  D. Develop a nurse/client contract for increasing the intake of calories and protein each day.

IV. Interventions to enhance adaptation and rehabilitation.

  A. Provide written and/or audiovisual materials on nutrition at client's level of education and understanding.

  B. Initiate early referral to dietitian for nutritional assessment and intervention, as indicated.

Evaluation

The oncology nurse systematically and regularly evaluates the client's and/or family's responses to the interventions to determine progress toward the achievement of expected outcomes. Relevant data are collected and actual findings are compared with expected findings. Nursing diagnoses, outcomes, and plans of care are reviewed and revised as necessary.

CACHEXIA

Theory

  I. Definition—a syndrome of progressive wasting associated with anorexia and metabolic alterations.

 II. Etiology of anorexia. Metabolically, cachexia appears to be mediated by cachectin or tumor necrosing factor (TNF), a cytokine protein produced by macrophages and the tumor that induces cachexia, anemia, and inflammation.

  A. May be primary—mediating factors are anorexia, decreased gluconeogenesis, alterations in glucose metabolism, increased metabolic rate, changed lipid metabolism, tumor versus host competition for ingested nutrients, and secretion of paraneoplastic substances from the tumor tissue.

  B. May be secondary—defined as weight loss and inanition based on mechanical factors or treatment-induced toxicities.

III. Risk factors.

  A. Disease-related.

     1. Cancer.

     2. Acquired immunodeficiency syndrome (AIDS).

     3. Infections, septic states, and inflammatory diseases.

  B. Treatment-related.

     1. Chemotherapy.

     2. Radiation therapy.

     3. Abdominal surgery.

  C. Situational.

     1. Psychological aspects of nutritional intake—cancer cachexia is viewed by some to be the hallmark of terminal illness, thus clients frequently "give up."

     2. Depression, inactivity, absence of an appetite, and poor performance status all affect the client's quality of life.

IV. Principles of medical management.
    A. Treatment of the underlying disease.
    B. Pharmacologic interventions.
        1. Megestrol acetate—has a dose-response effect.
        2. Metoclopramide at low doses to stimulate GI motility and decrease early satiety.
        3. Cannabinoid derivatives such as delta-9-tetrahydrocannabinol (THC) and Marinol to stimulate appetite.
        4. Metabolic inhibitors to induce anabolism.
        5. Dexamethasone and prednisolone to stimulate appetite and sense of well-being.
        6. Pentoxifylline—inhibits production of TNF.
    C. Total parenteral nutrition.
    D. Enteral feedings—oral or tube feedings.
V. Potential sequelae of cachexia.
    A. Increased morbidity and mortality (cause of death in 20%).
    B. Alterations in carbohydrate, protein, and lipid metabolism.
    C. Decreased tissue sensitivity to insulin and decreased insulin response to glucose administration.
    D. Impairment of immunocompetence, both humoral and cellular immunity.
    E. Poor wound healing and increased infection rates.
    F. Protein/calorie malnutrition with resultant weight loss, visceral and somatic protein depletion that compromises enzymatic, structural, and mechanical functions.
    G. Impaction due to lack of food intake and bulk and the effects of cancer treatments.

Assessment

I. History.
    A. Previous dietary patterns, food preferences, eating habits, type and quantity of food consumed, and history of anorexia with client/family.
    B. Patterns of anorexia and presence of fatigue and malaise.
        1. Onset, frequency, severity.
        2. Associated symptoms—food intolerances, taste abnormalities, mouth and throat pain, dysphagia.
        3. Other factors—precipitating, aggravating, alleviating factors.
    C. Previous self-care strategies.
        1. Ability to provide for own interventions to relieve anorexia.
        2. Use of food, nutritional supplements, and other remedies.
    D. Current or recent treatment for cancer and anticipated side effects.
    E. Associated ethnic, socioeconomic, emotional, and motivational factors that may affect the loss of weight.
II. Physical examination.
    A. Determine present weight and amount of total and recent weight loss.
    B. Assess for presence of dehydration and/or electrolyte imbalances.
    C. Assess for muscle atrophy, loss of fat deposits, and presence of edema.
    D. Perform anthropometric measurements or consult the nutritionalist.
        1. Tricep skin folds and midarm muscle circumference.
        2. Height and weight (weight loss >10% in previous 3 months is significant for diagnosis of protein/calorie malnutrition).

E. Review biochemical measurements.
   1. Visceral protein stores—serum albumin and total iron-binding capacity, electrolytes, and nitrogen balance.
   2. Lean body mass—collect 24-hour urine (three collections for accuracy) and calculate creatinine height index.
   3. Degree of anemia.
   4. Deficiencies in trace metals and vitamins, and glucose intolerance.
F. Immunologic measurements—calculate total lymphocyte count and perform skin sensitivity test.

Nursing Diagnoses

  I. Altered nutrition, less than body requirements.
 II. Risk for fluid volume deficit.
III. Risk for impaired skin integrity.
IV. Knowledge deficit.
 V. Fatigue.
VI. Powerlessness.
VII. Risk for caregiver role strain.

Outcome Identification

  I. Client consumes six to eight small feedings per day by mouth or by alternative route as tolerated.
 II. Client states the personal risk for complications related to cachexia and ways in which various cancer therapies may adversely affect nutritional reserves.
III. Family/significant other participates in measures to minimize risk of occurrence, severity, and complications of cachexia.
IV. Client states the changes in condition that require professional assistance and/or intervention.
   A. Weight loss of more than 1 to 2 pounds per day.
   B. Dehydration.
   C. Changes in skin integrity and wound healing, and infection.
   D. Inability to eat or drink.
   E. Any other area of concern for client's sense of well-being related to food intake.
 V. Client and family state awareness of resources in the community to assist with nutrition and caregiving support.

Planning and Implementation

I. See Anorexia, Planning and Interventions.

Evaluation

The oncology nurse systematically and regularly evaluates the client's and/or family's responses to the interventions to determine progress toward the achievement of expected outcomes. Relevant data are collected and actual findings are compared with expected findings. Nursing diagnoses, outcomes, and plans of care are reviewed and revised as necessary.

ASCITES

Theory

  I. Definition—abnormal accumulation of fluid in the abdominal cavity that is not reabsorbed into the systemic circulation.

II. Risk factors.
   A. Disease-related.
      1. Association with various tumors: ovarian, endometrial, breast, colon, gastric, pancreatic, and to a lesser extent mesothelioma, testicular, lung, lymphoma, sarcoma.
      2. As a result of liver metastasis.
   B. Treatment-related—previous radiation to the abdomen and/or surgical modification of venous or lymphatic channels.
III. Principles of medical management.
   A. Treatment of underlying cause.
   B. Diet and diuresis—usually only helpful when cause is due to cirrhosis.
   C. Removal of fluid by paracentesis.
   D. Obliteration of the intraperitoneal space using chemotherapy (belly bath) and/or instillation of radioactive colloids.
   E. Peritoneovenous shunting (LeVeen or Denver).
IV. Potential sequelae of progressive ascites.
   A. Discomfort, anorexia, early satiety, decreased bladder capacity, bowel obstruction, electrolyte imbalance, infection, respiratory compromise, edema, impaired skin integrity, abdominal distention, and weight gain.
   B. The appearance of ascites in advanced disease is prognostically grim. Palliation is usually all that can be offered and it needs to be done each time fluid reaccumulates. Life expectancy is a few months.

Assessment

I. History.
   A. Presence of risk factors.
   B. Pattern of ascites.
      1. Elicit subjective indicators—increasing abdominal girth, indigestion, early satiety, swollen ankles, easy fatigability, shortness of breath, constipation, and reduced bladder capacity.
      2. Review previous treatment strategies for ascites and current or recent treatment for cancer and anticipated side effects.
   C. Presence of self-care strategies.
      1. Ability to perform interventions to relieve or minimize effects of ascites.
      2. Willingness to self-monitor weight, girth, record-keeping.
II. Physical examination.
   A. Determine present weight and amount of weight gain, presence of distended abdomen, fluid wave, shifting dullness, bulging flanks, everted umbilicus, stretched skin, and presence of lower extremity edema and increased abdominal girth.
   B. Assess laboratory indicators—for presence of high level of carcinoembryonic antigen (>12 mg/mL), cytologic confirmation of the presence of malignant cells, chemistry confirmation, cytology examination result and character of transudate, as well as results of ultrasound and computed tomography examinations of abdomen.
   C. Assess client for associated ethnic, socioeconomic, emotional, and motivational factors that may influence care.

Nursing Diagnoses

I. Altered nutrition, less than body requirements.
II. Fluid volume excess.

    III. Risk for impaired skin integrity.
    IV. Risk for activity intolerance.
     V. Altered urinary elimination.
    VI. Pain, chronic.
   VII. Ineffective breathing pattern.
  VIII. Decreased cardiac output.
    IX. Self-care deficit, bathing, dressing and grooming, toileting.

Outcome Identification

     I. Client states the goals of interventions related to ascites.
    II. Client states the personal risk for potential recurrence of ascites and early symptoms that need to be reported to lessen extent of fluid accumulation and discomfort.
   III. Client participates in measures to minimize the discomfort associated with ascites including positioning and pain control.
   IV. Client and family state the changes in condition that require professional assistance and/or intervention.
      A. Weight gain of more than 2 pounds per day and/or increased abdominal girth.
      B. Acute respiratory distress, fever, or changes in level of pain.
      C. Edema noted in other body parts such as lower legs and feet.
    V. Client and family state awareness of resources in the community to assist with long-term care and client/family support.

Planning and Implementation

     I. Interventions to minimize the risk of occurrence, severity, or complications of ascites.
      A. Teach client/family to decrease sodium and increase protein intake.
      B. Maximize measures to promote comfort.
        1. Teach client/family to maintain a high-Fowler position.
        2. Employ positions to reduce edema.
        3. Avoid restrictive clothing.
        4. Remind of need for pain relief.
        5. Use methods to assist with activities as needed.
    II. Interventions to incorporate client/family in care.
      A. Encourage family to provide foods within dietary restrictions.
      B. Teach family methods to enhance calorie/protein content of foods and methods to enhance food intake.
      C. Teach family signs and symptoms of dehydration, infection, respiratory distress, and malnutrition.
      D. Teach family how to measure abdominal girth and weigh daily and how to assess changes such as fullness, bloating, and abdominal pressure.
   III. Interventions to enhance adaptation and rehabilitation.
      A. Provide written and audiovisual materials on care issues at client's level of education and understanding.
      B. Encourage importance of self-care recordkeeping such as diaries and logs.

Evaluation

    The oncology nurse systematically and regularly evaluates the client's and/or family's responses to the interventions to determine progress toward the achievement of expected outcomes. Relevant data are collected and actual findings are compared with expected findings. Nursing diagnoses, outcomes, and plans of care are reviewed and revised as necessary.

ELECTROLYTE IMBALANCES

Theory

I. Tumor or treatment-related metabolic disturbances frequently occur in clients with cancer.

II. Calcium (Ca++) imbalances
  A. Usual reference range: 4.5 to 5.5 mEq/L.
  B. Calcium is the fifth most abundant inorganic element in body, found in bone, with 99% in the form of insoluble crystals, 1% distributed between the body's intracellular and extracellular fluids, with 45% ionized in the serum, 45% bound by protein, and 10% found in insoluble complexes.
    1. Ionized Ca++—necessary for excitation of nerves, action of voluntary skeletal muscles, cardiac muscle, and involuntary muscles of the gut.
      a. If the body has too much ionized Ca++, there is decreased excitability of these tissues (hypercalcemia: >11 mg/dL).
      b. If there is too little ionized Ca++, there is increased excitability of nerves and muscles (hypocalcemia: <10 mg/dL).
    2. Since 45% of the Ca++ outside the bone is bound to albumin, it is important to correct the value of ionized Ca++ in the serum if the albumin is low.
  C. Causes of calcium imbalances.
    1. Hypercalcemia—secretion of parathyroid-related protein by tumor, secretion of other bone-resorbing substances by the tumor, decreased ability of the kidney's to clear Ca++ from the blood, and increased Ca++ absorption from the gut (see Chapter 17).
    2. Hypocalcemia.
      a. General causes.
        (1) Defect in parathyroid hormone (PTH).
        (2) Vitamin D dysfunction.
        (3) Multiple citrated blood transfusions.
        (4) Hyperventilation.
      b. Cancer-related causes.
        (1) Cisplatin-based chemotherapy.
        (2) Osteoblastic bone metastasis and oncogenic osteomalacia.
        (3) Metastatic spread into the parathyroid glands.
        (4) Tumor lysis syndrome (TLS).
  D. Clinical symptomatology of calcium imbalances depends on blood levels.
    1. Hypercalcemia.
      a. Calcium level 10 to 12 mg/dL—fatigue, lethargy, constipation, anorexia, nausea/vomiting, and polyuria.
      b. Calcium level higher than 12 mg/dL—stupor, altered mental status, coma, decreased deep tendon reflexes, increased cardiac contractility, oliguria, and renal failure.
    2. Hypocalcemia.
      a. Early—numbness, increased neuromuscular irritability, paresthesias of fingers and toes and perioral region.

  b. Late—clinical course varies.
    (1) From tetany of facial muscles in response to stimulation (Chvostek sign) and carpopedal spasm (Trousseau sign) to central nervous system abnormalities.
    (2) From petit mal to grand mal seizures.
    (3) From emotional disturbances to impairment of cognitive functions.
    (4) From laryngospasm and bronchospasms to possible death.
  c. Electrocardiogram changes.
    (1) Lengthening of the ST segment.
    (2) Lengthening of the QT interval.
    (3) Atrial and ventricular dysrhythmias.
E. Treatment of calcium imbalances.
  1. Hypercalcemia.
    a. Pharmacologic interventions—fluid repletion, diuretics, corticosteroids, calcitonin, mithramycin, biophosphonates, gallium nitrate, and antitumor treatment.
    b. Nonpharmacologic interventions—intravenous fluids, increased mobility, dialysis, and dietary restrictions.
  2. Hypocalcemia.
    a. If severe—intravenous calcium (calcium chloride or calcium gluconate).
    b. If chronic—oral calcium supplements with vitamin D.
III. Magnesium (Mg++) imbalances.
  A. Usual reference range 1.3 to 2.1 mEq/L.
  B. Fourth most abundant cation in the body.
  C. Second most abundant intracellular cation, with liver and muscle cells having highest concentration and 30 to 40% of dietary intake absorbed through the gastrointestinal tract with the bulk of the remainder found in the urine.
  D. Mg++ is a critical cofactor in regulating cellular calcium, hydrogen, sodium, and potassium pumps and in the phosphorylation of glucose.
  E. Hypomagnesemia frequently (40%) causes decreases in potassium and sodium levels.
  F. Causes of magnesium imbalances.
    1. Hypermagnesemia (>3.0 mg/dL)
      a. Renal failure.
      b. Adrenal insufficiency.
    2. Hypomagnesemia (<1.7 mg/dL).
      a. Cisplatin-induced renal wasting of Mg++.
      b. Use of diuretics, especially mannitol diuresis.
      c. Some antibiotics, especially aminoglycosides and amphotericin B.
      d. Any condition (e.g., liver failure) that potentiates nephrotoxicity.
      e. Other electrolyte abnormalities that contribute to hypomagnesemia.
        (1) Hypercalcemia and hyperaldosteronism.
        (2) Hypomagnesemia is accompanied by hypokalemia in 40%.
        (3) Hypophosphatemia is frequently associated with decreased Mg++ levels.
  G. Clinical symptomatology of magnesium imbalances.
    1. Hypermagnesemia.
      a. Lethargy, flushing, diaphoresis.
      b. Decreased blood pressure; slow weak pulse, and slow shallow respirations
      c. Diminished deep tendon reflexes.

    2. Hypomagnesemia.
       a. Neuromuscular and CNS symptoms comparable with those of hypocalcemia, including seizures.
  H. Treatment for magnesium imbalance.
    1. Hypermagnesemia—diuretics; volume expansion with saline and mannitol diuresis potentiate Mg++ wasting.
    2. Hypomagnesemia—magnesium sulfate given orally or intravenously.

IV. Sodium (Na+) imbalances.
  A. Usual reference range 135 to 145 mEq/L.
  B. Sodium is the major cation in the plasma and extracellular fluid and is regulated indirectly by alterations in the total body water content, accompanied by sensory receptors (osmoreceptors) that promote either the uptake of water or the excretion of urine.
  C. Serum osmolality is physiologically maintained between 286 and 294 mOsm and is accomplished through coordination with the central thirst mechanism, antidiuretic hormone (ADH), and renal sodium and water excretion.
  D. Sodium is the major determinant of serum osmolarity and tonicity.
  E. Causes of sodium imbalances.
    1. Hypernatremia (>160 mEq/L). Seen less frequently in clients with cancer.
       a. Inadequate intake of water and/or diabetes insipidus.
       b. Impaired renal function.
       c. Dehydration.
       d. Some medications (e.g., corticosteroids), antihypertensives (methyldopa, hydralazine, and reserpine).
    2. Hyponatremia (<120 mEq/L.). Most common electrolyte disorder in cancer.
       a. Syndrome of inappropriate antidiuretic hormone (SIADH) associated with lung cancer (see Chapter 17).
       b. Diuretic therapy, and some chemotherapeutic drugs (e.g., cyclophosphamide and vincristine).
  F. Clinical symptomatology of sodium imbalances.
    1. Hypernatremia.
       a. Pronounced polyuria and polydipsia.
       b. Low-grade fevers.
       c. Dry, sticky mucous membranes, flushed skin.
       d. Muscle weakness, diminished reflexes.
       e. Restlessness (irritability, disorientation), depression, lethargy.
       f. Intracranial bleeding.
       g. Convulsions, stupor, and coma.
    2. Hyponatremia.
       a. Mild; anorexia, headache, nausea and vomiting, myalgias and subtle neurologic symptoms.
       b. Severe (<115 mEq/dL)—obtundation, seizures, alterations in the mental status ranging from confusion to coma and death.
  G. Treatment of sodium imbalances (dependent on the degree/duration).
    1. Hypernatremia—should be corrected slowly over 2 to 3 days.
       a. Intravenous lysine vasopressin.
       b. If chronic; desmopressin by nasal route.
    2. Hyponatremia—correct cause (e.g., SIADH) which resolves the underly-

ing cause of excessive ADH production (e.g., chemotherapy for lung cancer and radiation therapy for brain metastasis).

    a. Water restriction to 500 mL/day.

    b. For acute onset, intravenous hypertonic saline and furosemide.

V. Potassium (K+) imbalances

  A. Usual reference range 3.5 to 5.0 mEq/L.

  B. Reciprocal relationship between K+ and Na+; a substantial intake of one element causes a corresponding decrease in the other, and the body has no efficient method for conserving K+.

  C. Causes of potassium imbalances.

    1. Hyperkalemia (>6 mEq/L).

      a. Dehydration.

      b. Compromised renal function.

      c. Acidosis resulting from sepsis.

      d. Myocardial infarction (MI).

      e. Burns.

      f. Ketoacidosis.

      g. Adrenal insufficiency (as steroids are tapered).

      h. Medications (e.g., indomethacin, K+ supplements, potassium-sparing diuretics, and any drug that causes renal toxicity—amphotericin B, methicillin, and tetracycline).

    2. Hypokalemia (<3 mEq/L)—usually results from multiple factors. Those with hypertension and congestive heart failure are at higher risk.

      a. Decreased dietary intake and potassium-free intravenous fluids.

      b. Increased GI losses—vomiting/gastric suction, urine, ileostomy, or diarrhea, which can result from antibiotic therapy; antacids, lactose intolerance, supplemental feedings, and infectious agents (*Clostridium difficile,* GI candidiasis).

      c. Drug therapies—insulin and glucose administration, loop and thiazide-type diuretics, mineralocorticosteroids, some antibiotics (penicillin, ampicillin, carbenicillin, ticarcillin), and some nephrotoxic antineoplastic agents (streptozocin, carmustine, and cisplatin).

  D. Clinical symptomatology of potassium imbalances.

    1. Hyperkalemia.

      a. Vague muscle weakness, malaise, paresthesias (face, tongue, feet, hands), muscle cramps, ascending flaccid paralysis.

      b. Bradycardia, dysarrythmias, electrocardiogram (ECG) changes—prolonged PR interval, wide QRS, tall, tented T wave, and ST depression.

      c. Diarrhea, colicky pain, and nausea and vomiting.

    2. Hypokalemia.

      a. Decreased reflexes, muscle weakness, paresthesias.

      b. Anorexia.

      c. Rapid/weak/irregular pulse, hypotension, mental confusion; if severe—ventricular fibrillation, respiratory paralysis, and cardiac arrest.

      d. ECG changes—flattened T wave, ST depression, U wave elevation.

  E. Treatment for potassium imbalances.

    1. Hyperkalemia—simultaneous hydration and diuresis to maintain urine output at 3 L/day. Intravenous solution of 50% glucose to raise plasma insulin levels, thereby causing an intracellular shift of intracellular K+

and/or sodium bicarbonate, and Kayexalate (orally/rectally) to promote excretion through the feces.

2. Hypokalemia—care given when receiving digitalis; may enhance its sensitivity.
   a. Intravenous potassium chloride supplementation—watch cardiac and renal function.
   b. Oral supplementation with medication and/or diet—fruits (raisins, dates, cantaloupe, bananas, apricots), vegetables (avocado, potato, tomato, carrots), orange juice, and milk.

Assessment

I. Identification of clients at risk for electrolyte imbalances of K+, Na+, Mg++, and Ca++.
   A. Determine risk for specific electrolyte imbalance.
   B. Establish patterns of occurrence—onset (rapid or slow) frequency, associated symptoms, precipitating factors, aggravating factors, and alleviating factors.
   C. Collaborate with physician as to etiology or causes of specific electrolyte imbalance.
   D. Be alert to medications that can potentiate specific electrolyte imbalances.
II. Physical examination.
   A. System review for clinical symptomatology of appropriate imbalance.
      1. Cardiovascular—heart rate (pattern/regularity), blood pressure, ECG if indicated.
      2. Neuromuscular—presence of fatigue, weakness, lethargy, cramping, myalgias and arthralgias, tremors, paresthesias and numbness, bone pain, changes in mentation, personality, concentration; confusion, and/or seizures.
      3. Renal—changes in elimination (increase or decrease in amount or frequency), weight gain, loss, calculi, or edema.
      4. GI—changes in appetite, food intake (amount/type), presence of nausea, vomiting, diarrhea, and/or other insensible losses or anorexia.
   B. Monitor laboratory data specific to electrolyte imbalance (may include other tests not listed as ordered by physician).
      1. Calcium imbalances—serum calcium, corrected serum calcium, albumin, blood urea nitrogen (BUN), creatinine levels, and serum potassium, sodium phosphorus, and blood coagulation levels.
      2. Magnesium imbalances—serum/urine magnesium, BUN, creatinine levels, potassium, calcium, phosphorus, and sodium.
      3. Sodium imbalances—serum/urine sodium, serum/urine osmolality, BUN, creatinine levels, thyroid function tests, potassium, chloride, serum pH, and antidiuretic hormone (ADH) level.
      4. Potassium imbalances—potassium, chloride, pH, sodium, serum glucose, BUN, and creatinine levels.
III. Psychosocial assessment.
   A. Explore anxiety-producing events and coping abilities.
   B. Attempt to identify strengths of client/family.

Nursing Diagnoses

I. Altered nutrition, less than body requirements.
II. Fluid volume deficit (regulatory failure).

III. Fluid volume excess.
IV. Fatigue.
 V. Impaired memory.
VI. Risk for altered tissue perfusion.
VII. Risk for injury.

Outcome Identification

 I. Client describes personal risk for specific electrolyte imbalances related to type of cancer and other conditions that may influence imbalance.
 II. Client participates in measures to minimize the risk of occurrence, severity, and complications of imbalances.
III. Client consumes foods and drinks that are indicated for specific electrolyte imbalance.
IV. Client and family list changes in the condition of the client that require professional assistance in management.
  A. Presence of new symptomatology and/or change in present condition.
  B. Weight loss or gain greater than 10% of body weight.
  C. Presence of signs and symptoms appropriate to the particular imbalance.

Planning and Implementation

 I. Interventions to minimize the risk of occurrence, severity, or complications of electrolyte imbalances.
  A. Individualize client/family teaching according to risk of specific imbalance and according to changes that need to be initiated by client/family in the plan of care.
  B. Modify diet accordingly—increasing or decreasing foods and drinks that may alter electrolyte level.
  C. Encourage compliance with the medication and diet regimen.
  D. Reinforce the need for frequent laboratory sampling.
  E. Provide written instructions and a list of signs and symptoms that need to be observed for and reported.
 II. Interventions to maximize safety.
  A. Assist client with ambulation, use of siderails or assistive devices and appropriate exercise as ordered (active/passive range of motion, isometrics).
  B. Recommend discontinuation of all over-the-counter medications that may interfere with therapeutic plan.
III. Interventions to monitor for complications of electrolyte imbalances.
  A. Observe for signs of dehydration, tremors, personality changes, and profound loss or gain in weight in a short time frame.
  B. Observe for untoward side effects that may be associated with rapid reversal or rebound of electrolyte imbalance.
IV. Interventions to incorporate client/family in care.
  A. Teach home management techniques to avoid or minimize electrolyte imbalances.
  B. Encourage the use of self-care diaries or logs.
  C. Teach importance of reporting critical changes in client condition to the physician, including presence of adverse or intensified pattern of vomiting and diarrhea, presence of mental changes, pain, dehydration, or other pathology.

Evaluation

The oncology nurse systematically and regularly evaluates the client's and/or family's responses to the interventions to determine progress toward the achievement of expected outcomes. Relevant data are collected and actual findings are compared with expected findings. Nursing diagnoses, outcomes, and plans of care are reviewed and revised as necessary.

BIBLIOGRAPHY

Aapro, M.S. (1995). Nutritional support of cancer patients. In M. Peckham, H. Pinedo, & U. Veronesi (eds.). *Oxford Textbook of Oncology* (vol 2). New York: Oxford University Press, p. 339.

Berg, D., & Bean, C. (1994). Anorexia and cachexia. In G.W. Wilkes, K. Ingeversen, & M.B. Burke (eds). *Oncology Nursing Drug Reference.* Boston: Jones & Bartlett, p. 339.

Brock, D., Fox, S., Gosling, G., et al. (1993). Testicular cancer. *Semin Oncol Nurs 9*(4), 224–236.

Camp-Sorrell D. Chemotherapy: Toxicity management. In S.L. Groenwald, M. Goodman, M. Frogge, C. Yarbo (eds.). *Cancer Nursing: Principles and Practice* (3rd ed.). Boston: Jones & Bartlett, pp. 331–365.

Clark, J.D., McGee, R.F., & Preston, R. (1992). Nursing management of responses in the cancer experience. In J.C. Clark & R.F. McGee (eds.). *Core Curriculum for Oncology Nursing* (2nd ed.). Philadelphia: W.B. Saunders, pp. 67–155.

DiSipio, L.B. (1995). Relieving xerostomia from radiation therapy. *Oncol Nurs Forum 22*(8), 1287.

Dodd, M.J., Larson, P.J., & Dibble, S.L. (1996). Randomized clinical trial of chlorhexidine versus placebo for prevention of oral mucositis in patients receiving chemotherapy. *Oncol Nurs Forum 23*(6), 921–927.

Goodman, M., Ladd, L.A., & Purl, S. (1993). Integumentary and mucous membrane alterations. In S.L. Groenwald, M. Goodman, M. Frogge, C. Yarbo (eds.). *Cancer Nursing: Principles and Practice* (3rd ed.). Boston: Jones & Bartlett, pp. 734–800.

Grant. M.M., & Rivera, L.M. (1995). Anorexia, cachexia, and dysphagia: The symptom experience. *Semin Oncol Nurs 11*(4), 258, 266–271.

Hanks, W., & Maguire, P.J. Pain and symptom control in advanced cancer. In M. Peckham, H. Pinedo, & U. Veronesi (eds.). *Oxford Textbook of Oncology* (vol. 2). New York: Oxford University Press, pp. 2424–2425.

Iwamoto, R.R., & Hockenberry-Eaton, M. (1995). Managing treatment related side effects of nausea and vomiting. *Cancer Pract 3*(4):203–206.

Lang-Klummer, J.M. (1993). Hypercalcemia. In S.L. Groenwald, M. Goodman, M. Frogge, C. Yarbo (eds.). *Cancer Nursing: Principles and Practice* (3rd ed.). Boston: Jones & Bartlett, pp. 644–661.

Lambersky, B.C., & Posner, M.C. (1994). Gastrointestinal toxicities. In J.M. Kirkwood, M.T. Lotze, J.M. Yasko (eds.). *Current Cancer Therapeutics.* Philadelphia: Current Medicine, pp. 254–261.

Lindsey, A.M. (1993). Hormonal disturbances. In S.L. Groenwald, M. Goodman, M. Frogge, C. Yarbo (eds.). *Cancer Nursing: Principles and Practice* (3rd ed.). Boston: Jones & Bartlett, pp. 662–674.

Lloyd, M.E. (1995). Oral medicine concerns of the BMT patient. In P.C. Buchsel, & M.B. Whedon (eds.). *Bone Marrow Transplantation: Administrative and Clinical Strategies.* Boston: Jones & Bartlett, p. 265.

Maxwell, M.B. (1993). Malignant effusions and edemas. In S.L. Groenwald, M. Goodman, M. Frogge, C. Yarbo (eds.). *Cancer Nursing: Principles and Practice* (3rd ed.). Boston: Jones & Bartlett, pp. 675–695.

McDermott, M. (1995). DAB: A three-drug combination provides alternative to 5-HT3 receptor drugs. *Oncol Nurs Forum 22*(4), 718.

McGuire, D.B., Altomonte, V., & Peterson, D.E., et al. (1993). Patterns of mucositis and pain in patients receiving preparative chemotherapy and bone marrow transplantation. *Oncol Nurs Forum 20*(10), 1493–1502.

Nelson, J.K., Moxness, K.E., Jensen, M.D., et al. (1994). Nutritional management of disease and disorders for adults. In J.K. Nelson, K.E. Moxness, M.D. Jensen, & C.F. Gastineau (eds.). *Mayo Clinic Diet Manual: A Handbook of Nutrition Practices* (7th ed.). St. Louis: C.V. Mosby, pp. 293–299.

Nelson, J.K., Moxness, K.E., Jensen, M.D., et al. (1994). Hospital diet progressions. In J.K. Nelson, K.E. Moxness, M.D. Jensen, & C.F. Gastineau (eds.). *Mayo Clinic Diet Manual: A Handbook of Nutrition Practices* (7th ed.). St. Louis: C.V. Mosby, p. 93.

Rhodes, V.A., Johnson, M.H., & McDaniel, R.W. (1995). Nausea, vomiting and retching: The management of the symptom experience. *Semin Oncol Nurs 11*(4), 256–265.

Rhodes, V.A., McDaniel, R.W., Simms, S.G., et al. (1995). Nurses' perceptions of antiemetic effectiveness. *Oncol Nurs Forum 22*(8), 1243–1252.

Skipper, A., Szeluga, D.J., & Groenwald, S.L. (1993). Nutritional disturbances. In S.L. Groenwald , M. Goodman, M. Frogge, C. Yarbo (eds). *Cancer Nursing: Principles and Practice* (3rd ed.). Boston: Jones & Bartlett, pp. 620–643.

Tombes, M.B., & Gallucci, B. *(*1993). The effects of hydrogen peroxide rinses on the normal oral mucosa. *Nurs Res 42*(6), 332–337.

Valdez, I.H., Wolff, A., Atkinson, J.C., et al. (1993). Use of pilocarpine during head and neck radiation therapy to reduce xerostomia and salivary dysfunction. *Cancer 71*(5), 1848–1851.

Van Oosterom, A.T., Dirix, L.Y., & Van Rijswijk, R. (1995). Metabolic disturbances. In Peckham, M., Pinedo, H., & Veronesi, U. (eds). *Oxford Textbook of Oncology (*1st ed., vol. 2). New York: Oxford University Press, p. 2207.

Alterations in Elimination

Annette W. Kuck, RN, MS, OCN
Elisa Ricciardi, RN, MS, CETN

INCONTINENCE

Theory

I. Definition.

A. Urinary incontinence—involuntary loss of urine that is sufficient to be a problem.

1. Stress—involuntary loss of urine during laughing, coughing, sneezing, or other physical activities that increase abdominal pressure.

2. Urge—involuntary loss of urine associated with an abrupt and strong desire to void.

3. Reflex—involuntary loss of urine with no sensation of urge voiding or bladder fullness.

4. Functional—state in which an individual experiences incontinence because of difficulty in reaching or inability to reach the toilet before urination.

5. Total—continuous loss of urine without distention or awareness of bladder fullness.

6. Urinary retention—chronic inability to void followed by involuntary voiding (overflow incontinence) caused by overdistention of the bladder.

B. Bowel incontinence—a change in normal bowel habits characterized by involuntary passage of stool at an inappropriate time and place.

II. Risk factors.

A. Disease-related.

1. Loss of ability to inhibit bladder or rectal contractions in clients with lesions in the cortex as a result of a cerebral vascular accident, multiple sclerosis, Parkinson disease, or primary or metastatic tumor.

2. Loss of bladder and bowel reflex contractions, which can occur in clients with suprasacral lesions of the spinal cord, spinal cord tumors, compression following radical pelvic surgery, or diabetic neuropathy.

3. Loss of sphincter competency, which affects the bladder's ability to store urine. The condition may be acquired after radical prostatectomy, radiation treatment, trauma, or sacral cord lesions.

4. Impaired or loss of sensation of the bladder caused by inflammation, chronic infection, and prolonged bladder distention.

5. Obstruction of the bladder caused by tumor, prostatic hyperplasia, or fecal impaction.

6. Immobility commonly associated with chronic degenerative disease.
7. Endocrine conditions that cloud the sensorium and induce diuresis, such as hyperglycemia and diabetes insipidus.
8. Inadequate rectal capacity or compliance.
9. Loss of functional ability, which often accompanies cognitive impairment in clients with central nervous system metastases, Alzheimer's disease, and dementia.

B. Treatment-related.
1. Surgical intervention that disrupts neural pathways, which may occur with abdominal perineal resection or radical prostatectomy.
2. Effects of radiation therapy on bladder and bowel can be an inflammatory reaction or can result in fibrosis or stenosis.
3. Chemotherapy agents, such as vincristine and ifosfamide, that cause neurotoxic side effects.
4. Fistula formation as a complication of surgery or radiation therapy.
5. Medications including anticholinergics, diuretics, narcotics, sedatives, hypnotics, tranquilizers, and laxatives.
6. Complications associated with indwelling catheters include urinary tract infections, urinary stones, epididymitis, scrotal abscess, urethritis, urethral erosion, fistula formation, and bladder cancer.

III. Principles of medical management.
A. Treatment of underlying condition affecting incontinence.
B. Surgical treatment such as bladder neck suspension, pubovaginal sling, artificial urinary sphincter, rectal sphincter repair, or fecal or urinary diversion.
C. Pharmacologic agents including anticholinergic, cholinergic, alpha-adrenergic blocking agents and estrogen to treat stress, urge, reflex, and overflow incontinence.
D. Bulking agents for bowel incontinence.
E. Dietary modifications by increasing fiber and fluid intake.
F. Bladder and or bowel training programs (e.g., biofeedback, electrostimulation, and intermittent catheterization).

IV. Potential sequelae of prolonged incontinence.
A. Perianal skin irritation and excoriation.
B. Changes in role relationship and lifestyle.
C. Embarrassment that may prevent search for medical attention.

Assessment

I. History.
A. Personal history
1. Cognitive ability.
2. Motivation to self-care in toileting.
3. Manual dexterity and mobility.
4. Living arrangements.
5. Identification of caregiver and degree of caregiver involvement.
6. Prescription and nonprescription medications.
B. Past and present patterns of elimination.
1. Precipitants of incontinence—caffeine and alcohol consumption, physical activity, surgery, trauma, and recent illnesses.
2. Urinary tract symptoms—nocturia, dysuria, hesitancy, enuresis, straining, poor stream.

    3. Duration of incontinence.

    4. Frequency and amount of continence and incontinence urinations.

    5. Previous treatments and its effects.

    6. Bowel habits and laxative use.

  II. Physical findings.

    A. Presence of abdominal masses.

    B. Palpation of full bladder.

    C. Pelvic organ prolapse.

    D. Presence of incontinence, odor, and perineal skin irritation or breakdown.

 III. Diagnostic testing.

    A. Urinalysis, culture and sensitivity to assess for hematuria, bacteruria, and glucosuria.

    B. Stool culture and sensitivity to rule out infection and *Clostridium difficile* infection.

    C. Presence and amount of post-voiding residual urine.

    D. Urodynamic and imaging studies (e.g., cystometrogram, voiding cystourethrogram, electromyogram to evaluate micturition and bladder filling and storing function).

    E. Cystoscopy to identify site of obstruction.

    F. Sigmoidoscopy, colonoscopy, barium enema, and anorectal physiology testing to examine the colon and rectum for the presence of disease and to test sphincter control.

Nursing Diagnoses

  I. Urinary incontinence.

    A. Incontinence, reflex.

    B. Incontinence, stress.

    C. Incontinence, urge.

    D. Incontinence, functional.

    E. Incontinence, total.

    F. Urinary retention.

  II. Bowel incontinence.

 III. Self-esteem disturbance.

 IV. Social isolation.

  V. Sleep pattern disturbance.

Outcome Identification

  I. Client describes appropriate actions when changes in elimination occur, such as urinary or fecal incontinence.

  II. Client recognizes the importance of adequate elimination for physiologic integrity.

 III. Client identifies factors that affect elimination such as diet, stress, physical activity, and neurogenic medications.

 IV. Client contacts an appropriate health care team member to determine etiology of incontinence and identify alternative measures for managing incontinence.

Planning and Implementation

  I. Interventions to minimize the risk of occurrence, severity, or complications of incontinence.

A. Determine cause of or contributing factors of incontinence.
B. Reduce environmental barriers to using toileting facilities.
C. Provide thorough perianal skin care.
   1. Assess perianal skin daily.
   2. Clean area after every voiding or bowel movement with soft washcloth and perianal cleanser, rinse thoroughly, and pat dry.
   3. Apply moisture barrier ointment or skin barrier after each incontinent episode.
   4. Apply a fecal drainage pouch if there are continuous or frequent episodes of bowel incontinence.
D. Implement appropriate behavioral techniques.
   1. Establish a routine schedule for voiding such as every 2 to 3 hours (habit training).
   2. Ask the client on a regular basis about voiding (prompt voiding).
   3. Teach the client to suppress the urge to void to rebuild bladder capacity (bladder retraining).
   4. Teach the client to exercise pelvic muscles twice a day.
E. Monitor intake, output, urine concentration, and intake/output ratio daily.
F. Design a bowel training program.
   1. Establish a consistent time for elimination each day.
   2. Use techniques to stimulate bowel evacuation such as digital stimulation, suppository.
   3. Monitor bowel elimination daily.
   4. Remove fecal impaction, if present.
   5. Recognize that bowel evacuation should occur when there is a sensation of rectal distention.
G. Determine present functional level and physical limitations.
H. Use internal and external catheters as a last method to manage incontinence.
II. Interventions to maintain optimal hydration and adequate nutrition.
A. Increase fluid intake to 2000 to 3000 mL/day, unless contraindicated.
B. Decrease fluid intake after 7:00 PM and provide minimal fluids during the night.
C. Reduce intake of caffeine beverages such as coffee, tea, and colas, and reduce intake of alcohol.
D. Avoid foods that provide a laxative effect or are gas-producing.
E. Include foods that increase the bulk of the stool.
III. Interventions to monitor the response of the client to symptom management.
A. Monitor subjective reports of the client and family of changes in the pattern of incontinence.
B. Monitor the client's compliance to the incontinence management program.
C. Monitor effectiveness of measures implemented to manage incontinence.
IV. Interventions to incorporate client and family in care.
A. Teach pelvic muscle exercises.
B. Teach proper use of devices to control incontinence.
C. Teach toileting programs (e.g., prompted voiding, bladder retraining).
D. Teach appropriate use of stool softeners, suppositories, and enemas.
E. Discuss the importance of increasing bulk and fluid intake in the diet.
F. Instruct on critical factors that needed to be reported to the physician.
   1. Signs and symptoms of urinary tract infections and fecal impaction.
   2. Changes in patterns of elimination.

Evaluation

The oncology nurse systematically and regularly evaluates the client's and/or family's responses to interventions to determine progress toward the achievement of expected outcomes. Relevant data are collected and actual findings are compared with expected findings. Nursing diagnoses, outcomes, and plans of care are reviewed and revised as needed.

CONSTIPATION

Theory

I. Definition—the infrequent passage of hard stool, often associated with abdominal and rectal pain. May also be associated with a feeling of incomplete evacuation following defecation.
   A. Primary—results from extrinsic factors such as decreased physical activity, lack of time or privacy for defecation, or low-fiber diet.
   B. Secondary—results from pathologic processes such as bowel obstruction and spinal cord compression or metabolic effects of hypercalcemia, hypokalemia, and hypothyroidism.
   C. Iatrogenic—follows use of pharmacologic agents such as analgesic opiates, chemotherapeutic agents, anticonvulsants, and some psychotropic medications.
II. Risk factors.
   A. Disease-related.
      1. Obstruction of bowel by tumor.
      2. Fluid and electrolyte imbalances—dehydration, hypercalcemia, and hypokalemia.
      3. Decreased physical activity and/or immobility.
      4. Mental confusion.
   B. Treatment-related.
      1. Manipulation of intestines during surgery.
      2. Surgical trauma to neurogenic pathways to intestines and/or rectum.
      3. Neurotoxic effects of cancer chemotherapeutic agents such as vincristine and vinblastine (Velban).
      4. Nutritional deficiencies such as decreased fiber, roughage, and fluid intake.
      5. Side effects of pharmacologic agents such as narcotics, analgesics, cholinergics, and antacids.
   C. Situational.
      1. Lack of privacy.
      2. Interference with usual bowel program.
      3. Failure to respond to defecation reflex because of pain, fatigue, social activities, or inability to reach the toilet.
      4. Depression, decreased physical activity, and treatment with anticholinergic medications.
III. Principles of medical management.
   A. Surgical correction of obstructive disease.
   B. Correction of fluid and electrolyte imbalances.
   C. Enemas or irrigations.
   D. Medications such as laxatives, stool softeners, and suppositories.
   E. Increased fiber in diet.

IV. Potential sequelae of constipation.
   A. Fecal impaction (also called dyschezia or terminal reservoir syndrome).
   B. Paralytic ileus.
   C. Intestinal obstruction.
   D. Laxative dependence.

Assessment

 I. History.
   A. Presence of risk factors.
   B. History of defining characteristics of constipation.
      1. Change in usual patterns of bowel elimination such as decreased frequency, hard stool, abdominal cramping, and increased use of laxatives.
      2. Date of last bowel movement.
      3. Change in factors contributing to bowel elimination such as activity level, fluid intake, dietary fiber intake, and/or laxative use.
      4. History of constipation and/or laxative use.
      5. Anxiety regarding bowel patterns.
      6. Perception of incomplete evacuation following defecation.
   C. Gastrointestinal symptoms—nausea, vomiting, and anorexia.
   D. Pattern of occurrence of constipation—onset; frequency; severity-associated symptoms; precipitating, aggravating, and alleviating factors.
   E. Perceived effectiveness of self-care measures to relieve constipation.
   F. Perceived impact of constipation on comfort, activities of daily living, and mood.
   G. History of rectal fissures or abscesses.
 II. Physical findings.
   A. Decreased or absent bowel sounds.
   B. Flatulence.
   C. Abdominal distention.
   D. Fecal impaction.
   E. Loss of appetite or early satiety.

Nursing Diagnoses

  I. Constipation.
 II. Constipation, colonic.
III. Constipation, perceived.

Outcome Identification

  I. Client describes appropriate actions when changes in elimination occur, such as constipation.
 II. Client recognizes the importance of adequate elimination for physiologic integrity.
III. Client identifies and manages factors that may affect elimination such as diet, stress, physical activity, and neurogenic conditions.
 IV. Client contacts an appropriate health team member when unable to relieve constipation through self-care measures.
  V. Client returns to normal pattern of bowel functioning.

Planning and Implementation

  I. Interventions to minimize risk and severity of constipation.

    A. Institute measures to maintain bowel elimination patterns.
        1. Encourage at least 3000 mL of fluid intake per day, unless contraindicated.
        2. Modify diet as tolerated to include high-fiber foods and roughage, with fresh fruits, vegetables, whole grains, and dried beans.
        3. Maintain or increase physical activity level.
        4. Establish a daily bowel program.
    B. Implement effective interventions usually used by client to alleviate constipation that are not contraindicated by health status.
    C. Implement orders for laxatives or enemas for relief of constipation.
    D. Initiate a prophylactic bowel regimen with narcotic or vinca alkaloid therapy (see Table 7–1).
  II. Interventions to maximize client safety.
    A. Check for impaction if symptoms warrant, such as decreased or absent bowel sounds, abdominal distention, and loss of appetite.
    B. Avoid digital rectal examinations if client is neutropenic and/or thrombocytopenic.
 III. Interventions to monitor for complications related to constipation.
    A. Assess for interference with deep breathing related to abdominal distention.
    B. Monitor indicators of social withdrawal related to flatulence and a focus on bowel elimination.
    C. Monitor untoward responses to symptom management.
        1. Abdominal cramping or diarrhea with laxatives.
        2. Rectal emptying and aggravation of constipation with enemas.
        3. Dehydration or decreased fluid intake, which reduces the effectiveness of stool softeners.
    D. Report critical changes to the physician.
        1. Abdominal distention.
        2. Fecal impaction.
        3. Bleeding.
        4. Absence of bowel sounds.
 IV. Implement strategies to enhance adaptation and rehabilitation.
    A. Encourage avoidance of laxative abuse with a combination of laxatives and stool softeners.
    B. Emphasize dietary control of constipation with foods high in fiber such as celery, bran, and whole wheat breads.
    C. Advise adoption of a daily fluid intake of 3000 mL, unless contraindicated.
    D. Advise adoption of a daily bowel program.
        1. Daily schedule for evacuation such as after meals when gastrocolic reflexes are active.
        2. Privacy.
        3. Medications such as stool softeners or expanders or natural laxative mixtures: avoidance of pharmaceutical laxatives if possible.
        4. Enemas or irrigation procedures if necessary.
  V. Interventions to incorporate client and family in care.
    A. Teach to control constipation through fluid intake, dietary control, and activity level.
    B. Inform of hazards of laxative dependence.
    C. Instruct to limit use of gas-producing foods such as cabbage, beans, green peppers, and onions in meal planning.

Evaluation

The oncology nurse systematically and regularly evaluates the client's and/or family's responses to interventions to determine progress toward the achievement of expected outcomes. Relevant data are collected and actual findings are compared with expected findings. Nursing diagnoses, outcomes, and plans of care are reviewed and revised as necessary.

DIARRHEA

Theory

I. Definition—an increase in the quantity, frequency, or fluid content of stool that is different than the usual pattern of bowel elimination.
   A. Classifications.
      1. Large volume—results from a larger-than-usual amount of water, intestinal secretion, or both in the intestine.
      2. Small volume—results from excessive intestinal mobility.
   B. Pathology—may be defined as acute or chronic, depending on underlying pathology.
   C. Mechanisms.
      1. Osmotic—unabsorbable substances in intestine draw water into intestinal lumen by osmosis, increasing the weight and volume of stool. Lactulose deficiency causes this type of diarrhea.
      2. Secretory—intestinal mucosa secretes excessive amounts of fluid and electrolytes. Bacteria such as *Escherichia coli* or *Clostridium difficile* can cause this type of diarrhea.
      3. Motile—caused by inflammatory disorder of the bowel, such as inflammatory bowel disease or radiation proctitis.
II. Risk factors.
   A. Disease-related.
      1. Obstruction of bowel from intrinsic or extrinsic tumor.
      2. Intestinal bacteria or viruses.
      3. Graft-versus-host disease in which immunocompetent cells of the allogeneic donor marrow recognize the normal gastrointestinal cells as "foreign" and initiate an immune reaction that leads to cell destruction of target tissues in the gut.
      4. Intestinal carcinoid tumors with liver metastases.
      5. Food intolerance or allergies.
   B. Treatment-related.
      1. Surgical resection of significant portions of bowel can cause fluid malabsorption syndrome.
      2. Radiation therapy to abdominal area causes increased cellular destruction in bowel lumen and increased intestinal motility.
      3. Chemotherapeutic agents can cause increased cellular destruction on bowel lumen and can heighten intestinal motility.
      4. Medications such as antibiotics, antacids, or laxatives.
      5. Nutritional therapies such as tube feedings and dietary supplements.
      6. Fecal impaction can create paradoxical diarrhea.
   C. Lifestyle-related.
      1. Increased stress and anxiety in presence of inadequate coping strategies.
      2. Changes in usual dietary habits such as increases in dietary fiber or other foods containing natural laxative properties.

III. Principles of medical management.
   A. Antidiarrheal or antispasmodic medications such as bismuth subsalicylate (Pepto-Bismol), loperamide (Imodium), or activated attapulgite (Kaopectate).
   B. Modification of associated therapy such radiation, chemotherapy, nutritional supplements, or antibiotics.
   C. Treatment of associated conditions such as *C. difficile* infection or graft-versus-host disease.
   D. Decompression or surgery for bowel obstruction.
   E. Manual disimpaction if white blood cell and platelet counts permit.
IV. Potential sequelae of prolonged diarrhea.
   A. Dehydration.
   B. Electrolyte imbalances such as hypokalemia or hyponatremia.
   C. Impaired skin integrity of perineal area.
   D. Decreased social interaction.

Assessment

I. History.
   A. Review of previous and current therapy for cancer.
   B. Review of prescription and nonprescription medications.
   C. Usual bowel pattern—frequency, color, amount, odor, and consistency of stool.
   D. Recent changes in factors contributing to usual bowel elimination patterns.
      1. Increased levels of stress.
      2. Dietary changes that increase bowel motility such as addition of fiber and roughage, fruit juices, coffee, alcohol, fried foods, or fatty foods.
   E. Known food or medication intolerance or allergies.
   F. Presence of flatus, cramping, abdominal pain, urgency to defecate, recent weight loss, decreased urinary output of 500 mL less than intake.
II. Physical examination.
   A. Hyperactive bowel sounds.
   B. Hard stool in rectum.
   C. Perineal skin irritation.
III. Psychosocial examination.
   A. Presence of fear.
   B. Presence of anxiety.
   C. Complaints of isolation.

Nursing Diagnoses

I. Diarrhea.
II. Risk for impaired tissue integrity.
III. Risk for fluid volume deficit.

Outcome Identification

I. Client describes appropriate actions when changes in elimination occur, such as diarrhea.
II. Client recognizes the importance of adequate elimination for physiologic integrity.
III. Client identifies and manages factors that may affect elimination such as diet, stress, physical activity, and neurogenic conditions.

IV. Client contacts an appropriate health care team member when diarrhea is severe, prolonged, or uncontrollable with self-care measures.

Planning and Implementation

I. Interventions to minimize risk of occurrence and severity of diarrhea.
   A. Modify dietary plan to avoid foods the client cannot tolerate.
   B. Decrease fiber and roughage.
   C. Encourage smaller meals eaten more frequently.
II. Implement strategies to decrease bowel motility.
   A. Serve foods and liquids at room temperature.
   B. Avoid coffee and alcohol.
   C. Avoid spicy, fried, or fatty foods and food additives.
   D. Teach strategies such as relaxation, distraction, or imagery to modify stress response.
III. Interventions to maximize client safety.
   A. Monitor level of weakness and fatigue.
   B. Provide assistance with ambulation and activities of daily living as indicated.
IV. Interventions to monitor for complications related to diarrhea.
   A. Assess the character of bowel movement at each stool or with a change in symptoms.
   B. Assess the perineal area every 8 hours or with a change in symptoms.
   C. Monitor intake and output ratio.
   D. Monitor for subtle changes in client affect, neuromuscular responses, activity level, and cognitive status as cues for potential electrolyte imbalances.
   E. Monitor changes in skin turgor.
   F. Report significant changes in condition or symptomatology to the physician.
V. Interventions to incorporate the client and family in care.
   A. Teach a perineal hygiene program to include cleansing perineal area with mild soap, rinsing thoroughly, patting area dry, and applying a skin barrier after each bowel movement.
   B. Teach dietary modifications to minimize diarrhea.
   C. Teach signs and symptoms related to complications of diarrhea to report to a member of the health care team.

Evaluation

The oncology nurse systematically and regularly evaluates the client's and/or family's responses to interventions to determine progress toward the achievement of expected outcomes. Relevant data are collected and actual findings are compared with expected findings. Nursing diagnoses, outcomes, and plans of care are reviewed and revised as necessary.

BOWEL OBSTRUCTION

Theory

I. Definition—narrowing of the intestinal lumen or interference with peristalsis.
   A. Mechanical obstruction—occurs in small intestines and accounts for 90% of all obstructions.
      1. Causes.
         a. Extrinsic lesions—adhesions of the peritoneum, hernias, and volvulus (twisting of the intestines).

    b. Intrinsic lesions—benign or malignant tumors, intussusception (telescoping of the intestines), an ischemic or inflammatory process that involves the bowel wall (such as inflammatory bowel disease or diverticulitis) and produces strictures, narrows the intestinal lumen, and impairs transit.

    c. Objects blocking the intestinal lumen, such as foreign bodies and fecal or barium impaction.

  2. Types.

    a. Simple—lumen is occluded in only one place and blood flow to abdomen is unchanged.

    b. Closed loop—lumen is blocked in two places.

    c. Strangulation—lumen is blocked and blood flow to some or all of the obstructed segment is restricted.

B. Nonmechanical obstruction.

  1. Definition—intestinal lumen is patent but neuromuscular dysfunction or a lack of intestinal blood flow inhibits peristalsis. Condition also called ileus or functional or adynamic obstruction.

  2. Causes.

    a. Intraabdominal.

      (1) Reflex inhibition associated with laparotomy and other abdominal surgeries or with trauma. The more the bowel is manipulated in surgery, the longer an ileus lasts. The length of surgery is not a factor in the development of ileus.

      (2) Inflammatory conditions such as peritonitis and pancreatitis.

      (3) Bowel ischemia as a result of mesenteric artery emboli or venous thrombosis.

    b. Extraabdominal.

      (1) Reflex inhibition related to fractures of the ribs, spine, or pelvis; kidney surgery; myocardial infarction; pneumonia; pulmonary embolus; electrolyte imbalances; metabolic imbalances such as septicemia.

      (2) Pharmacologic reflex inhibition can be caused by anticholinergics, ganglionic blockers, opiates, and chemotherapeutic agents.

      (3) Hypokalemia can cause slowed peristalsis leading to ileus.

C. Location.

  1. Small intestine obstructions occur due to:

    a. Postoperative intraabdominal adhesions. They can entrap a loop of intestine and contract causing strangulation. Adhesions can develop a few days postoperatively or many years later.

    b. Nonsurgical adhesions following an infection such as peritonitis or following radiation therapy. Nonsurgical adhesions can occur at any time following the infection or completion of radiation therapy.

    c. Inguinal and femoral hernias.

    d. Miscellaneous conditions such as cancer, telescoping, and inflammatory bowel disease.

  2. Large bowel obstructions occur most often in the sigmoid colon and are caused by:

    a. Cancer.

    b. Volvulus.

    c. Diverticulitis.

II. Risk factors.
   A. Disease-related.
      1. Obstruction of bowel by tumor. Most common tumors are ovarian cancer and colorectal cancers.
      2. Hernia.
      3. Inflammatory bowel disease.
      4. Gallstones.
      5. Peptic ulcers.
      6. Pancreatitis.
      7. Diverticular disease.
   B. Treatment-related.
      1. Manipulation of intestines during surgery.
      2. Surgical trauma to neurogenic pathways to intestines and/or rectum.
      3. Previous intestinal obstruction.
      4. Radiation therapy to abdominal area.
   C. Situational—ingestion of a foreign body.
III. Principles of medical management.
   A. Surgical correction of obstructive disease.
   B. Nothing by mouth (NPO).
   C. Abdominal decompression.
      1. Nasogastric suction.
      2. Percutaneous gastrostomy.
      3. Enema.
      4. Rectal tube.
      5. Sigmoidoscopy.
      6. Colonoscopy.
   D. Correction of fluid and electrolyte imbalances.
   E. Parenteral nutrition.
IV. Potential sequelae of bowel obstruction.
   A. Dehydration.
   B. Peritonitis.
   C. Bowel perforation.
   D. Hypotension.
   E. Hypovolemic or septic shock.

Assessment

I. History.
   A. Presence of risk factors.
   B. Symptoms.
      1. Abdominal pain and intestinal colic from intestinal stretching and pressure of peristalsis as the bowel tries to push its contents past the obstruction; can help identify the obstruction's type and severity.
         a. Small intestine obstructions—intermittent, crampy pain in the middle to upper abdomen that is temporarily relieved by vomiting.
         b. Large intestine obstructions—persistent crampy pain in the lower abdomen.
         c. Mechanical obstructions—crampy and spasmodic.
         d. Nonmechanical obstructions—diffuse, constant, and less intense pain that can be described as pressure or fullness.
         e. Partial obstructions—crampy pain after eating along with mild to moderate hypomotility.

   f. Complete bowel obstruction—pain intensifies and comes in waves or spasms.
   g. Strangulation—constant, intense pain that is intensified with movement.
2. Nausea and vomiting.
   a. Gastric outlet obstruction—sour emesis that is not bile-colored.
   b. Proximal small intestine obstruction—rapid onset, bitter, bile-stained emesis that may be projectile.
   c. Distal small intestine obstruction or colonic obstruction with an incompetent ileocecal valve—orange-brown malodorous feculent emesis.
3. Anorexia.
4. Constipation—may experience lack of bowel movements and flatus or may have paradoxical diarrhea (if partial blockage exists).
C. Past and present patterns of elimination.
   1. Any recent changes in stool consistency or bowel habits.
   2. Date and time of last bowel movement.
   3. Use of antacids, laxatives, or enemas.
D. Miscellaneous.
   1. Current medications.
   2. Endocrine history.
   3. Immunologic history.
   4. Diet.
II. Physical findings.
   A. Abdominal distention.
      1. The lower the obstruction, the longer it lasts; the more complete it is, the more severe the distention will be.
      2. Baseline measurement of abdominal girth should be obtained.
      3. Board-like abdomen may indicate peritonitis.
   B. Abnormal bowel sounds.
      1. Intermittent borborygmi (loud prolonged gurgles of hyperperistalsis).
      2. Mechanical obstruction—proximal to obstruction, high-pitched, tinkling, or hyperactive bowel sounds that may be heard in clusters or rushes. Distal to the obstruction, bowel sounds are hypoactive or absent.
      3. Nonmechanical—hypoactive, low-pitched gurgles or weak tinkles may be heard. Absent bowel sounds may indicate a paralytic ileus.
III. Diagnostic tests.
   A. Abdominal radiographs.
   B. Chest radiographs.
   C. Computed tomography scans of the abdomen.
   D. Contrast media studies.
      1. Oral barium—is not used until colonic obstruction is ruled out or if bowel perforation is suspected.
      2. Barium enema—is used to evaluate colonic obstruction.
   E. Endoscopy.

Nursing Diagnoses

I. Acute pain.
II. Risk for fluid volume deficit.

III. Risk for altered tissue perfusion.
IV. Risk for infection.
 V. Risk for altered nutrition, less than body requirements.

Outcome Identification

  I. Client describes appropriate action when changes in elimination occur such as bowel obstruction.
 II. Client recognizes the importance of adequate elimination for physiologic integrity.
III. Client identifies and manages factors that affect elimination such as diet, stress, physical activity, and neurogenic conditions.
IV. Client contacts an appropriate health care team member when symptoms of bowel obstruction occur.

Planning and Implementation

  I. Interventions to minimize risk and severity of bowel obstruction.
    A. Promote comfort.
      1. Pharmacologic.
        a. Opiate analgesics.
        b. Analgesic adjuncts.
        c. Smooth muscle relaxants.
        d. Antiemetics.
        e. Corticosteroids.
      2. Environmental.
        a. Relaxing environment.
        b. Back rubs or massage.
        c. Position on side and support with pillows.
    B. Administer fluid and electrolyte replacement therapy.
    C. Provide frequent oral care.
      1. Use moistened sponge sticks.
      2. Avoid lemon or glycerin swabs.
    D. Ambulate early and to the client's tolerance.
    E. Encourage deep breathing exercises.
 II. Interventions to maximize client safety.
    A. Elevate head of bed 45 degrees to improve ventilation and avoid aspiration.
    B. Provide care of nasogastric tube.
      1. Assess pressure around nostrils every shift.
      2. Apply a water-soluble lubricant to nasal mucosa.
      3. Irrigate the tube with normal saline.
III. Interventions to monitor for complications related to bowel obstruction.
    A. Assess for signs and symptoms of dehydration—dry mouth and lips, poor skin turgor, decreased urinary output.
    B. Assess for interference with deep breathing related to abdominal distention.
    C. Assess for signs and symptoms of peritonitis—board-like abdomen, increased pain on movement, shallow respirations, and tachycardia.
    D. Measure abdominal girth every shift.
    E. Monitor intake and output ratio, including gastric output.
    F. Monitor key laboratory values.
      1. Electrolytes—sodium, potassium, chloride levels.
      2. Renal function tests—blood urea nitrogen (BUN), creatinine levels.

3. Complete blood count—hemoglobin, hematocrit levels.
4. Arterial blood gases—bicarbonate level, arterial blood pH.
5. Serum enzymes—amylase, alkaline phosphatase, creatine kinase, and lactate dehydrogenase (LD) levels.

IV. Interventions to incorporate the client and family in care.
   A. Explain all treatments and their rationale.
   B. Instruct the client on deep breathing exercises.
   C. Instruct the client on interventions that reduce anxiety and provide comfort, such as relaxation techniques, mental imagery, and music.
   D. Instruct the client to breathe through the nose to decrease the amount of air swallowed.
   E. Teach signs and symptoms of bowel obstruction to report to the health care team.
   F. Teach signs and symptoms of infection to report to the health care team.

V. Report critical changes in client assessment parameters to the physician.
   A. Fever and chills.
   B. Local intense constant pain.
   C. Absence of bowel sounds after full 5 minutes of auscultation.
   D. Muscle guarding, rigidity, and rebound tenderness.
   E. Sudden worsening of client's condition.

Evaluation

The oncology nurse systematically and regularly evaluates the client's and/or family's responses to interventions to determine progress toward the achievement of expected outcomes. Relevant data are collected and actual findings are compared with expected findings. Nursing diagnoses, outcomes, and plans of care are reviewed and revised as necessary.

OSTOMIES, URINARY DIVERSIONS

Theory

I. Diversions.
   A. Fecal.
      1. Colostomy is a surgical creation of an opening between the colon and the abdominal wall.
         a. Types.
            (1) Temporary is indicated for bowel decompression in the presence of an obstructing tumor or fistulas involving the colon or rectum.
            (2) Permanent is indicated when the distal bowel, rectum, and anus are removed because of rectal cancer.
         b. Location of colostomy determines consistency and volume of output.
            (1) Cecostomy or ascending type produces semifluid to mushy stool that contains residual enzymes and occurs throughout the day.
            (2) Transverse type drains mushy stool at irregular intervals, usually after meals, which contain no enzymes.
            (3) Descending or sigmoid type produces soft to formed stool and can be regulated by irrigation.
         c. Stomas may be identified by the type of surgical construction: end, loop, or double-barrel.
            (1) End stoma is constructed by dividing the bowel and bringing the

    proximal end of the bowel through an opening in the abdominal wall.

        (a) Distal bowel segment is removed in abdominal perineal resection.

        (b) Distal bowel segment is sutured closed and left in place, called a Hartmann pouch, and continues to produce mucus from the rectum.

    (2) Loop stoma is constructed by bringing a loop of bowel out through an incision and stabilized on the abdomen.

        (a) Usually created in the transverse loop.

        (b) Temporary procedure to relieve an obstruction or as palliation in terminal cancer.

    (3) Double-barrel indicates two stomas side by side or apart from one another.

        (a) Distal stoma often referred to as a mucous fistula and produces mucus.

        (b) Proximal stoma produces stool.

  B. Urinary.

    1. Ileal conduit.

      a. Created from segment of small bowel. As the proximal end is sutured closed, the distal end is brought out through the abdominal wall. Stoma is created and the ureters are implanted into the small bowel segment.

      b. Commonly performed with radical cystectomy or radical cystoprostatectomy.

      c. Urine is produced almost continuously.

      d. As a freely refluxing system, there is high risk for chronic urinary tract infections, which increases the risk of stone formation.

    2. Continent diversions.

      a. Catheterizable internal reservoir constructed from ileum or large intestine, which stores up to 800 mL of urine.

II. Effects of treatment.

  A. Pelvic exenteration can result in a urinary diversion, fecal diversion, or both.

  B. Pelvic and abdominal radiation causes damage to the mucosa resulting in diarrhea and cystitis.

  C. Mucosal damage can occur when the stoma is located in the field of radiation treatment.

  D. Antineoplastic agents, such as 5-fluorouracil (5-FU), mitomycin C, and vincristine, can cause stomatitis, diarrhea, and constipation.

Assessment

I. Pertinent personal history.

  A. Type of surgery and stoma.

  B. Previous pelvic or abdominal radiation or chemotherapy treatments.

  C. Changes in patterns of elimination.

  D. Recurrent or chronic urinary tract infections.

  E. Difficulty in catheterizing a continent diversion.

  F. Diet habits and fluid consumption.

II. Physical findings.

  A. Characteristics of stoma and peristomal skin.

  B. Presence of leakage of urine from a continent diversion.

 C. Effectiveness of pouching system.

 D. Characteristics of effluent, that is, volume, consistency, and color.

Nursing Diagnoses

 I. Altered urinary elimination.

 II. Body image disturbance.

 III. Knowledge deficit.

 IV. Social isolation.

 V. Risk for impaired skin integrity.

 VI. Risk for sexual dysfunction.

Outcome Identification

 I. Client's stoma remains red and moist.

 II. Client manages care of ostomy/urinary diversion within his or her lifestyle.

 III. Client verbalizes feelings about the ostomy or urinary diversion and body image.

 IV. Client and significant other demonstrate confidence in their ability to resume previous sexual activities.

 V. Client contacts the wound, ostomy, continence nurse for ongoing evaluations and maintaining up-to-date equipment.

 VI. Client is aware of available support groups, such as the United Ostomy Association.

Planning and Implementation

 I. Interventions to minimize incidence and severity of complications associated with diversions.

  A. Stoma care.

   1. Stoma placement.

    a. Scars, bony prominences, skin creases or belt line are avoided.

    b. Site is marked while client is lying, standing, and sitting.

    c. Site is located within the borders of the rectus muscle.

   2. Appliance selection is based on type of effluent, abdominal contour, manual dexterity, patient preference, and cost.

   3. Change appliance every 5 days and as needed, for leakage or complaint of peristomal skin discomfort.

   4. Cut pouch opening so barrier clears stoma by 1/8 inch and protect exposed skin with skin barrier paste if needed.

   5. Gently remove pouch by pushing down on the skin while lifting up on the pouch.

   6. Cleanse peristomal skin with water and pat dry.

   7. Assess stoma and skin around stoma for erythema, dermatitis, bleeding, infection, stomal protrusion, retraction, herniation, and narrowing with each appliance change.

   8. Empty pouch when one third to one half full and before treatment.

  B. Management of diversion.

   1. Monitor volume, color, and consistency of effluent.

   2. Monitor functioning of new colostomies, which usually commences 3 to 5 days after surgery.

   3. Catheterize new continent diversions beginning about 3 to 4 weeks after surgery.

II. Interventions to monitor for side effects of treatment.
A. Cease irrigating colostomy until radiation or chemotherapy has been completed.
B. Protect stomal mucosa from trauma between daily radiation treatments.
C. Increase dietary fiber and fluid intake.
D. Encourage use of stool softeners if constipated.
E. Monitor intake, output, and color of stool and urine.
III. Implement strategies to enhance adaptation and rehabilitation.
A. Teach the client how to irrigate the colostomy as a management option for regulating function of a descending and sigmoid colostomy.
B. Teach the client measures to control gas and odor.
C. Teach ways to manage constipation and diarrhea.
D. Teach about the importance of adequate dietary fiber and fluid intake.
E. Discuss the signs and symptoms of urinary tract infections and the time at which to seek medical attention.
F. Inform about service resources available such as the United Ostomy Association.
G. Refer to the wound, ostomy, continence nurse for stoma marking and follow-up care.

Evaluation

The oncology nurse systematically and regularly evaluates the client's and/or family's responses to interventions to determine progress toward the achievement of expected outcomes. Relevant data are collected and actual findings are compared with expected findings. Nursing diagnoses, outcomes, and plans of care are reviewed and revised as necessary.

RENAL DYSFUNCTION

Theory

I. Definition—kidney impairment. Damage to the renal tubules, renal blood vessels, the interstitium or glomerulus of the kidney, leading to kidney dysfunction.
II. Risk factors.
A. Effects of disease.
1. Damaging casts and Bence Jones proteins are produced in multiple myeloma.
2. Compression by metastatic tumor can cause obstruction resulting in hydronephrosis.
3. Loss of ability by the kidneys to concentrate urine occurs in hypercalcemia of malignancy.
a. Hypercalcemia of malignancy occurs more commonly in cancers such as breast cancer with metastases; multiple myeloma; squamous cell cancer of the lung, head, or neck; renal cell cancer; lymphomas; and leukemia.
B. Treatment-related.
1. Radiation to renal structures can lead to permanent fibrosis and atrophy.
2. Precipitation of uric acid or calcium phosphate crystallization from lysis of tumor cells may result in obstruction or formation of stones.
3. Fluid and electrolyte imbalances caused by chemotherapy agents can have an indirect effect on kidney function and can lead to renal failure.

4. Direct effect by nephrotoxic agents such as antineoplastic agents (cisplatin, high-dose methotrexate, carmustine, streptozocin), aminoglycoside antibiotics, and amphotericin B.

Assessment

I. Pertinent personal history to identify risk factors.
   A. Advanced age.
   B. Diuretics, cardiac, and nephrotoxic medications.
   C. Type of malignancy.
   D. Comorbidities such as hypertension, diabetes insipidus.
   E. Previous pelvic or abdominal radiation or chemotherapy treatments.
   F. Renal stones.
   G. Preexisting renal dysfunction.
II. Physical findings.
   A. Cardiovascular—dysrhythmias, rapid thready pulse, orthostatic hypotension.
   B. Neurologic—lethargy, confusion.
   C. Poor skin turgor and dry mucous membranes.
   D. Gastrointestinal—nausea, vomiting, polydipsia.
   E. Genitourinary—nocturia, polyuria, oliguria, flank pain, dysuria.
III. Laboratory data.
   A. Serum creatinine and BUN levels reflect renal function.
   B. Creatinine clearance study is often done before implementing chemotherapy to assess renal function.
   C. Elevation of serum uric acid and calcium levels and a decrease in potassium and magnesium levels may suggest renal impairment.

Nursing Diagnoses

I. Risk for fluid volume deficit.
II. Risk for fluid volume excess.
III. Altered patterns of elimination.
IV. Knowledge deficit.

Outcome Identification

I. Client describes appropriate actions when changes occur in renal function.
II. Client recognizes the importance of renal function for physiologic integrity.
III. Client identifies and manages factors that may affect renal function, such as diet, medications, and physical activity.

Planning and Intervention

I. Interventions to monitor for incidence and risk of renal toxicity.
   A. Verify baseline renal function.
   B. Monitor intake and output closely.
      1. Observing urine output of less than 30 mL/hour may indicate renal impairment.
      2. Maintain a greater intake than output if the client is receiving diuretics unless contraindicated.
      3. Ensure aggressive hydration before, during, and after cisplatin administration.

   4. Maintain adequate fluid intake.
   5. Monitor for obstructive diuresis following the removal of obstruction.
      a. Urine output of greater than 2000 mL in 8 hours.
   6. Observe urine for stones.
C. Monitor vital signs and postural blood pressure.
D. Monitor laboratory data: serum creatinine, potassium, magnesium, sodium, creatinine clearance levels.
E. Record daily weights.
F. Maximize mobility.
   1. Change position every 2 hours.
   2. Perform passive range of motion exercises for patients on bed rest.
   3. Encourage weight-bearing and ambulation if able.
II. Interventions to incorporate client and family in care.
A. Instruct the client on importance of maintaining adequate hydration and safe weight bearing activity.
B. Teach the client signs and symptoms of hypercalcemia, dehydration, and obstruction and the appropriate time to seek medical attention.
C. Explain properties of medications prescribed.

Evaluation

   The oncology nurse systematically and regularly evaluates the client's and/or family's responses to interventions to determine progress toward the achievement of expected outcomes. Relevant data are collected and actual findings are compared with expected findings. Nursing diagnoses, outcomes, and plans of care are reviewed and revised as necessary.

BIBLIOGRAPHY

Agency for Health Care Policy and Research. (1996). *Managing Acute and Chronic Incontinence: Quick Reference Guide for Clinicians.* (AHCPR Publication No. 96-0686). Rockville, MD: United States Department of Health and Human Services.
Doughty, D., & Jackson, D. (1993). *Gastrointestinal Disorders.* St. Louis: Mosby-Year Book.
Hossan, E., & Striegel, A. (1993). Carcinoma of the bladder. *Semin Oncol Nurs 9*(4), 252–263.
Johnson, V., & Gary, A. (1995). Urinary incontinence: A review. *J Wound Ostomy Continence Nurs 1*(1), 8–15.
Kaplan, M. (1994). Hypercalcemia of malignancy: A review of advances in pathophysiology. *Oncol Nurs Forum 21*(6), 1039–1046.
Karlowicz, K. (1995). *Urologic Nursing Principles and Practice.* Philadelphia: W.B. Saunders.
McConnell, E.A. (1994). Loosening the grip of intestinal obstructions. *Nursing 24*(3), 32–42.
Marcio, J., Jorge, N., & Wexner, S. (1993). Etiology and management of fecal incontinence. *Dis Colon Rectum 36*(1), 77–97.
Ripamonti, C. (1994). Management of bowel obstruction in advanced cancer patients. *J Pain Symptom Manag 9*(3), 193–200.
Roberts, M.F. (1993). Diarrhea: A symptom. *Holist Nurs Pract 7*(2), 73–80.
Sangwan, Y., & Coller, J. (1994). Fecal incontinence. *Surg Clin North Am 74*(6), 1377–1398.
Walsh, B., Grunert, B., Teiford, G., & Otterson, M. (1995). Multidisciplinary management of altered body image in the patient with an ostomy. *J Wound Ostomy Continence Nurs 22*(9), 227–236.
Wright, P.S., & Thomas, S.L. (1995). Constipation and diarrhea: The neglected symptoms. *Semin Oncol Nurs 11*(4), 289–297.

PART FOUR

Cardiopulmonary Function

Alterations in Ventilation

Leslie V. Matthews, RN, MS, ANP, AOCN

ANATOMIC OR SURGICAL ALTERATIONS

Theory

I. Definition—inadequate ventilation or oxygenation due to anatomic or surgical alterations.
   A. Anatomic alterations.
      1. Space-occupying lesions within the lung itself or in the pleural space.
         a. Primary or metastatic cancer of the lung.
         b. Pneumothorax, abnormal accumulation of air within the pleural space; and/or hemothorax, abnormal accumulation of blood within the pleural space; empyema, abnormal accumulation of infected fluid or pus in the pleural space due to recent chest surgery, immunocompromise, or lung infections.
      2. Obstruction of tracheobronchial tree from primary or metastatic tumors or enlarged lymph nodes causing atelectasis.
      3. Compression of tracheobronchial tree from bronchospasm or laryngeal swelling from hypersensitivity reactions related to chemotherapy treatments or superior vena cava syndrome (SVCS).
   B. Surgical alterations.
      1. Thoracic surgery with closed chest drainage for removal of primary or metastatic cancer of the lung.
         a. Pneumonectomy—surgical removal of an entire lung.
         b. Lobectomy—removal of a lobe of the lung.
         c. Segmental resection—removal of one or more segments of a lung lobe.
         d. Wedge resection—removal of a small wedge-shaped localized area near the lung surface.
      2. Tracheostomy following head and neck surgery, and laryngectomy.
II. Risk factors.
   A. Primary or metastatic cancer of the lung.
   B. Recent surgery (especially thoracic or abdominal), immobility, or situations in which hypoventilation is likely.
   C. Chemotherapy with drugs known to cause allergic reactions (see Chapter 37).
   D. Cancers in which SVCS is associated (see Chapter 18).
   E. Thoracic or head and neck surgery.
      1. Primary or adjuvant tracheobronchial surgery.
      2. Surgery for palliation, tumor debulking.

     F. History of obstructive or restrictive pulmonary disease.

     G. History of cardiovascular disease.

III. Principles of medical management.

     A. Diagnostic tests.

       1. Chest x-ray examinations, computed tomography (CT) scans, magnetic resonance imaging (MRI).

       2. Arterial blood gases.

       3. Pulmonary function tests.

       4. Ventilation-perfusion scan.

       5. Bronchoscopy.

       6. Thoracentesis.

     B. Treatment strategies.

       1. Supplemental oxygen administration to facilitate adequate uptake of oxygen into the blood.

       2. Treatment aimed at the underlying disease process.

         a. Radiation therapy (RT) or chemotherapy for primary or metastatic cancer of the lung, or to reduce obstruction of the tracheobronchial tree.

         b. Thoracentesis to remove abnormal accumulated contents in pleural space; systemic antibiotic treatment for empyema.

         c. Treatment for anaphylactic/allergic reactions: stop drug, assess airway, give epinephrine, oxygen, vasopressors, intravenous fluid.

Assessment

  I. History.

     A. Cough, very common.

     B. Dyspnea, very common.

     C. Pain in chest.

     D. Ability to carry out activities of daily living.

     E. Tobacco use.

     F. Exercise/activity tolerance.

     G. Number of pillows used for sleep and comfort.

     H. Anxiety and apprehension.

     I. Presence of risk factors.

 II. Physical examination.

     A. Abnormal/altered breathing patterns.

       1. Tachypnea.

       2. Pursed-lip breathing.

       3. Use of accessory muscles of respiration.

     B. Abnormal breath sounds.

       1. Wheezes.

       2. Decreased or absent breath sounds.

     C. Sputum—amount, color, presence of blood.

     D. Cyanosis.

       1. Hypoxemia.

       2. Chronic obstructive pulmonary disease (COPD).

     E. Vital signs and pulse oximetry.

     F. Evaluate airway swelling, oropharyngeal swelling.

     G. Presence of enlarged lymph nodes or other masses in the head and neck area.

Nursing Diagnoses

   I. Ineffective airway clearance.

  II. Impaired gas exchange.

 III. Altered breathing patterns.

 IV. Activity intolerance.

   V. Pain.

 VI. Anxiety.

VII. Fatigue.

VIII. Knowledge deficit related to self-care management.

Outcome Identification

   I. Client utilizes measures to reduce or conserve energy expenditure.

  II. Client and/or family identify critical symptoms or changes in current status to report to health care providers.

 III. Identify correct procedures and precautions for oxygen use.

Planning and Implementation

   I. Interventions to minimize the risk of occurrence, severity, or complications of respiratory distress.
   - A. Employ measures to increase the ease and effectiveness of breathing and to promote physical comfort (use of pillows).
   - B. Incorporate measures to minimize the pain experience.
   - C. Utilize activity limitation and conservation of energy strategies.

  II. Interventions to maximize safety.
   - A. Encourage use of assistive devices as needed for ambulation, activities of daily living.
     1. Cane.
     2. Walker.
     3. Wheelchair.
   - B. Utilize activity limitation and conservation of energy strategies.
   - C. Use bedside rails, as appropriate.

 III. Interventions to monitor for complications.
   - A. Assess level of consciousness and mental status.
   - B. Assess heart rate and rhythm, respiratory effort, and vascular perfusion.
   - C. Critical changes should be reported to the physician.

 IV. Interventions to monitor response to management.
   - A. Assess respiratory rate, rhythm, and effort.
   - B. Assess for signs of respiratory impairment.
     1. Dyspnea.
     2. Dry persistent cough.
     3. Basilar rales.
     4. Tachypnea.
   - C. Monitor for adequate relief of symptoms.
     1. Subjective reports of client and family of:
        - a. Changes in the respiratory pattern.
        - b. Psychological responses to respiratory distress.

  V. Interventions to educate client and family regarding:
   - A. Activity limitation and conservation of energy strategies.
     1. Frequent rest periods.
     2. Easy-to-prepare meals.
     3. Often-used items within reach.

    B. Emergency care and available community resources.

    C. Signs and symptoms to report to the health care team.

Evaluation

The oncology nurse systematically and regularly evaluates the client's and/or family's responses to interventions to determine progress toward the achievement of expected outcomes. Relevant data are collected and actual findings are compared with expected findings. Nursing diagnoses, outcomes, and plans of care are reviewed and revised as necessary.

PULMONARY TOXICITY RELATED TO CANCER THERAPY

Theory

    I. Definition—parenchymal pulmonary disease caused by antineoplastic therapy, radiation, and chemotherapy.

  II. Classification.

    A. Radiation-induced pneumonitis.

      1. Subacute inflammatory response to radiation exposure to the lung.

      2. Toxic effects are proportionate to:

        a. Total radiation dose.

        b. Volume of lung tissue irradiated.

        c. Fractionation schedule.

        d. Concomitant administration of bleomycin.

    B. Chemotherapy-induced pulmonary fibrosis.

      1. Direct injury to parenchymal endothelial cell membranes of lung.

      2. Hypersensitivity reaction or immune complex–related reaction.

      3. Associated chemotherapy agents (Table 15–1).

 III. Risk factors.

    A. Radiation therapy.

      1. Occurs in 5 to 15% of all patients receiving RT.

      2. Chemotherapy given at the same time as RT.

      3. Previous RT.

      4. Steroid withdrawal.

      5. Tends to be more severe in the elderly.

    B. Chemotherapy-induced.

      1. Age more than 60 years old.

      2. Bleomycin cumulative dose higher than 400 units.

      3. Preexisting pulmonary disease (COPD).

      4. Smoking history.

      5. Concomitant or prior RT to lungs.

      6. Oxygen therapy at high concentration ($\geq 35\%$).

 IV. Principles of medical management.

    A. Radiation therapy–induced.

      1. Exclude other causes of pulmonary infiltrates—infection, recurrent tumors, or lymphangitic carcinomatosis.

      2. Mild symptoms managed with cough suppressants, antipyretics, and rest.

      3. Severe symptoms and impaired gas exchange.

        a. Administer prednisone until symptoms improve then taper slowly; pneumonitis may flare if taper is too rapid.

        b. Generally, only 50% respond to glucocorticoid therapy.

TABLE 15–1. **Chemotherapy-Induced Pulmonary Toxicity**

Drug	Risk Factors	Mechanism of Injury	Treatment
Bleomycin (Bleo)	Synergism with: Cisplatin Oxygen (>35%) Radiation therapy Cumulative dose >400 units Age >60 years	Endothelial swelling Pulmonary fibrosis Hypersensitivity reactions Direct injury from release of proteases	Assess for risk factors Monitor and limit cumulative dose Discontinue drug Steroids (indicated for Bleo hypersensitivity) Assess pulmonary status
Carmustine (BCNU)	Dose-related (>1500 mg/m^2) Increased risk with preexisting lung disease, smoking history	Pulmonary fibrosis Direct injury with toxic oxidant molecules	Assess for risk factors Discontinue drug Steroids not usually beneficial Assess pulmonary status
Mitomycin	Previous cytoxan or methotrexate administration Increased toxicity with radiation therapy (RT) High concentration O$_2$	Hypersensitivity reaction	Assess for risk factors Discontinue drug Steroids of some benefit Assess pulmonary status
Busulfan	Not considered dose-dependent Increased toxicity with RT/alkylating agents	Direct toxicity to epithelial lining Pulmonary fibrosis	Assess for risk factors Discontinue drug High-dose steroids Assess pulmonary status
Cyclophosphamide	Increased toxicity with: Cisplatin O$_2$ administration	Pulmonary damage from reactive oxygen metabolites	Assess for risk factors Discontinue drug Steroids of some benefit Assess pulmonary status
Methotrexate	Synergism with other agents possible	Direct damage unclear Hypersensitivity reaction	Discontinue drug Assess for capillary leak syndrome Steroids beneficial Assess pulmonary status

Adapted from Stover, D.E. Pulmonary toxicity. In V.T. DeVita Jr., S. Hellman, & S.A. Rosenberg (eds.). Cancer: Principles and Practice of Oncology (4th ed.). Philadelphia: J.B. Lippincott, 1993.

B. Chemotherapy-induced.
   1. Prevention is the best treatment by monitoring baseline pulmonary function tests (PFTs) and limiting cumulative dose of bleomycin to less than 400 units.
   2. Discontinuation of drug if dyspnea develops.
   3. Attempt to control symptoms with corticosteroids.

Assessment

I. History.
   A. Radiation therapy–induced pulmonary toxicity.
      1. Early, nonspecific symptoms include cough, dyspnea, and low-grade temperature.
      2. Occurs 6 to 12 weeks after completion of RT, although symptoms can range from 1 to 6 months after RT.
   B. Chemotherapy-induced pulmonary toxicity.
      1. Dyspnea is the cardinal symptom; also nonproductive cough, malaise, fatigue, and fever.
      2. Generally develops over weeks to months, but it can also develop quickly (within hours).
II. Physical examination.
   A. Radiation therapy–induced.
      1. Physical examination.
         a. Moist rales.
         b. Pleural friction rub.
         c. Evidence of pleural fluid heard over the area of irradiation.
         d. Tachypnea, cyanosis (late).
      2. Radiographic changes.
         a. Early—diffuse haziness.
         b. Late—infiltrates corresponding to the region of radiation exposure.
   B. Chemotherapy-induced.
      1. Physical examination.
         a. Results may be normal.
         b. End-inspiratory basilar rales.
         c. Tachypnea.
      2. Radiographic changes.
         a. Classic diffuse reticular pattern.
         b. Results may also be normal.
   C. Diagnostic tests and findings.
      1. Pulmonary function tests.
         a. Decreased lung volume.
         b. Decreased diffusion capacity.
      2. Arterial blood gases.
         a. Hypoxia.
         b. Hypocapnia and respiratory alkalosis.

Nursing Diagnoses

I. Impaired gas exchange.
II. Ineffective breathing pattern.
III. Pain.
IV. Fatigue.
V. Activity intolerance.

Outcome Identification

I. Client utilizes measures to reduce energy expenditure.
II. Client and/or family identify critical symptoms or changes in current status to report to health care providers.

Planning and Implementation

I. Interventions to monitor client status.
   A. Ensure that pulmonary function tests are performed before treatment.
   B. Assess respiratory rate, rhythm, and effort.
   C. Monitor cumulative doses of bleomycin and limit cumulative doses of bleomycin to less than 400 units.
   D. Assess for signs of pulmonary toxicity—dyspnea, dry persistent cough, basilar rales, and tachypnea.
   E. Monitor activities to minimize energy expenditure.
      1. Frequent rest periods.
      2. Easy-to-prepare meals.
      3. Often-used items within reach.
   F. Monitor for adequate relief of symptoms.
      1. Decreased pain.
      2. Increased comfort of breathing.

Evaluation

The oncology nurse systematically and regularly evaluates the client's and/or family's responses to interventions to determine progress toward the achievement of expected outcomes. Relevant data are collected and actual findings are compared with expected findings. Nursing diagnoses, outcomes, and plans of care are reviewed and revised as necessary.

DYSPNEA

Theory

I. Definition—a subjective sensation of difficulty breathing, the feeling of inability to get enough air, and the reaction to the sensation.
II. Risk factors.
   A. Disease-related.
      1. Tumors that impinge on respiratory structures and decrease the flow of air in and out of the lungs
      2. Conditions that increase metabolic demands such as fever, anemia, or infection.
      3. Cerebral metastasis that affects the respiratory center or stimulates the central and peripheral chemoreceptors.
      4. Metastatic effusions in the pleural space, cardiac space, or abdominal cavity that compromise lung expansion, gas exchange, or blood flow to the lungs.
      5. Coexisting pulmonary or cardiac disease that compromises lung expansion or blood flow to the lungs.
   B. Treatment-related.
      1. Incisional pain that may compromise lung expansion.
      2. Immediate (pneumonitis) and long-term (fibrosis) effects of radiation therapy to the lung fields.
      3. Antineoplastic agents that can cause pulmonary toxicity.
         a. For bleomycin, busulfan, nitrosureas, toxicity is dose-related.
         b. For methotrexate, toxicity is idiosyncratic and reversible.
      4. Anaphylactic reactions to antineoplastic agents and biologic response modifiers.

   5. Pneumothorax related to placement of vascular access catheters, fine-needle aspirations, or thoracentesis.
   C. Lifestyle-related.
      1. Strong emotional responses, particularly anxiety or anger contribute to the sensation of dyspnea.
      2. Tobacco use.
      3. Exposure to environmental toxic substances—asbestos, chromium, coal products, ionizing radiation, vinyl chloride, chloromethyl ethers.
III. Principles of medical management.
   A. Treatment of underlying disease with thoracentesis, radiation therapy, chemotherapy, antimicrobial medications.
   B. Pharmacologic agents.
      1. Increase air flow to the lungs—bronchodilators.
      2. Decrease local inflammation—steroids.
      3. Decrease pain and anxiety—narcotics, anxiolytics.
   C. Supplemental oxygen as indicated.
   D. Activity limitation, bronchial hygiene measures, appropriate positioning, relaxation training, and exercise as tolerated.

Assessment

   I. History.
      A. Presence of risk factors.
      B. Subjective complaints of shortness of breath, "can't catch breath," "smothering," uncomfortable breathing, anxiety, or panic.
      C. Pattern of dyspnea—onset, frequency, severity, associated symptoms, aggravating or alleviating factors.
      D. Impact of dyspnea on activities of daily living, lifestyle, relationships, role responsibilities.
  II. Physical findings.
      A. Tachypnea.
      B. Increased respiratory excursion.
      C. Use of accessory muscles with breathing.
      D. Retraction of intercostal spaces.
      E. Flaring of nostrils.
      F. Clubbing of digits caused by chronic hypoxemia.
      G. Cyanosis, pallor.
 III. Diagnostic tests and findings.
      A. Since the symptom is a subjective response, the client may not have abnormal findings or results.
      B. Complete blood count—hemoglobin deficiencies.
      C. Chest x-ray examination, CT—structural abnormalities.
      D. Pulmonary function tests.
      E. Bronchoscopic examination.
      F. Sputum or bronchial cultures.
      G. Arterial blood gas.

Nursing Diagnoses

   I. Impaired gas exchange.
  II. Ineffective breathing pattern.
 III. Fatigue.

IV. Pain.
 V. Potential for injury.

Outcome Identification

   I. Client lists signs and symptoms that should be reported to the health care team.
  II. Client describes interventions to aid in own comfort.
 III. Client describes correct procedures and precautions for oxygen use.
 IV. Client identifies strategies used to conserve energy.

Planning and Implementation

   I. Interventions are taught to increase the ease and effectiveness of breathing and to promote physical comfort.
      1. Utilize upright position with pillows as necessary.
      2. Lean forward with elbows on knees, table or pillows.
      3. Perform diaphragmatic breathing with slow exhalation; however, this type of breathing is not effective and may be harmful in clients with a history of pulmonary restrictive disease.
      4. Incorporate measures to minimize the pain experience.
      5. Utilize activity limitation and conservation of energy strategies.
      6. Encourage systematic relaxation techniques.
  II. Interventions to maximize safety.
      A. Encourage use of assistive devices as needed for ambulation, activities of daily living, such as cane, walker, wheelchair.
      B. Utilize activity limitation and conservation of energy strategies.
         1. Frequent rest periods.
         2. Use of ready-made meals.
         3. Often-used items within reach.
      C. Use bedside rails, as appropriate.
 III. Interventions to monitor for complications.
      A. Assess level of consciousness and mental status.
      B. Monitor intake and output.
      C. Assess heart rate and rhythm, respiratory effort, and vascular perfusion.
      D. Report critical changes to the physician.
         1. Unresponsiveness.
         2. Tachypnea, tachycardia.
         3. Acute pain.
 IV. Interventions to monitor response to management.
      A. Observe and report physical symptoms, such as decreased shortness of breath, increased energy, and ease of breathing.
      B. Monitor subjective reports of the client and family regarding:
         1. Changes in the pattern of dyspnea.
         2. Psychological responses to dyspnea.
  V. Interventions to educate patient and family.
      A. Teach activity limitation and conservation of energy strategies.
      B. Instruct in emergency care and available community resources.
      C. List signs and symptoms to report to the health care team.
         1. Increased pain.
         2. Increased difficulty in breathing.
         3. Nasal flaring.
         4. Skin changes (pallor, cyanosis).

Evaluation

The oncology nurse systematically and regularly evaluates the client's and/or family's responses to interventions to determine progress toward the achievement of expected outcomes. Relevant data are collected and actual findings are compared with expected findings. Nursing diagnoses, outcomes, and plans of care are reviewed and revised as necessary.

PLEURAL EFFUSIONS

Theory

    I. Definition—presence of abnormal amounts of fluid in the pleural space.

    II. Classification.

        A. Pleural effusion (benign) may be caused by:

            1. Increased hydrostatic pressure (congestive heart failure).

            2. Increased permeability in the microvascular circulation (infection, trauma).

            3. Increased negative pressure in the pleural space (atelectasis).

            4. Decreased oncotic pressure in the microvasculature (nephrotic syndrome, cirrhosis, hypoalbuminemia).

        B. Malignant pleural effusion, the presence of malignant cells in the pleura, may be caused by:

            1. Direct extension of primary lung tumor to the pleura or mediastinum or mesothelioma involving the pleura.

            2. Impaired lymphatic drainage from the pleural space resulting from obstruction caused by tumor.

            3. Increased permeability due to inflammation or disruption of the capillary endothelium.

            4. Altered mucosal lung or mediastinal tissue resulting from RT.

    III. Risk factors.

        A. Primary tumors of lung, breast, hematopoietic system.

        B. Prior pleural effusion.

        C. Radiation to the chest, thorax, or abdomen

        D. Surgical modification of venous or lymphatic vessels.

    IV. Principles of medical management.

        A. Diagnostic tests.

            1. Chest x-ray examination—blunting of costophrenic angle.

            2. Fluid accumulation.

            3. Thoracentesis—pleural fluid withdrawal of approximately 25 to 50 mL for accurate cytology testing and culture (to rule out infectious cause).

            4. Pleural biopsy—increases diagnostic yield when combined with cytologic studies.

        B. Therapeutic.

            1. Thoracentesis.

                a. May improve client comfort and relieve dyspnea.

                b. Reaccumulation of fluid is common.

                c. Potential for hypoproteinemia, pneumothorax, empyema, fluid loculation.

                d. Effective procedure for palliation, relief of acute respiratory distress.

2. Complete drainage via chest tube to continuous underwater-seal suction—promotes adherence of the visceral and parietal pleural surfaces by removal of accumulated fluid.
3. Sclerotherapy—instillation of sclerosing agents intrapleurally to produce mesothelial fibrosis using:
   a. Tetracycline, doxycycline.
   b. Nitrogen mustard, bleomycin.
   c. Talc.
   d. Lidocaine in the sclerosing agent solution helps decrease discomfort associated with procedure.
4. Parietal pleurectomy.
5. Open pleurectomy—historically has required thoracotomy.
6. Videothorascopic pleurectomy—using hydrodissection with an irrigation device entering into the pleural space; minimally invasive.
7. Chemotherapy and mediastinal radiation—may be effective in responsive tumors [lymphoma, small cell lung cancer (SCLC)].

Assessment

 I. History.
   A. Presence of risk factors.
      1. Breast or lung cancer.
      2. Previous treatment modalities.
   B. Symptoms—severity related to the speed of accumulation, not amount, and usually caused by pulmonary compression.
      1. Dyspnea.
      2. Cough usually dry and nonproductive.
      3. Chest pain.
 II. Physical examination.
   A. Tachypnea.
   B. Restricted chest wall expansion.
   C. Dullness to percussion.
   D. Diminished or absent breath sounds.
   E. Egophony on the affected side.
   F. Pleural friction rub.
   G. Fever.
   H. General manifestations.
      1. Compression atelectasis.
      2. Mediastinal shift, if pleural effusion severe.

Nursing Diagnoses

  I. Ineffective breathing pattern.
 II. Impaired gas exchange.
III. Anxiety.
IV. Pain.
 V. Potential for injury.

Outcome Identification

 I. Client and/or family describe signs and symptoms that should be reported to the health care team.

II. Client and/or family describe interventions to aid in client comfort.

III. Client and/or family identify correct procedures and precautions for oxygen use.

IV. Client and/or family describe strategies used to manage the pain that may be associated with pleural effusion.

Planning and Implementation

I. Interventions to decrease the severity of symptoms associated with pleural effusion.
   A. Teach measures to increase the ease and effectiveness of breathing and to promote physical comfort.
      1. Utilize upright position with pillows as necessary.
      2. Lean forward with elbows on knees, table, or pillows.
   B. Incorporate measures to minimize the pain experience (narcotic analgesia before chest tube insertion and as needed).
   C. Utilize relaxation techniques as indicated for anxiety.

II. Interventions to maximize safety.
   A. Encourage use of assistive devices as needed for ambulation, activities of daily living.
   B. Utilize activity limitation and conservation of energy strategies.
   C. Instruct family in use of and precautions related to oxygen therapy.

III. Interventions to monitor the consequences of therapy.
   A. Assess respiratory rate and rhythm, respiratory effort, and adventitious breath sounds.
   B. Assess characteristics of pain and relief measures.
   C. Monitor subjective response to drainage and rate of fluid reaccumulation.
   D. Report critical changes to the physician.
      1. Chest pain.
      2. Fever.
      3. Change in character of respiration.

IV. Interventions to educate client and family regarding:
   A. Activity limitation and conservation of energy strategies.
   B. Emergency care and available community resources.
   C. Signs and symptoms to report to the health care team.

V. Interventions to enhance adaptation or rehabilitation.
   A. Assist the patient to maintain a safe level of independence within the limitation of symptoms.
   B. Encourage the patient and family to express concerns.

Evaluation

The oncology nurse systematically and regularly evaluates the client's and/or family's responses to interventions to determine progress toward the achievement of expected outcomes. Relevant data are collected and actual findings are compared with expected findings. Nursing diagnoses, outcomes, and plans of care are reviewed and revised as necessary.

ANEMIA

Theory

I. Definition—symptom of abnormally low red blood cells (RBC), quality of hemoglobin (Hgb), and/or volume of packed cells.

A. World Health Organization (WHO) definition.
   1. Males—Hgb level less than 13.0 g; hematocrit (Hct) less than 42%.
   2. Females—Hgb level less than 12.0 g; Hct less than 36%.
II. Classification.
   A. Red cell morphology—size of RBC (microcytic, normocytic, or macrocytic).
   B. Amount of hemoglobin pigment (hypochromic, normochromic, hyperchromic).
III. Risk factors.
   A. Disease-related.
      1. Slow or persistent blood loss (gastrointestinal [GI] neoplasms, esophageal varices, peptic ulcer disease, acetylsalicylic acid/nonsteroidal antiinflammatory drugs [ASA/NSAIDs] ingestion) causing decreased red blood cell (RBC) volume.
      2. Primary malignancies of the marrow, tumor invasion of the marrow, or genetically transmitted red cell deficiencies (thalassemia) causing decreased quantity/quality of RBC production.
      3. Impaired absorption (postgastrectomy, celiac disease), inadequate intake (cachexia, alcoholism), or decreased utilization of iron, folic acid, vitamin K, or vitamin B_{12} causing decreased maturity and function of RBC.
      4. Autoimmune disorders associated with malignancy (multiple myeloma, chronic leukemias) causing increased destruction or sequestration of RBC.
      5. Acute or chronic renal disease causing decreased erythropoietin production.
   B. Treatment-related.
      1. Chemotherapy—destruction of rapidly dividing normal hematopoietic cells results in decreased production of RBC precursors and mature RBCs.
      2. Radiation therapy—destruction of RBC precursors in the radiation field.
      3. Pharmacologic agents—inhibit RBC production or cause decreased mineral and vitamin levels (oral contraceptives, estrogen, phenytoin, phenobarbital).
IV. Principles of medical management.
   A. Once the diagnosis is established, underlying cause must be identified and, if possible, corrected.
   B. Supplements such as iron, vitamins, folic acid.
   C. RBC transfusions are indicated when:
      1. Symptomatic anemia (dyspnea, tachycardia) occurs, regardless of the hematocrit.
      2. Client is actively bleeding.
      3. Hemoglobin level drops below 8 g/100 mL.
   D. Erythropoietin administration.
   E. Cessation of pharmacologic agents that interfere with red cell production or maturation.

Assessment

I. History.
   A. Signs and symptoms depend on:
      1. Rate at which anemia develops.
      2. Age of the individual.

  3. Individual's compensatory mechanisms.
  4. Activity level.
 B. Review history of:
  1. All medications, prescription and over-the-counter agents.
  2. Acute or chronic blood loss.
  3. Previous therapy for cancer.
  4. Signs and symptoms of anemia.
  5. Impact of anemia on activities of daily living (ADL), activity level, life-style.
 C. General manifestations of anemia.
  1. Easily fatigued.
  2. Dyspnea on exertion.
  3. Pallor (conjunctiva, nail beds, sclera).
  4. Weakness, listlessness.
  5. Headache.
  6. Hypotension.
  7. Tachycardia.
  8. Tachypnea.
 II. Physical findings.
 A. General appearance—pale, lethargic, or no overt signs, if anemia is mild.
 B. Vital signs—pulse and respiration may be increased in moderate to severe anemia; postural hypotension in severe anemia.
 C. Integument—pallor and dryness of the skin and mucous membranes; brittle, flattened, ridged, concave, or spoon-shaped nails (koilonychia); brittle, fine hair.
 D. Head, eyes, ears, nose, and throat (HEENT)—atrophy of the papillae of the tongue, smooth, shiny, beefy-red appearance; angular stomatitis or cheilitis; pale conjunctiva or sclera.
 E. Cardiovascular—tachycardia, mild cardiac enlargement; in severe anemia, functional systolic murmurs.
 F. Abdominal—hepatomegaly, splenomegaly.
 G. Neurologic—usually within normal limits (WNL); in severe anemia, confusion.
 III. Diagnostic tests and findings.
 A. Routine complete blood count (CBC) (with peripheral smear).
  1. Hgb level decreased.
  2. Hct level decreased.
  3. Mean corpuscular volume (MCV).
   a. Less than 80—microcytic.
   b. 80 to 100—normocytic.
   c. More than 100—macrocytic.
  4. Mean corpuscular hemoglobin concentration (MCHC).
   a. Low—hypochromic.
   b. Normal—normochromic.
  5. Reticulocyte count decreased.
  6. Chemistries.
   a. Iron level, total iron binding capacity (TIBC); ferritin, folate, vitamins B_{12} and K levels.
   b. Bilirubin level.

Nursing Diagnoses

 I. Fatigue.
 II. Activity intolerance.

III. Potential for injury.
IV. Knowledge deficit related to self-care.

Outcome Identification

I. Client lists signs and symptoms that should be reported to the health care team.
II. Client and/or family describe interventions to aid in client safety.
III. Client and/or family describe correct procedures and precautions for oxygen use.
IV. Client and/or family describe strategies to conserve energy.

Planning and Implementation

I. Interventions to decrease risk of complications of anemia
    A. Institute safety precautions.
        1. Avoid sudden changes in position such as from lying to sitting, sitting to standing.
        2. Assist with ambulation and self-care activities as needed.
        3. Teach patient to avoid hazardous activities such as driving if syncopal episodes are present.
        4. Assist client to conserve energy.
        5. Provide a nutritionally balanced diet and/or supplements.
    B. Educate the client and family regarding:
        1. Cause of anemia and treatment plan.
        2. Purpose, dosage, side effects, toxic effects of medication.
        3. Nutrition—counsel regarding specific needs.
        4. Activity—frequent rest periods as needed.
        5. Signs and symptoms related to complications of anemia or treatment to report to a member of a health care team.
            a. Change in mental status.
            b. Increased shortness of breath.
            c. Onset of active bleeding.
II. Interventions to monitor for complications related to anemia.
    A. Assess skin for evidence of inadequate oxygenation such as pallor, decreased capillary refill, or prolonged redness.
    B. Assess blood pressure in lying, standing, and sitting positions.
    C. Assess patient for evidence of side effects of therapy for anemia.
    D. Monitor occurrence of constipation or diarrhea related to iron supplements.

Evaluation

The oncology nurse systematically and regularly evaluates the client's and/or family's responses to interventions to determine progress toward the achievement of expected outcomes. Relevant data are collected and actual findings are compared with expected findings. Nursing diagnoses, outcomes, and plans of care are reviewed and revised as necessary.

BIBLIOGRAPHY

Clark, J.C., & McGee, R.F. (eds.) (1993). *Core Curriculum in Oncology Nursing* (2nd ed.). Philadelphia: W.B. Saunders.
Davey, S.S., & McCance, K.L. (1994). Alterations of pulmonary function. In McCance, K.L., & Huether, S.E. *Pathophysiology: The Biologic Basis for Disease in Adults and Children* (2nd ed.). St. Louis: Mosby-Year Book.

DeGowin, R.L. (1993). *Diagnostic Examination* (6th ed.). New York: McGraw-Hill, 1994.

DeVita, Jr., V.T., Hellman S., & Rosenberg S.A. (eds.). *Cancer: Principles and Practice of Oncology* (4th ed.). Philadelphia: J.B. Lippincott.

Ewald, G.A., & McKenzie, C.R. (eds.) (1995). *Manual of Medical Therapeutics* (28th ed.). Boston: Little, Brown.

Gross, J., & Johnson, B.L. (1993). *Handbook of Oncology Nursing* (2nd ed.). Sudbury, MA: Jones & Bartlett.

Groenwald, S.L., Frogge, M.H., Goodman, M., and Yarbro, C.H. (1993). *Cancer Nursing Principles and Practice* (3rd ed.). Sudbury, MA: Jones & Bartlett Publishers.

Pina, E.M., Harvey, J.C., Katariya, K., & Beattie, E.J. (1993). Malignant pleural effusions. In Harvey, J.C., & Beattie, E.J. (eds.). *Cancer Surgery.* Philadelphia: W.B. Saunders.

Stover, D.E. (1993). Pulmonary toxicity. In DeVita, Jr., V.T., Hellman, S., & Rosenberg, S.A. (eds.). *Cancer: Principles and Practice of Oncology* (4th ed.). Philadelphia: J.B. Lippincott, pp. 2362–2370.

Alterations in Circulation

Mary Mrozek-Orlowski, RN, MSN, AOCN

LYMPHEDEMA

Theory

I. Definition—difference in circumference of affected limb of greater than 1.5 cm compared with circumference of unaffected limb related to impaired lymphatic flow.
II. Pathophysiology.
   A. Scarring caused by surgical interruption of lymph flow in axilla or groin.
      1. Followed by interstitial fibrosis.
      2. May be enhanced by radiation therapy to affected area.
      3. Usually more extensive surgery or radiation worsens lymphedema.
      4. May be related to subclinical lymphangitis.
   B. Occurs in arms related to axillary lymph node dissection for breast cancer.
   C. Occurs in legs related to groin lymph node dissection for melanoma, soft tissue sarcoma, and eventually includes genitalia.
   D. Can occur with advanced or recurrent cancers, such as lymphoma; Kaposi's sarcoma; cancers of the prostate, ovary, and breast, where cancer cells obstruct lymph vessels.
III. Incidence.
   A. 5 to 10% occur in women undergoing modified radical mastectomy.
      1. Usually occurs within 1 year following surgery.
      2. Can occur as late as 20 years from surgery.
   B. 80% occur within 5 years of groin lymph node dissection.

Assessment

I. Risk factors.
   A. Infection in affected limb.
   B. Trauma.
   C. Inadequate muscle contraction.
   D. Obesity.
II. Inspection.
   A. Condition of skin.
   B. Mobility of extremity.
   C. Erythema or signs of infection.
   D. Impairment of circulation or constriction by clothing or jewelry.
III. Circumference of limb.
   A. Arm measured 5 and 10 cm above and below the olecranon process.
   B. Leg measurements done at the level of the calf.

C. Classification.
1. Mild—less than 3 cm difference.
2. Moderate—3 to 5 cm difference.
3. Severe—greater than 5 cm difference.

Nursing Diagnoses

I. Body image disturbance.
II. Risk for infection.
III. Chronic pain.
IV. Risk for impaired skin integrity.

Outcome Identification

I. Client verbalizes and demonstrates acceptance of body image.
II. Client verbalizes adequate information about prevention, early detection, and treatment of lymphedema.
III. Infection will be identified early.
IV. Pain will be prevented by early detection and prompt treatment of lymphedema.

Planning and Implementation

I. Prevention.
A. Nursing care designed to prevent lymphedema (Table 16–1).
B. Instruction on postoperative limb care and postsurgical exercises (Table 16–2).

TABLE 16–1. **Nursing Care of the Client with Axillary Lymph Node Dissection**

Nursing Care	Rationale/Comments
Ascertain from any client with breast cancer which side is the treated side. In a client with breast cancer, unless contraindicated, use the opposite side for a blood pressure, drawing blood, placing IVs or injections. If the client is in the hospital, put up a sign saying "Avoid BP or venipuncture in _____ arm."	The skin is the first line of defense against infection. A break in the skin increases the risk of infection
If the arm from the treated side must be used (in the case of bilateral breast cancer, the untreated arm in a cast, cellulitis of the untreated arm, or an emergency), proceed with caution. Monitor the arm for redness, heat, and infection. Some institutions require a physician's order before using affected arm.	A break in skin integrity increases the risk of infection
Teach lymph node dissection care to the patient. Remember that lymph node care needs to be taught to clients with groin node dissections at risk for lower extremity lymphedema. Stress that precautions need to be maintained throughout the patient's life.	Lymphedema has occurred as late as 10 years after axillary node dissection
Begin limited exercises (involving only the wrist and elbow) after surgery for axillary node dissection; delay exercises involving the shoulder until drains are removed.	Vigorous exercise begun too soon after surgery may increase seroma (fluid in lower axilla) development
For patients with lymphedema, consider physical therapy	May aid in lymph drainage from affected extremity

Adapted from Mrozek-Orlowski, M. (1996). Breast cancer. In M. Liebman & D. Camp-Sorrell (eds.). *Multimodal Therapy in Oncology Nursing.* St. Louis: Mosby-Year Book, pp. 119–132.

TABLE 16–2. **Client Education Guidelines for Clients with Axillary Lymph Node Dissection**

Numbness in the affected arm is common. Changes in sensation, sometimes described as "arm fall asleep" can happen over time. Hyperesthesias are also common.

Be cautious when shaving under your arm or your legs. Skin cuts may occur without your knowledge because of loss of sensation.

Begin stretching exercises about 24 hours after surgery, but limit the exercises to those that do not involve the shoulder if you have had an axillary node dissection. More strenuous exercises may begin a week or so after surgery, once the drains are removed.

Exercises are important to prevent stiffness.

Avoid carrying heavy loads with the affected arm.

Avoid having blood pressures taken, IVs placed, or injections in the affected arm, if you have had an axillary lymph node dissection.

Report any redness or warmth in the affected arm or leg to your doctor. These are signs of infection.

Do not cut your cuticles.

Prevent dry skin by using hand cream.

If your shoulder is still stiff and interferes with daily activities a month after axillary lymph node surgery, consult with your doctor about the possibility of physical therapy.

The exercises and massage may ease tightness in the shoulder.

Adapted from Mrozek-Orlowski, M. (1996). Breast Cancer. In M. Liebman & D. Camp-Sorrell (eds.). *Multimodal Therapy in Oncology Nursing.* St. Louis: Mosby-Year Book, pp. 119–132.

    C. Nutritional instruction including protein requirements.

    D. Teaching client signs and symptoms of infection.

II. Early detection and treatment.

    A. Measure arms or legs regularly.

    B. Elevate affected limb above the level of the heart when resting.

    C. Initiate massage therapy, if appropriate.

    D. Apply an elastic sleeve on the affected extremity, placed in the morning after edema is reduced.

    E. Use a sequential compression pump according to manufacturer's directions.

    F. Prevent dry skin with body lotion, avoiding breaks in skin on affected side.

III. Assess impact of lymphedema upon activities of daily living and general functioning

IV. Contact National Lymphedema Network, 2211 Post Street, Ste. 404, San Francisco, CA 94115; (800) 541-3259.

Evaluation

The oncology nurse systematically and regularly evaluates the client's and/or family's responses to interventions to determine progress toward the achievement of expected outcomes. Relevant data are collected and actual findings are compared with expected findings. Nursing diagnoses, outcomes, and plans of care are reviewed and revised as necessary.

CARDIOVASCULAR TOXICITY RELATED TO CANCER THERAPY

Theory

I. Definition—alteration in cardiac function, both conduction and function, related to cancer treatment.

II. Cardiotoxic drugs (Table 16–3).
   A. DNA intercalators such as doxorubicin, daunorubicin decrease contractibility of the heart leading to increased workload; hypertrophy results, related to direct insult of myofibrils
   B. High-dose fluorouracil may cause coronary artery spasm leading to ischemia and possible myocardial infarction.
   C. High-dose cyclophosphamide causes endothelial damage leading to myocardial necrosis.
   D. Taxines—mechanism is unknown but effect on heart is asymptomatic bradycardia.
III. Acuity.
   A. Acute reactions.
      1. Within 24 hours of drug administration.
      2. Self-limiting.
      3. Major changes such as arrhythmias warrant immediate drug discontinuation. Arrhythmias are usually transient so temporary discontinuation of therapy does not always require permanent cessation of therapy.
      4. Acute changes related to fluorouracil do require cessation of therapy, however.
   B. Subacute reactions.
      1. Begins several weeks after treatment.
      2. Usually reversible.
      3. Cancer treatment is not always stopped.
   C. Chronic reactions.
      1. Occurs with cumulative doses of agents such as anthracyclines that cause myocardial weakening.
      2. Characteristics (see Table 16–3).
      3. Treatment is stopped.
IV. Incidence.
   A. Acute and subacute reactions occur infrequently.
   B. Chronic reaction is related to cumulative doses of the drug.
V. Principles of medical management.
   A. Improve cardiac output.
   B. Reduce cardiac fluid load.

Assessment

I. Risk factors.
   A. Risk increases with:
      1. Additional doses of these agents over recommended lifetime dosage.
      2. Radiation therapy to left thorax.
   B. Multiple cardiotoxic drugs or high-dose therapy.
   C. High doses over short periods of time.
   D. Age.
      1. Children because of biologic differences, tissue sensitivity, and intensity of regimens.
      2. Elderly because of slower tissue self-repair mechanisms and cardiac disease.
   E. History of cardiac disease or hypertension.
   F. History of, or current, smoking.
II. Cardiac assessment.
   A. Assess results of ejection fraction and electrocardiogram if appropriate before administering drug.

B. Document total cumulative dosage of the cardiotoxic drug in client record.

C. Assess heart rate, rhythm, and regularity.

III. Laboratory values that interfere with cardiac function when abnormal.

A. Potassium.

B. Calcium.

C. Magnesium.

IV. Clinical manifestations of congestive heart failure.

A. Tachycardia.

B. Shortness of breath and nonproductive cough.

C. Neck vein distention and pedal edema.

D. Cardiomegaly.

E. Gallop heart rhythm.

F. Hepatomegaly.

Nursing Diagnoses

I. Risk for activity intolerance.

II. Decreased cardiac output.

III. Acute pain due to ischemia.

Outcome Identification

I. Client maintains activity level that allows normal daily activities as identified by the client.

II. Client's pain is controlled.

III. Client verbalizes adequate information regarding cardiac status.

Planning and Implementation

I. Prevention.

A. Consider changing agents when total dose nears total lifetime dosage.

B. Cardiac-protective iron chelating agents such as dexrazoxane (Zinecard) may be administered to prevent doxorubicin-induced cardiotoxicity in breast cancer patients with metastatic disease when those clients have received a dose greater than 300 mg/m^2.

C. Counsel client to participate in regular exercise.

D. Consider digoxin to improve heart contractibility if congestive heart failure is present.

II. Early detection and treatment.

A. When ejection fraction is less than 50 to 55% of institutional normal, consider reducing dosage or changing dosage.

B. Monitor results of regular multigated angiogram (MUGA) and electrocardiograms.

III. Treatment of congestive heart failure.

A. Administer and monitor effects of medications (e.g., diuretics, vasodilators, oxygen, and inotropic cardiac medications).

B. Initiate a low-sodium diet and other appropriate dietary changes.

IV. Client education.

A. Instruct the client regarding possible cardiotoxicities and that chronic toxicity may be irreversible.

B. Educate the client about signs and symptoms of congestive heart failure and other cardiac toxicities and the appropriate time at which to report them to the nurse or physician.

TABLE 16–3. **Cardiotoxic Drugs**

Drug	Incidence	Characteristics	Comment
DNA Intercalators			
Doxorubicin	Total dose <550 mg/m², incidence 0.1–1.2% Total dose >550 mg/m², incidence rises exponentially Total dose 1000 mg/m², incidence nearly 50%	ECG changes; nonspecific ST-T wave changes; premature ventricular and atrial contraction; low-voltage QRS changes and sinus tachycardia; decreased ejection fraction; cardiomyopathy with symptoms of congestive heart failure (CHF)	Chronic effects seen with cumulative doses may result in CHF Concomitant administration of other antineoplastics (e.g., cyclophosphamide) have been implicated as risk factors; however, the exact synergism is unclear
Daunorubicin	Total dose <600 mg/m², incidence 0–41% Total dose 1000 mg/m², incidence 12%		
Dactinomycin	Incidence rare Total dose >100 mg/m², with prior exposure to anthracyclines, transient ECG changes, incidence 28%		
Mitoxantrone	Total dose >160 mg/m², incidence 44% Without prior exposure to anthracyclines, incidence of decreased ejection fraction and CHF is 2.1–12.5%		

High-Dose Therapy

Cyclophosphamide	Not seen with cumulative doses or standard doses. Increased with high-dose therapy: >180–200 mg/kg/day × 4 days	Diminished QRS complex on ECG; cardiomegaly; pulmonary congestion	May result in acute lethal pericarditis and hemorrhagic myocardial necrosis
5-fluorouracil	Incidence 1.6%	Angina, palpitations, sweating, and/or syncope	May be treated prophylactically or therapeutically with long-acting nitrates or calcium channel blockers
Taxanes			
Paclitaxel	Incidence unknown	Asymptomatic bradycardia, hypotension, asymptomatic ventricular tachycardia, atypical chest pain	Toxicity has been documented as asymptomatic bradycardia (40–60 bpm), hypotension, asymptomatic ventricular tachycardia, and atypical chest pain. A baseline ECG, client history, and cardiac assessment should be performed before treatment; however, routine cardiac monitoring during infusion is not recommended

From Powel, L. (1996) Cancer Chemotherapy Guidelines and Recommendations for Practice. Pittsburgh, PA: Oncology Nursing Press, pp. 12–13.

  C. For clients with congestive heart failure, educate the client and family about energy conservation skills.

Evaluation

The oncology nurse systematically and regularly evaluates the client's and/or family's responses to interventions to determine progress toward the achievement of expected outcomes. Relevant data are collected and actual findings are compared with expected findings. Nursing diagnoses, outcomes, and plans of care are reviewed and revised as necessary.

EDEMA

Theory

  I. Definition—abnormal leakage of fluid from blood and lymph vessels leading to an excessive accumulation of fluid in the interstitial space. Fluid may be malignant or nonmalignant, as confirmed by cytology examination.
 II. Extracellular fluids separated by semipermeable membranes surround capillaries and cells, dividing them into interstitial and intravascular compartments. Normally, more fluid moves from intravascular to interstitial spaces than interstitial to intravascular. Lymphatic capillaries remove excess fluid and protein from the interstitial space, returning the fluid to the intravascular system.
III. Interruption of lymph flow, vascular obstruction, or other factors interfering with balance of fluid flow causes movement of fluids from intravascular to interstitial spaces, resulting in edema.
 IV. Causes of malignant edema (Table 16–4).
  V. Incidence.
      A. Difficult to assess because data unclear.
      B. Most data obtained when postmortem examinations were performed routinely.
 VI. Types.
      A. Pulmonary edema related to congestive heart failure.
      B. Ascites (see Chapter 13).
          1. Caused by malignant tumor cells studding the peritoneal cavity.
          2. Several pounds of weight may be gained.
      C. Sacral.
          1. Usually dependent edema from inactivity.
          2. Contributes to sacral skin breakdown.
      D. Lymphedema (see earlier).
VII. Principles of medical management.
      A. Treatment of disease.
      B. Diuretics—low-dose hydrochlorothiazide followed by spironolactone, using furosemide only if these other measures are unsuccessful.
      C. Electrolyte and albumin replacement.

Assessment

  I. Risk factors.
      A. Disease-related.
          1. Concurrent cardiac, renal, or liver disease causing fluid retention through congestive heart failure, renal or portal hypertension.

TABLE 16–4. **Causes of Malignant Edema (According to Underlying Physiologic Mechanism)**

Hydrostatic Pressure Abnormalities

Increased capillary fluid pressure
  Increased venous pressure
    Vein obstruction
     Tumor
     Thrombophlebitis
    Increased total volume with decreased cardiac output
    Fluid overload
  Sodium and water retention, increased aldosterone from:
    Decreased renal blood flow
     Renal failure
    Increased aldosterone
     Corticosteroid therapy
    Inability to metabolize aldosterone
     Liver metastasis

Oncotic Pressure Abnormalities

Decreased capillary oncotic pressure
  Loss of serum protein
    Anemia
    Bleeding
  Decreased protein intake
    Malnutrition
  Decreased albumin production
    Liver metastasis

Increased interstitial oncotic pressure
  Increased capillary permeability to protein
    Inflammatory reactions
     Seeding of cavity surfaces with tumor cells
     Infection
  Obstructed lymphatics: decreased removal of tissue fluid and protein
    Malignant disease
    Surgical removal of lymph nodes

From Maxwell, M. (1993). Malignant effusions and edemas. In S. Groenwald, M. Frogge, M. Goodman, & C. Yarbo (eds.). *Cancer Nursing: Principles and Practice.* Boston: Jones & Bartlett, p. 677.

    2. Allergic response causing interstitial fluid retention through histamine release.
    3. Septic shock causing interstitial fluid retention through histamine release.
B. Treatment-related.
    1. Surgical disruption of vascular and lymphatic channels.
    2. Radiation therapy causing inflammation of tissues and fibrosis of lymphatic channels within treatment field.
C. Medications such as estrogen or steroid therapy.
D. Lifestyle-related.
    1. Increased dietary sodium.
    2. Inadequate dietary protein.
E. Iatrogenic-related.
    1. Plasma expanders.
    2. Intravenous fluid therapy.
    3. Blood component therapy.

   II. Subjective findings.
    A. Presence of risk factors for edema.
    B. Patterns of previous edema—onset, frequency, location, severity; precipitating, aggravating, and alleviating factors; and associated factors.
    C. Impact of edema on activities of daily living; lifestyle; comfort; relationships; roles and responsibilities within the family, community, work, or school; and mood.
    D. Significance of edema in relation to disease and treatment.
   III. Objective findings.
    A. Local changes.
      1. Swelling.
        a. Edema of advanced cancer is often bilateral; unilateral edema suggests a treatable cause.
        b. Up to 10 pounds of fluid can accumulate in lower extremities before the condition is recognized as pitting edema.
      2. Warmth or coolness or discoloration of skin over edematous area.
      3. Diminished peripheral pulses in involved extremity.
      4. Nail blanching.
      5. Sensory changes (e.g., numbness, tingling, or pain).
    B. Motor changes.
      1. Altered range of motion.
      2. Pain on movement.
   IV. Laboratory tests.
    A. Abnormal serum electrolyte values related to sodium and water retention.
    B. Increased blood urea nitrogen (BUN) and serum creatinine values associated with renal failure.
    C. Decreased serum protein and albumin values associated with malnutrition and disease state.

Nursing Diagnoses

   I. Impaired skin integrity.
   II. Impaired physical mobility.
   III. Risk for self-care deficit.
   IV. Chronic pain.

Outcome Identification

   I. Client maintains intact skin.
   II. Client participates in activities of daily living, utilizing assistive devices as appropriate.
   III. Client reports pain control.
   IV. Client participates in exercise program to maintain physical mobility.

Planning and Implementation

   I. Refer to physical and occupational therapy for an exercise program to maintain mobility.
   II. Employ skin care measures that prevent skin breakdown.
    A. Skin lotion to avoid dry skin.
    B. Client positioning to prevent pressure points on bony areas.
   III. Teach nutritional measures.
    A. Sodium limitation.
    B. Improving protein intake with supplements.
   IV. Ensure elevation of extremities above heart level.

 V. Initiate client education.
   A. Instruct the client about a diet high in protein and low in sodium.
   B. Instruct the client about signs and symptoms of hyponatremia, if appropriate.
   C. Educate the client and family regarding measures to protect edematous areas.

Evaluation

The oncology nurse systematically and regularly evaluates the client's and/or family's responses to interventions to determine progress toward the achievement of expected outcomes. Relevant data are collected and actual findings are compared with expected findings. Nursing diagnoses, outcomes, and plans of care are reviewed and revised as necessary.

PERICARDIAL EFFUSION

Theory
   I. Definition—excessive accumulation of fluid within the pericardial sac that surrounds the heart.
  II. Pericardial metastasis results from lymphatic, hematogenous, or direct invasion of tumor cells to pericardium.
 III. Lymphatic and venous drainage obstructed by tumor or mediastinal lymph node involvement.
  IV. Radiation therapy, causing pericarditis and pericardial thickening, can contribute to effusion.
   V. During gradual accumulation, the pericardium can accommodate 4 L of fluid.
  VI. Rapid accumulation of only 150 to 200 mL of fluid can precipitate cardiac tamponade (see Chapter 18).
   A. Impaired hemodynamic function due to increased intrapericardial pressure resulting in decreased cardiac output and impaired venous return.
   B. Classified as a cardiac oncologic emergency.
 VII. Incidence.
   A. Reported in as many as 20% of cancer patients.
   B. Most cases are asymptomatic.
   C. Associated with cancers of:
      1. Lung (37%).
      2. Breast (22%).
      3. Hematologic system (leukemia and lymphoma, 17%).
      4. Sarcoma (4%).
      5. Melanoma (3%).
VIII. Principles of medical management.
   A. Pericardiocentesis.
      1. Performed using echocardiogram.
      2. Allows for pericardial drainage.
   B. Pericardiectomy and pericardial window.
      1. Requires general anesthesia.
      2. Useful for clients in whom conservative measures (pericardiocentesis) were unsuccessful.
   C. Sclerosing agents.
      1. Agents include 5-fluorouracil, thiotepa, cisplatin, bleomycin.
      2. Effusions recur in approximately 50% of patients.

   D. Radiation therapy.
      1. Used for lymphomas.
      2. 50% response rate.

Assessment

   I. Risk factors.
      A. Tuberculosis.
      B. Radiation therapy involving the cardiac fields.
      C. Coexisting pulmonary, cardiac, or liver disease.
  II. Subjective findings.
      A. Dyspnea.
      B. Cough.
      C. Chest pain.
      D. Orthopnea.
      E. Weakness.
      F. Dysphagia.
      G. Syncope.
      H. Palpitations.
 III. Objective findings.
      A. Pleural effusion.
      B. Tachycardia.
      C. Jugular venous distention.
      D. Hepatomegaly.
      E. Peripheral edema.
      F. Pulsus paradoxus (narrowing pulse pressure).
      G. Hypotension.
      H. Distant heart sounds related to fluid interfering with sounds.
      I. Pericardial rub.
  IV. Diagnostic and laboratory findings.
      A. Echocardiography (ECHO) is the fastest, most precise method for identify-
         ing and determining extent of effusion.
         1. Advantage—allows for evaluation of ventricular function.
         2. Disadvantage—may not be timely in a cardiac tamponade emergency.
      B. Abnormal electrocardiogram (ECG).
         1. Tachycardia.
         2. Premature contractions.
         3. Low QRS voltage.
         4. Nonspecific ST- and T-wave changes.
      C. Chest x-ray examination.
         1. Cardiomegaly.
         2. Not diagnostic.
      D. Pericardial fluid cytology examination.
         1. Bloody and exudative in appearance.
         2. Reveals tumor cells, but a false-negative result is possible.

Nursing Diagnoses

   I. Anxiety.
  II. Cardiac output, decreased.
 III. Activity intolerance.

IV. Sleep pattern disturbance.
 V. Altered tissue perfusion: cardiopulmonary.

Outcome Identification

  I. Client verbalizes signs and symptoms of pericardial effusion.
 II. Client participates in recommended treatment.
III. Client reports restful sleep.

Planning and Implementation

  I. Interventions to minimize risk of occurrence, severity, and complications of effusions.
    A. Elevate head of bed 45 degrees.
    B. Maintain cool environment.
    C. Report acute clinical changes.
      1. Respiratory distress.
      2. Changes in cardiac assessment.
      3. Distended neck veins.
 II. Interventions related to client education.
    A. Teach energy conservation.
    B. Inform client of safety measures regarding open fire and smoking around oxygen.
    C. Demonstrate relaxation techniques.
    D. Instruct on signs and symptoms of worsening effusion to report to the nurse or physician.

Evaluation

The oncology nurse systematically and regularly evaluates the client's and/or family's responses to interventions to determine progress toward the achievement of expected outcomes. Relevant data are collected and actual findings are compared with expected findings. Nursing diagnoses, outcomes, and plans of care are reviewed and revised as necessary.

THROMBOTIC EVENTS

Theory

  I. Definition—venous or arterial occlusion.
 II. Paraneoplastic syndrome
    A. Microangiopathic hemolytic anemia (MAHA) associated with thrombotic thrombocytopenic purpura (TTP).
    B. Thrombocytosis.
      1. Platelet count over $400,000/mm^3$.
      2. Appears to be an abnormality in regulation of megakaryocyte production.
III. Metastatic cancer.
    A. Trousseau syndrome, thrombotic events associated with gastrointestinal cancers, has long been recognized.
    B. Extremity thrombosis and pulmonary emboli.
    C. Found even without demonstrable cancer.
IV. Nonspecific thrombosis manifesting as pulmonary emboli or arterial occlusion.

V. Related to venous access devices (see Chapter 9).
VI. Disseminated intravascular coagulation (DIC) (see Chapter 17).
VII. Cancer treatments.
VIII. Incidence.
    A. Association due to MAHA difficult to ascertain because of confounding factors of DIC and undiagnosed cases.
    B. Thrombocytosis.
        1. Tumor cells appear to be associated with procoagulant activities.
            a. Depositing fibrin in tissues and acting late in clotting cascade, providing a surface for prothrombinase assembly.
            b. Microvasculature becomes hyperpermeable, allowing clotting proteins to leak into extravascular space.
            c. Procoagulants initiate clotting.
        2. Incidence is 30 to 40% of clients with:
            a. Cancers of breast, lung, and gastrointestinal tract.
            b. Leukemias.
            c. Hodgkin's and non-Hodgkin's lymphomas.
    C. Tamoxifen-associated thrombophlebitis has been reported.
IV. Principles of medical management.
    A. Anticoagulation utilizing heparin, low–molecular-weight heparin, coumadin, aspirin, or dipyridamole.
    B. Treat underlying disease such as breast cancer or leukemia.
    C. Thrombocytopheresis.

Assessment

I. Risk factors.
    A. Estrogen replacement therapy.
    B. Smoking history.
    C. Nonspecific gastrointestinal symptoms.
II. Subjective findings.
    A. Reports of bleeding as clotting factors are exhausted.
        1. Most often occurs late in the disease trajectory.
        2. Not helpful in diagnosis of malignancy except when associated with DIC.
    B. Pulmonary embolus.
        1. Chest pain.
        2. Shortness of breath.
    C. Venous occlusion.
        1. Pain in affected extremity.
        2. Reports of swelling and warmth in affected extremity.
    D. Arterial occlusion.
        1. Acute, abrupt pain in affected extremity.
        2. Reports of paleness in affected extremity.
III. Objective findings.
    A. Bruising or petechiae.
    B. Bleeding nose, bleeding from rectum, urinary tract.
    C. Pulmonary embolus.
        1. Decreased pulse oximetry.
        2. Increased respiratory rate.
        3. Shallow breaths as client guards against pain.
    D. Deep vein thrombosis.
        1. Swelling of extremity.
        2. Erythema.

   E. Arterial occlusion.
      1. Loss of pulse.
      2. Extremity coolness.
      3. Medical emergency because loss of the extremity is possible.
IV. Laboratory findings.
   A. MAHA—severe anemia (hemoglobin level 7 g/dL).
   B. Thrombocytosis—platelet count over 400,000/mm^3.
   C. Abnormal venogram result on affected extremity associated with venous thrombosis.
   D. Abnormal arteriogram result with arterial thrombosis.
   E. Abnormal ventilation/perfusion scan result with pulmonary embolus.
   F. Abnormal clotting factor levels such as fibrinopeptide A (FPA) and plasma fibrinogen are possible; however, the tests are not commonly used outside of suspected DIC.

Nursing Diagnoses

   I. Altered tissue perfusion: peripheral, cardiopulmonary.
  II. Risk for impaired skin integrity.
 III. Pain.
 IV. Activity intolerance.

Outcome Identification

   I. Client identifies early signs and symptoms of bleeding and clotting and reports them to health care providers.
  II. Client maintains compliance with anticoagulation therapy.
 III. Client's extremities are warm and of normal color.

Planning and Implementation

   I. Provide a safe environment (i.e., padded siderails on the hospital bed for a client at risk for bleeding).
  II. Respond quickly to arterial occlusion.
      A. Make immediate vascular surgery referral for possible surgery.
      B. Initiate pain control activities.
      C. Monitor arterial pulses in affected extremity.
 III. Manage treatment of venous occlusion.
      A. Monitor anticoagulant therapy.
         1. Partial thromboplastin time (PTT) for heparin therapy.
         2. Prothrombin time (PT) or international normalized ratio (INR) for coumadin therapy.
         3. Vitamin K therapy for abnormal coumadin level if indicated.
      B. Elevation of extremity to relieve edema.
 IV. Provide support for a client with pulmonary embolus.
      A. Monitor oxygen therapy.
      B. Initiate pain control activities.
  V. Initiate patient education.
      A. Relate instructions to signs of thrombosis or bleeding.
      B. Educate about self-injection if the client is using heparin at home.
      C. Educate about dietary restrictions in a patient receiving coumadin, such as avoiding leafy green vegetables high in vitamin K.
      D. Instruct patient to avoid situations that could alter skin integrity (e.g., straight razors).

E. Provide client with information about preventing lower extremity deep vein thrombosis (e.g., getting up and walking every 2 hours).

F. Related to smoking cessation.

Evaluation

The oncology nurse systematically and regularly evaluates the client's and/or family's responses to interventions to determine progress toward the achievement of expected outcomes. Relevant data are collected and actual findings are compared with expected findings. Nursing diagnoses, outcomes, and plans of care are reviewed and revised as necessary.

BIBLIOGRAPHY

Allen, A. (1992). The cardiotoxicity of chemotherapeutic drugs. In M.C. Perry (ed.). *The Chemotherapy Source Book.* Baltimore: Williams & Wilkins, pp. 582–597.

Baker, A.R., & Weber, J.S. (1993). Malignant ascites. In V.T. DeVita, Jr., S. Hellman, & S.A. Rosenberg (eds.). *Cancer: Principles and Practices of Oncology* (4th ed.). Philadelphia: J.B. Lippincott, pp. 2255–2261.

DeVita, Jr., V.T. Hellman, S., Rosenberg, S.A. (1993). *Cancer: Principles and Practices of Oncology* (4th ed.). Philadelphia: J.B. Lippincott.

Groenwald, S., Frogge, M., Goodman, M., & Yarbro, C. (1993). *Cancer Nursing: Principles and Practice.* Boston: Jones & Bartlett.

Kaszyk, L.K. (1986). Cardiac toxicity associated with cancer therapy. *Oncol Nurs Forum 13*(4), 81–88.

Knobf, M.D. (1985) Primary breast cancer: Physical consequences and rehabilitation. *Semi Oncol Nurs 1*, 214–224.

Graydon, J., Bubela, N., Irvine, D., & Vincent, L. (1995). Fatigue-reducing strategies used by patients receiving treatment for cancer. *Cancer Nurs 18*, 23–28.

Mrozek-Orlowski, M. (1996). Breast cancer. In M. Liebman & D. Camp–Sorrell (eds.). *Multimodal Therapy in Oncology Nursing.* St. Louis: C.V. Mosby, pp. 119–132.

Olopade, O.I., & Ultmann, J.E. (1991). Malignant effusions. *CA Cancer J Clin 41*(3), 166–179.

Powel, L. (1996). *Cancer Chemotherapy Guidelines and Recommendations for Practice.* Pittsburgh: Oncology Nursing Press, pp. 12–13.

Winningham, M.L., Nail, L., Burke, M. B., et al. (1994). Fatigue and the cancer experience: The state of the knowledge. *Oncol Nurs Forum 21*, 23–36.

Witte, C.L., Witte, M.H., Dumont, A.E. (1984). Pathophysiology of chronic edema, lymphedema, and fibrosis. In N. Staub, A.E. Taylor (eds.). *Edema.* New York: Raven Press, pp. 521–542.

Wujcik, D., & Downs, S. (1992). Bone marrow transplantation. *Crit Care Nurs Clin North Am 4*(1), 149–166.

PART FIVE

Oncologic Emergencies

Metabolic Emergencies

Joanne Peter Finley, RN, MS

DISSEMINATED INTRAVASCULAR COAGULATION

Theory

 I. Hemostasis is maintained through a balanced system of thrombosis and fibrinolysis (Fig. 17–1).
   A. The process of thrombosis is initiated through disruption of the endothelial membrane and/or tissue injury.
     1. Disruption of the endothelial membrane activates a cascade of clotting factors in the intrinsic pathway, resulting in coagulation.
     2. Tissue injury causes the release of tissue thromboplastin into the circulation and the activation of the extrinsic pathway, resulting in coagulation.
     3. Reactions that occur in the intrinsic and extrinsic pathways of coagulation are combined in a final common pathway.
   B. Fibrinolysis, the process by which the reactions that result in clotting are inhibited and developed clots are destroyed, is initiated by the formation of the fibrin clot.
     1. Plasmin is an enzyme that digests the components of the fibrin clot. D-dimer is an antigen that is formed when this occurs.
     2. The products of this reaction, fibrin-split products (FSPs) or fibrin-degradation products (FDPs), are released into the circulation and function as anticoagulants.
     3. FDPs are gradually cleared from the circulation in the reticuloendothelial system (RES).
 II. Definition—the inappropriate, accelerated, and systematic activation of the coagulation cascade, resulting in thrombosis and, subsequently, hemorrhage.
 III. In the presence of an underlying condition such as infection, malignancy, or trauma, the intrinsic and/or extrinsic pathway of the clotting cascade is triggered, thrombosis is accelerated, and fibrin clots are formed and deposited in the microcirculation.
 IV. The consumption of coagulation factors is greater than the ability of the body for replacement; therefore, coagulation is inhibited.
 V. In addition, fibrinolysis is initiated; FDPs are not removed effectively from the circulation, and an accumulation of these anticoagulant substances occurs.
 VI. Principles of medical management.
   A. Diagnostic tests (Table 17–1).
   B. Medical management of disseminated intravascular coagulation (DIC) is targeted to treatment of the underlying, predisposing conditions; replace-

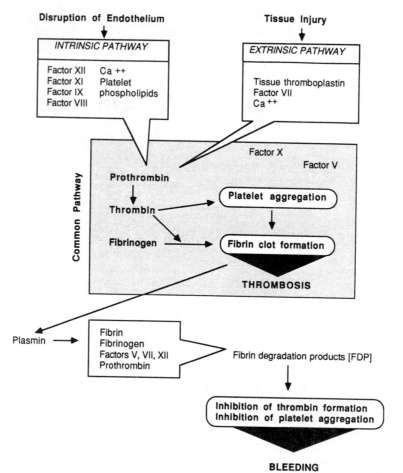

Figure 17–1. Physiology of thrombosis and fibrinolysis.

TABLE 17–1. **Laboratory Results With Disseminated Intravascular Coagulation**

Laboratory Test	Findings
D-dimer assay	Increased
Fibrin-degradation products	Increased
Prothrombin time (PT)	Increased
Partial thromboplastin time	Increased
Thrombin time	Increased
Fibrinogen	Decreased
Platelet count	Decreased
Hematocrit/hemoglobin	Decreased
Antithrombin III level	Decreased

ment of coagulation factors and platelets; and inhibition of the coagulation process.

1. Treatment of the underlying, predisposing condition such as chemotherapy for malignancy or antibiotics for infection.
2. Replacement of coagulation factors and platelets.
   a. Blood component therapy for abnormal hematologic parameters or active bleeding (see Chapter 9).
      (1) Cryoprecipitate provides fibrinogen and factor VIII.
      (2) Platelet concentrate.
      (3) Fresh frozen plasma provides plasma, fibrinogen, and other clotting factors; use of fresh frozen plasma may aggravate DIC since new clotting factors are added.
      (4) Packed red blood cells.
   b. Plasmapheresis to replace coagulation factors.
3. Inhibition of the coagulation or fibrinolytic process.
   a. Plasmapheresis removes triggers of coagulation.
   b. Acetylsalicylic acid (ASA) prevents clotting.
   c. Heparin interferes with thrombin production.
      (1) Use is considered controversial except in acute progranulocytic leukemia (APL).
      (2) Goal is to maintain partial thromboplastin time (PTT) at 1½ to 2 times normal levels.
      (3) Primary side effect is bleeding.
   d. ε-Aminocaproic acid (EACA) inhibits fibrinolysis.
      (1) Usually given with heparin.
      (2) Primary side effect is clotting.
   e. Antithrombin III inhibits procoagulants and fibrinolytic process.

Assessment

I. Identification of clients at risk.
   A. History of cancer—prostate, breast, colon, lung, or leukemia.
   B. Infection and sepsis (most common cause of DIC).
   C. History of cancer treatment—surgery, radiation, and chemotherapy.
   D. Trauma, burns, or shock.
   E. Pregnancy and obstetric complications.
   F. Presence of liver disease.
   G. Recent blood transfusion or hemolytic transfusion reaction.
II. Physical examination.
   A. Skin—petechiae, ecchymosis, purpura, acral cyanosis (blue/gray coloration of extremities), pallor, and bleeding from sites of invasive procedures.
   B. Gastrointestinal—abdominal distention, positive result of guaiac stool test, abdominal pain.
   C. Genitourinary—hematuria and decreased urinary output.
   D. Respiratory—dyspnea, hemoptysis, and tachypnea.
   E. Neurologic—restlessness, confusion, and lethargy.
   F. Musculoskeletal—joint pain, stiffness, and positive Homans's sign.
   G. Cardiovascular—tachycardia and diminished peripheral pulses.
III. Evaluation of laboratory data (see Table 17–1).

Nursing Diagnoses

I. Altered tissue perfusion.
II. Risk for injury: bleeding.

III. Fluid volume deficit.
IV. Impaired gas exchange.
V. Impaired skin integrity.
VI. Risk for injury.
VII. Pain.
VIII. Fear.

Outcome Identification

I. Client identifies personal risk factors for development of DIC.
II. Client lists critical signs and symptoms of DIC that should be reported immediately to the health care team.
III. Client describes self-care measures to maximize personal safety.

Planning and Implementation

I. Interventions to maximize safety for the client.
  A. Place bed in low position and siderails up.
  B. Clear pathways in room and hallways.
  C. Provide assistance as needed for activities of daily living.
  D. Minimize activities that trigger bleeding.
II. Interventions to decrease severity of symptoms associated with DIC.
  A. Apply direct pressure to sites of active bleeding.
  B. Elevate sites of active bleeding if possible.
  C. Apply pressure dressings or sandbags to sites of active bleeding.
  D. Administer pain medications as needed.
III. Interventions to monitor for sequelae of DIC and treatment.
  A. Monitor for signs and symptoms of progressive DIC.
    1. Tachycardia, hypotension, and cool, clammy, cyanotic skin.
    2. Anuria.
    3. Decreased mental status to coma.
    4. Changes in location, severity, or responses to pain.
    5. Changes in the depth, rate, or difficulty of respirations.
  B. Monitor for signs and symptoms of fluid overload.
IV. Interventions to monitor response of client to medical management.
  A. Monitor sites and amount of bleeding.
    1. Weigh dressings.
    2. Count peripads.
    3. Measure bloody drainage.
    4. Hematest urine, stool, and emesis.
  B. Monitor changes in laboratory values and report significant changes to physician.
  C. Assess tissue perfusion parameters—color, temperature, peripheral pulses.
  D. Monitor psychosocial responses of the client and family to critical illness.
V. Interventions to enhance adaptation and rehabilitation.
  A. Provide information about planned therapy and response to treatment at regular intervals.
  B. Listen to concerns and fears of the client and family.
VI. Interventions to incorporate the client and family in care.
  A. Instruct the client and family about critical signs and symptoms to report to the health care team—new sites of bleeding, changes in color of stool or urine, subjective changes in respiratory effort and effectiveness, and changes in mental status.

B. Instruct the client and family to save all urine, stool, and emesis.
C. Instruct the client and family in measures to prevent bleeding (see Chapter 12).

Evaluation

The oncology nurse systematically and regularly evaluates the client's and/or family's responses to interventions to determine progress toward the achievement of expected outcomes. Relevant data are collected and actual findings are compared with expected findings. Nursing diagnoses, outcomes, and plans of care are reviewed and revised as necessary.

SEPSIS

Theory

I. Sepsis is a systemic inflammatory response to pathogenic microorganisms and associated endotoxins in the blood.
  A. It usually presents with 2 or more of the following parameters.
    1. Temperature greater than 100.4°F.
    2. Heart rate greater than 90 beats per minute.
    3. Respiratory rate greater than 20 breaths per minute.
    4. White blood cell count greater than 12,000, or less than 4000, or greater than 10% bands.
II. Septic shock is manifested by hemodynamic instability and alterations in cellular metabolism caused by sepsis (Fig. 17–2).
III. Infectious agents.
  A. Gram-negative bacteria (*Escherichia coli, Klebsiella pneumoniae,* and *Pseudomonas aeruginosa*) are the most common cause of sepsis.
  B. Other organisms include fungi (*Candida* and *Aspergillus*), gram-positive bacteria, anaerobes, viruses, and protozoa.
  C. Most infections arise from endogenous flora of the client.
IV. Prognosis.
  A. Untreated bacteremia in neutropenia clients is fatal; septic shock is associated with a 50 to 70% mortality rate.
  B. Mortality is associated with causative organism, site of infection, and the level and duration of neutropenia.
V. Principles of medical management.
  A. Diagnostic tests.
    1. Blood culture—aerobic and anaerobic.
    2. Chest x-ray examination.
    3. Cultures of urine, throat, stool, sputum, and central venous catheters.
    4. Complete blood count.
    5. Prothrombin time (PT)/Partial thromboplastin time (PTT).
    6. Arterial blood gas values.
    7. Plasma lactate level.
      a. Degree of tissue hypoxia.
  B. Nonpharmacologic interventions.
    1. Fluid resuscitation—crystalloids (normal saline solution or lactated Ringer's solution) and colloids (albumin).
    2. Blood component therapy.
      a. Red blood cells.
      b. Granulocyte transfusions may be used if fever persists after broad-

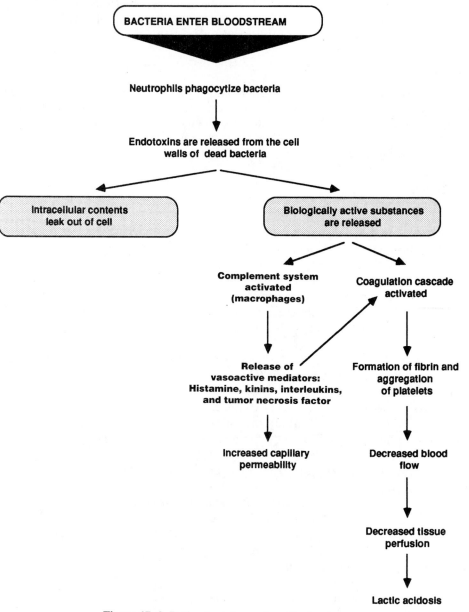

Figure 17–2. Pathophysiology of septic shock.

   spectrum antibiotic and antifungal therapy when prolonged neutropenia is expected.
3. Oxygen therapy progressing to ventilatory support as needed.
4. Central catheter or implantable port removal.
5. Nutritional support.
C. Pharmacologic interventions (see Chapter 10).
   1. Empiric antibiotics for first fever spike in neutropenia clients.
   2. If fever persists after 3- to 5-day course of antibiotics, antifungal therapy
      (amphotericin) may be initiated; rigors are major side effect.

    3. Dopamine—vasopressor that increases cardiac contractility, peripheral vascular resistance, and renal blood flow.

    4. Prostaglandin inhibitors.

    5. New treatments include.

       a. Mediator-specific therapies

       b. Antiendotoxin antibodies

Assessment

I. Identification of clients at risk.

  A. Neutropenia less than 1000 cells/mm^3.

  B. Age greater than 65 years.

  C. Prosthetic devices such as multilumen catheters, feeding tubes, and tracheostomy tubes.

  D. Malnutrition.

  E. Loss of skin or mucosal integrity.

  F. Diabetes.

II. Pertinent history.

  A. Recent chemotherapy, radiation therapy, or steroid therapy.

  B. Diagnosis of cancer such as leukemia, lymphoma, and multiple myeloma.

  C. Chronic disease such as diabetes mellitus and hepatic or renal disease.

  D. Splenectomy.

  E. Recent hospitalization.

III. Physical examination.

  A. Early signs and symptoms.

    1. Typical signs and symptoms of infection may be absent because of decreased or absent blood cells.

    2. Earliest signs—anxiety, restlessness, confusion, and decreased level of consciousness.

    3. Chills and fever.

    4. Tachypnea, rales, rhonchi, and wheezes.

    5. Tachycardia and widening pulse pressure.

    6. Warm, flushed skin.

    7. Anorexia.

  B. Late signs and symptoms.

    1. Disorientation and lethargy.

    2. Dyspnea, cyanosis, and increased pulmonary congestion.

    3. Tachycardia, thready pulse, and narrowing pulse pressure.

    4. Cool, clammy skin.

    5. Decreased or absent urinary output.

IV. Evaluation of laboratory data.

  A. Positive blood cultures.

  B. Decreased white blood cell count.

  C. Pulmonary infiltrates seen on chest x-ray examination.

  D. Prolonged PT and PTT.

  E. Elevated blood urea nitrogen (BUN) and creatinine levels.

  F. Respiratory alkalosis followed by metabolic acidosis.

  G. Elevated plasma lactate level.

Nursing Diagnoses

I. Altered tissue perfusion.

II. Fluid volume deficit.

III. Decreased cardiac output.
IV. Risk for injury.
 V. Pain.
VI. Hyperthermia.
VII. Altered protection.
VIII. Altered urinary elimination.

Outcome Identification

 I. Client describes personal risk factors for septic shock.
 II. Client lists critical signs and symptoms of septic shock that should be reported to a member of the health care team.
III. Client discusses strategies to decrease the risks of septic shock.

Planning and Implementation

 I. Interventions to maximize safety for the client.
   A. Assess environment for safety—bed in low position and siderails up.
   B. Orient client to time, place, and person.
   C. Maintain infection control measures—handwashing, oral care, perineal care, limitation of invasive procedures, and care of invasive equipment.
   D. Institute bleeding precautions.
 II. Interventions to decrease the severity of symptoms associated with septic shock.
   A. Report early signs and symptoms of septic shock to physician immediately.
   B. Obtain critical elements of diagnostic workup as ordered within a limited time frame.
   C. Initiate antibiotic or antifungal therapy immediately after ordered.
   D. Encourage client to turn, cough, and deep breathe to mobilize pulmonary secretions.
   E. Explain procedures, treatments, monitoring activities, and significance of changes in condition to decrease anxiety.
III. Interventions to monitor for sequelae of septic shock.
   A. Monitor vital signs (pulse, blood pressure, respirations, central venous pressure (CVP), and pulmonary artery (PA) pressure) at intervals dictated by clinical condition.
   B. Assess skin color, temperature, and capillary refill.
   C. Monitor intake and output.
   D. Weigh client each day.
   E. Assess potential sites of infection and obtain order for cultures of suspicious areas.
   F. Assess peripheral pulses.
   G. Monitor for signs and symptoms of complications of septic shock—DIC, adult respiratory distress syndrome.
IV. Interventions to monitor response to medical management.
   A. Monitor vital signs every 4 hours or more often as clinically indicated; report significant changes in vital signs (marked decrease in temperature, blood pressure, or pulse pressure or marked increase in pulse or respiratory rate) to the physician.
   B. Monitor changes in laboratory values and report significant changes (growth in cultures, increase in white blood count) to the physician.
   C. Monitor for signs and symptoms of fluid overload (weight gain, rales, edema).

V. Interventions to enhance adaptation and rehabilitation.
  A. Maintain bedrest for acutely ill client.
  B. Organize care activities to minimize energy expenditure and oxygen consumption.
  C. Encourage range of motion and isometric exercises.
  D. Reinforce principles of infection prevention and control in preparation for discharge.

Evaluation

The oncology nurse systematically and regularly evaluates the client's and/or family's responses to interventions to determine progress toward the achievement of expected outcomes. Relevant data are collected and actual findings are compared with expected findings. Nursing diagnoses, outcomes, and plans of care are reviewed and revised as necessary.

TUMOR LYSIS SYNDROME

Theory

  I. Definition—a metabolic imbalance that occurs with the rapid release of intracellular potassium, phosphorus, and nucleic acid into the blood as a result of tumor cell kill (Fig. 17–3).
 II. The syndrome includes:
  A. Hyperkalemia.
  B. Hyperphosphatemia.
  C. Hyperuricemia—results from conversion of nucleic acid to uric acid.

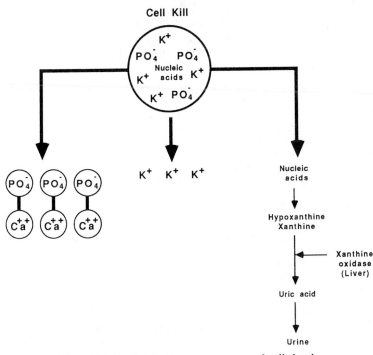

Figure 17–3. Metabolic consequences of cell death.

    D. Hypocalcemia—results from increased phosphorus binding to calcium to form calcium phosphate salts.

III. Potential effects of tumor lysis syndrome include:
    A. Renal failure—kidneys are the primary route of elimination for phosphorus, uric acid, and potassium.
    B. Cardiac arrhythmias.

IV. Principles of medical management.
    A. Diagnostic tests.
        1. Serum electrolytes (potassium, phosphorus, and calcium) and uric acid.
        2. Renal function studies—BUN and creatinine.
        3. Electrocardiography (ECG).
    B. Nonpharmacologic interventions.
        1. Intravenous hydration.
            a. Pre- and postcancer treatment.
        2. Hemapheresis.
        3. Dialysis.
        4. Potassium and phosphorus restrictions.
    C. Pharmacologic interventions.
        1. Allopurinol.
            a. Blocks xanthine oxidase to decrease uric acid production.
            b. Potential side effects—rash, fever, gastrointestinal upset, and diarrhea.
        2. Diuretics.
            a. Maintains urinary output.
            b. Potential side effects—dehydration.
            c. Usually maintained for 3 to 5 days after chemotherapy begins.
        3. Aluminum hydroxide.
            a. Binds dietary phosphate from small bowel.
            b. Potential side effect—constipation.
        4. Exchange resins such as sodium polystyrene sulfonate (Kayexalate).
            a. Decrease potassium levels.
            b. Potential side effects—hypokalemia, hypocalcemia, hypomagnesia, and constipation.
        5. Sodium bicarbonate—alkalinizes urine to increase solubility of uric acid.
            a. Potential side effects—metabolic alkalosis and hypocalcemia.

Assessment

I. Identification of clients at risk.
    A. Diagnosis of leukemia, lymphoma, or small-cell lung cancer.
    B. Diagnosis of tumors with a high growth fraction or elevated lactate dehydrogenase (LDH) level.
    C. Recent chemotherapy or radiation therapy for cancer.
    D. Concurrent renal or cardiac disease.

II. Physical examination.
    A. Early signs and symptoms.
        1. Neuromuscular—muscle weakness, twitching, paresthesia, lethargy, confusion, and fatigue.
        2. Cardiovascular—arrhythmias and bradycardia.
        3. Gastrointestinal—nausea, vomiting, anorexia, and diarrhea.
        4. Renal—oliguria, flank pain, hematuria, weight gain, and edema.

B. Late signs and symptoms.
   1. Seizures.
   2. Cardiac arrest.
   3. Acute renal failure.
III. Evaluation of laboratory data.
   A. Elevated BUN and serum creatinine levels.
   B. Elevated potassium and phosphorus levels.
   C. Decreased calcium and creatinine clearance.
   D. Elevated uric acid level.

Nursing Diagnoses

  I. Altered protection.
 II. Risk for injury.
III. Self-care deficit.
IV. Decreased cardiac output.
 V. Fluid volume excess.
VI. Altered nutrition: less than body requirements.

Outcome Identification

  I. Client describes personal risk factors for tumor lysis syndrome.
 II. Client participates in strategies to decrease the risk and severity of tumor lysis syndrome.
III. Client describes signs and symptoms of tumor lysis syndrome or side effects of treatment to report to the health care team.
IV. Client identifies emergency resources in the community.

Planning and Implementation

  I. Interventions to maximize safety for the client.
   A. Recognize clients at risk before initiation of treatment.
   B. Institute safety measures for changes in level of consciousness.
    1. Maintain bed in low position with siderails up.
    2. Place call light within reach.
    3. Evaluate client at regular intervals.
   C. Institute seizure precautions as calcium levels warrant.
   D. Place emergency equipment within access if severe hyperkalemia or hypocalcemia is present.
 II. Interventions to decrease incidence and severity of symptoms associated with tumor lysis syndrome.
   A. Teach the client and family about strategies to decrease the incidence of tumor lysis syndrome.
    1. Maintain adequate oral fluid intake.
    2. Take allopurinol as ordered by physician.
    3. Report signs and symptoms of tumor lysis syndrome to the health care team.
   B. Notify physician if pH of urine is less than 7.0.
   C. Consult with dietician to modify diet if renal dysfunction is present.
III. Interventions to monitor for sequelae of tumor lysis syndrome or treatment.
   A. Assess for symptoms of cardiac arrhythmias.
    1. Decrease in blood pressure.
    2. Increase in pulse rate.

    3. Irregular pulse, ECG changes.
    4. Chest pain.
    5. Shortness of breath.
  B. Assess for symptoms of renal failure.
    1. Decrease in urinary output to less than 600 mL/day.
    2. Changes in mental status.
    3. Anorexia, nausea, and vomiting.
    4. Diarrhea.
    5. Increase in weight.
  C. Assess for side effects of treatment (see section, Principles of medical management, Pharmacologic interventions, p. 324).
IV. Interventions to monitor response to medical management.
  A. Maintain strict intake and output. (Urine output should be greater than or equal to 100 mL/hr.)
  B. Weigh patient daily.
  C. Assess urine color and clarity.
  D. Report significant changes in laboratory values.

Evaluation

The oncology nurse systematically and regularly evaluates the client's and/or family's responses to interventions to determine progress toward the achievement of expected outcomes. Relevant data are collected and actual findings are compared with expected findings. Nursing diagnoses, outcomes, and plans of care are reviewed and revised as necessary.

ANAPHYLAXIS

Theory

  I. Anaphylaxis is an immediate hypersensitivity reaction that usually occurs within seconds to minutes. It is also known as a Type I reaction.
 II. Immediate hypersensitivity reactions are mediated by immunoglobulin E (IgE), which is produced by B lymphocytes (Fig. 17–4).
III. The antigen-specific IgE binds to mast cells and sensitizes them to the antigen.
IV. On subsequent exposure of the sensitized mast cell to the antigen, a series of reactions occur that result in degranulation of the mast cell and release of mediators of the hypersensitivity reaction (Table 17–2).
 V. Signs and symptoms of the immediate hypersensitivity reaction are a result of the effects of the mediators on target organs of the skin, lung, and gastrointestinal tract.
VI. Principles of medical management.
  A. Diagnostic tests.
    1. Intradermal skin tests.
    2. Test dose of agents.
      a. Administer small dose of agent that may cause anaphylaxis.
      b. Keep line open if agent given intravenously.
      c. Monitor for signs and symptoms of anaphylaxis (see section, Assessment, Physical examination, p. 324) for at least 15 minutes.
      d. If no reaction occurs, administer total dose as ordered by physician.
  B. Nonpharmacologic interventions.
    1. Intravenous fluid replacement.
    2. Oxygen therapy.

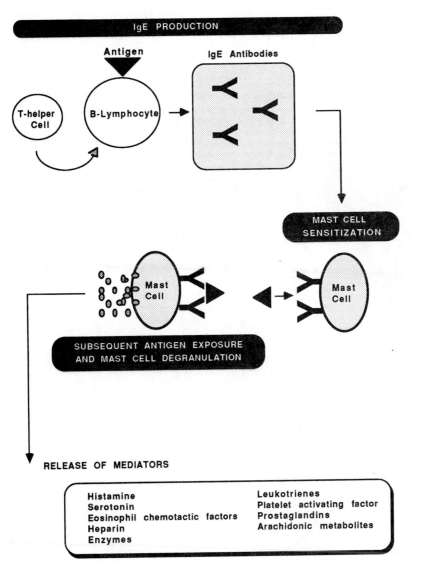

Figure 17–4. Immediate hypersensitivity reaction.

  3. Maintenance of patent airway.
     a. Intubation.
     b. Emergency tracheostomy if upper airway edema occurs.
  4. Hemodynamic monitoring.
  C. Pharmacologic interventions.
     1. Prophylaxis—diphenhydramine, prednisone, cimetidine, and acetamin-
        ophen.
     2. Emergency agents (Table 17–3).

Assessment

  I. Identification of clients at risk.
     A. Receiving antineoplastic agents such as L-asparaginase, bleomycin, cisplatin,
        or paclitaxel (Taxol).

TABLE 17–2. **Mediators of the Immediate Hypersensitivity Reaction**

Mediator	Action
Histamine	Contraction of smooth muscle Increased permeability of vessels Modulation of chemotaxis and prostaglandins
Serotonin	Contraction of smooth muscle Increased permeability of vessels
Eosinophil chemotactic factors	Attraction and deactivation of eosinophils and neutrophils
Heparin	Anticoagulation
Enzymes	Proteolysis, hydrolysis, and cleavage
Leukotrienes	Contraction of smooth muscle Increased permeability of vessels Modulation of histamine, prostaglandins, and chemotaxis
Platelet activating factor	Promotion of platelet aggregation and adhesion
Prostaglandins and arachidonic metabolites	Contraction and relaxation of smooth muscle Chemotaxis

B. Risk for anaphylaxis increases when agents are:
1. Crude preparations of the agent such as those used in Phase I studies.
2. Derived from bacteria such as L-asparaginase.
3. Given intravenously.
4. Given at high doses.
5. Given in successive doses.
C. Previous exposure to agent.

TABLE 17–3. **Pharmacologic Agents Used to Treat Anaphylaxis**

Agent	Results of Action	Nursing Implications
Epinephrine	Elevates blood pressure Dilates bronchi Constricts peripheral vessels Decreases itching	Monitor pulse rate, rhythm, and regularity
Diphenhydramine	Decreases itching Blocks histamine actions	Monitor for sudden decrease in blood pressure Encourage oral hygiene practices for dry mouth Teach client about safety issues associated with drowsiness
Hydrocortisone	Prevents delayed symptoms Inhibits synthesis of mediators of immune response	Take medication with food Report signs and symptoms of gastrointestinal distress to physician
Cimetidine	Decreases laryngeal edema Antagonizes H_2 receptors	Monitor for marked decrease in blood pressure
Aminophylline	Dilates bronchi	Monitor pulse rate, rhythm, and regularity
Dopamine	Increases cardiac contractility and peripheral vasculature resistance	Monitor blood pressure and catheter site

    D. Previous allergic reactions to agents such as foods, radiographic contrast media, blood products, insulin, opiates, and penicillins.

    E. Receiving biologic agents such as monoclonal antibodies.

II. Physical examination.

    A. Early signs and symptoms usually occur within 30 minutes.

        1. Integumentary—pruritus, urticaria, erythema, and angioedema.

        2. Cardiovascular—tightness in chest, flushing, dizziness, warmth, and hypotension.

        3. Gastrointestinal—nausea, vomiting, diarrhea, and abdominal discomfort.

        4. Respiratory—dyspnea and wheezing.

        5. Neurological—anxiety, feeling of doom, agitation, and dizziness.

    B. Late signs and symptoms.

        1. Cardiovascular—hypotension, tachycardia, chest pain, and arrhythmias.

        2. Respiratory—laryngeal edema, bronchospasm, and stridor.

        3. Neurologic—loss of consciousness.

III. Evaluation of laboratory data.

    A. Arterial blood gas values.

    B. IgE antibody level.

Nursing Diagnoses

  I. Alteration in comfort.

  II. Anxiety.

 III. Decreased cardiac output.

 IV. Fluid volume deficit.

  V. Ineffective breathing pattern.

 VI. Impaired skin integrity.

Outcome Identification

  I. Client identifies personal risk factors for anaphylactic reaction.

  II. Client describes signs and symptoms of anaphylaxis to report to the health care team: itching, hives, difficulty breathing, and anxiety.

 III. Client participates in strategies to decrease risk or severity of anaphylaxis.

    A. Avoids allergen.

    B. Informs care providers of allergy.

    C. Maintains emergency kit in environment in which potential exposure to an allergen may occur.

    D. Wears Medic Alert jewelry.

 IV. Client lists the location and telephone numbers of available community emergency services.

Planning and Implementation

  I. Interventions to maximize safety for the client.

    A. Have emergency agents and equipment within reach during administration of high-risk agents.

    B. Maintain free-flowing intravenous infusion when administering a potential allergen.

    C. Obtain baseline vital signs.

    D. Label medical record with allergy history.

    E. Remain with the client for 30 minutes after administering agent.

    F. If a reaction occurs, ask the client to remain in bed, put bed in low position, and raise siderails.

  II. Interventions to decrease severity of symptoms associated with anaphylaxis.

    A. At first sign of reaction.

      1. Stop flow of agent.

      2. Maintain intravenous infusion according to institutional protocol.

      3. Evaluate patency of airway, pulse, respirations, and blood pressure.

      4. Notify the physician of signs and symptoms observed and actions taken.

      5. Administer emergency drugs (see Table 17–3) as ordered by physician or per institutional protocol.

    B. Position the client to decrease respiratory distress symptoms (elevate head of bed).

    C. Position the client in supine position to perfuse vital organs.

 III. Interventions to monitor for sequelae of anaphylaxis or treatment.

    A. Observe for symptoms of respiratory distress.

      1. Increase in respiratory rate, rhythm, and effort.

      2. Presence of adventitious breath sounds.

      3. Changes in arterial blood gas values as ordered by physician.

    B. Observe for signs of fluid overload.

      1. Changes in weight greater than 5 pounds per day.

      2. Changes in intake and output ratio.

      3. Jugular neck vein distention.

    C. Observe for signs of anxiety.

      1. Remain with client during acute reaction.

      2. Be calm and confident while implementing emergency procedures.

      3. Explain the process and rationale for each procedure.

    D. Check for impaired skin integrity.

      1. Clip nails to decrease risk of scratching skin surfaces.

      2. Decrease pressure, friction, and shearing forces on skin surfaces.

      3. Encourage client to avoid scratching skin surfaces.

    E. Observe for cardiovascular collapse.

      1. Decrease in blood pressure.

      2. Increase in heart rate.

Evaluation

The oncology nurse systematically and regularly evaluates the client's and/or family's responses to interventions to determine progress toward the achievement of expected outcomes. Relevant data are collected and actual findings are compared with expected findings. Nursing diagnoses, outcomes, and plans of care are reviewed and revised as necessary.

HYPERCALCEMIA

Theory

    I. Normal levels of calcium are regulated by the action of the parathyroid gland (production of parathyroid hormone), gastrointestinal tract (absorption of vitamin D), and the kidneys (excretion) (Fig. 17–5).

    A. When calcium levels fall below normal, the parathyroid gland is stimulated to produce parathyroid hormone.

    B. Parathyroid hormone acts on the bone, a reservoir for calcium, and causes

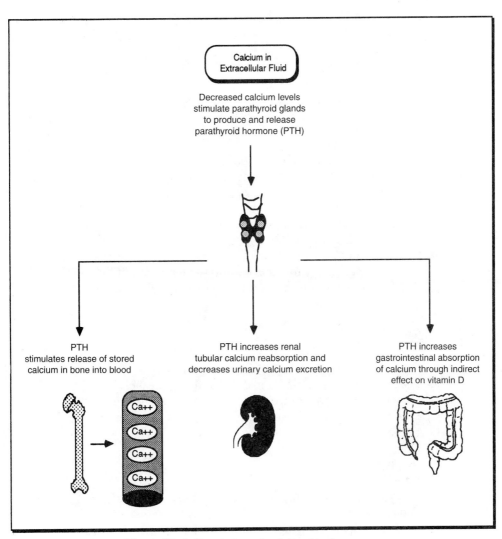

Calcium in
Extracellular Fluid

Decreased calcium levels
stimulate parathyroid glands
to produce and release
parathyroid hormone (PTH)

PTH
stimulates release of stored
calcium in bone into blood

PTH increases renal
tubular calcium reabsorption and
decreases urinary calcium excretion

PTH increases
gastrointestinal absorption
of calcium through indirect
effect on vitamin D

Ca++
Ca++
Ca++
Ca++

Figure 17–5. Regulation of calcium levels.

an increase in the amount of calcium released from the bone (resorption) into the circulation and ultimately the extracellular fluid.

   C. When calcium levels rise above normal, the kidney increases excretion of calcium to return the level to normal.

II. Hypercalcemia is defined as a serum calcium level greater than 11 mg/dL.

III. Potential causes of hypercalcemia among persons with cancer include:

   A. Increased bone resorption secondary to increased osteoclast activity because of humoral factors (tumor necrosis factor [TNF], interleukin) released by the tumor.

   B. Increased bone resorption secondary to direct tumor invasion of the bone.

   C. Decreased ability of the kidneys to clear calcium from the blood.

   D. Increased bone resorption secondary to prostaglandin secretion by tumor.

IV. Hypercalcemia occurs in 10 to 20% of persons with cancer and is the most common oncologic emergency.

V. Principles of medical management.
   A. Diagnostic tests.
      1. Serum and urine calcium.
      2. Serum potassium, sodium, and phosphorus.
      3. BUN and creatinine.
      4. ECG.
   B. Nonpharmacologic interventions.
      1. Administer intravenous fluids.
         a. Restore hydration.
         b. Increase the glomerular filtration rate.
         c. Treatment of choice for temporary improvement of symptoms.
         d. Normal saline is used.
      2. Maintain mobility.
      3. Institute dialysis if needed—provides rapid, temporary relief.
   C. Pharmacologic interventions.
      1. Administer antineoplastic therapy for primary and metastatic tumor.
      2. Administer drugs to lower serum calcium (Table 17–4).
      3. Discontinue agents that contribute to hypercalcemia—thiazide diuretics, estrogen therapy.

Assessment

  I. Identification of clients at risk.
   A. Diagnosis of breast, lung, renal, head, or neck cancer (80%).
   B. Diagnosis of multiple myeloma, lymphoma, and leukemia (20%).
   C. Primary hyperparathyroidism.
   D. Immobility.
   E. Dehydration.
   F. Renal dysfunction.
   G. Skeletal fractures.
   H. History of thiazide diuretic, lithium, and estrogen therapy.
   I. Older age.
 II. Physical examination—symptomatology related to the calcium level and the rapidity of onset.
   A. Early signs and symptoms.
      1. Cardiovascular—bradycardia, dysrhythmias, and increased digitalis sensitivity.
      2. Neuromuscular—fatigue, weakness, hyporeflexia, bone pain, lethargy, confusion, apathy, and personality changes.
      3. Gastrointestinal—anorexia, constipation, nausea, and vomiting.
      4. Renal—weight loss, renal calculi, polydipsia, and polyuria.
   B. Late signs and symptoms.
      1. Cardiovascular—heart block and cardiac arrest.
      2. Neuromuscular—stupor and coma.
      3. Gastrointestinal—ileus.
      4. Renal—renal failure.
III. Evaluation of laboratory data.
   A. Elevated serum calcium level (normal range, 8.5 to 10.5 mL/dL)

Corrected serum calcium =
   Measured serum calcium + (4.0 − serum albumin value) × 0.8

TABLE 17–4. **Pharmacologic Interventions for Hypercalcemia**

Agent	Action	Nursing Considerations
Furosemide	Blocks calcium reabsorption Inhibits sodium absorption	Monitor for signs of dehydration Monitor for signs of hypokalemia Weigh client daily
Prednisone	Inhibits bone resorption	Assess for signs of hyperglycemia Evaluate gastrointestinal symptoms Weigh client daily

Calcitonin	Inhibits bone resorption	Monitor for gastrointestinal
		  symptoms—nausea and vomiting
		Evaluate for signs and symptoms of
		  allergic reaction

Biphosphonates	Inhibit bone resorption	Evaluate renal function studies as
		  ordered by physician
		Monitor for gastrointestinal
		  symptoms

Gallium nitrate	Inhibits bone resorption	Evaluate renal function studies

Mithramycin	Inhibits bone resorption	Monitor for decrease in blood
		  pressure
		Assess for signs and symptoms of
		  thrombocytopenia
		Evaluate renal and hepatic function
		  studies as ordered by physician
		Use extravasation precautions with
		  administration

Indomethacin	Inhibits prostaglandin synthesis	Monitor for gastrointestinal
		  symptoms—nausea, pain, bleeding,
		  and vomiting
		Evaluate renal function studies as
		  ordered by physician
		Monitor intake and output ratio
		Evaluate central nervous system
		  reactions—depression, headache,
		  or increase in seizure activity or
		  Parkinson's symptoms

Phosphates	Inhibit bone resorption
	Limit calcium absorption from
	  gut
	Promote soft-tissue and
	  skeletal calcification
		Monitor for gastrointestinal
		  symptoms—nausea, vomiting, and
		  diarrhea
		Evaluate for signs of hypocalcemia
		Monitor for a decrease in blood
		  pressure
		Evaluate renal function studies as
		  ordered by physician
		Monitor intake and output ratio
		Monitor character of urine

    B. Decreased serum potassium, sodium, and phosphorus.
    C. Elevated BUN and creatinine levels.
    D. ECG changes.
       1. Dysrhythmias.
       2. Shortened QT interval.
       3. Broadened T wave.
       4. Increased PR interval.

Nursing Diagnoses

    I. Fluid volume deficit.

   II. Altered protection.

  III. Altered nutrition, less than body requirements.

  IV. Constipation.

   V. Impaired physical mobility.

  VI. Altered thought processes.

 VII. Risk for injury.

VIII. Pain.

  IX. Self-care deficit.

Outcome Identification

    I. Client identifies personal risk factors for hypercalcemia.

   II. Client describes signs and symptoms of hypercalcemia to report to the health care team—bone pain, changes in mental status or personality, nausea and vomiting.

  III. Client participates in strategies to decrease the risk or severity of hypercalcemia (i.e., hydration and safety measures).

  IV. Client describes community resources available for emergency care.

Planning and Implementation

    I. Interventions to maximize safety for the client.

      A. Maintain bed in low position with siderails up for clients with changes in mental status.

      B. Place call light within reach.

      C. Encourage the client to use assistive personnel or devices with ambulation.

      D. Use transfer devices and strategies for immobile clients to decrease risk of pathologic fractures.

   II. Interventions to decrease the incidence and severity of symptoms associated with hypercalcemia.

      A. Maintain level of mobility consistent with disease status and presenting symptoms.

         1. Full range of activity with assistive personnel or devices.

         2. Active range-of-motion exercises.

         3. Passive range-of-motion exercises.

         4. Weight-bearing activities such as standing at the bedside.

         5. Isometric exercises.

         6. Footboard.

         7. Referral to physical therapist.

      B. Implement measures to control pain (see Chapter 1).

      C. Encourage oral fluid intake.

      D. Recommend discontinuance of multivitamin preparations and antacids.

  III. Interventions to monitor response to medical management.

      A. Maintain urine output within prescribed range (usually 100–150 mL/hour) with IV fluids and diuretics.

      B. Maintain strict intake and output regimen.

      C. Check weight every day.

IV. Interventions to monitor for sequelae of hypercalcemia or treatment (see Table 17–4).
   A. Evaluate changes in character of pulse—decreased rate and irregular rhythm.
   B. Assess renal function—monitor intake and output, character of urine, laboratory tests as ordered by the physician, and daily weights.
   C. Evaluate changes in the character of pain—location, severity, aggravating and alleviating factors, and effect on activities of daily living.

Evaluation

The oncology nurse systematically and regularly evaluates the client's and/or family's responses to interventions to determine progress toward the achievement of expected outcomes. Relevant data are collected and actual findings are compared with expected findings. Nursing diagnoses, outcomes, and plans of care are reviewed and revised as necessary.

INAPPROPRIATE ANTIDIURETIC HORMONE SECRETION (SIADH)

Theory

I. Antidiuretic hormone (ADH) is released normally from the posterior pituitary in response to:
   A. Increased plasma osmolality.
   B. Decreased plasma volume.
II. ADH acts on the distal renal tubules and collecting ducts to increase permeability and thus increase water reabsorption.
III. Excess production of ADH from tumors or inappropriate stimulation of the posterior pituitary gland results in excessive water retention and dilutional hyponatremia.
IV. Principles of medical management.
   A. Diagnostic tests.
      1. Serum sodium.
      2. Serum osmolality.
      3. Urinary sodium.
      4. Urine osmolality.
      5. Water-loading test.
   B. Nonpharmacologic interventions.
      1. Fluid restriction (800 to 1000 mL/day).
         a. Used for mild to moderate SIADH (sodium level greater than 125 mg).
         b. Corrects decreased sodium level over 7 to 10 days.
         c. Not recommended for clients with chronic SIADH or severe symptoms.
      2. Hypertonic saline solution.
         a. Used for severe SIADH.
         b. Saline solution (3 to 5%) infused intravenously over 2 to 3 hours.
         c. Furosemide usually is given concurrently to increase fluid excretion.
   C. Pharmacologic interventions.
      1. Treat underlying pathology such as cancer or infection.
      2. Discontinue agents contributing to SIADH such as morphine, diuretics, or antidepressants.
      3. Administer other medications (Table 17–5).

TABLE 17–5. **Pharmacologic Agents Used to Treat SIADH**

Agent	Action	Nursing Implications
Demeclocycline	Interferes with antidiuretic hormone (ADH) action on tubules	Avoid offering medication with meals Assess female clients for pregnancy Assess clients for history of renal or liver disease Monitor urinary output Monitor for complaints of nausea or episodes of vomiting Teach clients to use sunglasses, sunscreen, long-sleeved clothing, hats, and avoidance of sun to decrease risks of photosensitivity Monitor for symptoms of diabetes insipidus Monitor for signs and symptoms of infection
Lithium	Interferes with ADH action	Monitor for complaints of nausea, vomiting, and anorexia Assess neurologic status—presence of tremors or weakness Assess cardiac status—pulse rate, regularity
Urea	Causes osmotic diuresis	Monitor for complications of nausea, vomiting, and anorexia

Assessment

I. Identification of clients at risk.
  A. Diagnosis of cancer of the lung, pancreas, duodenum, prostate, or brain, or Hodgkin's disease.
  B. Presence of pulmonary infections—pneumonia, abcesses, or tuberculosis.
  C. History of trauma, infection, or lesions of the central nervous system.
  D. History of previous cancer therapy.
  E. Treatment with cyclophosphamide, vincristine, cisplatin, thiazide diuretics, morphine, or antidepressants.
  F. Concurrent cardiac, renal, or hepatic diseases.
  G. Severe pain.
  H. Stress.
  I. Fear.
II. Physical examination.
  A. Early signs and symptoms.
    1. Constitutional—weakness and fatigue.
    2. Neurologic—confusion, irritability, weakness, headache, lethargy, and altered mental status.
    3. Gastrointestinal—nausea, vomiting, diarrhea, anorexia, thirst, and abdominal cramping.
    4. Renal—decreased urinary output and weight gain.
    5. Muscular—myalgias and muscle cramping.
  B. Late signs and symptoms.
    1. Progressive lethargy to coma.
    2. Seizure activity.
III. Evaluation of laboratory data.
  A. Serum sodium less than 130 mEq/L.
  B. Serum osmolality less than 280 mOsm/kg of water.
  C. Urinary sodium greater than 20 mEq/L.

   D. Urinary osmolality greater than 1400 mOsm/L.

   E. BUN and creatinine levels within normal ranges.

   F. Hypouricemia.

Nursing Diagnoses

   I. Fluid volume excess.

  II. Altered thought process.

 III. Potential for injury.

 IV. Altered nutrition: less than body requirements.

   V. Pain.

 VI. Altered urinary elimination.

VII. Altered oral mucous membrane.

Outcome Identification

   I. Client discusses personal risk factors for SIADH.

  II. Client participates in measures to decrease the severity of symptoms associated with SIADH.

 III. Client describes signs and symptoms to report to the health care team—weight gain greater than 5 pounds in 1 day, decrease in urinary output to less than 60 mL/hour, mental status changes, nausea, or any seizure activity.

 IV. Client demonstrates self-care skills related to monitoring and treatment of SIADH—measuring urinary output, administering medications, and taking weights.

  V. Client lists community resources available for emergency care.

Planning and Implementation

   I. Interventions to maximize safety for the client.

     A. Bed in low position and siderails up.

     B. Call light and personal items within reach.

     C. Assistance with activities of daily living as needed.

     D. Bed check device if client is confused.

     E. Use of rate regulator for intravenous infusions.

  II. Interventions to decrease the severity of symptoms associated with SIADH.

     A. Thirst secondary to fluid restriction.

       1. Assist the client to divide amount of fluids between day, evening, and night hours.

       2. Offer sugarfree candy or gum to stimulate salivation.

       3. Rinse mouth with water every 2 hours.

       4. Monitor intravenous fluid intake.

     B. Neurologic changes.

       1. Orient to person, time, and place as needed.

       2. Use environmental cues such as calendars and clocks.

       3. Implement seizure precautions (Table 17–6).

 III. Interventions to monitor for sequelae of SIADH or treatment.

     A. Observe for fluid overload.

       1. Weigh client daily.

       2. Maintain strict intake and output records.

       3. Test urine for specific gravity.

TABLE 17–6. **Seizure Precautions**

Remain with patient
Alter environment to promote safety
Loosen tight clothing
Turn client's head to side
Monitor for respiratory distress
Monitor for another seizure before complete recovery from previous seizure

---

   B. Monitor for electrolyte abnormalities.
     1. Monitor vital signs.
     2. Evaluate for changes in mental status.
     3. Assess for signs and symptoms of hypokalemia.
     4. Assess for signs and symptoms of hyponatremia.
     5. Monitor laboratory data (electrolyte values and osmolality of serum and urine) as ordered by the physician.
   C. Monitor for side effects of pharmacologic therapy (see Table 17–5).

Evaluation

The oncology nurse systematically and regularly evaluates the client's and/or family's responses to interventions to determine progress toward the achievement of expected outcomes. Relevant data are collected and actual findings are compared with expected findings. Nursing diagnoses, outcomes, and plans of care are reviewed and revised as necessary.

BIBLIOGRAPHY

Arrambide K., & Toto, R.D. (1993). Tumor lysis syndrome. *Semin Nephrol 13*(3), 273–280.
Batcheller, J. (1994). Syndrome of inappropriate antidiuretic hormone secretion. *Crit Care Nurs Clin North Am 6*(4), 687–692.
Bell, T. (1993). Disseminated intravascular coagulation. Clinical complexities of aberrant coagulation. *Crit Care Nurs Clin North Am 5*(3), 389–410.
Bick, R.L. (1994). Disseminated intravascular coagulation. Objective criteria for diagnosis and management. *Med Clin North Am 78*(3), 511–543.
Bone, R.C. (1994). Sepsis and its complications: The clinical problem. *Crit Care Med 22*(7), S8–S12.
Brown, K.K. (1994). Septic shock: How to stop the deadly cascade. *AJN 94*(9), 20–26.
Bryce, J. (1994). SIADH. Recognizing and treating syndrome of inappropriate antidiuretic hormone secretion. *Nursing 24*(4), 33.
Bunn, P.A., & Ridgway, E.C. (1993). Paraneoplastic syndromes. In V.T. DeVita, Jr., S. Hellman, & S.A. Rosenberg (eds.). *Cancer: Principles & Practice of Oncology* (4th ed.). Philadelphia: J.B. Lippincott.
Cordisco, M.E. (1994). Fighting DIC. *RN 57*(8), 36–40.
Dabrow, M.B., & Wilkins, J.C. (1993). Hematologic emergencies. *Postgrad Med 93*(5), 193–202.
Dunn, D.L. (1994). Gram-negative bacterial sepsis and sepsis syndrome. *Surg Clin North Am 74*(3), 621–635.
Ferguson, K.L., & Brown, L. (1996). Bacteremia and sepsis. *Emerg Med Clin North Am 14*(1), 185–194.
Hall, T.G., & Schaiff, R.A. (1993). Update on the medical treatment of hypercalcemia of malignancy. *Clin Pharm 12*, 117–125.
Hande, K.R., & Garrow, G.C. (1993). Acute tumor lysis syndrome in patients with high-grade non-Hodgkin's lymphoma. *Am J Med 94*, 133–139.
Hazinski, M.F. (1994). Mediator-specific therapies for the systemic inflammatory response syndrome, sepsis, severe sepsis, and septic shock. *Crit Care Nurs Clin North Am 6*(2), 309–319.
Hoigne, R., Schlumberger, H.P., Vervloet, D., & Zoppi, M. (1993). Epidemiology of allergic drug reactions. *Monogr Allergy. 31,* 147–170.
Jones, D.P., Mahmoud, H., & Chesney, R.W. (1995). Tumor lysis syndrome: Pathogenesis and management. *Pediatr Nephrol 9*(2), 206–212.
Kaplan, M. (1994). Hypercalcemia of malignancy: A review of advances in pathophysiology. *Oncol Nurs Forum 21*(6), 1039–1048.

Kemp, S.F., Lockey, R.F., Wolf, B.L., et al. (1995). Anaphylaxis: A review of 266 cases. *Arch Intern Med 155*, 1749–1754.

Kurtz, A. (1993). Disseminated intravascular coagulation with leukemia patients. *Cancer Nurs 16*(6), 456–463.

Lynn, W.A., & Cohen, J. (1995). Management of septic shock. *J Infect 30*, 207–212.

McCoy-Adabody, A.M., & Borger, D.L. (1996). Selected critical care complications of cancer therapy. *AACN Clin Issues 7*(1), 26–36.

Oncology Nursing Society. (1992). *Cancer Chemotherapy Guidelines: Recommendations for the Management of Vesicant Extravasation, Hypersensitivity, and Anaphylaxis.* Pittsburgh: Oncology Nursing Society.

Pimentel, L. (1993). Medical complications of oncologic disease. *Emerg Med Clin North Am 11*(2), 407–419.

Shelton, B.K. (1994). Disorders of hemostasis in sepsis. *Crit Care Nurs Clin North Am 6*(2), 373–387.

Singer, F.R., & Minoofar, P.N. (1995). Biphosphonates in the treatment of disorders of mineral metabolism. *Adv Endocrinol Metab 6*, 259–288.

Sriskandan, S., & Cohen, J. (1995). The pathogenesis of septic shock. *J Infect 30*, 201–206.

Stucky, L.A. (1993). Acute tumor lysis syndrome: Assessment and nursing implications. *Oncol Nurs Forum 20*(1), 49–59.

Suffredini, A.F. (1994). Current prospects for the treatment of clinical sepsis. *Crit Care Med 22*(7), S12–S18.

Theriault, R.L. (1993). Hypercalcemia of malignancy: Pathophysiology and implications for treatment. *Oncology 7*(1), 47–55.

Vassilopoulou-Sellin, R. (1995). Current approaches for hypercalcemia. *Cope* Jan./Feb., 10–11.

Yucha, C.B., & Toto, K.H. (1994). Calcium and phosphorus derangements. *Crit Care Nurs Clin North Am 6*(4), 747–759.

Structural Emergencies

Jane C. Hunter, RN, MN, OCN

INCREASED INTRACRANIAL PRESSURE

Theory

   I. The intracranial cavity is a nonexpandable chamber that contains:
     A. Brain tissue.
     B. Vascular tissue.
     C. Cerebrospinal fluid.
  II. An increase in intracranial pressure can result when the volume of any of the three components increases.
 III. Primary or metastatic tumors within the intracranial cavity can result in increased intracranial pressure by:
     A. Displacement of brain tissue.
     B. Edema of brain tissue.
     C. Obstruction of cerebrospinal fluid flow.
     D. Increased vascularity associated with tumor growth.
 IV. Principles of medical management.
     A. Diagnostic tests.
        1. Computed tomography (CT) scan.
        2. Magnetic resonance imaging (MRI).
        3. Cerebral angiography—determines if impression from CT scan or MRI is a vascular abnormality or tumor.
        4. Myelography—determines if drop metastases are present.
        5. CT-guided needle biopsy—obtains a tissue diagnosis without open craniotomy.
        6. Positron-emission tomography (PET)—limited use in brain tumor diagnosis as compared with CT and MRI.
     B. Nonpharmacologic interventions.
        1. Surgery.
          a. Complete resection of primary tumor or single brain metastasis.
          b. Tumor bulk reduction with decompression.
            (1) Provides symptomatic relief.
            (2) Is contraindicated with multiple, small intracranial tumors.
          c. Shunt placement—provides an alternate pathway for cerebrospinal fluid.
        2. Radiation therapy.
          a. Primary treatment or palliative treatment for metastatic disease, depending on radiosensitivity of tumor.

      b. Adjuvant treatment with either surgery or chemotherapy.

      c. Specialized radiation therapy approaches for brain metastases.

         (1) Stereotactic external radiation—gamma knife and linear accelerator.

         (2) Brachytherapy.

  C. Pharmacologic interventions.

    1. Chemotherapy for primary or metastatic tumor.

      a. Most antineoplastic agents do not cross blood-brain barrier; nitrosoureas and procarbazine are exceptions.

      b. Regional drug delivery such as intra-arterial, intrathecal, or intratumor drug administration circumvents blood-brain barrier.

      c. Preliminary reports from clinical studies show tumor regression with intravenous administration of conventional chemotherapy such as cisplatin, etoposide, and vinblastin. Effect on overall control of brain metastases is unknown.

    2. Corticosteroids.

      a. Used to decrease inflammation—60 to 80% of clients show decrease in symptoms.

      b. Begins before radiation therapy and may be tapered.

      c. May require maintenance doses for residual tumor and dependence may develop from long-term use.

    3. Osmotherapy.

      a. Reduces intracellular water of brain and total water of body

      b. Mannitol and diuretics may be used.

    4. Fluid restriction.

    5. Anticonvulsants—if seizures begin.

    6. Barbiturates

Assessment

  I. Identification of clients at risk.

    A. Clients with cancers of the lung, breast, testicles, thyroid, stomach, or kidney, or those with melanoma.

    B. Clients with primary tumors of brain or spinal cord.

    C. Clients with a diagnosis of leukemia or neuroblastoma.

  II. Physical examination—signs and symptoms depend on volume and location of abnormality.

    A. Early signs and symptoms.

      1. Headaches.

        a. Early morning headache may be bilateral and located in occipital or frontal areas.

        b. Headache may be initiated or aggravated by Valsalva maneuver, coughing, or bending.

      2. Neurologic.

        a. Blurred vision.

        b. Diplopia.

        c. Decreased visual fields.

        d. Extremity drifts.

        e. Lethargy, apathy, confusion, restlessness.

      3. Gastrointestinal—loss of appetite, nausea, and occasional vomiting.

B. Late signs and symptoms.
 1. Cardiovascular—bradycardia and widening pulse pressure.
 2. Respiratory—slow, shallow respirations; tachypnea; and Cheyne-Stokes respirations.
 3. Neurologic—decreased ability to concentrate; decreased level of consciousness; personality changes; hemiplegia; hemiparesis; seizures; pupillary changes; papilledema.
 4. Abnormal posturing.
 5. Temperature elevations.

Nursing Diagnoses

   I. Alteration in tissue perfusion: cerebral.
  II. Alteration in sensory perception.
 III. Altered thought processes.
 IV. Ineffective breathing pattern.
  V. Impaired verbal communication.
 VI. Impaired physical mobility.
 VII. Risk for injury.
VIII. Pain.
  IX. Anxiety.
   X. Knowledge deficit.

Outcome Identification

   I. Client or family identifies signs and symptoms of increased intracranial pressure to report to health care team.
  II. Client participates in strategies to maximize safety and comfort within the acute care setting and at home.
 III. Client participates in decision-making regarding treatment and subsequent care needs.
 IV. Client describes community resources available for rehabilitation and support.

Planning and Implementation

   I. Interventions to maximize safety for the client.
      A. Maintain bed rest with increasing intracranial pressure and progressive symptoms; elevate head of bed.
      B. Keep bed in lowest position and siderails elevated.
      C. Develop a daily schedule of activities with appropriate rest periods.
      D. Use assistive devices as needed.
  II. Interventions to decrease severity of symptoms associated with increased intracranial pressure.
      A. Instruct the client to avoid Valsalva maneuver.
         1. Administer stool softeners as ordered to prevent constipation and straining.
         2. Administer antiemetics as ordered to prevent vomiting.
         3. Implement measures to control discomfort from headaches.
         4. Instruct client to be passive during turning and repositioning.
      B. Implement measures to decrease stress.
         1. Maintain a calm environment.

    2. Minimize external stimulation—light, noise, touch, and temperature extremes.

    3. Encourage calmness during interactions between the client and others.

    4. Teach stress reduction strategies to client and family.

  C. Monitor activities and positioning to minimize increased intracranial pressure.

    1. Elevate head of bed 30 degrees to promote venous drainage.

    2. Avoid isometric muscle contractions.

    3. Avoid positions that rotate the head or extend or flex the neck.

    4. Avoid lying in prone position or activities that exert pressure on the abdomen.

III. Interventions to monitor for sequelae of increased intracranial pressure.

  A. Monitor blood pressure for widening pulse pressure; pulse for decrease in rate; and respirations for changes in rate, pattern, or effort.

  B. Assess for changes in levels of consciousness with each client contact.

  C. Monitor for sensory or motor changes—changes in visual acuity, pupil reactions, verbal expression; decrease in muscle strength, coordination, and movement.

  D. Assess for presence of associated symptoms such as nausea, vomiting, and headache.

IV. Interventions to enhance adaptation and rehabilitation.

  A. Assist the client and family to set realistic goals to maintain optimal activity and self-care levels within limitations imposed by disease.

  B. Assist the client and family to assess physical environment in acute care setting and home and make appropriate changes to promote safety.

    1. Encourage having major living area on ground level in the home.

    2. Remove scatter rugs from floors.

    3. Encourage use of rubber-soled, tie shoes and assistive devices as needed.

    4. Orient the client to person, time, and place as needed.

  C. Refer to appropriate supportive services.

    1. Physical therapy for activity program and use of assistive devices.

    2. Social services for support, financial evaluation, and community services.

Evaluation

    The oncology nurse systematically and regularly evaluates the client's and/or family's responses to interventions to determine progress toward the achievement of expected outcomes. Relevant data are collected and actual findings are compared with expected findings. Nursing diagnoses, outcomes, and plans of care are reviewed and revised as necessary.

SPINAL CORD COMPRESSION

Theory

  I. Spinal cord is a cylindrical body of nervous tissue that occupies the upper two thirds of the vertebral canal.

 II. Spinal cord has motor, sensory, and autonomic functions.

III. Compression of the spinal cord may occur as a result of tumor invasion of the vertebrae and subsequent collapse on the spinal cord; tumor invasion of the spinal canal and resulting increased pressure; or primary tumors of the spinal cord.

IV. Compression of the spinal cord can result in minor changes in motor, sensory, and autonomic function to complete paralysis.

V. Principles of medical management.

A. Diagnostic tests.

1. Spinal x-ray examinations—show bone abnormalities or soft-tissue masses.

2. Bone scan—identifies metastases to vertebral bodies.

3. MRI—increasingly used as main tool to diagnose and localize spinal metastases.

4. CT scan.

5. Myelogram—used with or without CT scan when MRI is nondiagnostic.

B. Nonpharmacologic interventions.

1. Radiation therapy.

a. Used as most common treatment for epidural metastases and cord compression.

b. Used alone when no evidence of spinal instability is present and tumor is known to be radiosensitive.

c. Given over several weeks to a total dose of 3000 to 4000 cGy.

2. Surgery.

a. Used if tumor is not responsive to radiation therapy.

b. Used if recurrent tumor is in an area previously treated with radiation therapy.

c. Used to decompress area by laminectomy or resection of a vertebral body.

3. Surgery followed by radiation therapy.

C. Pharmacologic interventions.

1. Steroids.

a. Reduce spinal cord edema and pain.

b. May have oncolytic effect on certain tumors.

2. Antineoplastic agents.

a. Used as an adjuvant treatment to radiation and/or surgery for tumors responsive to antineoplastics such as lymphomas, germ cell tumors, and neuroblastoma.

b. Used if recurrence of tumor is at a site of previous surgery or radiation therapy.

c. Used as treatment of choice in children and infants because radiation therapy can inhibit growth.

3. Analgesics—more than 95% of patients with spinal cord compression have pain (see Chapter 10).

Assessment

I. Identification of clients at risk.

A. Cancers that have a natural history for metastasizing to the bone—breast, lung, prostate, kidney, and myeloma.

B. Cancers that metastasize to the spinal cord—lymphoma, seminoma, and neuroblastoma.

C. Primary cancers of the spinal cord—ependymoma, astrocytoma, and glioma.

II. Pertinent history.

A. Type of primary tumor.

B. Time since onset of symptoms, and level and degree of compression.

III. Physical examination—presenting signs and symptoms vary with the location and severity of the compression.
  A. Early signs and symptoms.
    1. Neck or back pain—always requires prompt evaluation in a client with cancer. Back pain is first symptom in 96% of patients. May be local, radicular, or both.
      a. Local—constant, dull and aching; usually progressive.
      b. Radicular—may be constant or initiated with movement.
      c. Pain usually worse when sitting up.
      d. Pain exacerbated by straining, coughing, or flexion of neck.
    2. Motor weakness or dysfunction.
    3. Loss of sensation for light touch, pain, or temperature.
    4. Sexual impotence.
  B. Late signs and symptoms.
    1. Loss of sensation for deep pressure and position.
    2. Incontinence or retention of urine or stool.
    3. Paralysis.
    4. Muscle atrophy.

Nursing Diagnoses

  I. Pain.
  II. Impaired physical mobility.
  III. Alteration in sensory perception: tactile.
  IV. Constipation.
  V. Urinary retention.
  VI. Sexual dysfunction.
  VII. Risk for impaired skin integrity.
  VIII. Body image disturbance.
  IX. Altered role performance.
  X. Knowledge deficit.

Outcome Identification

  I. Client lists signs and symptoms that should be reported to the health care team.
    A. Changes in bowel or bladder patterns.
    B. Characteristics of pain, sensory and motor function.
    C. Changes in skin integrity.
    D. Changes in sexual function.
  II. Client describes strategies to minimize sequelae of spinal cord compression and treatment.
  III. Client and family participate in rehabilitation program designed to promote adaptation to residual limitations associated with spinal cord compression.
  IV. Client and family identify community resources available for assistance and support.

Planning and Implementation

  I. Interventions to maximize safety for the client.
    A. Mobilize the client according to findings of stable or unstable spine (Table 18–1).

TABLE 18–1. **Mobility Interventions**

Unstable Spine	Stable Spine
Place sandbags on either side of the head to limit movement	Initiate range-of-motion exercises after physical therapy evaluation and with a physician order
Use cervical collar to support cervical spine	Instruct client/family in isometric exercises
Support head and neck during all movement	Provide personal assistance with ambulation
Use no pillows	Instruct client/family in use of assistive devices with ambulation
Maintain alignment when turning or positioning	Maintain proper alignment while in bed, turning, or positioning
Use a log roll, pull sheet, or transfer board when turning or positioning	
Place client on special bed as indicated: Stryker frame or CircOlectric bed	

B. Instruct the client and family to assess pressure and temperature of objects coming in contact with the client's areas of compromised feeling or sensation.
II. Interventions to decrease the severity of symptoms associated with spinal cord compression.
   A. Assist the client to positions of comfort with maintenance of proper body alignment.
   B. Institute nonpharmacologic methods of pain control (see Chapter 1).
   C. Institute a bowel and bladder program (Table 18–2).

TABLE 18–2. **Elements of a Bowel and Bladder Program**

Bowel Program	Bladder Program
Provide high-fiber diet: 15–30 g of fiber/day	Include foods in diet to maintain urinary pH of less than 7
Offer oral intake of 3000 mL fluid/day	Avoid foods that produce alkaline urine such as citrus fruits
Use bedside commode or toilet for all bowel movements	Schedule times for voiding—every 2–3 hr
Schedule bowel movement at same time each day	Palpate bladder after voiding to evaluate retention
Offer a hot drink 30 min before scheduled bowel movement	Monitor fluid intake
Use stool softeners such as mineral oil or dioctyl sodium sulfosuccinate (DSS)	Decrease fluid intake after 7:00 PM
Monitor for signs and symptoms of fecal impaction	Monitor for signs and symptoms of urinary tract infection
If Laxatives Are Needed	*If Catheterization Is Needed*
Use stimulant to defecation such as a glycerin suppository	Teach client/family intermittent self-catheterization
Use chemical stimulant such as bisacodyl (Dulcolax), castor oil, senna concentrate (Senokot), or cascara	

III. Interventions to monitor for sequelae of spinal cord compression or treatment.
   A. Monitor for progression of motor or sensory deficits every 8 hours (Table 18–3).
      1. Decrease in muscle strength.
      2. Decrease in coordination.
      3. Decrease in perception of temperature, touch, and position.
   B. Monitor bowel and bladder elimination patterns and effectiveness.
      1. Record intake and output every 8 hours.
      2. Palpate for bladder distention if interval between voidings increases.
      3. Record frequency and characteristics of stool with each bowel movement.
      4. Conduct gentle digital rectal examination to check for impaction if no bowel movement within 3 days.
   C. Assess changes in location, character, and associated aggravating and alleviating factors of pain.
IV. Interventions to enhance adaptation and rehabilitation.
   A. Inform client and family of changes in the condition of the client.
   B. Initiate a consultation with physical and occupational therapy as soon as the spine has been stabilized.
   C. Assist client to maintain a safe level of independence within the limitations imposed by the cord compression.
   D. Encourage client and family to express concerns about the effect of residual limitations on activities of daily living and lifestyle.
   E. Use PLISSIT model to address changes in sexual function (see Chapter 6).

Evaluation

The oncology nurse systematically and regularly evaluates the client's and/or family's responses to interventions to determine progress toward the achievement of expected outcomes. Relevant data are collected and actual findings are compared with expected findings. Nursing diagnoses, outcomes, and plans of care are reviewed and revised as necessary.

TABLE 18–3. **Assessment of Motor and Sensory Functions**

Function	Assessment Techniques
Muscle strength	Upper extremities: ask client to grip your finger as firmly as possible
	Lower extremities: ask client to resist plantar flexion of his/her feet
Coordination of hands and feet	Ask client to touch each finger to his/her thumb in rapid sequence
	Ask client to turn hand over and back as quickly as possible
	Ask client to tap your hand as quickly as possible with the ball of each foot
Sensory perception	Touch client along length of extremities and trunk with the blunt and sharp end of a safety pin and ask client to identify as either "sharp" or "dull"
	Ask client to report the sensation of touch when touched with a wisp of cotton
	Move one of the client's fingers and ask if the finger is being moved up or down
	Touch skin of client with test tube of hot water and then cold water; ask the client to describe the temperature

SUPERIOR VENA CAVA SYNDROME

Theory

I. The superior vena cava (SVC) is a thin-walled major vessel that carries venous drainage from the head, neck, upper extremities, and upper thorax to the heart.

II. The SVC is located in the mediastinum and is surrounded by the rigid structures of the sternum, trachea, and vertebrae, and the aorta, right bronchus, lymph nodes, and pulmonary artery.

III. The SVC is a low-pressure vessel that is easily compressed; compression can occur from direct tumor invasion, enlarged lymph nodes, or a thrombus within the vessel.

IV. When obstruction of the SVC occurs, venous return to the heart from the head, neck, thorax, and upper extremities is impaired.
   1. Venous pressure increases.
   2. Cardiac output decreases.

V. Principles of medical management.
   A. Goals of treatment include treatment of the underlying cause and of presenting symptoms.
   B. Treatment and prognosis are determined by the histologic diagnosis of the primary tumor.
   C. Diagnostic tests.
      1. Chest x-ray examination—positive findings associated with superior vena cava syndrome (SVCS) include mass, pleural effusion, and superior mediastinal widening.
      2. CT scan.
      3. Additional tests to determine the histologic diagnosis of the primary condition—bronchoscopy, bone marrow biopsy, mediastinoscopy, thoracentesis, sputum specimen, and needle biopsy of palpable lymph nodes.
   D. Nonpharmacologic interventions.
      1. Radiation therapy—the primary treatment for SVCS if client has non-small cell cancer of the lung or a histologic diagnosis cannot be made.
      2. Removal of central venous catheter in catheter-induced SVCS if the thrombus cannot be lysed with urokinase or streptokinase.
      3. Oxygen therapy.
      4. Percutaneous transluminal angioplasty using balloon technique.
      5. Insertion of expandable wire stents to open and maintain patency of SVC.
   E. Pharmacologic interventions.
      1. Antineoplastic therapy alone in clients who have had previous mediastinal radiation therapy.
      2. Antineoplastic therapy in conjunction with radiation therapy.
      3. Steroids.
      4. Diuretics.
      5. Thrombolytic therapy.

Assessment

I. Identification of clients at risk.
   A. Presence of lymphoma involving the mediastinum, germ cell tumors, cancers of the lung and breast, and Kaposi's sarcoma.
   B. Presence of central venous catheters and pacemakers.

C. Previous radiation therapy to the mediastinum.

D. Associated conditions such as histoplasmosis, benign tumors, and aortic aneurysm.

II. Physical examination.

A. Early signs and symptoms of SVCS.

1. Facial swelling upon arising in the morning.
2. Redness and edema in conjunctivae and around the eyes.
3. Swelling of the neck and arms.
4. Neck and thoracic vein distention.
5. Dyspnea—most common symptom.
6. Nonproductive cough.
7. Hoarseness.
8. Cyanosis of upper torso.
9. Stridor.

B. Late signs and symptoms of SVCS.

1. Headache.
2. Irritability.
3. Visual disturbances.
4. Dizziness.
5. Changes in mental status.

III. Evaluation of laboratory data—assess available laboratory data against previous and normal values.

A. Arterial blood gases.
B. Electrolytes.
C. Kidney function.
D. CBC.
E. Coagulation studies.

Nursing Diagnoses

I. Ineffective airway clearance.
II. Deceased cardiac output.
III. Altered tissue perfusion: cardiopulmonary.
IV. Anxiety.
V. Knowledge deficit.

Outcome Identification

I. Client identifies critical signs and symptoms to report to the health care team.
II. Client describes plans for continued follow-up care.
III. Client participates in decision-making about care, discharge planning, and life activities.
IV. Client identifies community resources and services for assistance and support.

Planning and Implementation

I. Interventions to maximize safety for the client.

A. Provide for environmental safety—bed in low position, siderails up, and call light and personal items within reach.

B. Avoid venipunctures, intravenous fluid administration, or measurement of blood pressure in the upper extremities.

C. Take blood pressure in lower extremities.

D. Assist client with ambulation as needed.

E. Remove rings and restrictive clothing.

II. Interventions to decrease severity of symptoms associated with SVCS.
   A. Elevate head of bed to decrease dyspnea.
   B. Instruct the client to avoid the Valsalva maneuver or other activities that cause straining.
   C. Apply pressure to sites of invasive procedures in the upper body.
   D. Space care activities to decrease energy expenditure.
   E. Maintain lower extremities in a dependent position.
   F. Explain care procedures in clear, simple terms to decrease anxiety.
   G. Reassure the client that close monitoring will occur.
   H. Encourage client to ask questions about care measures and/or changes in condition.
III. Interventions to monitor the sequelae of SVCS or treatment.
   A. Assess for progressive respiratory distress.
      1. Increased respiratory rate with stridor.
      2. Increased anxiety.
      3. Presence of adventitious breath sounds.
      4. Increased subjective complaints of difficulty breathing.
   B. Monitor for signs of progressive edema.
      1. Increased swelling in face, arms, or neck.
      2. Increased venous distention of neck or thorax.
   C. Monitor for changes in tissue perfusion.
      1. Decreased or absent peripheral pulses.
      2. Decrease in blood pressure—systolic pressure less than 90 mm Hg.
      3. Pale or cyanotic skin of the face, extremities, or nail beds.
   D. Assess for changes in neurologic/mental status:
      1. Decrease in orientation to person, place, and time.
      2. Increased confusion.
      3. Presence of lethargy.
      4. Increased dizziness or blurred vision.
      5. Increase in severity of headaches.
   E. Monitor for signs and symptoms of side effects of anticoagulant therapy—petechiae, ecchymoses, bleeding of gums, nose, urinary tract, or gastrointestinal system.
   F. Monitor for signs and symptoms of steroid therapy—weakness of involuntary muscles, mood swings, steroid-induced glycosuria, dyspepsia, or insomnia.
IV. Interventions to enhance adaptation and rehabilitation from SVCS.
   A. Reassure the client that changes in physical appearance will subside as SVCS resolves.
   B. Assist the client to plan activities that include continued treatment of disease and management of possible side effects of treatment.
   C. Explain changes in status to client and family after each assessment.

Evaluation

The oncology nurse systematically and regularly evaluates the client's and/or family's responses to interventions to determine progress toward the achievement of expected outcomes. Relevant data are collected and actual findings are compared with expected findings. Nursing diagnoses, outcomes, and plans of care are reviewed and revised as necessary.

CARDIAC TAMPONADE

Theory

I. The pericardium is a two-layered sac surrounding the heart.
  A. The space between the two layers is the pericardial cavity.
  B. The cavity normally is filled with 50 mL of fluid.
II. An increase in the intrapericardiac pressure may occur due to:
  A. Fluid accumulation in the pericardial sac.
  B. Direct or metastatic tumor invasion to the pericardial sac.
  C. Fibrosis of the pericardial sac related to radiation therapy.
III. As intrapericardiac pressure increases:
  A. Left ventricular filling decreases.
  B. The ability of the heart to pump decreases.
  C. Cardiac output decreases.
  D. Impaired systemic perfusion occurs.
IV. Principles of medical management.
  A. Diagnostic tests.
    1. Chest x-ray examination—enlarged pericardial silhouette.
    2. CT scan—pleural effusion, masses, or pericardial thickening.
    3. Echocardiography (ECHO)—most precise diagnostic test; two echoes are seen with tamponade.
    4. Electrocardiography (ECG)—tachycardia, premature contractions, and electrical alternans.
    5. Pericardiocentesis and cytology testing of fluid.
      a. Bloody fluid associated with positive cytology test result.
      b. Cytology testing has a significant false-negative rate.
  B. Nonpharmacologic interventions.
    1. Pericardiocentesis—temporary removal of excess pericardial fluid.
    2. Pericardial window—surgical opening of the pericardium to allow fluid drainage.
    3. Total pericardectomy—removal of the pericardial sac for clients with constrictive or chronic pericarditis.
    4. Radiation therapy—radiation to radiosensitive tumors of the pericardium; contraindicated in radiation pericarditis.
  C. Pharmacologic interventions.
    1. Pericardial sclerosis—instillation through a pericardial catheter of chemicals (tetracycline, thiotepa, bleomycin are among those used) causing inflammation and subsequent fibrosis.
    2. Systemic antineoplastic therapy.
    3. Corticosteroids—temporary reduction of inflammation of constrictive pericarditis.

Assessment

I. Identification of clients at risk.
  A. Clients with primary tumors of the heart, including mesothelioma and sarcomas (rare).
  B. Clients with metastatic tumors to the pericardium—lung, breast, gastrointestinal tract, leukemia, Hodgkin's or non-Hodgkin's lymphoma, sarcoma, or melanoma.
  C. Clients who have received more than 4000 cGy of radiation to a field in which the heart is included.

   D. Clients with acquired immunodeficiency syndrome (AIDS)-related Kaposi's sarcoma.
 II. Physical examination.
   A. Early signs and symptoms.
     1. Retrosternal chest pain relieved by leaning forward and intensified when lying supine.
     2. Dyspnea.
     3. Cough.
     4. Muffled heart sounds.
     5. Weak or absent apical pulse.
     6. Anxiety and agitation.
     7. Hiccups.
   B. Late signs and symptoms.
     1. Tachycardia.
     2. Tachypnea.
     3. Decreased systolic pressure and rising diastolic pressure (narrow pulse pressure).
     4. Pulsus paradoxus greater than 10 mm Hg—classic for cardiac tamponade.
     5. Increased central venous pressure (CVP).
     6. Altered levels of consciousness.
     7. Oliguria.
     8. Peripheral edema.
III. Evaluation of laboratory data—review laboratory data and compare results with previous values and normal parameters.
   A. Arterial blood gas (ABG) values.
   B. Electrolyte values.

Nursing Diagnoses

  I. Decreased cardiac output.
 II. Ineffective breathing pattern.
III. Altered tissue perfusion: cardiopulmonary.
IV. Pain.
 V. Anxiety.
VI. Knowledge deficit related to cardiac tamponade and its management.

Outcome Identification

  I. Client identifies signs and symptoms to be reported to the health care team.
 II. Client describes the effects of cardiac tamponade or treatment on activities of daily living and lifestyle.
III. Client discusses need and plans for continued follow-up.

Planning and Implementation

  I. Interventions to maximize safety for the client.
   A. Assist the client with activities of daily living and ambulation as needed.
   B. Keep bed in low position and with siderails up.
 II. Interventions to decrease severity of symptoms associated with cardiac tamponade.
   A. Elevate head of bed to position of comfort to minimize shortness of breath.
   B. Monitor response to oxygen therapy as ordered by the physician.

   C. Institute nonpharmacologic measures to relieve pain (see Chapter 1).
   D. Plan care activities to minimize energy expenditure and allow for rest periods.
   E. Explain procedures to the client and family to decrease anxiety.
III. Interventions to monitor for sequelae of cardiac tamponade.
   A. Monitor blood pressure, pulse, respirations for narrowing pulse pressure, paradoxical pulse, arrhythmias, and respiratory distress.
   B. Maintain an accurate intake and output record.
   C. Assess level of consciousness for changes in behavior, orientation, and awareness.
   D. Monitor subjective complaints of the client about pain and shortness of breath.
   E. Assess character and amount of drainage from pericardial catheter, if present.
   F. Assess catheter site for signs and symptoms of infection.
   G. Evaluate extremities for peripheral edema.
IV. Interventions to enhance adaptation and rehabilitation.
   A. Encourage the client and family to communicate concerns about condition and treatment to a member of the health care team.
   B. Include the client and family in planning and implementation of care if health status permits and participation is not stressful to client and family.

Evaluation

The oncology nurse systematically and regularly evaluates the client's and/or family's responses to interventions to determine progress toward the achievement of expected outcomes. Relevant data are collected and actual findings are compared with expected findings. Nursing diagnoses, outcomes, and plans of care are reviewed and revised as necessary.

BIBLIOGRAPHY

Boyer, C.L. (1993). Three cancer complications that can't wait. *Nurs 93 23*(10), 34–41.
Broderson, J.M. (1995). Surgical options for brain tumor treatment. *Crit Care Nurs Clin North Am 9*(1), 91–101.
Clezki, J., & Macklis, R.M. (1995). The palliative role of radiotherapy in the management of the cancer patient. *Semin Oncol 22*(2[suppl 3]), 82–90.
Critical differences: Superior vena cava syndrome. (1993). Am J Nurs 93(2), 52.
Davies, P.S. (1995). Neoplastic cardiac tamponade. In C. Miaskowski, & K.V. Gettrust (eds.). *Oncology Nursing: Plans and Care for Specialty Practice.* Albany: Delmar Publishers, pp. 279–285.
Delaney, T.F., & Oldfield, E.H. (1993). Spinal cord compression. In V.T. DeVita, Jr., S. Hellman, S. Rosenberg (eds.). *Cancer: Principles and Practice of Oncology* (4th ed., vol. II). Philadelphia: J.B. Lippincott, pp. 2118–2127.
Dietz, K.A., & Flaherty, A.M. (1993). Oncologic emergencies. In S.L. Groenwald, M.H. Frogge, M. Goodman, et al. (eds.). *Cancer Nursing: Principles and Practice* (3rd ed.). Boston: Jones & Bartlett, pp. 800–839.
Dunne-Daly, C.F. (1994). Radiation therapy for oncologic emergencies. *Cancer Nurs 17*(6), 516–527.
Ewer, M.S., & Benjamin, R.S. (1993). Cardiac complications. In J.F. Holland, E. Frei, R.C. Blast, et al. (eds.). *Cancer Medicine* (3rd ed., vol II). Philadelphia: Lea & Febiger, pp. 2332–2335.
Gates, M.L. (1995). Superior vena cava syndrome. In C. Miaskowski, & K.V. Gettrust (eds.). *Oncology Nursing: Plans of Care for Specialty Practice.* Albany: Delmar Publishers, pp. 315–323.
Held, J.L. (1994). Identifying spinal cord compression: Find out how to assess for and manage this oncologic emergency. *Nurs 94 24*(5), 28.
Held, J.L., & Peahota, A. (1993). Nursing care of the patient with spinal cord compression. *Oncol Nurs Forum 20*(10), 1507–1514.
Henson, J.W., & Posner, J.B. (1993). Neurological complications. In J.F. Holland, E. Frei, R.C. Blast, et al. (eds.). *Cancer Medicine* (3rd ed., vol II). Philadelphia: Lea & Febiger, pp. 2268–2273.
Kuric, J. (1995). Spinal cord tumors. *Crit Care Nurs Clin North Am 7*(1), 151–156.
Levin, V.A., Gutin, P.H., & Leibel, S. (1993). Neoplasms of the central nervous system. In V.T. DeVita,

Jr., S. Hellman, & S.A. Rosenberg (eds.). *Cancer: Principles and Practice of Oncology* (4th ed., vol II). Philadelphia: J.B. Lippincott, pp. 1679–1700.

Morris, J.C., Holland, J.F. (1993). Oncologic emergencies. In J.F. Holland, E. Frei, R.C. Blast, et al. (eds.). *Cancer Medicine* (3rd ed., vol II). Philadelphia: Lea & Febiger, pp. 245–251.

O'Hanlon-Nichols, T. (1996). Clinical snapshot: Intracranial tumors. *Am J Nurs* 96(4), 38–39.

Pass, H.I. (1993). Management of malignant pleural and pericardial effusions. In V.T. DeVita, Jr., S. Hellman, S.A. Rosenberg (eds.). *Cancer: Principles and Practice of Oncology* (4th ed., vol II). Philadelphia: J.B. Lippincott, pp. 2251–2253.

Peterson, R. (1993). A nursing intervention for early detection of spinal cord compressions in patients with cancer. *Cancer Nurs* 16(2), 113–116.

Reese, K. (1995). Spinal cord compression. In C. Miaskowski & K.V. Gettrust (eds.). *Oncology Nursing: Plans of Care for Specialty Practice.* Albany: Delmar Publishers, pp. 303–314.

Schafer, S.L. (1993). Oncologic complication. In S.E. Otto (ed.). *Oncology Nursing.* St. Louis: C.V. Mosby, pp. 399–429.

Spinal-cord compression: Early detection may avert paralysis. (1993). *Am J Nurs* 93(1), 56.

Uaje, C., Kahsen, K., & Parish, L. (1996). Oncology emergencies. *Crit Care Nurs Q* 18(4), 26–34.

Vos, H.R. (1993). Making headway with intracranial hypertension. *Am J Nurs* 93(2), 28–35.

Wegmann, J.A. (1993). Central nervous system cancers. In S.L. Groenwald, M.H. Frogg, M. Goodman, & C.H. Yarbro (eds.). *Cancer Nursing: Principles and Practice* (3rd ed.). Boston: Jones & Bartlett, pp. 959–983.

Wright, D.C., Delaney, T.F., & Buckner, J.C. (1993). Treatment of metastatic cancer. In V.T. DeVita, Jr., S. Hellman, & S.A. Rosenberg (eds.). *Cancer: Principles and Practice of Oncology* (4th ed., vol. II). Philadelphia: J.B. Lippincott, pp. 2173–2185.

Wright, J.E., & Shelton, B.R. (1993). *Desk Reference for Critical Care Nursing.* Boston: Jones & Bartlett, pp. 271–288.

Yahalon, J. (1993). Superior vena cava syndrome. In V.T. DeVita, Jr., S. Hellman, & S. Rosenberg (eds.). *Cancer: Principles and Practice of Oncology* (4th ed., vol. II). Philadelphia: J.B. Lippincott, pp. 2111–2118.

PART SIX

Scientific Basis
for Practice

19

Carcinogenesis

Deborah Lowe Volker, RN, MA, OCN

I. What is cancer?
  A. Definition—a malignant disease characterized by:
    1. A series of cellular, genetic aberrations that cause abnormal cell proliferation.
    2. Unchecked local growth (tumor formation) and invasion of surrounding tissue.
    3. Ability to metastasize (e.g., spread in a noncontiguous fashion to form secondary sites).
  B. Pathology—cancer arises due to cumulative alterations in a cell's genes.
    1. Proto-oncogenes—the genetic portion of the deoxyribonucleic acid (DNA) that regulates normal cell growth and repair; mutation may allow cells to proliferate beyond normal body needs.
    2. Tumor suppressor genes (also termed *antioncogenes*)—the genetic portion of the DNA that stops cell division; mutation may allow cells to proliferate beyond normal body needs.
    3. Oncogenes.
      a. Abnormal, mutated genes responsible for the transformation of a normal cell into a cancer cell.
      b. May arise from mutations in proto-oncogenes, tumor suppressor genes, or other genes that repair cellular DNA.
      c. Different types of oncogenes may act together to induce cancers. For example,
        (1) p53 tumor suppressor gene—normally functions to stop cell proliferation, which allows DNA damage to be repaired.
          (a) When mutated, p53 restraint on cell proliferation is lost.
          (b) p53 mutations occur in about one half of all human cancers; most common in colorectal, lung, and breast cancers.
        (2) *Ras* family of proto-oncogenes—normally function to promote cellular growth.
          (a) When mutated, *ras* oncogenes may allow cells to proliferate unrestrained.
          (b) *Ras* oncogenes are the most frequently detected oncogenes in human cancers; most common in pancreatic, colorectal, and thyroid cancers.

d. Clinical implications.
(1) Presence of certain oncogenes may have diagnostic and prognostic value.
(2) Prevention of gene mutation is one focus of chemoprevention clinical trials.
(3) Understanding of genetic changes may result in new targets for treatment.

C. Carcinogenesis—refers to the process by which cancer arises. Likely involves a series of multiple steps or cellular changes over time (Fig. 19–1). The three-stage theory of causation (carcinogenesis) is the most widely used explanation of the process by which a normal cell is transformed into a cancer cell.

1. Initiation—a carcinogen (cancer-causing agent) damages the DNA by changing a specific gene; this gene may then:
   a. Undergo repair (thus, no initiation occurs).
   b. Become permanently changed (mutated) but not cause cancer unless subsequently exposed to threshold levels of cancer promoters.
   c. Become transformed (mutated) and produce a cancer cell line if the initiator is a complete carcinogen (acts as both an initiator and a promoter).

2. Promotion.
   a. Definition of promotion—process by which carcinogens are subsequently introduced, resulting in one of the following changes.
      (1) Reversible damage to the proliferation mechanism of the cell; the effects of promoting factors may be inhibited by:
         (a) Cancer-reversing agents; clinical studies may include use of antiproliferatives (retinoids, hormone inhibitors, antiinflammatory agents), antioxidants (vitamins, A, C, and E; carotenoids, selenium), or protease inhibitors.
         (b) Host characteristics such as an effective immune system.
         (c) Time or dose limits on the exposure to the promoter.
      (2) Irreversible damage to the proliferation mechanism, resulting in cancer cell transformation.
   b. Characteristics of promoting factors.
      (1) Can induce tumors in initiated cells.
      (2) Will not cause tumors when applied *before* the initiating factor.
      (3) Have a threshold level—if a subthreshold dose or widely spaced doses are given, no effect occurs.
      (4) May also be initiators (cigarette smoke, asbestos, alcohol).
   c. Time frame.
      (1) Time between exposure to initiators and promoters and development of cancer is quite variable.
      (2) May depend upon dosage and length of exposure.

3. Progression.
   a. Invasion—cells continue to divide; increased bulk, pressure, and secretion of enzymes result in local spread and invasion of surrounding structures (exception: carcinoma in situ—malignancy limited to the epithelium; has not yet invaded the basement membrane [underlying tissue]).
   b. Neovascularization—formation of new blood vessels.
      (1) Increases nutrients to tumor cells; seems to contribute to progression.

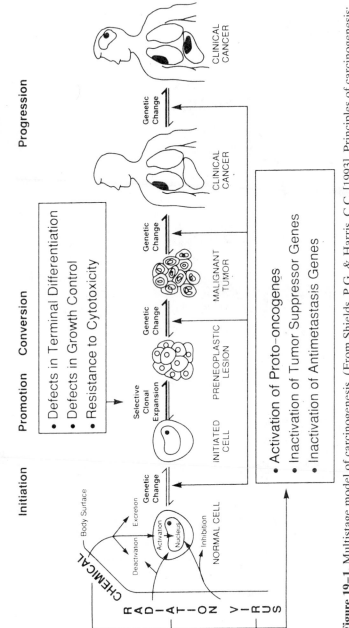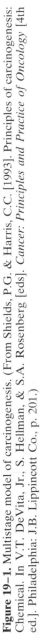

Figure 19-1. Multistage model of carcinogenesis. (From Shields, P.G. & Harris, C.C. [1993]. Principles of carcinogenesis: Chemical. In V.T. DeVita, Jr., S. Hellman, & S.A. Rosenberg [eds]. *Cancer: Principles and Practice of Oncology* [4th ed.]. Philadelphia: J.B. Lippincott Co., p. 201.)

(2) Tumor angiogenesis—refers to a tumor's ability to stimulate the proliferation of new blood vessels from the host. Permits rapid growth of tumor cells and increases risk of metastases.

(3) Modulated by a number of factors, including tumor angiogenesis factor (TAF), and fibroblast growth factors (FGF).

(4) Clinical implication—antiangiogenesis factors may be useful in treating solid tumors.

c. Metastasis—the production of secondary tumors at distant sites. (Fig. 19–2).

(1) Routes of metastasis—cells may spread by:

(a) Seeding throughout a body cavity such as the peritoneal cavity.

(b) Dissemination via the lymphatic system—entrapment may occur in the first lymph node encountered, or cells may bypass the first node and reach more distant sites ("skip metastasis").

(c) Dissemination via blood capillaries and veins; most metastases form by this method; proposed mechanism:

i. Migration of metastatic cells to the periphery of the primary tumor.

ii. Penetration of the extracellular matrix of the tumor by enzymes and other factors.

iii. Penetration of surrounding blood vessel walls.

iv. Dissemination into the bloodstream.

v. Interaction with host factors (platelets, lymphocytes).

vi. Formation of clusters or emboli.

Formation of a Metastasis

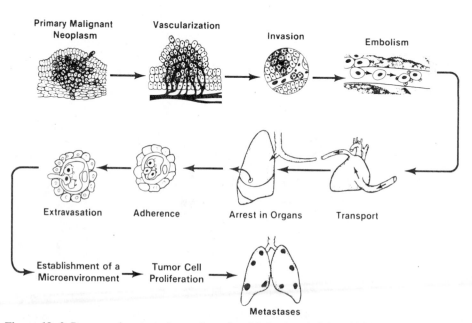

Figure 19–2. Process of metastasis consists of multiple sequential and highly selective steps. (From Fidler, I.J. & Nicolson, G.L. [1987]. The process of cancer invasion and metastasis. *Cancer Bull* 39[3], 127.)

       vii. Adherence to blood vessel walls in distant organ.

      viii. Localized growth stimulated by growth factors.

       ix. Extravasation out of blood vessel into adjacent tissue.

        x. Proliferation of the metastatic deposit of cells.

       xi. Formation of a supporting vascular system via angiogenesis (secretion of TAF).

  (2) Sites.

    (a) Most common—bone, lung, liver, and central nervous system.

    (b) Predilection for certain tumors to metastasize to specific sites may be influenced by:

       i. Patterns of blood flow.

      ii. Cell receptors and genes that direct the cell to travel to specific sites.

     iii. Necessary growth factors, which can be elicited only in selected organs.

  (3) Clinical implications.

    (a) Metastasis is the major cause of death from cancer.

    (b) Most tumors have begun to metastasize at the time of detection.

  d. Heterogeneity—refers to differences among individual cells within a tumor; degree of heterogeneity increases as the tumor grows (Fig. 19–3).

  (1) Differences include:

    (a) Genetic composition.

    (b) Invasiveness.

    (c) Growth rate.

    (d) Hormonal responsiveness.

    (e) Metastatic potential.

    (f) Susceptibility to antineoplastic therapy.

  (2) Heterogeneity is caused by random mutations during tumor progression.

  (3) Clinical implications—can cause tumors to be highly resistant to any one specific therapy.

II. What causes cancer (carcinogenesis)?

  A. Exposure to carcinogens.

    1. Exposure to radiation—cellular DNA damaged by a physical release of energy.

      a. Ionizing radiation.

       (1) Damage to the cell by this source:

         (a) Is usually repaired and no mutation results.

         (b) May give rise to a malignancy when damage affects proto-oncogenes or tumor suppressor genes.

         (c) Depends on numerous factors.

           i. Level of tissue oxygenation—well-oxygenated cells are more radiosensitive.

          ii. Genetic composition—certain genetic disorders, particularly those associated with inefficient DNA repair mechanisms, increase risk.

         iii. Age—children, fetuses, and elderly are at higher risk.

         iv. Cell-cycle phase (Fig. 19–4)—G_2 more sensitive than S or G_1.

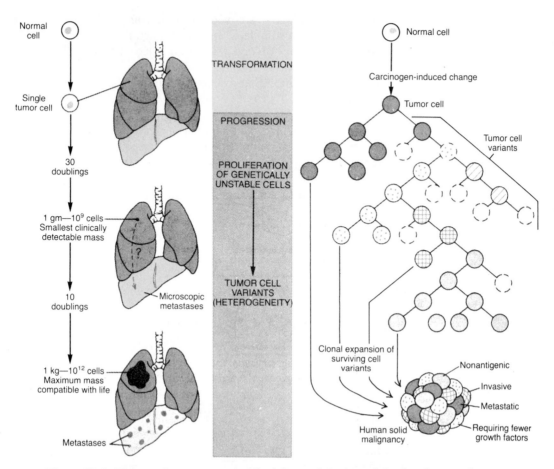

Figure 19–3. Biology of tumor growth. The left panel depicts minimal estimates of tumor cell doublings that precede the formation of clinically detectable tumor mass. It is evident that by the time a solid tumor is detected, it has already completed a major portion of its life cycle as measured by cell doublings. The right panel illustrates clonal evolution of tumors and generation of tumor cell heterogeneity. New subclones arise from the descendants of the original transformed cell, and with progressive growth the tumor mass becomes enriched for those variants that are more adept at evading host defenses and are likely to be more aggressive. (Modified from Tannock, I.F. [1983]. Biology of tumor growth. *Hosp Pract* 18:81.)

v. Degree of differentiation—immature cells most vulnerable.

vi. Cell proliferation rate—cells with high mitotic index most vulnerable.

vii. Tissue type—hematopoietic and gastrointestinal tissue very sensitive.

viii. Total dose and rate of dose—the higher the cumulative dose and dose rate, the greater the likelihood of mutation.

(2) Most exposure is from natural, unavoidable sources.

(3) Examples of ionizing radiation.

(a) Diagnostic or therapeutic sources—diagnostic radiographs, radiation therapy, radioisotopes used in diagnostic imaging.

(b) Cosmic rays.

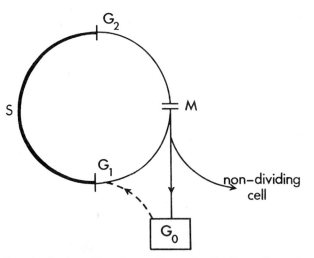

Figure 19–4. Cell cycle. In the cell cycle, continuously dividing cells go from one mitosis (M) to the next, passing through G_1, S (DNA synthesis phase), and G_2. Some cells leave the cycle temporarily, entering a G_0 state from which they can be rescued by appropriate mitogenic stimuli. Other cells leave the cycle permanently, entering terminal differentiation. (From Baserga, R. [1993]. Principles of molecular cell biology of cancer: The cell cycle. In V.T. DeVita, Jr., S. Hellman, & S.A. Rosenberg [eds.]. *Cancer: Principles and Practice of Oncology* [4th ed.]. Philadelphia: J.B. Lippincott Co., p. 61.)

        (c) Radioactive ground minerals and gases—radon gas, radium, uranium.

    (4) Cancers linked to exposure to ionizing radiation include:

        (a) Skin cancer.

        (b) Leukemia (particularly acute myelogenous leukemia [AML] and chronic myelogenous leukemia [CML]).

        (c) Lung cancer.

        (d) Thyroid cancer.

        (e) Breast cancer.

        (f) Osteosarcoma.

  b. Ultraviolet radiation (UVR)—is a complete carcinogen.

    (1) Sources of UVR.

        (a) Sunlight.

        (b) Tanning salons.

        (c) Industrial sources—welding arcs and germicidal lights.

    (2) Risk of carcinogenesis by UVR is increased by:

        (a) Prolonged exposure as a result of occupational or recreational activities.

        (b) Hereditary diseases characterized by inefficient DNA repair mechanisms (examples—xeroderma pigmentosum, ataxia telangiectasia).

        (c) Skin pigmentation—the greater the amount of melanin, the greater is the protection against UVR.

    (3) Skin cancers most commonly associated with UVR include:

        (a) Melanoma.

        (b) Basal cell carcinoma.

        (c) Squamous cell carcinoma.

2. Chemical carcinogens—chemical substances that alter DNA (Table 19–1); examples include:
   a. Alkylating antineoplastic agents—cyclophosphamide, nitrogen mustard, melphalan, busulfan, nitrosoureas.
   b. Aromatic hydrocarbons—soot, pitch, coal tar, benzene.
   c. Organic compounds—vinyl chloride, isopropyl oil.
   d. Tobacco products—cigarette smoke, chewing tobacco, snuff.
   e. Inorganic compounds—chromates, asbestos, nickel.
   f. Plant and microbial products—*Senecio* alkaloids in herbal teas and medicines, aflatoxin B, betel nuts, griseofulvin, cycasin, safrol.

TABLE 19–1. **Chemicals and Mixtures That are Carcinogenic or Probably Carcinogenic in Humans**

Agent	Site
Lifestyle/Personal Choice Exposure	
Tobacco	Lung, pancreas, oral cavity and pharynx, larynx, urinary tract
Tobacco quids and betel nut	Oral mucosa
Ethanol with smoking	Esophagus
Industrial Exposure	
Arsenic compounds	Skin, lungs
p-Biphenylamine and o-nitrobiphenyl	Urinary bladder
Asbestos	Pleura, peritoneum, lung
Asbestos with cigarette smoking	Synergistic increase in lung
Benzidine (4,4'-diaminobiphenyl)	Urinary bladder
Bis(chloromethyl) ether	Lung
Bis(2-chloroethyl) sulfide	Respiratory tract
Chromium compounds	Lung
2(or β)-Naphthylamine	Urinary bladder
Nickel compounds	Lungs, nasal sinuses
Soots, tars, oils	Skin, lungs
Vinyl chloride	Liver mesenchyme
Radon gas (radiation)	Lung
Radon gas with cigarette smoking	Synergistic increase in lung
Drugs and Therapeutic Exposure	
N,N-Bis(2-chloroethyl)-2-naphthylamine (Chlornaphazine)	Urinary bladder
Cancer chemotherapy regimens (alkylating agents)	Leukemias, lymphomas, solid tumors
Diethylstilbestrol	Vagina
Estrogen	Breast, uterus
Phenacetin	Renal pelvis
Psoralen with ultraviolet radiation	Skin

From Lieberman, M.W. & Lebovitz, R.M. (1990). Neoplasia. In J.M. Kissane (ed.). *Anderson's Pathology* (9th ed.). St. Louis: C.V. Mosby Co., p. 596.

   g. Hormones—estrogens and diethylstilbestrol.
   h. Others—chromium, polychlorinated biphenyls (PCBs), some insecticides, and fungicides.
   3. Viruses (Table 19–2).
   a. Infect DNA, resulting in proto-oncogene changes and cell mutation.
   b. Effects modified by:
      (1) Age—the very young and elderly are more susceptible.
      (2) Immunocompetence—many viruses are oncogenic only if the host is immunocompromised.
B. Compromised immune system.
   1. Immune surveillance against cancer—theory that proposes recognition and destruction of cancer cells by the immune system.
   2. Surveillance occurs via recognition of tumor-associated antigens (TAAs) that mark some cancer cells as foreign.
   3. Immune response may fail because of:
   a. Constitutional factors.
      (1) Age—an immature or senescent immune system.
      (2) Tumor burden.
         (a) Too little—insufficient to stimulate response.
         (b) Too much—overwhelms the immune system.
      (3) Cancer cells may:
         (a) Shed substances that:
            i. Suppress immune activity.
            ii. Shield the cell from recognition.
            iii. Resemble normal cells and thus escape detection.
         (b) Invade the bone marrow, resulting in decreased production of lymphocytes.
         (c) Become coated with fibrin and escape detection.
   b. Iatrogenic factors.
      (1) Immunosuppressive drug therapy—incidence of malignancy increases with use of glucocorticosteroids, alkylating agents, azathioprine, cyclosporine.
      (2) Radiation-induced suppression of immune response.
   4. Immune surveillance theory is limited because:
   a. Association between immunosuppression and cancers is inconsistent.
   b. Most cancers associated with immunosuppression are hematologic malignancies associated with Epstein-Barr virus.
   c. Certain animal model findings contradict the theory.

TABLE 19–2. **Human Viruses Strongly Associated With Cancer**

Virus	Type of Cancer
Human T-cell leukemia virus type I (HTLV-1)	Adult T-cell leukemia (ATL)
Hepatitis B virus (HBV)	Hepatocellular carcinoma
Epstein-Barr virus (EBV)	Burkitt's lymphoma Nasopharyngeal cancer (NPC)
Human papillomavirus (HPV)	Cervical and genital cancer

Benchimol, S. (1992). Viruses and cancer. In. I.F. Tannock & R.P. Hill (eds.). *The Basic Science of Oncology* (2nd ed.). New York: McGraw-Hill, p. 89.

C. Genetic predisposition—predisposition to certain cancers may be inherited; mechanism is unclear in most cases, although some are linked to inheritance of dominant antioncogenes; examples:
   1. Familial polyposis coli.
   2. Multiple endocrine neoplasia.
   3. Dysplastic nevus syndrome.
   4. Neurofibromatosis.
   5. Wilms' tumor.
   6. Retinoblastoma.
   7. Xeroderma pigmentosum.
   8. Ataxia telangiectasia.
   9. Fanconi anemia.

III. What are the characteristics of cancer cells?
   A. Microscopic studies show structural changes in cancer cells (Fig. 19–5) that are described in pathologic terms such as:
      1. Pleomorphism—cells are variable in size and shape.
         a. Some are unusually large; others are too small.
         b. Multiple nuclei can be present.
      2. Hyperchromatism—nuclear chromatin more pronounced upon staining.
      3. Polymorphism—nucleus enlarged and variable in shape.
      4. Aneuploidy—unusual numbers of chromosomes present.
      5. Abnormal chromosome arrangements.
         a. Translocations—exchange of material between chromosomes.
         b. Deletions—loss of chromosome segments.
         c. Amplification—additional genes.
         d. Aneuploidy—abnormal number of chromosomes
   B. Biochemical studies show differences in cell metabolism and products such as:
      1. Cell membrane changes.
         a. Production of surface enzymes that may aid in invasion and metastasis.

Nuclear hyperchromatism   Prominent   Mitotic   Pleomorphism
High nucleus:cytoplasm ratio nucleoli   activity

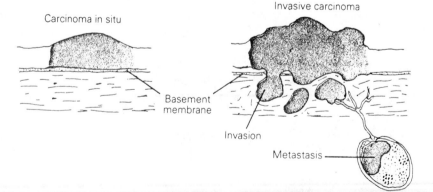

Carcinoma in situ

Invasive carcinoma

Basement membrane

Invasion

Metastasis

Lymph node

Figure 19–5. Features of malignant neoplasms. (From Lefkowitch, J.H. [1989]. *Histopathology of Disease.* New York: Churchill Livingstone, p. 17.)

    b. Loss of glycoproteins that normally aid in cell-to-cell adhesion and organization.

    c. Loss of antigens that otherwise label the cell as "self."

    d. Production of new tumor-associated antigens that mark the cell as "non-self"; examples:

        (1) Oncofetal antigens—antigens that are expressed by certain normal cells during fetal development but are subsequently repressed; may reappear when cell becomes malignant; examples:

            (a) Carcinoembryonic antigen (CEA)—may be elevated in colorectal, breast, lung, liver, pancreatic, and gynecological cancers.

            (b) α-fetoprotein (AFP)—may be elevated in hepatocellular, testicular, lung, pancreatic, and ovarian cancers.

        (2) Placental antigens—antigens normally produced by the placenta such as:

            (a) Human chorionic gonadotropin (HCG) and human placental lactogen (HPL), which usually are associated with gynecological cancers.

        (3) Differentiation antigens, which are found in normal differentiating tissue; associated with acute lymphocytic leukemia (ALL), chronic lymphocytic leukemia (CLL), and lymphoblastic lymphoma.

        (4) Lineage-associated determination antigens such as CA-125, which is associated with ovarian cancer.

        (5) Viral antigens—appear in certain cancers associated with viral origins.

    e. Clinical usefulness—certain tumor antigens may be used as *tumor markers* (Table 19–3), biochemical substances synthesized and released by tumor cells; may be used as indicators of tumor presence but may also be present in a variety of benign conditions; most tumor markers lack specificity to cancer.

  2. Abnormal glycolysis—higher rate of anaerobic glycolysis, making the cell less dependent on oxygen.

  3. Abnormal production of substances that give rise to paraneoplastic syndromes (signs or symptoms that occur in a client with cancer but are not due directly to the local effects of the tumor (Table 19–4).

    a. Hormone or hormone-like substances, especially from nonendocrine cells.

    b. Procoagulant materials that affect the clotting mechanism.

C. Cell kinetic (growth and division) studies show:

  1. Loss of contact inhibition (the normal inhibition of cell movement and division once in contact with other cell) (Figure 19–6).

  2. Defect in cell-to-cell recognition and adhesion—cancer cells do not recognize and adhere to each other as well as normal cells do.

  3. Increased mitotic index (the proportion of cells in a tissue that are in mitosis at any given time).

    a. Large numbers of mitotic cells reflect the higher proliferative activity of the tumor.

    b. A high mitotic index is not unique to cancer; however, normal cells in, for example, the gastrointestinal system, bone marrow, and hair follicles have a rapid rate of cell turnover and thus a high mitotic index.

  4. Abnormal cell differentiation.

    a. Differentiation—refers to the extent to which tumor cells resemble comparable normal cells, both morphologically and functionally.

        (1) Grade—an evaluation of the degree of differentiation of the malignant cells.

TABLE 19–3. **Selected Tumor Markers and Applications in Diagnostic Medicine**

Tumor Marker	Exemplary Malignant Neoplasms	Commonly Associated Nonneoplastic Diseases
Hormones		
Human chorionic gonadotropin (hCG)	Gestational trophoblastic disease, gonadal germ cell tumors	Pregnancy
Calcitonin	Medullary cancer of thyroid	———
Catecholamines and metabolites	Pheochromocytoma	———
Oncofetal Antigens		
Alpha-fetoprotein (AFP)	Hepatocellular carcinoma, gonadal germ cell tumors (especially endodermal sinus tumor)	Cirrhosis, toxic liver injury, hepatitis
Carcinoembryonic antigen (CEA)	Adenocarcinomas of colon, pancreas, stomach, lung, breast, ovary	Pancreatitis, inflammatory bowel disease, hepatitis, cirrhosis, tobacco abuse
Isoenzymes		
Prostatic acid phosphatase	Adenocarcinoma of prostate	Prostatitis; nodular prostatic hyperplasia
Neuron-specific enolase	Small-cell carcinoma of lung; neuroblastoma	———
Specific Proteins		
Prostate-specific antigen (PSA)	Adenocarcinoma of prostate	Nodular prostatic hyperplasia, prostatitis
Immunoglobulin (monoclonal)	Multiple myeloma	Monoclonal gammopathy of unknown significance
CA 125	Epithelial ovarian neoplasms	Menstruation, pregnancy, peritonitis
CA-19-9	Adenocarcinoma of pancreas or colon	Pancreatitis; ulcerative colitis

From Pfeifer, J.D. & Wick, M.R. (1995). The pathologic evaluation of neoplastic disease. In G. Murphy, W. Lawrence, & R.E. Lenhard (eds.). *American Cancer Society Textbook of Clinical Oncology* (2nd ed.). Atlanta: American Cancer Society, p. 92.

(a) Grading criteria vary greatly for different tumors; based on degree to which tumor cells resemble their normal counterpart.
(b) Often characterized as grade I, II, III, or IV.
(c) Grade I—well differentiated; also termed *low grade.*
(d) Grade IV—poorly differentiated; also termed *high grade.*
(2) Benign tumors—composed of well-differentiated cells; tend to resemble the mature, functionally normal cells of the tissue of origin.
(3) Malignant tumors—may be composed of cells that range from well-differentiated to undifferentiated, primitive cells.
(4) Anaplasia, or lack of differentiation, is:
(a) A hallmark of malignancy.
(b) The result of proliferation of transformed cells that do not mature.
(c) Not a result of "dedifferentiation" (a reversion of the maturational process).

TABLE 19–4. **Paraneoplastic Syndromes**

Clinical Syndromes	Major Forms of Underlying Cancer	Causal Mechanism
Endocrinopathies		
Cushing's syndrome	Small cell carcinoma of lung Pancreatic carcinoma Neural tumors	ACTH or ACTH-like substance
Syndrome of inappropriate antidiuretic hormone secretion (SIADH)	Small cell carcinoma of lung Intracranial neoplasms	Antidiuretic hormone or atrial natriuretic hormones
Hypercalcemia	Squamous cell carcinoma of lung Breast carcinoma Renal carcinoma Adult T-cell leukemia/ lymphoma Ovarian carcinoma	Parathyroid hormone–related peptide TGF-α, TNF-α, IL-1
Hypoglycemia	Fibrosarcoma Other mesenchymal sarcomas Hepatocellular carcinoma	Insulin or insulin-like substance
Carcinoid syndrome	Bronchial adenoma (carcinoid) Pancreatic carcinoma Gastric carcinoma	Serotonin, bradykinin, ? histamine
Polycythemia	Renal carcinoma Cerebellar hemangioma Hepatocellular carcinoma	Erythropoietin
Nerve and Muscle Syndromes		
Myasthenia	Bronchogenic carcinoma	? Immunologic, ? toxic
Disorders of the central and peripheral nervous systems	Breast carcinoma	
Dermatologic Disorders		
Acanthosis nigricans	Gastric carcinoma Lung carcinoma Uterine carcinoma	? Immunologic, ? secretion of epidermal growth factor
Dermatomyositis	Bronchogenic, breast carcinoma	? Immunologic, ? toxic
Osseous, Articular, and Soft Tissue Changes		
Hypertrophic osteoarthropathy and clubbing of the fingers	Bronchogenic carcinoma	Unknown
Vascular and Hematologic Changes		
Venous thrombosis (Trousseau's phenomenon)	Pancreatic carcinoma Bronchogenic carcinoma Other cancers	Tumor products (mucins) that activate clotting
Nonbacterial thrombotic endocarditis	Advanced cancers	Hypercoagulability

Table continues on following page

TABLE 19–4. **Paraneoplastic Syndromes** (*Continued*)

Clinical Syndromes	Major Forms of Underlying Cancer	Causal Mechanism
Anemia	Thymic neoplasms	Unknown
Others		
Nephrotic syndrome	Various cancers	Tumor antigens, immune complexes

From Cotran, R.S., Kumar, V., & Robbins, S.L. (1994). *Robbins Pathologic Basis of Disease* (5th ed.). Philadelphia: W.B. Saunders Co., p. 296.

     b. Functional changes.
        (1) The greater the degree of differentiation of a cell, the more likely it will have some of the functional capabilities of its normal counterpart.
        (2) The more anaplastic the tumor, the less likely any specialized function will be present.
   5. Growth characteristics—the length of time required for a tumor to become clinically detectable is influenced by:
     a. Growth fraction—the fraction of proliferating cells in the tumor.
        (1) Normal tissue.
           (a) Growth fraction is variable, depending on type of tissue.
           (b) Example—intestinal epithelium contains approximately 16% actively proliferating cells; central nervous system cells are nonproliferating.
        (2) Type of malignancy.
           (a) Growth fraction also is variable, depending on type of cancer; for example:
              i. In many solid tumors, 1 to 8% of cells are actively proliferating.
              ii. In very aggressive, rapidly growing tumors, 20 to 30% of cells are actively proliferating.
     b. Tumor volume-doubling time.
        (1) The time within which the total cancer cell population doubles.
        (2) Average volume-doubling time of most primary tumors—8 to 12 weeks, with a range of 11 to 90 weeks.
        (3) Influencing variables.
           (a) Tumor type—most tumors have a high proportion of nonproliferating cells.
           (b) Vascularity.
               i. Supplies necessary nutrients and removes wastes.
              ii. Varies within tumor (Fig. 19–7).
     c. Center is poorly vascular; hence, slower growing.
     d. Periphery is more vascular; hence, increased growth.
        (1) Cell loss by:
           (a) Continuous shedding from the primary tumor.
           (b) Death caused by toxic products released from other necrotic cells within the tumor.
     e. Hormone levels.
        (1) Certain cancers (that arise from hormone-dependent tissue) require hormones for growth.
        (2) Reduction in hormone levels reduces tumor growth.
        (3) Increased hormone levels promote growth.

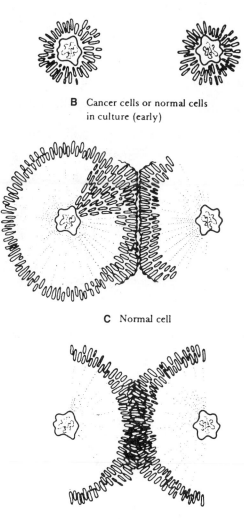

A Cancer cells or normal cells

B Cancer cells or normal cells in culture (early)

C Normal cell

D Cancer cells

Figure 19–6. Impaired contact inhibition of cancer cells. (From Groenwald, S.L. [1993]. Differences between normal and cancer cells. In S.L. Groenwald, M.H. Frogge, M. Goodman, & C.H. Yarbro [eds.]. *Cancer Nursing: Principles and Practice* [3rd ed.]. Boston: Jones & Bartlett, p. 50.)

    f. Gompertzian growth—refers to a hypothetical growth curve over the lifetime of an "average" tumor (Fig. 19–8).

      (1) Growth increases exponentially at first (tumor growth doubles constantly over time).

      (2) Growth then slows owing to hypoxia, decreased availability of nutrients and growth factors, toxins, and faulty cell-to-cell communication.

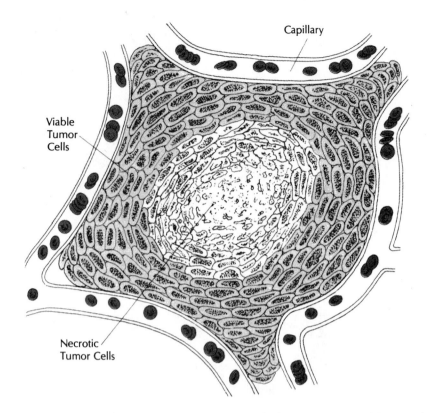

Figure 19–7. In many tumors, viable tissue and necrotic tissue are arranged in one of two patterns: cylindrical or nodular. Both patterns appear to reflect the presence or absence of proximate vascular support. The nodular pattern is depicted here. Viable tissue lies around the outer margins of the nodule, near surrounding vessels, whereas the center is necrotic. (Reproduced with permission. Tannock, I.F. [1983]. Biology of tumor growth. *Hosp Pract* 18[4], 86. Illustration by Nancy Lou Makris.)

      g. Clinical conclusions (see Fig. 19–3).
        (1) Tumor growth rates vary widely.
        (2) Smallest clinically detectable mass equals:
          (a) One gram in weight.
          (b) One cubic centimeter in diameter.
          (c) One billion cells.
          (d) Approximately 30 tumor volume-doubling times.
        (3) Growth from 1 g to 1 kg (potentially lethal size) requires only 10 more doublings.
        (4) Tumors increase in size because the rate of cell production exceeds rate of cell death.
    D. Tumor growth patterns (Fig. 19–9).
      1. Noncancerous and precancerous growth changes.
        a. Hypertrophy.
          (1) An increase in the size of cells.
          (2) Can result from hormonal stimulation, increased workload, or compensation as a consequence of functional loss of other tissue.
        b. Hyperplasia.
          (1) A reversible increase in the number of cells in a tissue.
          (2) Can result from hormonal stimulation (during pregnancy).

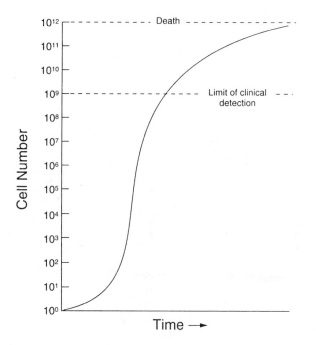

Figure 19–8. The Gompertzian growth curve. During the early stages of development, growth is exponential. As a tumor enlarges, its growth slows. By the time a tumor becomes large enough to cause symptoms and be clinically detectable, most of its growth has already occurred, and the exponential phase is over. (From Fleming, I.D., Brady, L.W., & Cooper, M.R. [1995]. Basis for major current therapies for cancer. In G. Murphy, W. Lawrence, & R.E. Lenhard [eds.]. *American Cancer Society Textbook of Clinical Oncology* [2nd ed.]. Atlanta: American Cancer Society, Inc., p. 114.)

   (3) Abnormal hyperplastic changes such as those associated with chronic irritation can lead to increased risk of malignancy.
 c. Metaplasia.
   (1) Reversible process involving replacement of one mature cell type by another mature cell type not usually found in the involved tissue.
   (2) Initiated by chronic irritation, inflammation, vitamin deficiency, or other pathologic process.
   (3) Example—replacement of columnar epithelial cells in respiratory passages of smokers with squamous cell epithelium.
 4. Dysplasia.
   (1) Alteration in normal adult cells.
   (2) Characterized by variations in size, shape, and organization.
   (3) Can result from chronic irritation or inflammation.
   (4) Smokers may exhibit dysplastic changes in respiratory tissues and oral mucosa.
   (5) Possible reversible if stimulant is removed.
   (6) Strongly associated with subsequent neoplastic changes.
 2. Hyperplasia, metaplasia, and dysplasia are not neoplastic per se, but may precede the development of cancer.
 3. Cancerous conditions.
 a. Anaplasia.
   (1) The cytologic and positional disorganization of cells.
   (2) Degree of anaplastic changes may vary.
   (3) Most often used to describe malignancy.

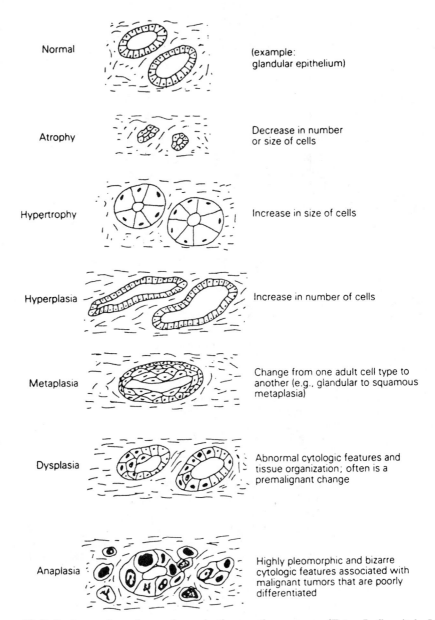

| Normal | | (example: glandular epithelium) |

| Atrophy | | Decrease in number or size of cells |

| Hypertrophy | | Increase in size of cells |

| Hyperplasia | | Increase in number of cells |

| Metaplasia | | Change from one adult cell type to another (e.g., glandular to squamous metaplasia) |

| Dysplasia | | Abnormal cytologic features and tissue organization; often is a premalignant change |

| Anaplasia | | Highly pleomorphic and bizarre cytologic features associated with malignant tumors that are poorly differentiated |

Figure 19–9. Features of reactive and neoplastic growth processes. (From Lefkowitch, J.H. [1989]. *Histopathology of Disease.* New York: Churchill Livingstone, p. 160.)

       b. *Neoplasm* versus *tumor.*
         (1) Interchangeable terms.
         (2) Refers to abnormal growth of tissue that serves no function and continues to grow unchecked once the stimulus is removed.
         (3) Can be benign or malignant.
       c. *Cancer*—common term for all malignancies.
       d. Differences between benign and malignant neoplasms (Table 19–5).
   E. Tumor nomenclature.
       1. Usually named according to tissue of origin (numerous exceptions exist).

TABLE 19–5. **Classifications of Human Tumors by Tissue Type**

Tissue of Origin	Benign	Malignant
Epithelium		
Surface epithelium (nonglandular)	Papilloma	Carcinoma (squamous cell, epidermoid, transitional cell)
Glandular epithelium	Adenoma	Adenocarcinoma
Basal layer of epidermis	———	Basal cell carcinoma
Trophoblasts of placental villi	Hydatidiform mole	Choriocarcinoma
Connective tissue		
Fibrous tissue	Fibroma	Fibrosarcoma
Cartilage	Chondroma	Chondrosarcoma
Bone	Osteoma	Osteosarcoma
Smooth muscle	Leiomyoma	Leiomyosarcoma
Striated muscle	Rhabdomyoma	Rhabdomyosarcoma
Fat	Lipoma	Liposarcoma
Endothelial tissue and its derivatives		
Blood vessels	Hemangioma	Hemangiosarcoma
Lymph vessels	Lymphangioma	Lymphangiosarcoma
Bone marrow		
Granulocytes	———	Myelocytic leukemia
Erythrocytes	Polycythemia vera	Erythrocytic leukemia
Lymphocytes	Infectious mononucleosis	Lymphocytic leukemia
Plasma cells	———	Multiple myeloma
Monocytes	———	Monocytic leukemia
Endothelial lining	———	Ewing's sarcoma
Lymphoid tissue		Non-Hodgkin's malignant lymphomas Lymphocytic type Histiocytic type Undifferentiated, pleomorphic type Undifferentiated, Burkitt type
Thymus	———	Thymoma
Neural tissue and its derivatives		
Glial tissue	"Benign" gliomas (some ependymomas and oligodendrogliomas are considered nonmalignant)	Glioblastoma multiforme, medulloblastoma, astrocytoma, ependymoma, oligodendroglioma
Meninges	Meningioma	Meningeal sarcoma
Neuronal cells	Ganglioneuroma	Neuroblastoma
Nerve sheath	Neurilemmoma	Neurilemmal sarcoma (schwannoma)
Nerve sheath	Neurofibroma	Neurofibrosarcoma
Melanocytes	Pigmented nevus (mole)	Malignant melanoma
Adrenal medulla	Pheochromocytoma	Malignant pheochromocytoma
Retina	———	Retinoblastoma
Specialized nerve endings	Carcinoid tumors	Carcinoid tumors
Mixed tumors derived from more than one cell type		
Embryonic kidney	———	Nephroblastoma (Wilms' tumor)
Gonadal tissue	Teratoma	Teratocarcinoma
Gonadal tissue	———	Embryonal carcinoma with choriocarcinoma

2. Benign tumors.
    a. Labeled by adding the suffix *-oma* to the tissue of origin.
    b. Examples:
        (1) Lipoma—benign tumor composed of lipid cells.
        (2) Adenoma—benign tumor composed of glandular cells.
3. Malignant tumors.
    a. Classified according to:
        (1) Tissue of origin.
        (2) Biologic behavior.
        (3) Anatomic site.
        (4) Degree of cell differentiation.
    b. Carcinomas.
        (1) Arise in epithelial tissue.
        (2) Prefixes describe specific type of epithelial tissue.
            (a) *Adeno-*.
                i. Describes tumors arising from glandular epithelium (columnar).
                ii. Organ of origin also included.
                iii. Example—pancreatic adenocarcinoma (a malignant epithelial neoplasm located in the pancreas).
            (b) *Squamous.*
                i. Describes tumors arising from squamous epithelium.
                ii. Organ of origin is included.
                iii. Example—squamous cell carcinoma of the skin.
    c. Sarcomas.
        (1) Originate in connective tissue.
        (2) Prefixes for specific connective tissue sarcomas include:
            (a) *Osteo*—arising from bone.
            (b) *Chondro*—arising from cartilage.
            (c) *Lipo*—arising from fat.
            (d) *Rhabdo*—arising from skeletal muscle.
            (e) *Leiomyo*—arising from smooth muscle.
    d. Hematologic malignancies.
        (1) Leukemias.
            (a) Arise from hematopoietic cells.
            (b) Classified according to cell type and maturity.
            (c) *Lympho-* denotes leukemia of lymphoid origin.
            (d) *Myelo-* denotes leukemia of myeloid origin.
        (2) Lymphomas.
            (a) Malignancies of the lymphocyte.
            (b) Subclassified as:
                i. Hodgkin's disease.
                ii. Non-Hodgkin's lymphoma.
        (3) Multiple myeloma—arises from the plasma cell (B lymphocyte) line.
IV. What are the implications of diagnosis and staging on treatment goals and strategies?
    A. Decisions related to the treatment are made after review of the clinical, pathologic, laboratory, and diagnostic data by a multidisciplinary team of cancer specialists.
    B. Key factors to evaluate before making a treatment decision.
        1. Site of cancer.
            a. Review of client history.
            b. Physical examination.
            c. Radiologic examination.
            d. Laboratory data.

2. Histologic type and grade of cancer.
   a. Diagnosis of cancer is determined by tissue biopsy.
      (1) Incisional biopsy.
         (a) Aspiration.
         (b) Fine-needle biopsy—removal of a core of tissue.
         (c) Punch biopsy—removal of tissue from the core of the tumor.
      (2) Excisional biopsy—removal of tissue with client under general or local anesthesia.
         (a) Provides an opportunity to remove the entire lesion.
         (b) Serves as a mechanism for removal of an adequate sample of tissue for diagnosis.
      (3) Cytology—examination of fluid containing cells that have been shed.
         (a) A positive result from cytology examination may be adequate for diagnosis.
         (b) A negative result from cytology examination is inconclusive, and additional attempts to obtain tissue for diagnosis are indicated.
   b. Biopsy confirmation is important in that proof of a diagnosis is mandated by insurance companies for coverage.
   c. Tissue biopsy allows for histopathologic grading of tumor.
3. Extent of disease or stage of cancer.
   a. Knowledge of the usual pattern of spread of specific cancers provides guidelines for the staging workup.
   b. Obtaining an extensive history and physical examination is initial step of the staging procedure.
   c. Tests selected for the staging procedure are designed to evaluate the extent of local disease and potential sites of metastatic disease.
      (1) Noninvasive procedures such as x-ray examinations, computed tomographic (CT) scans, magnetic resonance imaging (MRI), and ultrasound.
      (2) Invasive procedures such as exploratory laparotomy.
   d. Staging systems.
      (1) A uniform system for staging.
         (a) Allows comparisons of treatment results across client populations.
         (b) Serves as an aid to indicate appropriate and standard therapy.
      (2) TNM—most widely accepted system for staging.
         (a) T—extent of primary *t*umor.
         (b) N—absence or presence and extent of regional lymph *n*ode metastasis.
         (c) M—absence or presence of distant *m*etastases.
         (d) Addition of numbers after each letter indicate the extent of disease; the higher the number, the more advanced the disease.
         (e) Addition of prefixes to the TNM indicate the timing of the staging (only cTNM and pTNM are most typically used).
            i. cTNM: *C*linical classification made before treatment; based on results of physical examination, radiologic studies, biopsy.
            ii. pTNM: *P*athologic classification based on information obtained via surgical exploration.
            iii. rTNM: *R*etreatment classification used after disease-free interval and further treatment is planned.
            iv. aTNM: *A*utopsy classification done after death when complete pathologic evaluation is made.

(3) Disease stage is typically divided into four classifications, with I the earliest stage and IV the most extensive disease. But many other disease-specific systems exist. Examples:
  (a) Colon cancer: Duke classification.
    i. Based on depth of bowel wall penetration and number of positive lymph nodes.
    ii. Stage A—confined to bowel wall.
    iii. Stage B—spread beyond bowel wall.
    iv. Stage C—lymph node metastases present.
  (b) Hodgkin's disease: Ann Arbor system.
    i. Based on anatomic spread and systemic symptoms.
    ii. Stage I—single lymph node or region.
    iii. Stage II—two or more lymph node regions on same side of diaphragm.
    iv. Stage III—lymph node involvement on both sides of the diaphragm.
    v. Stage IV—widely disseminated disease
    vi. All stages—A means no symptoms; B means symptoms such as fever, night sweats, weight loss.
4. General health status of the client.
  a. Physical examination.
  b. Additional radiologic and laboratory tests are conducted to determine the ability of the client to withstand the demands of and potential consequences of the proposed therapies.
  c. Evaluation of pulmonary, renal, liver, gastrointestinal, and cardiac function are often obtained.
  d. Host performance scales (Table 19–6).
5. Types of therapy.
  a. Primary treatment—major modality used to treat the cancer.
  b. Adjuvant therapy—therapy given *after* the primary treatment to control potential or known sites of metastasis.
  c. Neoadjuvant treatment—adjuvant therapy given *before* the primary treatment to control potential or known sites of metastasis.
  d. Prophylactic treatment—treated directed to a sanctuary site when the risk for developing cancer at the site is high.
6. Goals of therapy.
  a. Cure—eradication of cancer cells in the body.
    (1) Maximal risk of recurrence of disease usually occurs within the first 2 years after primary treatment.
    (2) Clients who have been diagnosed with one cancer may be at higher risk for the development of another cancer that shares similar causative factors, such as breast and endometrial cancers; lung, head, neck, and esophageal cancers.
    (3) Continued annual follow-up is required for evaluation of the presence of recurrence and late effects of treatment.
  b. Control—containment of the growth of cancer cells without complete eradication.
  c. Palliation—comfort and relief of symptoms when the possibility of cure is hopeless.
    (1) Treatment may include any of the therapeutic modalities.
    (2) Treatment course generally is shorter than treatment given with curative intent.
C. Treatment may include single and multimodal approaches.
  1. Single-modality approach.
    a. Reserved for clients with small local disease and without evidence of predilection for metastasis.

TABLE 19–6. **Host Performance Scales**

American Joint Committee on Cancer

H	The physical state (performance scale) of the client, considering all cofactors determined at the time of stage classification and subsequent follow-up examinations
H0	Normal activity
H1	Symptomatic and ambulatory; cares for self
H2	Ambulatory more than 50% of time; occasionally needs assistance
H3	Ambulatory 50% or less of the time; nursing care needed
H4	Bedridden; hospitalization may be needed

Karnofsky Scale: Criteria of Performance Status (PS)

Able to perform normal activity; requires no care	100	Normal; no complaints or evidence of disease
	90	Able to perform normal activity; minor signs and symptoms of disease
	80	Able to perform normal activity with effort; some signs and symptoms of disease
Unable to work; able to live at home and care for most personal needs; requires varying amount of assistance	70	Cares for self; unable to perform normal activity or to do active work
	60	Requires occasional assistance but is able to care for most of own needs
	50	Requires considerable and frequent medical care
Unable to care for self; requires equivalent of institutional or hospital care; disease may be progressing rapidly	40	Requires special care and assistance; disabled
	30	Hospitalization indicated, although death not imminent; severely disabled
	20	Hospitalization necessary; active supportive treatment required; very sick
	10	Fatal processes progressing rapidly; moribund
	0	Dead

Eastern Cooperative Oncology Group Scale (ECOG)

0	Fully active; able to perform all predisease activities without restriction
1	Restricted in physically strenuous activity but ambulatory and able to perform work of a light or a sedentary nature
2	Ambulatory and capable of all self-care but unable to perform any work activities; up and about more than 50% of waking hours
3	Capable of only limited self-care; confined to bed or chair 50% or more of waking hours
4	Completely disabled; cannot carry on any self-care; totally confined to bed or chair

       b. Examples of cancers for which single-modality treatment is appropriate—early skin cancer, colon cancer, head and neck cancers, and leukemia.
    2. Multimodal approach.
       a. Reserved for clients with bulky tumors or a high likelihood of having or actually having metastatic disease.
       b. Surgery, radiation therapy, chemotherapy, and biotherapy may be combined sequentially or given concurrently.
       c. Examples of cancers for which multimodal treatment is appropriate—breast cancer, lymphoma, lung cancer, and endometrial cancer.
  D. Evaluation of response to treatment.
    1. Complete response—absence of signs and symptoms of cancer for at least 1 month.

2. Partial response.
   a. A 50% or more reduction in the sum of the products of the greater and lesser diameters of all measured lesions.
   b. Lasts at least 1 month, and
   c. Without the development of any new lesions during therapy.
3. Progression.
   a. A 25% or more increase in the sum of the products of the greater and lesser diameters of all measured lesions, or
   b. Development of any new lesions.

V. How are these concepts related to nursing care?
   A. Form the basis for client teaching about prevention and health promotion. (See Chapter 40.)
      1. Avoidance of known carcinogens at known locations.
         a. Home. (See Table 19–1 for specific substances.)
         b. Occupational sites, especially those with:
            (1) Asbestos.
            (2) Carcinogenic chemicals.
            (3) Sun.
            (4) Tobacco (smoke-free work environment).
         c. Recreational areas in activities including the sun, tanning booths.
      2. Emphasis on health promotion and lifestyle choices.
         a. Smoking cessation.
         b. Dietary choices.
         c. Methods to avoid sexually transmitted viral carcinogens.
         d. Screening and follow-up monitoring when at risk for familial carcinogenesis.
         e. Self-examination for early cancer detection.
            (1) Breasts.
            (2) Testes.
            (3) Skin.
            (4) Oral cavity.
            (5) Vulvar area.
         f. Other screening activities (according to American Cancer Society guidelines, see Chapter 41).
      3. Investigative potential of reversing agents (e.g., chemoprevention trials).
      4. Emphasis on reversibility of cellular changes (as appropriate); behavior or lifestyle changes *can* make a difference.
      5. Clarification of misconceptions about carcinogenic potential of screening and diagnostic radiologic examinations.
         a. Average yearly exposure to natural, background radiation—0.7 to 1.5 mGy.
         b. Biologic effects often not apparent until 1000-mGy dose (1 Gy) incurred.
         c. Approximate doses for common radiographic procedures.
            (1) Chest radiograph—0.08 mGy.
            (2) Mammography—2–9 mGy/2 films.
         d. Carcinogenic risk from diagnostic procedures is extremely small.
      6. Emphasis on risk of *not* undergoing screening radiography (i.e., undetected cancer).
   B. Form the basis of client teaching about cancer diagnoses.
      1. Pathology examination necessary for cancer diagnosis.
      2. Cytological examinations.
         a. Detection before palpable lesion is present.
         b. Promotion of chance for early cure.

         3. Tumor-associated antigens are used as tumor markers:
            a. At time of diagnosis.
            b. During treatment.
            c. After treatment to monitor recurrence or progression.
         4. Radiologic examinations are necessary for detection of micrometastases.
   C. Form the basis of client teaching about treatment.
         1. High mitotic index of certain cancer cells renders them more susceptible to cytotoxic effects of chemotherapeutic agents.
         2. Stable cells (bone, neural tissue) are less sensitive to effects of chemotherapy because of lower mitotic index.
         3. Use of hyperoxygenation procedures are based on principles of cell sensitivity to radiation effects.
         4. Tumor heterogeneity explains the necessity for:
            a. Intense initial treatment.
            b. Subsequent repeated treatments, with a variety of drugs.
            c. Failures in treatment of metastases.
         5. Adjuvant therapy is used for presumed micrometastases to kill the last remaining cancer cells.
         6. Use of hormonal manipulation for tumors is effective only in hormone-dependent tissues.
         7. Use of fractionated radiation therapy is to minimize damage to healthy tissue while achieving a lethal effect to malignant cells.
         8. Carcinogenic potential of alkylating chemotherapeutic agents and radiation therapy necessitates long-term client follow-up to detect iatrogenic malignancies.
   D. Form the basis for understanding treatment side effects.
         1. Chemotherapy and radiation therapy are nonselective between malignant and normal cells.
         2. Effect on normal cells (especially rapidly dividing cells) accounts for treatment-related side effects (myelosuppression, alopecia, mucositis, nausea and vomiting, diarrhea, dysphagia).
   E. Account for paraneoplastic syndromes.
         1. Related clinical problems are based on ectopic production of hormones and other substances by the malignant cells.
         2. Hormones are atypical of the tissue that gives rise to the tumor, resulting in clinical syndromes (endocrine, coagulant).
   F. Form the basis for client teaching and follow-up to detect metastasis.
         1. Likelihood of metastasis at time of diagnosis may necessitate:
            a. Extensive diagnostic workup.
            b. Systemic approach to therapy.
            c. Adjuvant therapy.
         2. Potential for disease recurrence via metastasis necessitates frequent and long-term follow-up.
VI. What are the implications for the professional development of the nurse?
   A. Promotes understanding of terminology and nomenclature necessary for client teaching and interdisciplinary communication or collaboration.
   B. Promotes understanding of cancer prevention and early detection.
   C. Forms basis for understanding the rationale for treatment protocols, timing of treatment, and diagnostic follow-up.
   D. Enhances understanding of reasons for intensity of initial treatment protocols.
   E. Forms basis for understanding current research and trends in care.
   F. Forms basis for understanding and initiating cancer nursing research.
   G. Promotes understanding of prognostic implications of disease.

H. Enhances participation in identification and discussion of ethical issues related to disease and treatment.

BIBLIOGRAPHY

Cotran, R.S., Kumar, V., & Robbins, S.L. (1994). *Robbins Pathologic Basis of Disease* (5th ed.). Philadelphia: W.B. Saunders.

Fidler, I.J., & Ellis, L.M. (1994). The implications of angiogenesis for the biology and therapy of cancer metastasis. *Cell 79*(2), 185–188.

Greenwald, P., Kelloff, G., Burch-Whitman, C., et al. (1995). Chemoprevention. *CA Cancer J Clin 45*(1), 31–49.

Greenwald, P., Kramer, B.S., & Weed, D.L. (1995). *Cancer Prevention and Control.* New York: Marcel Dekker.

Kelley, M. J., & Johnson, B.E. (1994). Genetic mechanisms of solid tumor oncogenesis. *Adv Intern Med 39*, 93–122.

Maxwell, M.B. (1993). Principles of treatment planning. In S.L. Groenwald, M.H. Frogge, M. Goodman, & C.H. Yarbro (eds.). *Cancer Nursing: Principles and Practice* (3rd ed.). Boston: Jones & Bartlett, pp. 208–221.

Mendelsohn, J., Howley, P.M., Israel, M.A., & Liotta, L.A. (1995). *The Molecular Basis of Cancer.* Philadelphia: W.B. Saunders.

Pamies, R.J., & Crawford, D.T. (1996). Tumor markers: An update. *Med Clin North Am 80*(1), 185–199.

Ponder, B.A.J., & Waring, M.J. (1995). *The Genetics of Cancer.* Boston: Kluwer Academic Publishers.

Ruddon, R.W. (1995). *Cancer Biology* (3rd ed.). New York: Oxford University Press.

Stanley, L.A. (1995). Molecular aspects of chemical carcinogenesis: The role of oncogenes and tumor suppressor genes. *Toxicology 96*(3), 173–194.

Templeton, D.J., & Weinberg, R.A. (1995). Principles of cancer biology. In G. Murphy, W. Lawrence, & R.E. Lenhard (eds.). *American Cancer Society Textbook of Clinical Oncology* (2nd ed.). Atlanta: American Cancer Society, pp. 164–177.

Weisburger, J.H., & Williams, G.M. (1995). Causes of cancer. In G. Murphy, W. Lawrence, & R.E. Lenhard (eds.). *American Cancer Society Textbook of Clinical Oncology* (2nd ed.). Atlanta: American Cancer Society, pp. 10–39.

Immunology

Lynne Brophy, RN, MSN

THEORY

I. Immune system is an interactive network that has four functions.
   A. Protection—it protects the body against infection.
   B. Surveillance—recognition and destruction of foreign substances by recognition of antigens on the cell surface.
   C. Homeostasis through destruction of abnormal and malignant cells and worn, damaged, or mutated cells.
   D. Regulation through augmentation and depression of immune responses.
II. Components of the immune system.
   A. Composed of organs, cells, and cytokines, protein messengers that cells secrete.
   B. White blood cells are responsible for the majority of immune system activities.
   C. Lymphoid organs act as nonspecific defenses and stimulate inflammation when invaded.
      1. Two primary organs include bone marrow, in which blood cells mature, and thymus, in which T cells mature.
      2. Secondary organs serve as storage, filters, and circulation routes for lymphocytes and may be the site of their activation and include:
         a. Lymph nodes, which are a type of sewage processing plant for the body. They drain and filter extracellular fluid and waste.
         b. Lymph vessels.
         c. The spleen, which removes aging or abnormally shaped blood cells from the circulation and stores and filters antigens and antibodies.
         d. The tonsils, which are lymphoid tissue.
   D. Cells of the immune system are created in the bone marrow.
      1. Blood cell development or hematopoiesis begins with a single cell, the pluripotent stem cell.
      2. The pluripotent stem cell divides to produce undifferentiated stem cells that are committed to one of two cell lineages or pathways:
         a. Myeloid stem cells, which mature into red blood cells, and platelets.
         b. Lymphoid stem cells, which mature into six types of white blood cells falling into two categories.
            (1) Granulocytes contain toxic granules in their cytoplasm used to digest cells that have been phagocytized.
               (a) Basophils, which represent 0.4% of the white blood cell population.

(b) Eosinophils, which represent 2.3% of the white blood cell population.

(c) Neutrophils, which represent 62% of the white blood cell population.

(2) Agranulocytes do not contain toxic granules and represent 35.3% of the white blood cell population.

(a) T lymphocytes—which mature in the thymus gland, thus the name T lymphocytes; constitute 70 to 80% of the lymphocyte population.

(b) B lymphocytes—first discovered in an anatomic location called the bursa of Fabricius in birds, thus the name B lymphocytes; constitute 5 to 15% of the lymphocyte population.

(c) Monocytes—which represent 5.3% of the white blood cell population and come in three types: mobile monocytes; mobile mature monocytes, called macrophages; and nonmobile mature monocytes, called tissue macrophages.

III. Functions of white blood cells.

A. White blood cells are the functional cells for inflammation and immunity.

B. Activities of each type of white blood cell are summarized in Table 20–1.

C. Generally, all white blood cells are capable of movement and recognition.

1. Movement.

a. White blood cells have the ability to move about the body, traveling into the bloodstream through lymphatic drainage.

b. White blood cells can move by diapedesis (or changing shape to move through a small space in a vessel or lymph channel wall) and out of the lymph system.

c. Circulating granulocytes live 4 to 8 hours in the blood. They are viable an additional 4 to 5 days when they inhabit the tissues.

d. In the circulation, white blood cells are like security guards, sensitive to foreign material and cells.

2. Recognition.

a. When the immune system is healthy, white blood cells act against proteins recognized as abnormal or foreign, including:

(1) Abnormal host cells.

(2) Infected host cells.

(3) Foreign cells.

(4) Pathogens.

IV. Responses of the immune system are categorized as innate or acquired. Both parts are interwoven and occur simultaneously.

A. Innate or natural or nonspecific immunity does not have the ability to target specific pathogens and includes:

1. Mechanical barriers—intact skin and mucous membranes, and cilia lining the respiratory tract.

2. Chemical barriers—saliva, sweat, gastric acid, and digestive enzymes.

3. Fever, which results from the hypothalamus being stimulated by interleukin-1 when it is released by activated macrophages, lymphocytes, neutrophils, and natural killer (NK) cells during the inflammatory response, infection, or other exposure to antigen.

4. Phagocytosis, which destroys the majority of bacteria, viruses, and other pathogens or foreign materials invading the body.

a. Performed by neutrophils and macrophages.

b. Involves the neutrophil or macrophage engulfing and destroying a foreign substance in the bloodstream, lymph system, or tissue.

c. Can begin as a result of chemotaxis. Chemotaxis occurs when tissue is

TABLE 20–1. **General Leukocyte Functions**

Leukocyte	Function
Basophils	Secretion of histamine, kinins, and heparin in areas of tissue injury or invasion Interacts with IgE for stimulation of degranulation in the presence of allergens
B lymphocyte	Sensitization to specific antigen Retention of sensitization Synthesis and secretion of antibodies directed against the specific antigen
Cytotoxic/cytolytic T lymphocyte	MHC-restricted recognition and destruction of nonself cells from other human beings or animals
Eosinophil	Limited phagocytic action during helminth infestations Secretes cytokines to limit inflammatory responses Elevated serum levels during and after allergic reaction
Helper/inducer T lymphocyte	Synthesis and secretion of a variety of immune-boosting cytokines
Macrophage	Recognition of nonself cells Antigen processing and antigen presentation Phagocytosis (specific and nonspecific) Promotion of T-cell activation
Monocyte	Maturation into macrophage Limited phagocytic activity
Mast cells	Located outside many of the capillaries in the body Secretion of mediators of inflammatory response within tissues
Natural killer cells	Recognition of nonself cells Destruction of unhealthy self cells Protection against cancer development
Neutrophils	Nonspecific phagocytosis
Suppressor T lymphocyte	Synthesis and secretion of a variety of immunosuppressive cytokines Modulates immune activity

Modified from Workman, M.L. (1995). Essential concepts of inflammation and immunity. *Crit Care Nurs Clin North Am* 7(4), 603.

invaded and becomes inflamed. Many different chemical and protein substances are produced in the area. These substances fall into three categories.

(1) Bacterial toxins released before and after phagocytosis.

(2) Particles of destroyed inflamed tissue.

(3) Complement (to be discussed later in this chapter).

5. The reticuloendothelial system (RES)—a system of phagocytes, named when it was believed that macrophages were derived from endothelial cells.

   a. Composed of:

      (1) Monocytes—circulating monocytes live 10 to 20 hours. A portion of monocytes mature into circulating macrophages.

      (2) Macrophages, the mature form of monocytes. A portion of monocytes travel to the tissues and mature into macrophages. Tissue or fixed macrophages survey the surrounding tissue for invaders.

b. Once an invading pathogen or other foreign substance is identified by the RES, it is phagocytized.
  (1) If an invading pathogen is not destroyed in the tissues, it can move into the lymph system and travel to a lymph node to be destroyed by a tissue macrophage there.
  (2) Tissue macrophages are present in various blood and lymph filtering sites in the body and at points where pathogens frequently enter the body. These sites are presented in Table 20–2.
6. Inflammation—foreign invaders not destroyed by phagocytosis can cause tissue injury. Trauma, chemicals, burns, and many other events can also cause tissue injury. When tissue injury occurs, specific chemicals and proteins are secreted in response. This process is called *inflammation.*
  a. The purpose of inflammation is to provide nonspecific defense against foreign invaders.
  b. Inflammation is a catalyst for destruction of invaders and repair of tissue.
    (1) Types of invaders that can stimulate inflammation include pathogens; allergens; another person's tissue (e.g., donated bone marrow, a kidney); and a man-made, foreign material (e.g., a Hickman catheter).
  c. Degree of inflammatory response is based on:
    (1) Degree of "foreignness" of the invader.
    (2) Intensity of exposure to foreign material.
    (3) Size and chemical makeup of the invader.
    (4) Complexity of the molecule: the more complex, the greater the immune response.
    (5) Severity of the invasion or injury.
    (6) Duration of exposure.
    (7) Size of exposure.
  d. Stages of inflammation.
    (1) Stage I—the vascular stage.
      (a) Nonmobile macrophages, which dwell in the tissue, immediately begin phagocytizing a foreign body after it has invaded the tissues.
      (b) Basophils, eosinophils, and mast cells at the site of inflammation release the following vasoactive amines from the cytoplasmic granules: histamine, bradykinin, prostaglandins, serotonin, leukotriene, and heparin.
      (c) Together, these vasoactive amines isolate the section of inflamed tissue to prevent any infection from spreading.

TABLE 20–2. **Locations of Specific Tissue Macrophages**

Macrophage	**Tissue Location**
Alveolar macrophages	Lung
Histiocytes	Skin and other connective tissues
Kupffer's cells	Liver
Mesangial cells	Kidney
Microglial cells	Central nervous system
Peritoneal macrophages	Peritoneal cavity
Synovial type-A cells	Joints

From Workman, M.L. (1995). Essential concepts of inflammation and immunity. *Crit Care Nurs Clin North Am 7*(4), 606.

      i. Heparin coagulates blood and body fluids in the area.

      ii. Histamine constricts small blood vessels, decreasing blood flow out of the area.

      iii. Bradykinins dilate arterioles and with serotonin increase capillary permeability, producing the leakage of plasma proteins into the extracellular space.

      iv. Prostaglandins respond to stimulation by tumor necrosis factor alpha (TNF-alpha) and interleukin-1 to produce fever.

      v. Amines activate macrophages, which then produce colony stimulating factors and TNF-alpha and interleukin-1, stimulating the brain to produce localized warmth at the site of invasion and fever, an inhospitable environment for bacterial growth.

      vi. These vasoactive amines dilate the capillaries in the area of inflammation, allowing neutrophils, chemotaxins, and colony stimulating factors to move through the blood vessel wall to the site of inflammation.

      vii. Because of these physiologic responses, the tissue becomes red, swollen, tender, and warm.

(2) Stage II—cellular exudate stage.

  (a) Large quantities of neutrophils move into the inflamed areas of tissue from the bloodstream.

  (b) The serum neutrophil count rises four- to five-fold to 10,000 to 25,000/mm^3.

  (c) The increased production of neutrophils by the bone marrow is stimulated by cytokines (IL-3, G-CSF, and GM-CSF) secreted by cells responding to invasion and participating in the process of inflammation.

  (d) As more fluid moves to the inflamed area, the host may experience a loss of function of that area (such as a finger) as it becomes more swollen and painful (due to pressure and injury).

(3) Stage III—regeneration and repair.

  (a) After neutrophils have begun to migrate to the site of inflammation, monocytes follow and increase at a slower pace because of the smaller number of monocytes present in the body.

  (b) Gradually, through increased production, the number of monocytes present at the site of inflammation becomes greater than the number of neutrophils. Monocytes process antigens they have phagocytized and present these antigens to other sections of the immune system involved in specific immunity.

(4) Stage IV—increased production of granulocytes and monocytes by the bone marrow.

B. Acquired or specific immunity.

  1. Begins with antigen that is phagocytized by a macrophage and is presented to B lymphocytes or T lymphocytes and T helper cells.

    a. Each antigen is unique because of its peculiar combination of proteins and polysaccharides.

    b. In order to be antigenic and recognized by a B or T lymphocyte as nonself, two characteristics must exist.

      (1) The antigen must be of high molecular weight.

      (2) On the surface of each antigen must be a pattern of recurring molecules called *epitopes.*

(a) Epitopes, which serve as identifiers, are formed by genes within the organism.

(b) The genes that pattern the epitope compose the major histocompatibility complex (MHC). In humans, the MHC is referred to as the human leukocyte antigen complex.

2. B cell or humoral immunity.

   a. B lymphocytes dwell in lymphoid tissue, waiting for macrophages to bring antigens to the as yet unused B lymphocyte for processing.

   b. Each B-cell lymphocyte develops to recognize only one type of antigen. This characteristic is called *specificity*. Once specificity develops, three processes occur in this particular B-cell line.

      (1) Specific B-cell lymphocytes are produced at a fast pace.

      (2) Some specified B-cell lymphocytes differentiate to become plasma cells. Each specialized plasma cell produces one specific antibody; these committed, highly differentiated cells are not phagocytic.

      (3) Some specialized B-cell lymphocytes become memory cells and exist in the body capable of recognizing a particular antigen at future exposures and producing plasma cells to generate abundant antibody specific to the antigen.

   c. Some of antibodies circulate in the bloodstream in addition to the site of invasion.

   d. Antibodies protect the body from invasion by direct action on invading substances and activation of complement.

      (1) Direct action on invaders can take place in three ways and is not usually strong enough to stop invasion of pathogens.

         (a) Lysis or rupture of the invading cell membrane.

         (b) Agglutination or clumping of large particles with antigens on the surfaces. This clump can become large enough to become insoluble and to precipitate.

         (c) Neutralization occurs when a cell is inactivated by antibodies covering the cell by adhering to antigens on its surface.

      (2) Complement is an interactive network of approximately 20 unique proteins present in plasma.

         (a) Complement proteins have the ability to leak out of the vascular spaces into tissue.

         (b) When an antibody adheres to an antigen, a portion of the antibody changes, making it possible for a preliminary complement protein to bind to the antibody.

         (c) Once the first complement protein (C1) binds to the antibody, a cascade of reactions, which create enzymes, takes place, resulting in five therapeutic effects.

            i. Phagocytosis is stimulated when one of the products of the complement cascade interacts with neutrophils and macrophages, enticing them to phagocytize antigen-antibody complexes. This process is called *opsonization.*

            ii. Another product of the complement cascade, the lytic complex, is able to rupture the cell membranes of foreign cells.

            iii. Complement products make the outer coatings of invading cells sticky, resulting in agglutination.

            iv. Complement products change the structures of some viruses, making them nonvirulent.

            v. Complement products encourage basophils and mast

cells to release histamines in the blood, which aids in the process of inflammation.

3. T-cell immunity or cell-mediated immunity is the second type of immune response.

   a. When antigens are exposed to antibodies in the bloodstream they are presented to T cells (or T lymphocytes) by macrophages.

   b. T lymphocytes specific to the antigen are produced and they are referred to as *activated T cells.*

   c. These activated T cells are released into lymphatic fluid from the bloodstream. Then they move back and forth from the lymphatic ducts to the blood vessels.

   d. T lymphocyte memory cells are also produced and are able to respond more quickly in producing more activated T lymphocytes when exposed to the same antigen in the future.

   e. Antigens can also attach to the membranes of T lymphocytes.

   f. There are three types of T lymphocytes that work within the immune system.

     (1) Helper T cells, the largest subgroup of T cells, regulate the majority of immune system functions, as described in Figure 20–1. They do this through the secretion of lymphokines, which:

       (a) Stimulate production and maturation of cytotoxic T cells.

       (b) Stimulate production and maturation of suppressor T cells.

       (c) Activate macrophages.

     (2) Cytotoxic T cells or natural killer cells (NK cells) are capable of directly attacking other cells and destroying them.

       (a) NK cells bind to the antigens on the surface of cells that they recognize. After binding to the cells, the NK cell secretes a substance called *perforins,* which creates a hole in the membrane of the cell.

       (b) The NK cell then releases cytotoxic substances into the cells, which results in swelling and then disintegration of the cell.

       (c) NK cells have the ability to destroy cancer cells and cells foreign to the body, such as transplanted cells, including donor bone marrow.

       (d) NK cells are able to recognize tumor cells not processed by phagocytes.

       (e) NK cells are also able to eliminate target cells through a process called antibody-dependent cell-mediated cytotoxicity.

         i. NK cells bind antibodies to their surfaces.

         ii. When the antibodies are attached, cytotoxic enzymes that destroy tumor cells are secreted.

         iii. This activity is important in preventing the growth and spread of tumors.

     (3) Suppressor T cells are able to turn off the functioning of both cytotoxic and helper T cells.

   g. T lymphocytes are also able to recognize and bind to antigen.

     (1) T lymphocytes cannot read epitopes until the molecule is phagocytized and digested and its antigens are linked with the MHC antigens on the surface of the natural killer T lymphocytes.

     (2) Some molecules resist digestion by phagocytes and therefore may never be read by T lymphocytes.

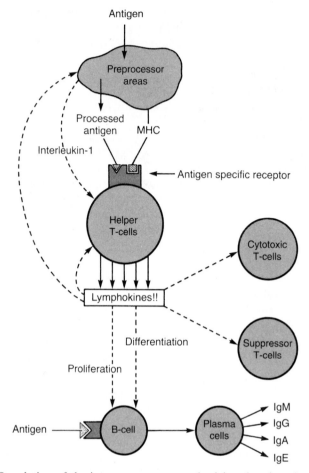

Figure 20–1. Regulation of the immune system, emphasizing the pivotal role of the helper T cells. (From Guyton, A.C. [1992]. *Human Physiology and Mechanisms of Disease* [5th ed.]. Philadelphia: W.B. Saunders Co., p. 266.)

      h. If T lymphocytes are reduced in number or are not functioning well, invading cells and proteins may never be recognized.

V. Communication methods used by the immune system.

  A. Cytokines are proteins produced by cells and secreted to communicate a message to another cell.

    1. Examples of cytokines.

      a. Interleukins.

      b. Lymphokines.

      c. Monokines.

      d. Interferons.

      e. Tumor necrosis factor, alpha and beta.

      f. Transforming growth factor.

    2. Cytokines have a short half-life.

    3. Cytokines can exert their effects even when present in very small quantities.

      a. They bind to receptors on cell membranes and exert their effects.

      b. They induce growth and differentiation of lymphocytes.

      c. They are the communication mechanism between the immune system and the neuroendocrine system.

        (1) For example, interleukin-1 induces fever by stimulating the temperature-regulating section of the hypothalamus.

VI. The immune system plays a role in preventing carcinogenesis.

    A. The immune system, specifically the T-cell lymphocytes, macrophages, and antibodies, are able to recognize and destroy abnormal cells that have the potential to become cancer cells.

      1. These abnormal cells are identified by T-cell recognition of the antigens on the cell's surface.

    B. Cells that are potentially cancerous develop in the body on a regular basis and should be eliminated before they develop into tumors.

    C. When a person is malnourished, elderly, chronically ill, immunosuppressed, or under significant stress, the immune system can fail to recognize and destroy abnormal cells and cancer can develop. However, not all persons fitting into one or more of these categories develop cancer.

BIBLIOGRAPHY

Gallucci, B., & McCarthy, D. (1995). The Immune System. In P. Trahan Reiger (ed.). *Biotherapy: A Comprehensive Nursing Overview*. Boston: Jones & Bartlett, pp. 15–42.

Guyton, A.C. (1992). *Human Physiology and Mechanisms of Disease* (5th ed.). Philadelphia: W.B. Saunders.

Kuby, J. (1992). *Immunology*. New York: W.H. Freeman and Company.

Pfeifer, K.A. (1994). Pathophysiology. In S.E. Otto (ed.). *Oncology Nursing* (2nd ed.). St. Louis: C.V. Mosby, pp. 3–19.

Sahai, J., & Louie, S.G. (1993, July). Overview of the immune and hematopoietic systems. *Am J Hosp Pharm 50*(7Suppl. 3), 4–9.

Workman, M.L. (1995). Essential concepts of inflammation and immunity. *Crit Care Nurs Clin North Am 7*(4), 601–615.

Wujcik, D. (1995). Hematopoietic growth factors. In P. Trahan Reiger (ed.). *Biotherapy: A Comprehensive Nursing Overview*. Boston: Jones & Bartlett, pp. 113–133.

21

Genetics

Kathleen A. Calzone, RN, MSN

Theory

I. Organization and function of genetic material.
   A. Chromosomes are threadlike structures that contain genetic information.
      1. There are 46 chromosomes in the human body, which are made up of 23 chromosome pairs, one copy from each parent.
   B. Genes are individual units of hereditary information, which are located at a specific position on the chromosome.
      1. Genes consist of a sequence of deoxyribonucleic acid (DNA) that codes for a specific protein.
      2. Genes consist primarily of exons and introns.
         a. *Exons* are protein-coding segments of a gene.
         b. *Introns* are nonprotein-coding segments of a gene.
   C. Nucleic acids consist of bases and a sugar and phosphate group. There are two types of nucleic acids.
      1. DNA comprises two nucleotide chains, running in opposite directions, that are held together by hydrogen bonds, which are coiled around one another to form a double helix.
         a. In DNA there are two types of bases, purines and pyrimidines.
            (1) Two types of purines, adenine (A) and guanine (G).
            (2) Two types of pyrimidines, thymine (T) and cytosine (C).
         b. DNA base pairs are complementary, A attaches to T, and G attaches to C.
      2. RNA (ribonucleic acid) consists of a single nucleotide chain that represents a complementary copy of a strand of DNA.
         a. In RNA the bases are the same as DNA except that the base uracil (U) replaces thymine (T).
         b. *Transcription* refers to the process of making RNA from DNA.
         c. *Translation* refers to the process of making proteins from RNA.
         d. *Proteins* consist of chains of amino acids. Sequence of the amino acids determines the function of the protein.
         e. Three primary types of RNA.
            (1) Messenger RNA (mRNA) contains information about the order of the amino acids in a protein.
            (2) Transfer RNA (tRNA) brings the amino acids to the site of protein synthesis.
            (3) Ribosomal RNA (rRNA) provides the structural support for the protein in addition to other functions.

II. Basic mechanisms of carcinogenesis, mutations, and heredity.
  A. Cancer has a multifactorial etiology with several genetic, environmental, and personal factors interacting to produce a malignancy.
  B. Genetic alterations are at the very core of cancer development, although most cancer is not the result of an inherited germline alteration.
    1. Most cancer is associated with genetic alterations that occur in single cells sometime during the life of an individual.
    2. A malignant tumor arises after a series of genetic mutations have accumulated.
  C. Genetic alterations that are acquired are associated with exogenous or indigenous factors. For example, carcinogens are thought to operate by causing genetic alterations.
  D. A malignant tumor is derived from a series of genetic alterations in genes that control cell growth and proliferation.
    1. Types of regulatory genes
      a. Proto-oncogenes are essential for normal cell growth and regulation. Alterations occurring in proto-oncogenes result in oncogene activation, which can result in uncontrolled cell growth.
      b. Tumor suppressor genes function as regulators of cell growth. Some tumor suppressor genes appear to play a role in cell cycle regulation, whereas others have a role in DNA repair.
        (1) Many genes responsible for familial cancer syndromes appear to be tumor suppressor genes.
      c. Mismatch repair genes correct DNA replication errors.
      d. Apoptosis genes activate a program that leads to cell death.
      e. Telomerase genes have a role in cellular aging through the telomeres, which are the ends of the chromosome.
        (1) As cells age, telomerase is normally repressed and the telomeres are progressively lost.
        (2) In cancer, telomerase is reactivated, which keeps the telomeres intact and increases the likelihood of cancer by facilitating cell immortalization.
    2. *Knudson "two hit" hypothesis* refers to the inactivation of both copies of a given regulatory gene. Because all individuals are born with two copies of almost every gene, both functioning copies of the gene must be inactivated for cancer to occur.
    3. Mutations are variations in the sequence of DNA.
      a. Categories of mutations.
        (1) Genetic alterations are usually acquired; however, in someone with a genetic predisposition to cancer a mutation has been inherited in the germline.
          (a) *Somatic* refers to acquired genetic alterations.
          (b) *Germline* refers to inherited genetic alterations.
      b. Types of mutations.
        (1) Pathologic.
          (a) Missense mutations are single-base pair changes that result in the substitution of one amino acid for another in the protein being constructed. If the substituted amino acid is critical to the function of the protein, carriers are at high risk for developing disease.
          (b) RNA-negative mutations result in the absence of RNA transcribed from a gene copy.

(c) Nonsense mutations change an amino acid signal into a signal to stop adding amino acids to a growing protein. Nonsense mutations result in a truncated, presumably nonfunctional protein.

(d) Frameshift mutations occur when one or more bases are added to the normal sequence. Usually, frameshift mutations result in the generation of a stop signal not far from the region of the mutation, resulting in a shortened form of the protein.

(e) Splicing mutations occur when DNA that should be removed from the coding sequence is retained, or DNA that should not be added is spliced in, resulting in frameshift mutations.

(2) Nonpathologic.

(a) Polymorphisms are changes in the DNA sequence of a gene that are not disease related and that occur at variable frequency in the general population.

E. Mendelian inheritance.

1. Dominant inheritance requires only one altered copy of a gene to result in cancer susceptibility (Fig. 21–1).

2. Recessive inheritance requires two altered copies of a gene, one from each parent, to result in cancer susceptibility (Fig. 21–2).

III. Key technical characteristics of predisposition genetic testing.

A. Techniques for identifying mutations.

1. Single strand confirmation polymorphism analysis (SSCP).

a. A sequence change into DNA alters the size and/or shape of a DNA fragment, which can be detected by SSCP on a gel.

b. An altered gene produces a band that is different than a normal gene.

c. SSCP easily detects insertions or deletions of four or more bases of DNA; however, mutations that change one base for another without altering the length of the DNA fragment are difficult to detect.

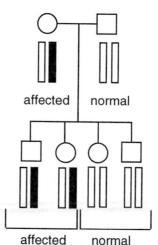

affected   normal

affected   normal

Figure 21–1. Autosomal dominant inheritance.

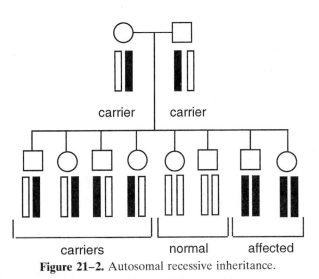

Figure 21–2. Autosomal recessive inheritance.

2. Heteroduplex analysis adds some sensitivity to SSCP by increasing the likelihood of seeing changes on a gel.
3. *Protein truncation assay* refers to an analysis of coding DNA, which is directly translated in the laboratory into protein.
   a. Shortened proteins can then be detected on a gel, based on the mobility differences between larger and smaller proteins.
   b. Protein truncation assay is sensitive for the detection of alterations in which the sequence change results in a shortened form of the protein but does not detect other types of alterations.
4. Direct sequencing determines the sequence of both copies of the gene being tested and detects all sequence changes in the regions being analyzed.
   a. Direct sequencing detects all sequence changes in the regions being analyzed but misses alterations that are outside the coding region and results in absence of RNA transcribed from a gene.
B. Considerations in genetic testing laboratory selection.
   1. Laboratories where genetic testing is performed should meet the following criteria:
      a. Clinical Laboratory Improvement Act (CLIA)–approved laboratory.
      b. Laboratory Director certified by the American Board of Medical Genetics.
IV. Common hereditary cancer syndromes and cancer susceptibility genes.
   A. The common hereditary cancer syndromes, clinical manifestations, inheritance patterns, and genes are outlined in Table 21–1.
   B. Indications for cancer predisposition testing.
      1. Criteria for predisposition genetic testing vary, depending upon the gene tested.
         a. The universal criteria for predisposition genetic testing include:
            (1) Confirmed family history consistent with the hereditary cancer syndrome.
            (2) Informed consent by the client to be tested.
            (3) A test that can be interpreted once performed.

TABLE 21–1. **Common Hereditary Cancer Syndromes and Cancer Susceptibility Genes**

Syndrome	Clinical Manifestations	Gene	Mode of Inheritance
Ataxia telangiectasia	Cerebral ataxia, oculocutaneous telangiectasias, radiation hypersensitivity, leukemia, lymphoma, breast cancer, and other solid tumors	ATM	Autosomal recessive
Beckwith-Wiedemann syndrome	Wilms' tumor, adrenal carcinomas, hepatoblastomas	Linked to 11p15	Autosomal dominant
Breast/ovarian cancer syndrome	Breast cancer, ovarian cancer, prostate cancer, colon cancer	BRCA1	Autosomal dominant
Breast/ovarian cancer syndrome	Breast cancer (male and female), ovarian cancer, prostate, pancreatic	BRCA2	Autosomal dominant
Cowden disease	Multiple mucocutaneous lesions, vitiligo, angiomas, benign proliferative disease of multiple organ systems, breast cancer, thyroid cancer, colonic neoplasms	CD1	Autosomal dominant
Familial adenomatous polyposis (Gardner syndrome)	Colon polyposis (adenomas), desmoid tumors, osteomas, thyroid cancer, hepatoblastoma	APC	Autosomal dominant
Fanconi anemia	Leukemia, esophageal cancer, hepatoma	FAC FAA	Autosomal recessive
Gorlin syndrome	Basal cell carcinoma, brain tumors, ovarian cancer	PTCH	Autosomal dominant
Hereditary nonpolyposis colorectal cancer (Lynch syndrome)	GI cancers, cancer of endometrium, ovary, ureter	MSH2 MLH1 PMS1 PMS2	Autosomal dominant
Li-Fraumeni syndrome	Breast cancer, sarcoma, brain tumors, leukemia, adrenocortical carcinoma	p53	Autosomal dominant
Melanoma	Melanoma	p16, CDK4	Autosomal dominant
Muir-Torre syndrome	GI and GU cancers, skin, breast cancer, benign breast tumors	MSH2 MLH1	Autosomal dominant
Multiple endocrine neoplasm type I	Pancreatic cancer, pituitary adenomas	Linked to chromosome 11q	Autosomal dominant
Multiple endocrine neoplasm type II	Thyroid cancer, pheochromocytoma	RET	Autosomal dominant
Neurofibromatosis	Neurofibromatosis, pheochromocytomas, optic gliomas	NF1	Autosomal dominant
Prostate cancer	Prostate	Linked to chromosome 1q	Autosomal dominant
Retinoblastoma	Retinoblastoma, osteosarcoma	RB1	Autosomal dominant
von Hippel-Lindau	Hemangioblastoma, renal cell cancer, pheochromocytomas	VHL	Autosomal dominant

TABLE 21–1. **Common Hereditary Cancer Syndromes and Cancer Susceptibility Genes** (*Continued*)

Syndrome	Clinical Manifestations	Gene	Mode of Inheritance
Wilms' tumor	Wilms' tumor	WT1	Autosomal dominant
Xeroderma pigmentosum	Skin cancer, melanoma, leukemia	RAD2	Autosomal recessive

2. Not every client is appropriate for predisposition genetic testing for inherited cancer susceptibility.

C. Outcomes for cancer predisposition testing.

1. Predictive value of a negative test result varies depending upon whether there is a known genetic alteration in the family.

   a. A negative test result in the presence of a known genetic alteration indicates that the client is within the general population risk of cancer associated with that branch of the family.

      (1) However, family history from the other parent still influences the risk of developing cancer.

   b. A negative result with no known family genetic alteration can occur because of one of the following:

      (1) Identifying an alteration in a cancer susceptibility gene may not be possible due to the limited sensitivity of the techniques used.

      (2) The function of the gene can be affected by an alteration in a different gene.

      (3) The cancer in the family may be associated with a cancer susceptibility gene other than the one tested.

      (4) The cancer in the family is not the result of a germline genetic alteration.

2. Predictive value of a positive test result varies depending upon the type of genetic alteration identified and the degree of certainty that the function of the gene has been affected.

   a. *Penetrance* refers to the cancer risks associated with the specific genetic alteration. Penetrance may be different for different genetic alterations in the same cancer susceptibility gene.

V. Potential therapeutic interventions.

A. Somatic gene therapy.

1. Introduction of a functioning gene into the somatic cells to replace missing or defective genes or to provide a new cellular function.

2. Investigational trials using somatic gene therapy for a variety of cancers are ongoing.

B. Germline gene therapy.

1. Introduction of a functioning gene into the egg or sperm to prevent transmission of a genetic alteration.

2. Germline gene therapy is not available. Germline gene therapy raises several ethical, legal, and social concerns.

VI. Medical management issues associated with the care of individuals harboring a cancer susceptibility gene.

A. The management of cancer risk falls into four basic categories.

1. Surveillance, which is monitoring to detect cancer as early as possible, when the chances for cure are greatest.

2. Prophylactic surgery is the removal of as much of the tissue at risk as possible to reduce the risk of developing a cancer.

    3. Chemoprevention involves taking a medicine, vitamin, or other substance to reduce the risk of cancer.
    4. Risk avoidance is the avoidance of exposures that may increase the risk of certain cancers. The extent to which this strategy is successful is unknown.
  B. Insufficient data exist regarding the benefits and limitations of all cancer risk management strategies in individuals at high risk for cancer because of an alteration in a cancer susceptibility gene.
VII. Ethical, legal, and social issues involved in predisposition testing for inherited cancer susceptibility.
  A. Predisposition genetic testing can have profound psychological consequences.
    1. Survivor guilt is often observed in clients who have not inherited the genetic alteration that is present in other close family members.
    2. Transmitter guilt is often observed when a family members passes on the genetic alteration to one of their offspring.
    3. Heightened anxiety can result when clients learn that they are at a substantially increased risk for developing cancer or another primary lesion.
    4. Depression and anger can occur regardless of genetic status.
    5. Personal identity issues result because genetic information involves the very essence of who and what we are as individuals.
    6. Regret of previous decisions can occur in clients who have made major decisions based upon their perceived cancer risk and testing results are inconsistent with what they had previously thought.
    7. Uncertainty occurs because predisposition genetic testing does not provide information about if or when cancer develops. In many instances there is no proven prevention strategy.
    8. Intrafamilial issues arise because predisposition genetic testing affects all family members. These issues include but are not limited to:
      a. Coercion regarding testing, disclosure of testing results, and cancer risk management approaches.
      b. Role alterations for spouses, because they are not at risk physically by the genetic information.
    9. Stigmatization can occur both within the family and within the individual's social network.
  B. Predisposition genetic testing also has social implications.
    1. Financial considerations.
      a. Predisposition genetic testing is very expensive. Little information is available about the likelihood that insurers will cover testing and counseling while not using the results against the client.
      b. Insurers may be reluctant to cover enhanced surveillance programs that have no proven efficacy.
      c. Insurers may not be willing to cover the expense of prophylactic surgery that has no proven benefit.
    2. Availability and quality assurance of laboratory testing is not certain because there is no regulation beyond CLIA approval for molecular laboratories performing testing.
    3. Availability and quality assurance of genetic counseling are of concern given the small number of trained providers in cancer genetics.
  C. Legal issues for the client undergoing testing.
    1. Insurance discrimination can occur for those harboring an altered cancer susceptibility gene because they may be considered as having a preexisting condition or may be too high a risk to insure.
      a. Health insurance.
      b. Life insurance.
      c. Disability insurance.

2. State and federal legislative approaches have already been proposed or enacted, depending upon the issue and state.

3. Self-insured employers are exempt from state laws and regulations on health insurance because of the Employee Retirement Income Security Act of 1974 (ERISA), which governs employer pension plans as well as other benefits.

4. Individuals may face discrimination from employers.

   a. In March 1995, the United States Equal Employment Opportunity Commission released guidelines on the definition of "disability" under the Americans with Disabilities Act (ADA), which is now extended to include discrimination based on genetic information. This set of guidelines is not law, but simply is an interpretation of the language of the ADA and may be overturned in a court of law.

5. Risk of discrimination can also occur with education and housing.

D. Genetic technology raises legal liability issues for the health care provider.

   1. Privacy and confidentiality.

      a. Clinical genetic testing results are placed in the medical record, although such placement may place the client at risk for insurance discrimination.

   2. All health care providers have a duty to uphold the standard of care in cancer genetics.

      a. Disclose benefits and risks of predisposition genetic testing (informed consent).

      b. Keep genetic information confidential unless given permission.

         (1) Health care providers may have a duty to inform clients regarding their potential for increased cancer risk due to an inherited susceptibility and the availability of predisposition genetic testing.

VIII. Key issues required for informed consent.

A. Components associated with informed consent for predisposition genetic testing.

   1. Purpose of the genetic test.

   2. Motivation for testing.

   3. Risks of genetic testing.

      a. Psychological distress.

      b. Discrimination.

      c. Social issues.

   4. Benefits of genetic testing.

      a. Enhanced cancer risk management.

      b. Reproductive decision-making.

      c. Relief of uncertainty.

   5. Limitations of genetic testing.

   6. Inheritance pattern of the gene being tested.

      a. Risk of misidentified paternity.

   7. Accuracy and sensitivity of genetic testing method.

   8. Outcomes of genetic testing.

      a. Predictive value of a negative test result.

      b. Predictive value of a positive test result.

   9. Confidentiality of genetic testing results.

   10. Possibility of discrimination.

   11. Alternatives for cancer risk assessment besides genetic testing.

   12. Cancer risk management strategies if the client is found to have an alteration in a cancer susceptibility gene.

      a. Efficacy of surveillance strategies.

      b. Efficacy of prevention strategies.

13. Cost of testing.
    a. Professional genetic counseling fees.
    b. Genetic testing fees.
    c. Potential of insurance reimbursement for counseling and testing fees.
14. Right to refuse.
15. Testing in children.

Assessment

I. Assessment of a client with a family history of cancer.
    A. Pedigree refers to the development of a family tree (Fig. 21–3).
        1. Components of a pedigree.
            a. Bilineal three-generation family history.
            b. Cancer history of each family member including:
                (1) Primary site.
                (2) Age at diagnosis.
                (3) Laterality in paired organs such as breasts, eyes.
            c. Previous prophylactic surgery to reduce cancer risk.

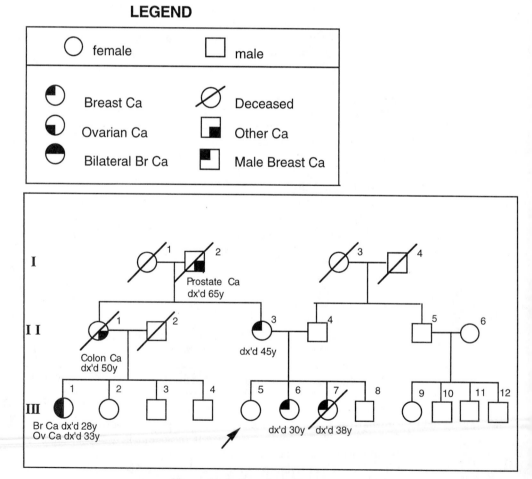

Figure 21–3. Sample pedigree.

      d. Other health problems.
      e. Racial and ethnic background.
      f. Consanguinity.
      g. Pregnancy loss.
      h. Birth defects.
      i. Early infant death.
      j. Environmental and occupational exposures.
   2. Confirmation of the family history.
      a. Documentation is essential for all reported cancers by pathology records or the equivalent because there is often confusion in a family about the primary site and age at diagnosis of cancer.
B. Personal health history.
   1. Complete review of systems.
   2. Cancer history.
   3. Risk factor history including exposures to environmental or occupational carcinogens.
   4. Current surveillance plan.
C. Psychosocial history.
   1. Perception of cancer risk.
   2. Beliefs about etiology of cancer in the family.
   3. Prior mental illness.
   4. Current support mechanisms.
   5. Previous patterns of stress management.
   6. Motivation for cancer risk assessment and/or predisposition genetic testing.
   7. Insurance and employment status.

Nursing Diagnoses

  I. Knowledge deficit of cancer genetics and predisposition genetic testing.
 II. Altered health maintenance.
III. Ineffective individual coping.
IV. Altered family processes.

Outcome Identification

    I. Client and/or family, consistent with cultural, educational, and emotional status, describe the:
    A. Genetic pattern of cancer.
    B. Risks and benefits of predisposition genetic testing.
    C. Alternatives for cancer risk management.
   II. Client identifies factors that may decrease or increase cancer risk.
 III. Client describes cancer warning signals and the cancer risk management alternatives.
 IV. Client describes health promotion activities.
  V. Client identifies the agencies in which cancer risk management services can be obtained.
 VI. Client describes and demonstrates self-examination procedures.
VII. Client and/or family, consistent with cultural, physical, and psychosocial domain:
    A. Identify personal and community resources that enhance coping.
    B. Use identified coping strategies that lead to effective outcomes.
    C. Participate in care and decision-making.

   D. Identify alternatives for coping when existing strategies are ineffective.
   E. Establish contact with a member of the health care team as needed.
   F. Communicate feelings about inherited cancer susceptibility.
IV. Family and the significant other, consistent with the cultural, physical, and psychosocial domain:
   A. Identify personal and community resources that enhance coping.
   B. Use identified coping strategies that lead to effective outcomes.
   C. Participate in care and decision-making.
   D. Identify alternatives for coping when existing strategies are ineffective.
   E. Establish contact with a member of the health care team as needed.
   F. Communicate feelings about inherited cancer susceptibility.

Planning and Implementation

I. Interventions to assist the client and family to understand cancer genetics and predisposition genetic testing.
   A. Describe the organization and function of genetic material and the role of genetics in carcinogenesis.
   B. Assess the client's beliefs about the etiology of cancer in the family and correct misconceptions.
   C. Describe the process for cancer risk evaluation and predisposition genetic testing.
   D. Discuss the risks and benefits of predisposition genetic testing.
II. Interventions to decrease perceived and definite barriers to cancer risk management.
   A. Educate and monitor the performance of self-examination techniques.
   B. Provide education on the benefits of cancer risk management.
   C. Facilitate the reimbursement for cancer risk management procedures.
   D. Encourage communication regarding fears and concerns.
III. Interventions to enhance coping and adaptation.
   A. Refer the client and/or family to community support services.
   B. Refer the client and/or family to professional counseling services when indicated.
   C. Encourage the use of coping strategies that have previously been effective.

Evaluation

   The oncology nurse systematically and regularly evaluates the client's and/or family's responses to interventions to determine progress toward the achievement of expected outcomes. Relevant data are collected and actual findings are compared with expected findings. Nursing diagnoses, outcomes, and plans of care are reviewed and revised as necessary.

BIBLIOGRAPHY

American Society of Clinical Oncology. (1996). Genetic testing for cancer susceptibility. *J Clin Oncol* *14*, 1730–1736.
American Society of Human Genetics. (1996). Statement on informed consent for genetic research. *Am J Hum Genet 59*, 471–474.
Andrews, L., Fullerton, J.E., Holtzman, N.A., Motulsky, A.G. (eds.). (1994). *Assessing Genetic Risks: Implications for Health and Social Policy* (Institute of Medicine Executive Summary). Washington D.C.: National Academy Press.
Carroll-Johnson, R. (ed.). (1995). The genetic revolution: Promise and predicament for oncology nurses. *Oncol Nurs Forum 22*(suppl. 2), 3–39.

Collins, F.S., & Galas, D. (1993). A new five-year plan for the U.S. human genome project. *Science 262*, 43–46.

Geller, G., Botkin, J.R., Green, M.J., et al. (1977). Genetic testing for susceptibility to adult onset cancer: The process and content of informed consent. *JAMA 277*, 1467–1474.

Hoffman, D.E., & Wulfsberg, E.A. (1995). Testing children for genetic predispositions: Is it in their best interest? *J Law, Med Ethics 23*, 331–344.

Holtzman, N. (1992). The diffusion of new genetic tests for predicting disease. *FASEB J 6*, 2806–2812.

Hudson, K.L., Rothenburg, K.H., Andrews, L.B., et al. (1995). Genetic discrimination and health insurance: An urgent need for reform. *Science 270*, 391–393.

International Society of Nurses in Genetics (ISONG). (1996). Statement of genetics clinical nursing practice.

Knudson, A.G. (1993). All in the (cancer) family. *Nat Genet 5*, 103–104.

Lessick, M., & Williams, J. (1994). The Human Genome Project: Implications for nursing. *Med Surg Nurs 3*, 49–58.

National Advisory Council for Human Genome Research. (1994). Statement on the use of DNA testing for presymptomatic identification of cancer risk. *JAMA 271*, 785.

NIH-DOE Working Group on Ethical, Legal and Social Implications of Human Genome Research. (1993). *Genetic Information and Health Insurance: Report on the Task Force on Genetic Information and Insurance*. NIH Publication No. 93–3686. Bethesda, MD.

Rothenberg, K.H. (1995). Genetic information and health insurance: State legislative approaches. *J Law Med and Ethics 23*, 312–319.

Scanlon, C., & Fibison, W. (1995). *Managing Genetic Information: Implications for Nursing Education*. Washington, D.C.: American Nurses' Association.

Schnieder, K.A. (1994). *Counseling about Cancer: Strategies for Genetic Counselors*. Dennisport: Massachusetts Graphic Illusions.

Strauss-Tranin, A. (ed.). (1997). Genetics and cancer. *Sem Oncol Nurs 12*, 67–144.

U.S. Equal Employment Opportunity Commission. (1995). Compliance Manual Section 902: *Definition of the Term "Disability."* Washington, D.C.

Weber, B.L. (1996). Genetic testing for breast cancer. *Sci Med 3*, 12–21.

Weinberg, R.A. (1994). Oncogenes and tumor suppressor genes. *CA Cancer J Clin 44*, 160–170.

Nursing Care of the Client With Breast Cancer

Marge Bernice, RN, MS, OCN
Nina Entrekin, RN, MN, OCN

Theory

I. Physiology and pathophysiology associated with breast cancer.
   A. Anatomy of the breast (Fig. 22–1).
      1. Adult female breast lies on the anterior chest wall between the sternum and midaxillary line from the second to sixth ribs.
      2. The breast parenchyma is divided into 15 to 20 lobes.
      3. Each lobe contains 20 to 40 lobules and is connected by duct to the nipple surface.
      4. The breast's most biologically active component is the terminal ductal-lobular unit (TDLU).
      5. The stroma and subcutaneous tissue of the breast are comprised of connective tissue, nerves, blood vessels, lymphatic vessels, and fat.
      6. Lymphatic fluid flows outward toward the lymph nodes with the majority flowing to the axillary nodes (Fig. 22–2).
   B. Histopathology.
      1. Noninvasive breast cancers.
         a. Also called in-situ cancer or "precancer."
         b. Confined to the duct or lobule.
         c. Not capable of spreading to other parts of body.
         d. Ductal carcinoma in situ (DCIS).
            (1) Also referred to as intraductal.
            (2) Usually is not palpable and is detected only by mammogram or as an incidental finding in biopsy of another lesion.
            (3) Comedo subtype is more prone to recurrence and evolution to invasive carcinoma.
         e. Lobular carcinoma in situ (LCIS).
            (1) Also called lobular neoplasia.
            (2) Considered a marker for increased risk of invasive breast cancer in either breast rather than a premalignant lesion.
            (3) No distinguishing characteristics, usually an incidental finding in biopsy, not detected by mammogram or clinical examination.
      2. Invasive breast cancers.
         a. Also referred to as infiltrating.
         b. No longer completely contained within the duct or lobule and has grown into surrounding tissue.

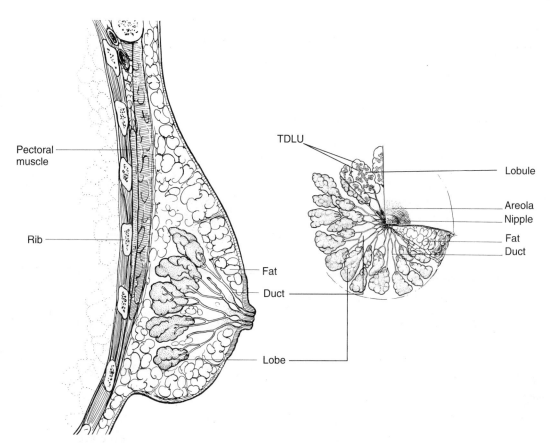

Figure 22–1. Anatomy of the breast (TDLU = terminal ductal-lobular unit). (Redrawn from National Cancer Institute. [1984]. *The Breast Cancer Digest:* A Guide to Medical Care, Emotional Support, Educational Programs, and Resources [2nd ed.]. NIH Pub. No. 84–1691. Bethesda, MD: p. 5.)

    c. Capable of spreading to other parts of the body.
    d. Invasive ductal carcinoma.
        (1) Most common type, accounts for approximately 70% of all breast cancers.
        (2) May be mixed with other types.
    e. Invasive lobular carcinoma.
        (1) Accounts for approximately 10% of all breast cancers.
        (2) Commonly multicentric.
    f. Other types.
        (1) Include tubular, papillary, mucinous, medullary.
        (2) Occur less frequently, typically have more favorable prognosis.
    g. Special manifestations.
        (1) Inflammatory.
            (a) Usually presents with inflammation, erythema, pain, induration, skin thickening, and edema due to invasion of dermal lymphatics.
            (b) Breast changes are dramatic and diffuse; often there is no dominant mass.

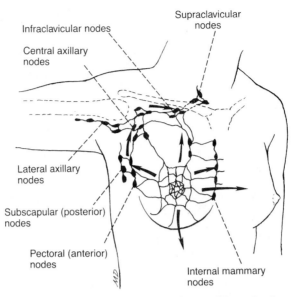

Figure 22–2. Routes of lymphatic drainage from the breast. (From Luckman, J. & Sorenson, K.C. [1987]. *Medical-Surgical Nursing: A Psychophysiologic Approach* [3rd ed]. Philadelphia: W.B. Saunders, p. 1809.)

      (2) Paget's disease.
          (a) Eczematoid lesion of nipple areolar complex.
          (b) Usually associated with another cancer in the breast.
  3. Hormone receptors.
    a. Estrogen receptor (ER) and progesterone receptor (PR) assays are routinely done on the primary tumor specimen.
    b. Determines whether tumor is sensitive to hormones; information helps guide decisions regarding systemic treatment.
    c. In general, receptor-negative tumors have a slightly worse prognosis and rarely respond to hormone treatments.
  4. Prognostic factors.
    a. Tumor size—larger tumors are associated with a poorer prognosis.
    b. Nuclear grade—high-grade, poorly differentiated tumors have a worse prognosis.
    c. Lymph node involvement—increased number of positive lymph nodes is associated with a worse outcome.
    d. Hormone receptor status—ER- and PR-negative tumors are associated with a less favorable prognosis.
    e. Histologic type—inflammatory breast cancer carries the least favorable prognosis; noninvasive cancers have an excellent prognosis.
    f. Proliferative indices—tumors with abnormal complement of deoxyribonucleic acid (DNA) (aneuploid) and/or high S-phase fraction (SPF) (large proportion of rapidly multiplying cells) are associated with a worse prognosis.
    g. Other factors under investigation include oncogenes (e.g., HER-2/neu, c-erb-B-2), tumor suppressor genes, epidermal growth factor (EGF), cathepsin D, heat shock protein, nm23, p53.

C. Metastatic patterns.
   1. Regional spread.
      a. Axillary nodes.
         (1) Receive most of lymph leaving the breast.
         (2) Test positive at diagnosis in approximately 45% of clients.
         (3) Likelihood of involvement increases with primary tumor size.
      b. Internal mammary nodes.
         (1) Test positive at diagnosis in approximately 22% of clients.
         (2) Likelihood of involvement increases with inner quadrant or central primary tumors.
   2. Distant spread.
      a. Metastases may occur via hematogenous or lymphatic pathways.
      b. Most common sites of metastasis are bone, lung, liver, brain.
D. Epidemiology.
   1. Most common cancer in women.
   2. Accounts for 31% of all cancer in women.
   3. Accounts for 17% of all cancer deaths in women.
   4. Incidence rates have increased approximately 1% per year over the past 50 years.
   5. Increase in incidence is largely, but not fully, attributable to increase in screening/early detection.
   6. Death rate essentially stable since 1930 despite increasing incidence due to modest improvement in 5-year survival rates.

II. Principles of medical management.
   A. Screening and diagnostic procedures.
      1. Screening procedures (Table 22–1).
         a. Breast self examination (BSE)—recommended monthly for all women over 20 years of age.
         b. Clinical breast examination (CBE).
         c. Mammography.
            (1) 30% reduction in breast cancer mortality in women over 50 years of age receiving regular screening; 17% reduction in mortality in women in their 40s who receive regular screening.
            (2) American Cancer Society (ACS) recommends annual mammograms for women age 40 and over. The National Cancer Institute (NCI) recommends screening every one to two years for women age 40 and over.
            (3) Federal law (Mammography Quality Standards Act) requires that all mammography facilities be certified.

TABLE 22–1. **American Cancer Society Recommendations for Breast Cancer Screening**

Age Group	Examination	Frequency
20–39	Breast self-examination	Monthly
	Clinical breast examination	Every 3 years
40 and older	Breast self-examination	Monthly
	Clinical breast examination	Annually
	Mammography	Annually

    d. Mammography, BSE, and CBE are complementary screening modalities to be used in combination rather than singly.
2. Adjunctive imaging procedures.
    a. Ultrasonography.
        (1) Uses high-frequency sound waves to create an image.
        (2) Distinguishes cystic from solid masses.
    b. Galactography.
        (1) Injection of contrast medium into the duct.
        (2) Useful in delineating the anatomy of the affected duct in cases of a spontaneous single-duct nipple discharge.
3. Investigational imaging methods.
    a. Magnetic resonance imaging (MRI).
        (1) Uses magnetic field to create an image.
        (2) Useful in women with silicone breast implants.
    b. Digital mammography.
        (1) Achieves higher resolution by computerizing, enhancing, and recreating image.
    c. Computer-aided diagnosis (CAD).
        (1) Computerized analysis of mammogram used by the radiologist as a "second opinion."
        (2) May improve sensitivity and specificity of mammogram analysis.
    d. Positron emission tomography (PET).
        (1) Measures glucose utilization by tissue.
        (2) May be useful in distinguishing benign from malignant masses, assessing tumor response to treatment, and evaluating axillary lymph nodes.
    e. Scintimammography.
        (1) Nuclear medicine imaging using Technetium-99m sestamibi as a radiolabeled tracer.
        (2) May be useful in differentiating low- and high-risk lesions.
4. Biopsy procedures (Table 22–2).
    a. Pathologic evaluation is required to make the diagnosis of breast cancer.
    b. Considerations for method of biopsy include size and location of lesion, likelihood of malignancy, potential for follow-up, cost, and client preference.
    c. Two-step approach separates biopsy from definitive surgery and is preferred because it allows the client an opportunity to explore treatment alternatives after the diagnosis of cancer is made.
    d. Fine needle aspiration—thin needle (21–27 gauge) is inserted into the

TABLE 22–2. **Breast Biopsy Techniques**

Type of Biopsy	Method of Analysis	Palpable Lesion	Nonpalpable Lesion
Needle	Cytology	Fine-needle aspiration (FNA)	Stereotactic FNA
	Histology	Core biopsy	Stereotactic core biopsy (SCB)
Open	Histology	Incisional/excisional biopsy	Needle localization breast biopsy (NLBB)

mass, material is aspirated by negative pressure and is smeared on a slide for cytologic analysis.

    e. Needle core biopsy—needle with large lumen (usually 14 gauge) is used to remove a core of tissue for histologic analysis.

    f. Incisional biopsy—surgical removal of a portion of tumor through skin incision.

    g. Excisional biopsy—surgical removal of entire tumor, generally with margin of normal tissue, through a skin incision.

    h. Nonpalpable lesions must be localized under ultrasound or mammographic guidance before biopsy.

    i. Stereotactic localization involves use of specially designed computerized mammography equipment to calculate the location of a nonpalpable abnormality for needle aspiration or biopsy.

    j. Needle localization can be performed by a radiologist to locate and mark a nonpalpable abnormality for the surgeon before open biopsy.

B. Staging methods and procedures.

  1. Staging workup may include:

    a. Chest radiograph.

    b. Liver scan.

    c. Bone scan.

  2. Staging classification.

    a. Stage 0—carcinoma in situ.

    b. Stage I—tumor diameter under 1 cm with negative nodes.

    c. Stage II—tumor diameter under 2 cm with positive axillary nodes, 2 to 5 cm with negative or positive axillary nodes, or over 5 cm with negative nodes.

    d. Stage III—tumor diameter over 5 cm with positive nodes, tumor of any size with direct extension to chest wall or skin, positive internal mammary nodes, or axillary lymph nodes that are fixed.

    e. Stage IV—any distant metastasis.

C. Treatment strategies.

  1. Individualized treatment is based on multiple factors including stage, histologic type, prognostic indicators, hormone receptors, and patient factors.

  2. Breast cancer management usually involves both local and systemic treatment.

  3. Local treatments.

    a. Goal is to remove or destroy cancer cells in the breast area.

    b. Surgical treatments (Table 22–3).

      (1) Mastectomy—removes entire breast.

      (2) Breast conservation therapy (BCT)—preserves breast by removing only the tumor and surrounding tissue and is always followed by radiation therapy to the breast (Table 22–4).

      (3) Standard surgical procedures for invasive cancer include axillary node dissection (surgical procedures for noninvasive cancers typically do not).

      (4) BCT and modified radical mastectomy have equivalent 5-year survival rates for early breast cancers.

      (5) National Cancer Institute (NCI) 1990 Consensus Conference concluded that BCT is appropriate for majority of women with Stage I and II breast cancer and is preferable because it preserves the breast.

TABLE 22–3. **Breast Cancer Surgical Procedures**

Breast-Conserving Surgeries*

Lumpectomy	Excision of tumor with margin of healthy tissue
Segmental resection (tylectomy, quadrantectomy, partial mastectomy)	Excision of tumor with wider margin of healthy tissue

Mastectomies

Subcutaneous mastectomy**	Removes all breast tissue except overlying skin and nipple areolar complex
Total mastectomy	Complete removal of all breast tissue including skin, gland, areola
Modified radical mastectomy	Removal of above plus axillary lymph node dissection (level of dissection varies with technique)
Radical mastectomy	Removal of above plus underlying pectoral muscles

*Usually in conjunction with axillary node dissection via second incision when surgery is done for invasive cancer.
**Not used in cancer treatment because breast tissue is incompletely removed.

(6) Contraindications to BCT (Table 22–5).
(7) Breast reconstruction.
   (a) Surgically recreates breast mound after mastectomy.
   (b) May be immediate (at same time as mastectomy) or delayed (6 months or more following surgery).
   (c) Procedures are covered by most insurance carriers.
   (d) Options include techniques using implants or muscle flaps (Table 22–6).
   (e) Use of silicone gel implants has been restricted by the Food

TABLE 22–4. **Surgical Options for Early-Stage Breast Cancer**

	Breast Conservation Therapy	Modified Radical Mastectomy
Removes the malignant tumor and a small amount of normal tissue from breast	X	
Removes the entire breast		X
Removes some lymph nodes from underarm	X	X
Includes radiation treatment after surgery	X	

Adapted from Virginia M. Pressler, M.D. with permission.

TABLE 22–5. **Contraindications to Breast Conservation Treatment**

First- and second-trimester pregnancy

Two or more gross malignancies in separate quadrants of breast

Diffuse microcalcifications that are suspicious or indeterminate

Prior therapeutic radiation to the breast

History of collagen vascular disease

Large tumor in a relatively small breast

Data from Winchester, D.P., & Cox, J.D. [1992]. Standards for breast conservation treatment. *CA 42*, 9–10.

TABLE 22–6. **Techniques of Breast Reconstruction**

Technique	Advantages	Disadvantages
Implant Methods		
Implant—saline or silicone implant can be placed beneath the pectoralis major muscle if there is sufficient skin available	Simpler, less costly procedures with shorter surgical and recovery times compared with flap methods	Capsular contraction (formation of scar tissue around implant) and infection are possible complications
Tissue expander—expander is placed beneath the pectoralis major muscle; expander is inflated with saline solution at regular intervals to gradually stretch the skin until desired size achieved; expander is removed and replaced with implant.		Cannot be performed on previously irradiated tissue
		Results in less natural breast contour
		Long-term effects of silicone implants unknown
Flap Methods		
Latissimus dorsi flap—muscle, fat, and skin from upper back is rotated around to chest wall with or without implant to recreate breast mound.	Use of autologous tissue: Avoids implant complications and concerns	Technically more difficult and costly procedures with longer surgical and recovery time
Transverse rectus abdominis myocutaneous (TRAM) flap—a portion of rectus abdominis muscle with skin and subcutaneous fat from lower abdomen is transported to chest; removal of abdominal fat results in "tummy tuck"	Results in a more natural texture and shape TRAM flap method provides added benefit of "tummy tuck"	Decreased muscle strength in area from which flap is taken; abdominal hernia is a possible complication of TRAM flap
Free flap—microvascular transfer of muscle and skin from a distant site (usually gluteus) to chest wall and anastomosis of blood vessels to internal mammary artery		Necrosis and seroma are possible complications

and Drug Administration (FDA) because possible safety concerns; can be implanted only in clients taking part in FDA-approved studies.
  (f) Techniques for nipple areolar reconstruction include skin grafting from thigh crease or opposite nipple, permanent tattooing.
  c. Radiation therapy.
    (1) Primary therapy is usually initiated 2 to 4 weeks after segmental resection when incisions have healed and shoulder range of motion is adequate.
    (2) Total of 6000 cGy administered—4500 to 5000 cGy to entire breast, usually followed by 1000 to 1500 cGy to the tumor site by interstitial iridium-192 implants or an electron beam "boost."
    (3) Possible immediate side effects are edema, tenderness, skin changes, and fatigue.
    (4) Long-term effects may include hyperpigmentation, soft tissue fibrosis, rib fractures, pneumonitis, brachial plexopathy.
    (5) May be administered before, sequentially with, or following chemotherapy.
    (6) May be administered as an adjunctive treatment for clients with tumor close to the chest wall, locally advanced tumors, or tumors from recurrent or inflammatory breast cancer.
    (7) May be administered to specific sites of bone metastasis for palliation of pain.
  4. Systemic treatments.
    a. Goal is to destroy or control overt or occult cancer cells anywhere in the body.
    b. Treatment recommendations are individualized and based on factors such as stage, nodal, menopausal, and hormone receptor status.
    c. Chemotherapy.
      (1) Single-agent treatment.
        (a) Doxorubicin hydrochloride (Adriamycin) is the most active single agent.
        (b) Cyclophosphamide (Cytoxan) is the most active alkylating a agent.
        (c) Paclitaxel (Taxol) and docetaxel (Taxotere) are new agents (taxoids) for treatment of anthracycline-resistant recurrent or metastatic breast cancer.
      (2) Combination drug regimens, rather than single agents, are more commonly used.
        (a) Combinations of "first-line" drugs are used to treat breast cancer: cyclophosphamide, doxorubicin, methotrexate and 5-fluorouracil (Table 22–7).
        (b) 20 to 30% of clients who become resistant to first-line drugs often respond to second-line agents: ifosfamide, cisplatin, carboplatin, etoposide, mitomycin C, vinblastine, paclitaxel, docetaxel.
      (3) Optimal regimen and treatment duration has not yet been demonstrated.
      (4) Neoadjuvant chemotherapy treatment may be given to reduce the size of the tumor before surgery.

TABLE 22–7. **Chemotherapeutic Regimens Commonly Used in Breast Cancer**

CMF

AC

FAC

CMFVP

ACMF

A = doxorubicin, V = vincristine, P = prednisone, F = 5-fluorouracil, M = methotrexate, C = cyclophosphamide

(5) Dose intensification—administration of doses much higher than conventional dose treatment in an effort to overcome tumor cell drug resistance and improve response; dose-intensive regimens require hematopoietic support via autologous bone marrow transplant (ABMT), peripheral blood progenitor cell (PBPC) infusion, or colony-stimulating factor (CSF) injection.

d. Hormonal therapy.

(1) ER and PR test results predict those clients likely to respond to hormonal therapy.

(a) Overall response rate of 65% in women with high-positive ER test results.

(b) Only 10% response rate in those with negative ER test results.

(c) PR test result is positive in approximately 75% of ER-positive tumors; may be a more accurate predictor.

  i. If both ER and PR test results are positive, a 77% response rate has been observed.

  ii. If both ER and PR test results are negative, only a 5% response rate has been observed.

(2) Additive therapies modify the action of specific hormones.

(a) Tamoxifen (Nolvadex) is a synthetic "anti-estrogen" that blocks the binding of estrogen to ERs, thus inhibiting cancer growth; first-line oral agent.

(b) Estrogen (diethylstilbestrol, ethinyl estradiol) are second-line oral agents; mechanism of action not fully understood.

(c) Progestins (megestrol acetate, medroxyprogesterone acetate) are second-line agents that act by inhibiting estrogen stimulation of breast cancer cells.

(d) Androgens (fluoxymesterone) inhibit endogenous hormone release; infrequently used agents for second-line treatment of recurrent hormone-responsive tumors.

(3) Ablative therapies inhibit the production or effect of specific hormones.

(a) Ovarian ablation may be achieved by surgery (oophorectomy), ovarian radiation, or chemically with GnRH inhibitors such as leuprolide (Lupron), buserelin, and goserelin (Zoladex).

(b) Adrenal ablation may be achieved by surgery (adrenalectomy), or chemically with aminoglutethimide (Cytadren) or anastrozole (Arimidex).

     5. Standard therapies by stage.
       a. Stage 0 (noninvasive cancers).
         (1) Ductal carcinoma in situ (DCIS)—total mastectomy without lymph node removal *or* lumpectomy followed by radiation therapy.
         (2) Lobular carcinoma in situ (LCIS)—close clinical surveillance (no treatment) *or* bilateral total mastectomy without lymph node removal *or* enrollment in clinical trial evaluating tamoxifen to prevent development of invasive cancer.
       b. Stages I and II.
         (1) Lumpectomy and axillary node dissection followed by radiation therapy *or* modified radical mastectomy, *plus*
         (2) Adjuvant systemic treatment with tamoxifen or chemotherapy based on hormone receptor status and individual prognostic factors.
       c. Stage III.
         (1) Modified radical mastectomy *or* radical mastectomy with radiation therapy pre- or postoperatively, *plus*
         (2) Systemic treatment with chemotherapy or hormone therapy (may be given preoperatively if very large tumor or fixed nodes).
       d. Stage IV.
         (1) Systemic chemotherapy or hormone therapy, *plus*
         (2) Local treatments as needed for palliation.
  D. Survival.
     1. By stage.
       a. Local stage (confined to the breast)—96% with 5-year survival; 58% of cancers diagnosed at this stage.
       b. Regional stage (spread to surrounding tissue)—75% with 5-year survival; 32% of cancers diagnosed at this stage.
       c. Distant stage (metastasis present)—20% with 5-year survival; only 6% are diagnosed at this stage.
     2. By number of positive axillary nodes.
       a. 0 positive nodes—65 to 70% with 10-year survival.
       b. 1 to 3 positive nodes—48 to 63% with 10-year survival.
       c. 4 to 9 positive nodes—28% with 10-year survival.
       d. More than 10 positive nodes—18% with 10-year survival.

Assessment

  I. Pertinent personal and family history.
    A. Primary risk factors.
     1. Sex—more than 99% of all breast cancer cases occur in women.
     2. Age—risk increases over age 50 years.
     3. Personal history of breast cancer—15% develop breast cancer in the opposite breast.
     4. Family history of breast cancer.
       a. Two- to three-fold increased risk in women with a first-degree relative with breast cancer.
       b. Risk is further increased if the first-degree relative developed breast cancer premenopausally and/or bilaterally.
       c. Genetically determined breast cancers.
         (1) Account for less than 5% of all cases.

(2) Are more likely to be bilateral, occur at younger ages, and appear in multiple family members over three or more generations.

(3) Mutated BRCA-1 gene (on chromosome 17) is linked to an increased risk of breast and ovarian cancers.

(4) BRCA-2 (on chromosome 13) is believed to convey increased breast cancer risk.

B. Secondary risk factors.

1. Parity—risk is increased in women who have never had children; risk may be increased further in women who had their first child after age 30.

2. Prolonged hormone stimulation.

   a. Early menarche (before age 12).

   b. Late menopause (after age 50).

   c. Long-term use of exogenous estrogens may be a tumor-promoting factor.

3. Atypical hyperplasia on previous breast biopsy.

4. Exposure to excessive ionizing radiation such as from multiple fluoroscopies or radiation for mastitis, chest acne, or Hodgkin's disease.

5. History of endometrial, ovarian, or colon cancer.

C. Women with a high-risk profile account for only one third of all cases of breast cancer; the majority of women with breast cancer have no identifiable risk factors.

D. Role of environmental, lifestyle, and dietary factors is under investigation.

II. Physical examination.

A. Early signs and symptoms.

1. Early—usually asymptomatic.

2. Majority present with painless lump or thickening in the breast.

   a. 90% are discovered by the client rather than her health provider.

   b. 50% occur in the upper outer quadrant of the breast (more breast tissue in this quadrant).

   c. Less than 25% of all breast lumps are malignant.

B. Late signs and symptoms.

1. Primary tumor changes.

   a. Dimpling of the skin.

   b. Nipple retraction or deviation.

   c. Asymmetry of breasts.

   d. Peau d'orange skin—skin edema with prominent pores (appearance similar to the peel of an orange) resulting from obstructed lymphatic drainage.

   e. Bloody discharge from the nipple.

   f. Ulceration of the breast.

2. Nodal involvement.

   a. Firm, enlarged axillary lymph nodes.

   b. Palpable supraclavicular nodes.

3. Distant metastasis.

   a. Pain in shoulder, hip, lower back, or pelvis.

   b. Persistent cough.

   c. Anorexia or unexplained weight loss.

   d. Digestive disturbances.

   e. Persistent dizziness or blurred vision.

   f. Headache.

   g. Difficulty walking.

III. Laboratory data specific to breast cancer.
   A. Pathology report of breast lesion.
   B. Baseline biologic tumor marker profile may be obtained in some settings.
      1. Carcinoembryonic antigen (CEA).
      2. CA 15-3.
   C. Complete blood count.
   D. Liver chemistry results.

Nursing Diagnoses

   I. Knowledge deficit of disease process, treatment options, side effects, and self-care.
   II. Ineffective individual coping.
   III. Decisional conflict.
   IV. Body image disturbance.
   V. Impaired physical mobility.
   VI. Sensory/perceptual alterations (kinesthetic).
   VII. Altered sexuality patterns.
   VIII. Altered tissue perfusion (peripheral).
   IX. Risk for infection.

Outcome Identification

   I. Client describes the state of the disease and therapy at a level consistent with her cultural and educational background and emotional status.
   II. Client participates in the decision-making process pertaining to the plan of care to the extent desired or possible.
   III. Client identifies appropriate community and personal resources that provide information, facilitate coping, and assist with changes in body image and sexuality (e.g., Reach to Recovery, Look Good Feel Better, and local support groups).
   IV. Client describes the schedule for ongoing therapy and long-term follow-up care.
   V. Client communicates feelings about living with cancer and body image changes.
   VI. Client lists measures to prevent infection and lymphedema.
   VII. Client identifies the signs and symptoms of infection.
   VIII. Client practices exercises to regain full mobility of the affected shoulder and arm.
   IX. Client engages in open communication with significant other regarding changes in sexuality.

Planning and Implementation

   I. Interventions to maximize safety for the client.
   A. Prevent fluid accumulation under the chest wall incision by maintaining patency of surgical drains.
      1. Drains are left in for approximately 1 week or until output is less than 30 mL/24 hours.
      2. Client is usually discharged with drain in place; teach her how to strip tubing, empty drain reservoir, measure and record output.

    B. Promote venous lymphatic drainage.
       1. Elevate affected arm with the hand higher than the elbow and the elbow higher than the shoulder to facilitate venous drainage.
       2. Place a sign on the bed advising that no blood pressure readings, injections, or blood testing should be done on the affected arm.
    C. Adduct arm in the first 24 hours to minimize tension on suture lines.
    D. Promote functional recovery of arm and shoulder.
       1. Perform limited exercise for the first 24 hours (squeezing ball, wrist and elbow flexion and extension).
       2. Encourage the client to use the affected arm for activities of daily living (eating, hair brushing).
       3. Begin active range of motion exercises, usually on the second to third day or as ordered by the physician (Fig. 22–3).
  II. Interventions to increase knowledge and facilitate treatment decision-making.
    A. Explain treatment options in a nonjudgmental way and at the client's level of understanding.
    B. Encourage discussion regarding potential physical and emotional changes resulting from treatment and her personal values and beliefs as they are related to treatment options.
 III. Interventions to monitor for unique side effects of treatment for breast cancer.
    A. Teach the client to measure the circumference of the affected arm and to notify the physician if it is increased.
    B. Inform the client about altered arm and breast sensations (numbness and tingling of arm, lack of sensation on chest wall, phantom breast sensation after mastectomy) that may persist for several years.
    C. Assess for menopausal symptoms (hot flashes, vaginal dryness) that may be associated with adjuvant endocrine therapy or chemotherapy-induced ovarian failure.
    D. Interventions to monitor for and manage side effects of surgery, chemotherapy, and radiation (see Chapters 34, 35, and 37).
 IV. Interventions to enhance adaptation and rehabilitation.
    A. Promote communication between the physician and client; alert the physician to the client's concerns about breast cancer and its treatment.
    B. Assess coping abilities, support systems, feelings about body image, sexual identity, role relationships; see the Chapter 6 discussion on sexual dysfunction for interventions to manage problems with sexuality.
    C. Discuss breast prostheses, where permanent ones can be obtained, names of contact persons at the stores, costs, insurance coverage; information has been compiled by Reach to Recovery volunteers in local communities.
    D. Prepare client for long-term follow-up, with office visits every 3 months for the first 2 to 3 years, every 6 months for the next 2 to 3 years, and then at least annually
    E. Teach the client with a mastectomy the importance of examining the mastectomy incision and chest wall as well as practicing BSE of the remaining breast, teach the client with BCT how to recognize changes in BSE (breast will feel different after radiation).
    F. Teach the client and family precautions to take with the affected arm to prevent trauma and infection, which can lead to lymphedema (Table 22–8; see also Chapter 16).
  V. Interventions to incorporate the client and family in care.
    A. Assess psychological status of spouse or significant other—level of distress, ability to serve as support system.

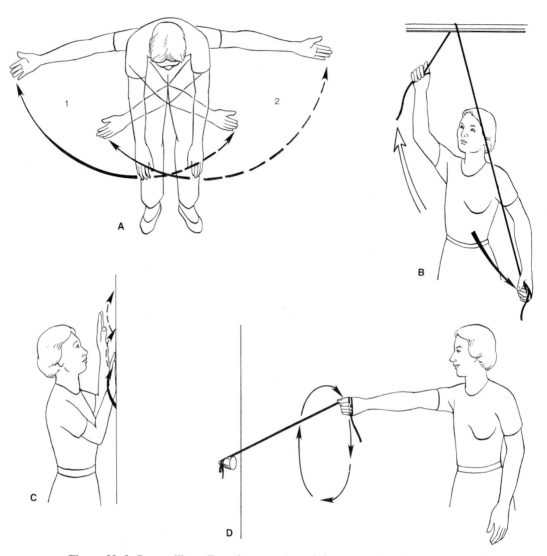

Figure 22–3. Post-axillary dissection exercises. (*A*) Arm swings. Stand with feet 8 inches apart. Bend forward from waist, allowing arms to hang toward floor. Swing both arms up to sides to reach shoulder level. Swing back to center, then cross arms at center. Do not bend elbows. If possible, do this and other exercises in front of mirror to ensure even posture and correct motion. (*B*) Pulley motion. Using affected arm, toss 6-foot rope over a shower curtain rod or over top of a door. Grasp one end of rope in each hand. Slowly raise affected arm as far as comfortable by pulling down on the rope on opposite side. Keep raised arm close to your head. Reverse to raise unaffected arm by lowering the affected arm. Repeat. (*C*) Hand wall climbing. Stand facing wall with toes 6 to 12 inches from wall. Bend elbows and place palms against wall at shoulder level. Gradually move both hands up the wall parallel to each other until incisional pulling or pain occurs. (Mark that spot on wall to measure progress.) Work hands down to shoulder level. Move closer to wall as height of reach improves. (*D*) Rope turning. Tie rope to door handle. Hold rope in hand of affected side. Back away from door until arm is extended away from body, parallel to floor. Swing rope in as wide a circle as possible. Increase size of the circle as mobility returns. (From Luckman, J. & Sorenson, K.C. [1987]. *Medical-Surgical Nursing: a Psychophysiologic Approach* [3rd ed]. Philadelphia: W.B. Saunders, p. 1823.)

TABLE 22–8. **Precautions to Prevent Lymphedema**

Avoid burns while cooking

Avoid sunburns

Have all injections, vaccinations, blood samples, and blood pressure tests done on the other arm whenever possible

Use an electric razor with a narrow head for underarm shaving to reduce the risk of nicks or scratches

Carry heavy packages or handbags on the other arm

Wash cuts promptly, treat with antibacterial medication, and cover with a sterile dressing; check often for redness, soreness, or other signs of infection

Never cut cuticles; use hand cream or lotion

Wear watches or jewelry loosely, if at all, on the treated arm

Wear protective gloves when gardening and when using strong detergents

Use a thimble when sewing

Avoid harsh chemicals and abrasive compounds

Use insect repellent to avoid bites and stings

Avoid elastic cuffs on blouses and nightgowns

From (1990) *After Breast Cancer: a Guide to Followup Care.* NIH Pub. No. 90–2400.

B. Include significant others in teaching (e.g., about surgical drain care, range of motion exercises).
C. Teach female first-degree relatives of client the importance of regular breast cancer screening.

Evaluation

The oncology nurse systematically and regularly evaluates the client's and/or family's responses to interventions to determine progress toward the achievement of expected outcomes. Relevant data are collected and actual findings are compared with expected findings. Nursing diagnoses, outcomes, and plans of care are reviewed and revised as necessary.

BIBLIOGRAPHY

American Cancer Society. (1996). *Breast Cancer Facts and Figures.* Pub. No. 8610. Atlanta: American Cancer Society.

Bilodeau, B.A., & Degner, L.F. (1996). Information needs, sources of information and decisional roles in women with breast cancer. *Oncol Nurs Forum 23,* 691–999.

Breast cancer screening for women ages 40–49. NIH Consensus Statement 1997, January 21–23; 15(1).

Chapman, D.D., & Goodman, M. (1997). Breast cancer. In S.L. Groenwald, M.H. Frogge, M. Goodman, & C.H. Yarbro (eds.). *Cancer Nursing: Principles and Practice* (4th ed.). Boston: Jones & Bartlett, pp. 916–979.

Donegan, W.L., & Spratt, J.S. (eds.). (1995). *Cancer of the Breast* (4th ed.). Philadelphia: W.B. Saunders .

Dow, K.H. (ed.). (1996). *Contemporary Issues in Breast Cancer.* Boston: Jones & Bartlett.

Engelking, C. (ed-in-chief), & Kalinowski, B.H. (guest ed.). (1995). *A Comprehensive Guide to Breast Cancer Treatment: Current Issues and Controversies.* (Monograph.) New York: Triclinica Communications.

Harris, J.R., Lippman, M.E., Morrow, M., & Hellman, S. (eds.). (1996). *Disease of the Breast.* Philadelphia: Lippincott-Raven.

Harris, J.R., Lippman, M.E., Veronesi, U., & Willett, W. (1992a). Breast cancer: First of three parts. *N Engl J Med 327,* 319–328.

Harris, J.R., Lippman M.E., Veronesi, U., & Willette, W. (1992b). Breast cancer: Second of three parts. *N Engl J Med 327,* 390–398.

Harris, J.R., Lippman, M.D., Veronesi, U., & Willette, W. (1992c). Breast cancer: Third of three parts. *N Engl J Med 327,* 473–480.

Hortobagyi, G.N., & Buzdar, A.U. (1995). Current status of adjuvant systemic therapy for primary breast cancer: Progress and controversy. *CA 45*, 199–226.

Knobf, M.T. (1994). Treatment options for early stage breast cancer. *Medsurg Nurs 3*, 249–328.

Knobf, M.T. (1996). Breast cancers. In R. McCorkle, M. Grant, M.F. Stromborg, & S.B. Baird (eds.). *Cancer Nursing: A Comprehensive Textbook* (2nd ed.). Philadelphia: W.B. Saunders, pp. 547–610.

Leitch, A.M., Dodd, G.D., Costanza, M., et al. (1997). American Cancer Society guidelines for the early detection of breast cancer: Update 1997. *CA 47*, 150–153.

Love, S.M. (1995). *Dr. Susan Love's Breast Book* (2nd ed.). Reading, MA: Addison-Wesley.

Moore, M.P., & Kinne, D.W. (1995). Surgical management of primary invasive breast cancer. *CA 45*, 279–288.

Stoll, B.A. (ed.) (1995). *Reducing Breast Cancer Risk in Women*. Dordrecht, The Netherlands: Kluwer Academic.

Treatment of early-stage breast cancer. NIH Consens Dev Conf Consens Statement 1990, June 18–21; *8*(6).

Winchester, D.P., & Cox, J.D. (1992). Standards for breast-conservation treatment. *CA 42*, 134–162.

Nursing Care of the Client With Cancer of the Urinary System

Julena Lind, RN, MN

KIDNEY CANCER

Theory

I. Physiology and pathophysiology of cancer of the kidney.
   A. Anatomic placement of a kidney (Figs. 23–1 and 23–2).
   B. Primary function.
      1. Pair of organs approximately 4½ inches long lying behind the peritoneum in a mass of fatty tissue.
      2. Consists chiefly of nephrons (parenchyma) in which urine is secreted, collected, and discharged into a main cavity (renal pelvis) and then conveyed by the ureters to the bladder.
   C. Changes associated with cancer—excessive cell production results in growth into adjacent organs and gradual loss of function in the affected kidney.
   D. Two major types of kidney cancer.
      1. Renal cell (also called hypernephroma or adenocarcinoma of the kidney).
         a. Most common—75 to 85% of all kidney tumors.
         b. Occurs in parenchyma.
         c. Often associated with paraneoplastic syndromes (e.g., inappropriate secretion of parathyroid hormone, ACTH, and erythropoietin).
      2. Cancer of the renal pelvis.
         a. Comprises 5 to 9% of all kidney tumors.
         b. Generally arises from epithelial tissue anywhere in renal pelvis; may be multifocal.
         c. Because of the relative infrequent occurrence, cancer of the renal pelvis will not be discussed in this text.
      3. Renal cell cancers tend to grow toward the medullary portion of the kidney and spread in direct extrusion to the renal vein and sometimes into the vena cava.
      4. Between 30% and 50% of kidney cancers have metastasized by the time of diagnosis; mean survival time with metastasis is approximately 4 months.
   E. Trends in epidemiology.
      1. Kidney cancer is relatively rare in the United States (US), accounting for only 3% of all cancers.
      2. A slight steady increase in kidney cancer among males has been reported; 2:1 male predominance.

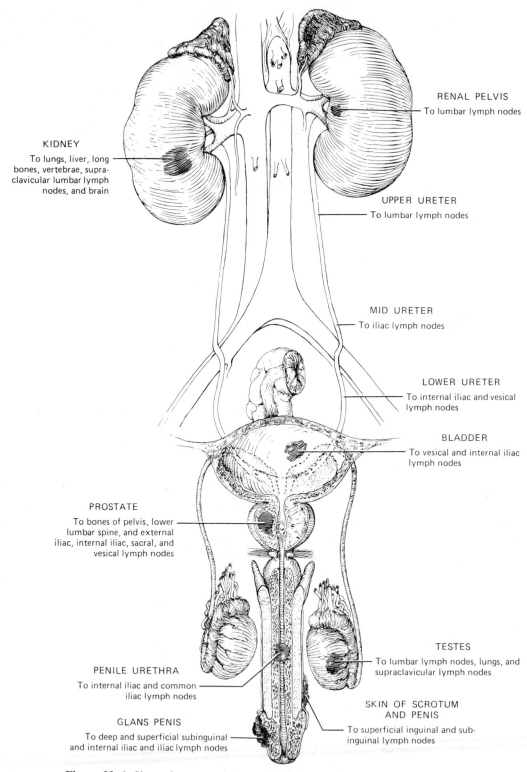

KIDNEY
To lungs, liver, long bones, vertebrae, supra-clavicular lumbar lymph nodes, and brain

RENAL PELVIS
To lumbar lymph nodes

UPPER URETER
To lumbar lymph nodes

MID URETER
To iliac lymph nodes

LOWER URETER
To internal iliac and vesical lymph nodes

BLADDER
To vesical and internal iliac lymph nodes

PROSTATE
To bones of pelvis, lower lumbar spine, and external iliac, internal iliac, sacral, and vesical lymph nodes

TESTES
To lumbar lymph nodes, lungs, and supraclavicular lymph nodes

PENILE URETHRA
To internal iliac and common iliac lymph nodes

SKIN OF SCROTUM AND PENIS
To superficial inguinal and sub-inguinal lymph nodes

GLANS PENIS
To deep and superficial subinguinal and internal iliac and iliac lymph nodes

Figure 23–1. Sites of tumor origin and metastases in the male. (Modified from Johnson, D.E., Swanson, D.A., & von Eschenbach, A.C. [1987]. Tumors of the genitourinary tract. In E.A. Tanagho & J.W. McAninch [eds.]. *Smith's General Urology* [12th ed.]. San Mateo, CA: Appleton & Lange, p. 332.)

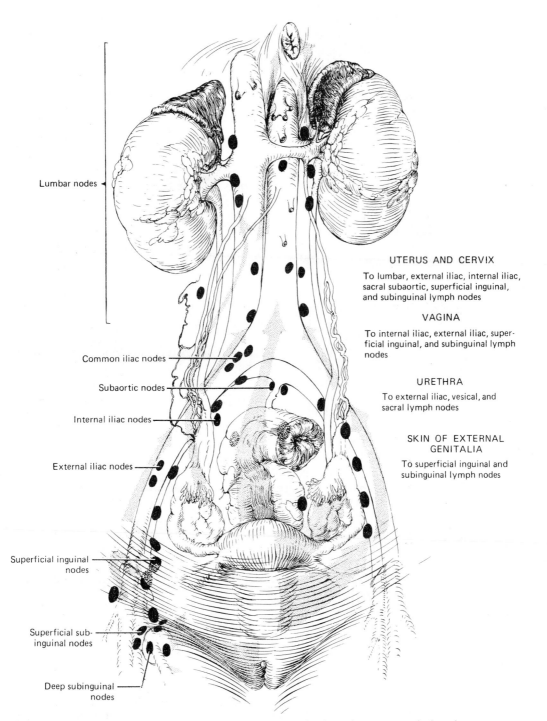

Lumbar nodes

Common iliac nodes

Subaortic nodes

Internal iliac nodes

External iliac nodes

Superficial inguinal nodes

Superficial sub-inguinal nodes

Deep subinguinal nodes

UTERUS AND CERVIX

To lumbar, external iliac, internal iliac, sacral subaortic, superficial inguinal, and subinguinal lymph nodes

VAGINA

To internal iliac, external iliac, superficial inguinal, and subinguinal lymph nodes

URETHRA

To external iliac, vesical, and sacral lymph nodes

SKIN OF EXTERNAL GENITALIA

To superficial inguinal and subinguinal lymph nodes

Figure 23–2. Anatomic relationships and sites of lymph nodes for urinary tumors in females. (Modified from Johnson, D.E., Swanson, D.A., & von Eschenbach, A.C. [1987]. Tumors of the genitourinary tract. In E.A. Tanagho & J.W. McAninch [eds.]. *Smith's General Urology* [12th ed.]. San Mateo, CA: Appleton & Lange, p. 333.)

3. Cigarette smoking is the most definitive risk factor with approximately 25 to 30% of cases attributable to smoking.
4. A genetic link, renal cell cancer has a (rare) familial form in which there is translocation in the short arm of chromosome 3.
5. Average age at diagnosis is 55 to 60 years.
6. Geographic differences in incidence.
   a. Scandinavian countries have a relatively high incidence (renal cell cancer accounts for 11% of all cancers).
   b. Japan has a low incidence.
   c. United States and Western European countries have an intermediate risk.
II. Principles of medical management.
   A. Screening and diagnostic tests—no screening tests are available for kidney cancer; diagnostic tests include:
      1. Kidney, ureter, and bladder (KUB) radiography (Table 23–1).
      2. Nephrotomography.
      3. Excretory urography (test of choice) (Table 23–1).
      4. Retrograde urography (Table 23–1).
      5. Renal ultrasound.
      6. Renal computerized tomography (CT).
      7. Renal angiography.
      8. Magnetic resonance imaging (MRI).
   B. Staging methods and procedures.
      1. Based on factors that influence survival—regional lymph node involvement, invasion through the renal capsule, extension to contiguous organs, and distant metastases.
      2. Size of the primary tumor is not correlated strongly with survival and may not be a significant factor in staging.
      3. Systems most often used for classifying renal cell carcinoma—Robson's classification, and the TNM system (Tables 23–2 and 23–3).
   C. Treatment strategies.
      1. Renal cell cancer is usually treated by surgical removal via a radical nephrectomy, including removal of the lymph nodes in the renal hilar area.
         a. Nephron-sparing surgery now being accepted more often in situations when radical nephrectomy would leave a client anephric.
         b. Palliative nephrectomy sometimes being done for selected clients with metastatic disease who have severe disability from associated local symptoms.
      2. Regional lymphadenectomy remains controversial, because the impact on survival is not clear.
      3. Radiotherapy and chemotherapy.
         a. Renal cell cancers are usually radioresistant.
         b. Metastatic bone pain can be treated by radiotherapy.
         c. Adjuvant chemotherapy has not improved survival.
      4. Treatment of advanced disease.
         a. Approximately 30% have metastases at diagnosis.
         b. Adjunctive or palliative nephrectomy has been used.
         c. Hormonal therapy, using progesterone such as medroxyprogesterone acetate (Depo-Provera) or megestrol acetate (Megace), testosterone, or antiestrogens such as tamoxifen, has been used.
         d. Biotherapy.
            (1) High doses of interleukin-2 (IL-2) and large number of lymphokine-activated killer cells (LAK) have shown promise in treating metastatic renal cancer, but with significant toxicities.

TABLE 23–1. **Urologic Diagnostic Tests and Nursing Interventions**

Test	Preparation	Nursing Interventions
X-ray examination of kidneys, ureter, bladder (KUB)	None—plain film of abdomen	Explain client will lie flat on x-ray examination table Do not schedule after barium studies (will obscure kidneys)
Excretory urography	Dye is excreted unchanged by kidneys; therefore hydration is important, followed by nothing by mouth 6 to 8 hr before test Dye is injected intravenously; anaphylactic or allergic reaction to dye may occur; may premedicate with antihistamines	Assess history of allergy to iodine dyes or contrast media before test; pretesting may be indicated Use of iodine dyes may be contraindicated in clients with severe renal or hepatic disease or clinical hypersensitivity (severe allergies, asthma) Have emergency equipment and personnel available before injection (anaphylaxis and cardiovascular reactions may occur) and 30–60 min after test (delayed reactions) Observe for adverse reactions to dye—angina, chest pain, arrhythmias, hypotension, dizziness, blurred vision, headache, fever, convulsions, dyspnea, rhinitis, laryngitis, nausea
Retrograde urography	General anesthesia or narcotic analgesia may be used; cystoscope is inserted; iodinated dye is injected via urethral catheter Laxatives at bedtime before test may be used to cleanse bowel	Observe for reaction to anesthetic or analgesic Monitor for bleeding, symptoms of urinary tract infections, dysuria, or difficulty voiding after test

425

TABLE 23–2. **Robson's Renal Cell Cancer Classification**

Stage I:	Tumor is confined within the kidney parenchyma (no involvement of perinephric fat, renal vein, or regional lymph nodes).
Stage II:	Tumor involves the perinephric fat but is confined within Gerota's fascia (including the adrenal).
Stage IIIA:	Tumor involves the main renal vein or inferior vena cava.
Stage IIIB:	Tumor involves regional lymph nodes.
Stage IIIC:	Tumor involves both local vessels and regional lymph nodes.
Stage IVA:	Tumor involves adjacent organs other than the adrenal (colon, pancreas, etc.).
Stage IVB:	Distant metastases.

From Dreicer, R., & Williams, R.D. (1995). Renal parenchymal neoplasms. In E.A. Tanagho & J.W. McAninch (eds.), *Smith's General Urology* (14th ed.). Norwalk, CT: Appleton & Lange, p. 376.

        (2) Interleukin-2 (IL-2) in combination with alpha interferon has demonstrated improved response rates with much lower toxicity (as compared with IL-2 with LAK).
    D. Five-year survival rate:
        1. Stages I and II—50 to 70%.
        2. Stage III—approximately 50%.
        3. Stage IV—less than 10%.

Assessment

  I. Pertinent client and family history.
    A. Carcinogens linked to kidney cancer.
        1. Cigarette smoking, nicotine, and coal tars.
        2. Exposure to cadmium, lead pigment in colored printing ink, and asbestos.
        3. Heavy use of analgesics, specifically phenacetin-containing products, increases the risk of cancer of the renal pelvis.
    B. Association between renal cell cancer and obesity in women was first identified in 1974.

TABLE 23–3. **TNM Renal Cell Classification**

Primary Tumor (T)

(All sizes measured in greatest dimension)

TX:	Primary tumor cannot be assessed.
T0:	No evidence of primary tumor.
T1:	Tumor 2.5 cm or less limited to the kidney.
T2:	Tumor more than 2.5 cm limited to the kidney.
T3:	Tumor extends into major veins or invades adrenal gland or perinephric tissues but not beyond Gerota's fascia.
	T3a: Tumor invades adrenal gland or perinephric tissues but not beyond Gerota's fascia.
	T3b: Tumor grossly extends into renal vein(s) or vena cava.
T4:	Tumor invades beyond Gerota's fascia.

Regional Lymph Nodes (N)

NX:	Regional lymph nodes cannot be assessed.
N0:	No regional lymph node metastasis.
N1:	Metastasis in a single lymph node 2 cm or less.
N2:	Metastasis in a single lymph node, greater than 2 cm but not more than 5 cm or multiple nodes none greater than 5 cm.
N3:	Metastasis in a lymph node greater than 5 cm.

Distant Metastases (M)

MX:	Presence of distant metastasis cannot be assessed.
M0:	No distant metastasis.
M1:	Distant metastasis.

Stage Grouping

Stage I:	T1	N0	M0
Stage II:	T2	N0	M0
Stage III:	T1	N1	M0
	T2	N1	M0
	T3a	N0,N1	M0
	T3b	N0,N1	M0
Stage IV:	T4	Any N	M0
	Any T	N2,N3	M0
	Any T	Any N	M1

From Dreicer, R., & Williams, R.D. (1995). Renal parenchymal neoplasms. In E.A. Tanagho & J.W. McAninch (eds.). *Smith's General Urology* (14th ed.). Norwalk, CT: Appleton & Lange, p. 377.

II. Physical examination.
   A. In 40% of people with renal cell cancer the initial, but not early, sign is gross hematuria.
   B. Pain (dull, aching) and a palpable abdominal mass are late signs.
   C. More generalized late signs—fever, weight loss, elevated erythrocyte sedimentation rate (ESR), and/or anemia.
III. Evaluation of diagnostic data.
   A. Gross hematuria found on urinalysis.
   B. Elevated ESR.
   C. Obstruction or blockage related to tumor presence as demonstrated in excretory urogram.
   D. Differential diagnosis of renal cysts versus neoplasms demonstrated by nephrotomogram and/or renal ultrasound.

Nursing Diagnoses

   I. Ineffective airway clearance.
  II. Risk for fluid volume deficit.
 III. Pain.
  IV. Constipation.
   V. Knowledge deficit.
  VI. Anxiety.

Outcome Identification

   I. Client demonstrates normal respiratory status postoperatively.
  II. Client's urine volume is normal.
 III. Client verbalizes an understanding of disease and rationale for treatment.
  IV. Client experiences pain relief.
   V. Client resumes normal bowel functioning postoperatively.
  VI. Client explains care at home following discharge including:
   A. Lists signs of abdominal distention.
   B. Describes the importance of liberal oral fluid intake (up to 2500 mL/day).
   C. Describes the importance of a low-fat diet.
   D. Lists phenacetin-containing drugs.
   E. Cites strategies to deal with fatigue or other responses to biotherapy.
   F. Lists resources—local American Cancer Society branch.
 VII. Client participates in follow-up care.
   A. Verbalizes the schedule for follow-up appointments and the rationale for blood pressure checks, excretory urogram, chest x-ray examinations, and other diagnostic tests.
   B. Reports signs and symptoms of recurrence—abdominal or flank pain, hematuria, bone pain, respiratory changes.
   C. Reports signs and symptoms of renal dysfunction—decreased urine output, fluid retention, hypertension.

Planning and Implementation

   I. Interventions to maximize safety.
   A. Prevention of atelectasis and pneumonia.
     1. Because of the close proximity of the nephrectomy incision to the diaphragm, deep breathing and coughing can be extremely uncomfortable.

    2. Clients should be taught proper splinting and instructed to take at least 10 deep breaths every hour while awake.

    3. Incentive spirometer and intermittent positive pressure breathing may be beneficial.

B. Observation for signs of hemorrhage.

    1. Bleeding is a danger (but not a frequently observed complication) after nephrectomy because the kidney is highly vascular.

    2. Acute massive hemorrhage is manifested by profuse drainage and distention at the suture line or by internal bleeding.

    3. The nephrectomy dressing and underlying sheet should be examined frequently for blood.

    4. Observe for signs of excessive bleeding and vital signs for internal hemorrhage.

C. Monitor urine output postoperatively for volume of at least 30 mL/hour.

D. Maintenance of water seal drainage for chest tubes if thoracoabdominal incision is used.

II. Interventions to decrease severity of symptoms associated with treatment.

A. Pain relief measures.

    1. Pain can be severe after nephrectomy because of incisional pain and muscular aches and pains (related to lithotomy position on operative table).

    2. Pain medication should be given on a regular basis and titrated to the needs of the client (see Chapter 10).

B. Prevention and observation for paralytic ileus.

    1. Paralytic ileus occurs fairly commonly after nephrectomy (kidneys are retroperitoneal; thus the intestines are manipulated in surgery).

    2. Ambulation and encouragement to turn from side to side may help promote peristalsis and increase comfort.

    3. Observe for abdominal distention and auscultate bowel sounds frequently.

C. Prevention of loss of function of remaining kidney.

    1. Teach the client and family the importance of continuing liberal oral intake (up to 3000 mL/day).

    2. Teach the client and family to avoid potentially nephrotoxic drugs (e.g., nonsteroidal anti-inflammatory drugs [NSAIDs]) without first checking with the physician or nurse.

    3. Teach the client and family to avoid activity that would injure the remaining kidney (e.g., contact sports).

    4. Teach the client and family signs and symptoms of urinary tract infection.

III. Interventions to promote well-being at home.

A. Teach the client and family follow-up monitoring.

    1. Frequent blood pressure and renal function tests to monitor function of remaining kidney.

    2. Schedule tests.

        a. Excretory urography to detect contralateral tumors.

        b. Chest x-ray examination to rule out lung metastases.

        c. Bone scans to detect bony metastasis.

B. Teach the client and family to report signs of respiratory distress, hemoptysis, pain, or pathologic fracture of an extremity (related to bony metastasis).

C. Teach client and family to observe for flu-like symptoms and medicate with acetaminophen; and use energy-sparing strategies if receiving IL-2 and alpha interferon.

Evaluation

The oncology nurse systematically and regularly evaluates the client's and/or family's responses to interventions to determine progress toward the achievement of expected outcomes. Relevant data are collected and actual findings are compared with expected findings. Nursing diagnoses, outcomes, and plans of care are reviewed and revised as necessary.

BLADDER CANCER

Theory

I. Physiology and pathophysiology associated with bladder cancer.
   A. Anatomy of the bladder.
      1. Consists of a membranous sac that serves as temporary retainer for urine, which is then discharged through the urethra.
      2. In men, in addition to the local lymph nodes, critical adjacent structures include the prostate, seminal vesicles, urethra, and nerves at the base of the penis (see Figure 23–1).
      3. In women the critical adjacent structures include the uterus, ovaries, fallopian tubes, urethra, and local lymph nodes (see Figure 23–2).
   B. Changes associated with cancer.
      1. Proliferation of abnormal tissue in one or more places inside the bladder.
      2. Clinical changes—bleeding if the tumor has produced a bladder wall lesion and, occasionally, urethral obstruction.
   C. Major types of bladder cancer.
      1. In North America 90 to 95% of bladder tumors are transitional cell carcinomas.
         a. Transitional cell tumors arise in the epithelial layer of the bladder, which rests on the basement membrane.
         b. If the basement membrane remains intact, metastasis to the vascular or lymphatic system is unlikely.
         c. Within the transitional cell classification, the tumors are further subdivided—carcinoma in situ (confined to urothelial lining), papillary infiltrating, papillary noninfiltrating, and solid tumors.
            (1) Papillary tumors have a propensity for recurrence.
            (2) Transitional cell tumors are usually multifocal.
            (3) High recurrence and multicentricity necessitate aggressive follow-up.
      2. Squamous cell carcinoma account for 6 to 8% of bladder cancers.
      3. Adenocarcinomas are rare (2%).
   D. Metastatic patterns.
      1. Many of these tumors arise on floor of bladder and can involve one or both ureteral orifices.
      2. Most important prognostic feature—depth of penetration into the bladder wall; the deeper the penetration, the greater is the risk of metastases.
      3. Some tumors spread rapidly to the pelvic lymph nodes; others grow slowly and spread into the pelvic tissues.
      4. Metastasis takes place via direct extension from the muscle of the bladder into the perivesical fat (or serosa).
         a. Tumor can obstruct ureters or bladder neck.
         b. Can spread by direct extension to involve other adjacent structures such as the sigmoid colon, rectum, prostate, uterus, or vagina.

5. The grade (or degree of tumor cell differentiation) is a key predictor of the aggressive nature of the cancer.

E. Trends in epidemiology.
  1. The incidence of bladder cancer has been gradually increasing over the past 30 years in most industrialized countries. The reason is not known.
  2. The rate of diagnosis in the localized stage has increased over the past 20 years because of improved diagnostic tests and the trend to classify as malignant papillomas that were once classified as benign.
  3. A higher male-to-female ratio: approximately 4:1.
  4. Bladder cancer occurs twice as often in smokers as nonsmokers.
  5. Estimated that smoking responsible for 40 to 50% of deaths from bladder cancer.

II. Principles of medical management.
  A. Screening and diagnostic tests.
    1. No good early screening test for bladder cancer exists.
    2. Urinary cytology—for best results specimens are obtained from late morning or early afternoon urine.
    3. Bladder washings provide even more reliable results.
    4. Flow cytometry—technique used to examine the deoxyribonucleic acid content of urinary cells; useful in identifying high-grade, high-stage tumors.
    5. Excretory urography (intravenous pyelography)—done before cystoscopy to help evaluate the upper tracts (Table 23–1).
    6. Cystoscopy—for tumor visualization, for possible biopsy, and to allow bimanual examination of the bladder (to determine fixation and extent of tumor).
    7. Imaging.
      a. Computerized tomography (CT)—aids in defining the extent of local tumor and in identifying pelvic lymph node metastasis.
      b. Transurethral ultrasound—used to define local extension and the degree of involvement of the bladder wall.
      c. MRI—to distinguish the tumor from the normal bladder wall and to identify the presence of pelvic lymph node involvement.
  B. Staging methods and procedures.
    1. Most common systems used in the United States—Jewett/Marshall and the TNM system developed by the American Joint Committee on Cancer (Tables 23–4 and 23–5).

TABLE 23–4. **Bladder Stage Groupings**

Jewett/Marshall Stage	Stage	TNM Classification
CIS, 0	0	Tis N0 M0; Ta N0 M0
A	I	T1 N0 M0
B1	II	T2 N0 M0
B2, C	III	T3a N0 M0; T3b N0 M0
D1, D2	IV Any N, M1	T4 N0 M0; Any T, N1, N2, N3 M0; Any T

Data from Lieskovsky, G., Alhlering, T., & Skinner, D.G. (1988). Diagnosis and staging of bladder cancer. In D.G. Skinner & G. Lieskovsky (eds.). *Diagnosis and Management of Genitourinary Cancer.* Philadelphia, W.B. Saunders, p. 267.

TABLE 23–5. **TNM Bladder Classification**

T = Primary Tumor

TX	Primary tumor cannot be assessed
T0	No evidence of primary tumor
Tis	Carinoma-in-situ
Ta	Noninvasive papillary carcinoma
T1	Tumor invades submucosa/lamina propria
T2	Tumor invades superficial muscle
T3a	Tumor invades deep muscle
T3b	Tumor invades perivesical fat
T4	Tumor invades adjacent organs

N = Regional Lymph Nodes (Below Aortic Bifurcation)

NX	Regional lymph nodes cannot be assessed.
N0	No regional lymph node metastasis
N1	Metastasis in single node <2 cm
N2	Metastasis in single node >2 cm but <5 cm, or multiple nodes <5 cm
N3	Metastasis in nodes >5 cm

M = Distant Metastases

MX	Presence of distant metastasis cannot be assessed
M0	No distant metastasis
M1	Distant metastasis

Used with permission of the American Joint Committee on Cancer (AJCC®), Chicago, Illinois. The original source for this material is the AJCC® *Manual for Staging of Cancer,* 4th edition (1992), published by Lippincott-Raven Publishers, Philadelphia.

2. Another factor often considered in treatment but not actually included in the staging systems—grade of the tumor (grades 1, 2, 3, 4); refers to the degree of tumor cell differentiation and helps to determine the aggressiveness of therapy.

C. Standard therapies.

1. Carcinoma in situ is usually treated by fulguration and administration of intravesical thiotepa or radical cystectomy.

2. Superficial low-grade tumors are treated by transurethral surgery with resection and fulguration (if multiple small lesions are found).

   a. Because the chance of recurrence is so great, intravesical chemotherapy has been used; most common drugs are thiotepa, doxorubicin, Bacillus Calmette-Guérin (BCG), or mitomycin C.

   b. Small superficial bladder tumors also have been treated with laser therapy.

   c. Superficial recurrences are managed by repeated transurethral resections and intravesical chemotherapy.

3. Radical cystectomy with urinary diversion.

   a. Treatment of choice for cure of high-stage, high-grade tumors, which need more aggressive treatment because of the invasion to the bladder muscle.

   b. In men, includes excision of the bladder with the perivesical fat, attached peritoneum, and entire prostate and seminal vesicles.

c. Aggressive surgery in women includes removal of the bladder and entire urethra; the uterus, ovaries, fallopian tubes, and anterior wall of the vagina (not all surgeons remove the reproductive organs); pelvic lymph node dissection also may be performed.

d. Types of urinary diversions (see Chapter 14).

    (1) Ileal conduit (Fig. 23–3)—well-known urinary diversion performed with cystectomy.

        (a) Portion of the terminal end of the ileum is isolated, the proximal end is closed, the distal end is brought out through a hole in the abdominal wall and is sutured to the skin, creating a stoma.

        (b) Ureters are implanted into the ileal segment, urine flows into the conduit, and peristalsis propels urine out through the stoma.

    (2) Continent ileal reservoir (Fig. 23–4)—technique that provides an intraabdominal pouch for storage of urine.

        (a) Typically has nipple valves created to maintain and prevent ureteral reflux.

        (b) No external collecting device is needed; urine remains in the reservoir until client self-catheterizes through stoma, usually with 16-French or 18 red Robinson catheter.

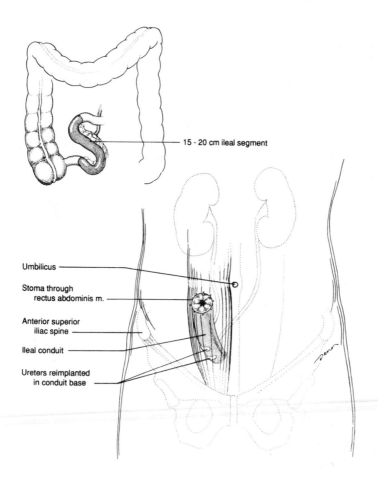

15 - 20 cm ileal segment

Umbilicus

Stoma through
rectus abdominis m.

Anterior superior
iliac spine

Ileal conduit

Ureters reimplanted
in conduit base

Figure 23–3. Urinary diversion using a segment of ileum. As short a segment as possible is used, and it is usually positioned in the right lower quadrant of the abdomen in an isoperistaltic direction. (From Carroll, P.R., & Barbour, S. [1992]. Urinary diversion and bladder substitution. In E. Tanagho & J. McAninch (eds.). *Smith's General Urology* [13th ed.]. Norwalk, CT: Appleton & Lange, p. 427.)

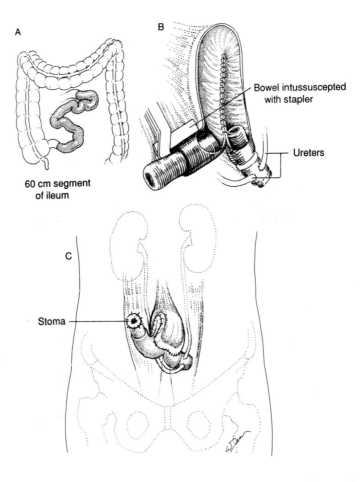

A

B

Bowel intussuscepted
with stapler

Ureters

60 cm segment
of ileum

C

Stoma

Figure 23–4. Kock Pouch urinary reservoir. (*A*) Shaded area indicates section of small intestine selected for reservoir construction. (*B*) Afferent (nonrefluxing) limb for ureteral implantation and efferent limb (with nipple valve) for stoma created by using stapling devices. (*C*) Completed reservoir with the efferent limb drawn through the abdominal wall and stoma created. (From Carroll, P.R., & Barbour, S. [1992]. Urinary diversion and bladder substitution. In E. Tanagho & J. McAninch (eds.). *Smith's General Urology* [13th ed.]. Norwalk, CT: Appleton & Lange, p. 432.)

    e. Radical cystectomy can damage the nerves responsible for erectile ability; therefore in many centers a penile prosthesis is implanted at the time of surgery or soon thereafter.

  4. Radiation therapy.

    a. Definitive radiotherapy—according to some experts, can cure approximately 16 to 30% of clients with invasive bladder cancer, a rate less than surgery; however, often used in countries other than United States.

    b. Preoperative radiation—used to decrease both pelvic lymph node recurrence and dissemination during surgical excision.

  5. Advanced bladder cancer is often treated with single agent or combination chemotherapy.

    a. Single-agent therapy has demonstrated limited success with cisplatin proving the most effective agent.

    b. Combination chemotherapy—complete responses with M-VAC (methotrexate, vincristine, doxorubicin, and cisplatin); other combinations include doxorubicin and cyclophosphamide; doxorubicin and cisplatin; doxorubicin and 5-fluorouracil; methotrexate and cyclophosphamide plus cisplatin.

 D. Trends in survival show an increase in survival rates (Table 23–6).

TABLE 23–6. **Bladder Cancer Survival**

Stage	Percentage
Localized	92
Regional	48
Distant	8
All stages	80

From American Cancer Society. (Jan., 1995). *Cancer Facts and Figures—1995*. Atlanta: American Cancer Society.

Assessment

I. Pertinent personal and family history.
   A. Four major variables are related to bladder cancer incidence.
      1. Race—age-adjusted bladder cancer rate in white men in the U.S. is twice the rate of black men.
      2. Gender—in whites the male-female ratio is 4:1.
      3. Age—most tumors occur in men over 50 years old.
      4. Geographic location—areas with a high incidence of bladder cancer include Africa and Egypt (attributed to the parasite *Schistosoma haematobium;* higher rate of squamous cell type); more prevalent in highly industrialized urban areas than rural areas.
   B. Assess occupational risks—exposure to dyes, rubber, leather, paint, and organic chemicals (latency period may be 20 years).
   C. Determine smoking history—rate is twice as high in smokers versus non-smokers.
   D. Artificial sweeteners act as both initiators and promoters in rats, but risk in humans is inconclusive.
II. Physical examination.
   A. Early signs and symptoms.
      1. Gross painless hematuria—most common presenting symptom but not usually considered an early sign.
      2. Irritability of the bladder (dysuria, urinary frequency, urgency, and burning on urination)—common.
   B. Later signs and symptoms.
      1. If the tumor is large, compression of the internal urethral orifice may occur and cause decrease in force and caliber of the stream.
      2. Obstruction of the ureters can cause flank pain and result in hydronephrosis.
III. Laboratory data.
   A. DNA flow cytometry of urine specimen (higher DNA content indicates more aggressive tumor).
   B. Serum carcinoembryonic antigen (CEA) levels are moderately elevated in 50% of late stage bladder cancer cases.

Nursing Diagnoses

I. Knowledge deficit.
II. Risk for infection (pyelonephritis).

III. Pain.
IV. Risk for impaired skin integrity.
V. Body image disturbance.
VI. Fluid volume deficit.
VII. Sexual dysfunction.

Outcome Identification

I. Client verbalizes an understanding of disease and rationale and outcomes of treatment.
II. Client explains the preoperative regimen; describes antibiotic regimen and sources of obtaining medications.
III. Client does not develop urinary tract infection.
IV. Client experiences pain relief.
V. Client's urine volume is normal.
VI. Client explains care at home following discharge including:
   A. Describes a viable stoma (i.e., pink and moist).
   B. Describes desired urinary output (>30 mL/hour).
   C. Lists the signs and symptoms of urinary tract infection and measures to prevent it.
   D. Describes strategies to prevent ammonia salt encrustation.
   E. Demonstrates pouch change.
   F. Describes the use of skin barriers.
   G. Demonstrates the steps of peristomal skin care.
   H. Describes potential changes in sexual functioning.
VII. Client describes schedule and rationale for aggressive follow-up care (as frequent as every 2 to 4 months for the first 3 years).
VIII. Client identifies selected resources—enterostomal therapy, home care, and support services (CanSurmount, American Cancer Society).

Planning and Implementation

I. Interventions to maximize safety for the client.
   A. Teach the client and family the importance of a low-residue diet 2 days before surgery, followed by clear liquid diet on the day before surgery.
   B. Teach the client and family the importance of using the prescribed antibiotics and cathartics before surgery (incomplete adherence to the preoperative regimen increases the risk of infection); unlike a fecal diversion that is subject to an adynamic ileus, the urinary diversion should produce urine from the time of surgery.
      1. Maintain current input and output records; the urinary flow should be rather continuous.
      2. Monitor for significant imbalances in weight and electrolyte values.
      3. Monitor for bleeding.
   C. Participate with or initiate referral to enterostomal therapist to assist in marking preoperative stomal site to avoid skin folds, scars, bony prominences, and belt lines that interfere with adherence of appliance.
      1. Consider vocational and recreational activities and visibility to the client when lying, sitting, standing.
      2. Preferable site is 3 inches in diameter, without folds or prominences, and slightly convex.

    D. Monitor signs of urinary tract infection—elevated temperature, flank pain, malodorous urine, and/or hematuria.

    E. Attach straight drainage bag to pouch when the client is in bed or at bedtime to prevent infections and damage to stomal tissue.

II. Interventions to decrease severity of symptoms (pain) associated with the disease and/or treatment.

    A. After evaluation of pain status, medicate client routinely for pain.

    B. Splint abdomen with pillow when the client is coughing.

    C. Position with pillows when turning the client.

III. Interventions to monitor for unique side effects of treatment.

    A. Monitor and document color of stoma through a clear pouch.

        1. Color of the intestinal stomal tissue can be compared to the mucosal lining of the mouth.

        2. Stoma may bleed when rubbed because of the capillaries in the area.

        3. Ideally, stoma should protude ½ to ¾ inch above the skin to allow the urine to drain into the aperture of the appliance.

        4. Normal color of the stoma is a deep pink to dark red; a dusky appearance ranging from purple to black may develop if circulation is seriously impaired.

    B. Assess the client for signs of peritonitis related to anastomotic leak.

        1. Abdominal distention or tenderness.

        2. Elevated temperature.

        3. Sudden decrease in urinary output or presence of abdominal wound drainage.

    C. Monitor urinary output—at least 30 mL/hour.

        1. Monitor for blood—should be clear within 2 days postoperatively.

        2. Decreased urine output may be a sign of obstruction of urinary drainage or renal failure.

        3. Stomal edema is normal in the early postoperative period.

        4. Edema should not interfere with stomal functioning, but a larger opening in appliances is needed initially to prevent pressure or constriction of the stoma.

        5. Edema should resolve during the first 1 or 2 weeks after surgery.

    D. Monitor placement of stents (usually in place 7 to 10 days postoperatively).

    E. Maintain patent nasogastric suction for 2 to 3 days postoperatively.

IV. Interventions to enhance adaptation and rehabilitation.

    A. Assess the client and family for signs of readiness to learn self-care of the stoma.

        1. Write all instructions.

        2. Encourage the client to observe pouch change and gradually to participate in self-care.

        3. Encourage the client and family to empty the pouch when ⅓ full.

        4. Follow-up with phone calls after discharge.

        5. Refer to the home health nursing agency if indicated.

    B. Teach the client and family care of the stoma and schedule return demonstrations until proper technique is achieved.

    C. Teach the client and family preventive elements of care (Table 23–7).

        1. Ways to avoid malodorous urine.

            a. Avoid ingestion of large quantities of alkaline liquids such as carbonated beverages.

            b. Drink fluids with high vitamin C content.

TABLE 23–7. **Management of Common Ileal Conduit Problems**

Problem	Interventions
Urinary odor	Avoid rubber pouch Soak appliance in vinegar/water 1:4
Rash around stoma or under pouch	Dry and powder skin except under adhesive Use a skin barrier, e.g., Stomahesive
Macerated skin around stoma	Dry skin and apply a hydroponic skin barrier Decrease size of pouch opening
Crystals on or around stoma	Apply vinegar compresses on stoma and inside pouch
Ulcerated stoma	Enlarge pouch opening Consult enterostomal therapist if not partially healed in 1 week
Monilial infection following antibiotic therapy	Dry skin and apply nystatin powder Encourage oral fluids
Hyperplasia of skin around stoma	Decrease pouch opening size
Fistula	Revision of stoma at new site

      c. Clean reusable pouch regularly with soap and water, rinsing with vinegar if desired.

      d. Avoid foods (e.g., fish, asparagus) that cause urinary odors.

  2. Ways to prevent urinary tract infection.

      a. Drink at least 2 L of fluid per day.

      b. Use straight drainage bag at bedtime and clean the system each morning.

  3. Ways to prevent ammonia salt encrustation—ingest food and fluid (cranberry juice) that keep the urine acid.

  4. Ways to prevent peristomal skin breakdown.

      a. Use a skin barrier if irritation is present.

      b. Use appropriate stoma opening in the barrier and the pouch.

      c. Remove pouch if burning or itching occurs.

      d. Change pouch on a regular basis (e.g., every 3 to 7 days).

      e. Do not use preparations that are greasy or that contain benzoin or alcohol on irritated skin.

  D. Arrange preoperative and/or postoperative visit by rehabilitated client with similar diversion.

Evaluation

    The oncology nurse systematically and regularly evaluates the client's and/or family's responses to interventions to determine progress toward the achievement of expected outcomes. Relevant data is collected and actual findings are compared with expected findings. Nursing diagnoses, outcomes, and plans of care are reviewed and revised as necessary.

PROSTATE CANCER

Theory

  I. Physiology and pathophysiology associated with prostatic cancer.

    A. Anatomy and physiology—the prostate is:

1. A small, firm organ made of glands and musculature enclosed in a fibrous capsule.
2. Approximately the size of a walnut (4 to 6 cm long).
3. Located posterior to the symphysis pubis, inferior to the bladder, and in front of the rectum (see Fig. 23–1).
4. Inverted so that the base is at the neck of the bladder, and is penetrated by a portion of the urethra (prostatic urethra).
5. Controlled by sex hormones (growth and function).
6. A secondary sex organ that secretes a component of seminal fluid.

B. Pathophysiology and metastatic patterns.
1. 95% are adenocarcinomas.
2. More common in the posterior lobe, although some researchers believe that the tumors are multifocal.
3. Grows and spreads locally to the seminal vesicles, bladder, and peritoneum (see Fig. 23–1).
4. Varies in histology and differentiation; most prostatic tumors are extremely slow-growing and indolent, but an unusually wide range of biologic malignancy exists.
5. May be detected accidentally and may never grow and spread (a minority of tumors).
6. Spreads via the blood vessels and lymphatic system.
   a. Spreads into the perineural lymphatics, involving the seminal vesicles and the sacral, external iliac, and lumbar lymph nodes.
   b. One third of men with early cancer have evidence of metastases to the pelvic lymph nodes.
   c. Clients with widespread cancer often have scalene or supraclavicular node involvement.
   d. Hematogenous spread of prostatic cancer typically involves the lung, liver, kidneys, and bones.

C. Trends in epidemiology.
1. A significant relative rise in incidence in past 10 years, probably the result of increased detection by prostatic specific antigen (PSA).
2. Accounts for approximately 30% of all cancer in men.
3. A significant increase in survival in white men, possibly because of improved screening.
4. Risk factors.
   a. Age.
      (1) More than 14% of men age 50 have cancer of prostate.
      (2) Some theorize that prostate cancer is normal part of the aging process since 95% of men who die over the age of 90 years have some foci of disease in the prostate at autopsy.
   b. Ethnicity.
      (1) Asians are at low risk; however, incidence increases markedly in those who adapt Western habits, particularly dietary ones.
      (2) Highest rate of prostatic cancer in the world is among African Americans; much lower in African blacks.

II. Principles of medical management.
A. Screening tests.
1. The digital rectal examination (DRE) is the most effective method of early detection. Rectal examination may reveal a small asymptomatic nodule (50% of prostatic nodules are malignant).

2. ACS recommends: annual digital examination for men over 40 years old, annual PSA test for men over 50 years old. If either is suspicious, transrectal ultrasound examination.

B. Diagnostic tests.
   1. Rectal examination by which the prostate may be palpated for firm, hard lesions.
   2. Biopsy.
      a. Fine-needle aspiration—perineal or transrectal; transrectal preferred.
      b. Open—in selected cases (i.e., if size of prostate demands removal).
   3. Histologic diagnosis—may be found in asymptomatic specimens removed for benign prostatic hypertrophy.
   4. Cytologic examination of urine and expressed prostatic fluid (result of which is positive in as many as 85% of men with prostate cancer).
   5. CT scans to diagnose pelvic lymph node involvement.
   6. MRI to determine involvement of the seminal vesicles and changes in the contour of the prostate.
   7. Laboratory studies.
      a. Acid phosphatase—elevated serum levels; trauma to prostate causes release into bloodstream.
         (1) Wait 48 hours after rectal examination or catheterization to draw serum for acid phosphatase study.
         (2) Elevated acid phosphatase level in a client suspected of having prostatic cancer may indicate metastatic disease.
      b. Prostatic acid phosphatase level can be measured by radioimmunoassay; 80% of men with stage D have increased levels.
      c. Alkaline phosphatase—elevated serum level.
         (1) Elevated in presence of bone metastasis.
         (2) Many clients with cancer of prostate have bone metastasis on presentation.
      d. PSA—increased levels may be significant as an adjunct in differential diagnosis or as a marker for disease progression.

C. Staging methods and procedures.
   1. Staging workup may include:
      a. Gleason pathologic grade with prostatic acid phosphatase level to help predict disease extension.
      b. Transrectal ultrasound and PSA to identify extracapsular extension and tumor volume.
      c. Chest x-ray examination to assess hilar node, lung, and rib involvement.
      d. Excretory urogram (see Table 23–1) to detect obstruction caused by pelvic lymph node metastasis or direct invasion by tumor.
      e. Liver scan and brain scan to detect distant metastases.
      f. CT scan to detect presence of pelvic lymph nodes.
      g. Bone scans to test for metastases to bones.
   2. Staging systems (Tables 23–8, 23–9, 23–10).

D. Standard therapies described by staging system (Jewett).
   1. Stage A.
      a. Because clients with untreated, well-differentiated, low-grade tumors are generally thought to have a 15-year survival rate comparable to that of men of the same age without prostate cancer, the disease may be left untreated.
         (1) Age of client and morbidity of treatment must be considered;

TABLE 23–8. **TNM Prostate Classification**

T = Primary Tumor

TX: Primary tumor cannot be assessed

T0:   No evidence of primary tumor

T1:   Clinically inapparent tumor not palpable or visible by imaging

T1a: Tumor incidental histologic finding in 5% or less of tissue resected

T1b: Tumor incidental histologic finding in more than 5% of tissue resected

T1c: Tumor identified by needle biopsy (e.g., because of elevated PSA).

T2:   Tumor confined within prostate*

T2a: Tumor involves half of a lobe or less

T2b: Tumor involves more than half of a lobe, but not both lobes

T2c: Tumor involves both lobes

T3:   Tumor extends through the prostatic capsule†

T3a: Unilateral extracapsular extension

T3b: Bilateral extracapsular extension

T3c: Tumor invades seminal vesicle(s)

T4:   Tumor is fixed or invades adjacent structures other than seminal vesicles

T4a: Tumor invades any of: bladder neck, external sphincter, or rectum

T4b: Tumor invades levator muscles and/or is fixed to pelvic wall

N = Regional Lymph Nodes

Regional lymph nodes are the nodes of the true pelvis, which essentially are the pelvic nodes below the bifurcation of the common iliac arteries. They include the following groups (laterality does not affect the N classification): pelvic (NOS), hypogastric, obturator, iliac (internal, external, NOS), periprostatic, and sacral (lateral, presacral, promontory [Gerota's], or NOS). Distant lymph nodes are outside the confines of the true pelvis and their involvement constitutes distant metastasis. They can be imaged using ultrasound, computed tomography, magnetic resonance imaging, or lymphangiography, and include: aortic (para-aortic, periaortic, lumbar), common iliac, inguinal, superficial inguinal (femoral), supraclavicular, cervical, scalene, and retroperitoneal (NOS) nodes.

NX: Regional lymph nodes cannot be assessed

N0:   No regional lymph node metastasis

N1:   Metastasis in a single lymph node, 2 cm or less in greatest dimension

N2:   Metastasis in a single lymph node, more than 2 cm but not more than 5 cm in greatest dimension; or multiple lymph node metastases, none more than 5 cm in greatest dimension

N3:   Metastasis in a lymph node more than 5 cm in greatest dimension

M = Distant Metastasis‡

MX: Presence of distant metastasis cannot be assessed

M0:   No distant metastasis

M1:   Distant metastasis

M1a: Nonregional lymph node(s)

M1b: Bone(s)

M1c: Other site(s)

Histopathologic Grade

GX: Grade cannot be assessed

G1:   Well differentiated (slight anaplasia)

TABLE 23–8. **TNM Prostate Classification** (*Continued*)

G2:	Moderately differentiated (moderate anaplasia)
G3–4:	Poorly differentiated or undifferentiated (marked anaplasia)

NOS, not otherwise specified.
*Tumor found in one or both lobes by needle biopsy, but not palpable or visible by imaging, is classified as T1c.
†Invasion into the prostatic apex or into (but not beyond) the prostatic capsule is not classified as T3, but as T2.
‡When more than one site of metastasis is present, the most advanced category (pM1c) is used.
From Montie, J.E. Staging of prostate cancer: Current TNM classification and future prospects for prognostic factors. *Cancer 75*(7suppl), 1814–1818, 1996. Copyright © 1996 American Cancer Society. Reprinted by permission of Wiley-Liss, Inc., subsidiary of John Wiley & Sons, Inc.

younger men with longer overall life expectancy often advised to seek more aggressive treatment.
    b. Common treatment for well-differentiated stage A tumors is radical perineal or retropubic prostatectomy, usually with pelvic lymphadenectomy.
    c. Radiation, with curative intent, also is used; should be delayed 4 to 6 weeks after transurethral resection to decrease incidence of stricture.
  2. Stage B.
    a. Surgery—radical prostatectomy for cure (with or without postoperative radiotherapy).
      (1) Perineal approach is generally treatment of choice.
      (2) Retropubic approach may be associated with lower incidence of urethral stricture formation.
      (3) Suprapubic approach may be used.
      (4) Walsh technique for radical retropubic prostatectomy minimizes

TABLE 23–9. **AJCC Stage Groupings of Prostate Cancer**

Stage 0
T1a, N0, M0, G1
Stage I
T1a, N0, M0, G2, 3–4
T1b, N0, M0, any G
T1c, N0, M0, any G
T1, N0, M0, any G
Stage II
T2, N0, M0, any G
Stage III
T3, N0, M0, any G
Stage IV
T4, N0, M0, any G
any T, N1, M0, any G
any T, N2, M0, any G
any T, N3, M0, any G
any T, any N, M1, any G

Used with permission of the American Joint Committee on Cancer (AJCC®), Chicago, Illinois. The original source for this material is the AJCC® *Manual for Staging of Cancer*, 4th edition (1992), published by Lippincott-Raven Publishers, Philadelphia.

TABLE 23–10. **Jewett Staging System of Prostate Cancer**

Stage A
Stage A is clinically undetectable tumor confined to the prostate gland and is an
  incidental finding at prostatic surgery
    Substage A1: well-differentiated with focal involvement, usually left untreated
    Substage A2: moderately or poorly differentiated or involves multiple foci in the gland
Stage B
Stage B is tumor confined to the prostate gland
    Substage B0: nonpalpable, PSA-detected
    Substage B1: single nodule in one lobe of the prostate
    Substage B2: more extensive involvement of one lobe or involvement of both lobes
Stage C
Stage C is a tumor clinically localized to the periprostatic area but extending through the
  prostatic capsule; seminal vesicles may be involved
    Substage C1: clinical extracapsular extension
    Substage C2: extracapsular tumor producing bladder outlet or ureteral obstruction
Stage D
Stage D is metastatic disease
    Substage D0: clinically localized disease (prostate only) but persistently elevated
      enzymatic serum acid phosphatase titers
    Substage D1: regional lymph nodes only
    Substage D2: distant lymph nodes, metastases to bone or visceral organs
    Substage D3: D2 prostate cancer patients who relapsed after adequate endocrine
      therapy

Used with permission of the American Joint Committee on Cancer (AJCC®), Chicago, Illinois. The
original source for this material is the AJCC® *Manual for Staging of Cancer,* 4th edition (1992),
published by Lippincott-Raven Publishers, Philadelphia.

damage to pelvic nerves needed to achieve erection and preserve potency.
  (5) Complications associated with surgical treatment.
      (a) Impotence, 60 to 90% with standard procedure, 25 to 60%
          with Walsh procedure.
      (b) Incontinence or dribbling (in 6 to 30% of patients).
      (c) Stricture formation in urethra.
  b. Lymph node dissection usually performed with prostatectomy.
  c. Radiation therapy is becoming more widely used.
    (1) Reported lower incidence of impotence than with surgery.
    (2) Types of radiation used.
      (a) External beam therapy of 6000 to 7000 cGy to extended
          field—25 to 30% have gradual loss of erectile function within
          6 to 12 months.
      (b) Interstitial implants (temporary or permanent)—lower inci-
          dence of impotence reported than with external beam source.
    (3) Complications associated with radiation therapy.
      (a) Acute cystitis.
      (b) Proctitis.
      (c) Impotence.
  3. Stage C.
    a. External beam radiation therapy, started 4 to 6 weeks after transure-
       thral resection.
    b. Radical prostatectomy usually with pelvic lymphadenectomy in highly
       selected patients.

    c. Symptomatic treatment because some stage C patients have urinary symptoms; can be done by radiation, radical surgery, transurethral radical prostatectomy (TURP), or hormonal manipulation.

4. Stage D.
    a. Hormonal manipulation—to counter effects of male hormones (androgens); prompt initiation for palliation may prevent or alleviate symptoms.
       (1) Orchiectomy—surgical removal of testicles; used for prompt response, for clients unreliable in taking medications, or for clients in whom side effects of estrogens contraindicate continued use.
       (2) Luteinizing hormone-releasing hormones (LHRH analogues; e.g., leuprolide, goserelin)—decrease production of testosterone; may produce fewer side effects than estrogens, used with flutamide to reduce "flare."
       (3) Antiandrogens (cyproterone acetate, megestrol acetate, flutamide)—interferes with intracellular androgen activity; effects may be delayed 1 to 2 months.
       (4) Estrogen therapy—generally diethylstilbestrol (DES), results in decreased pain, weight gain, decreased tumor size, decreased urinary symptoms.
       (5) Complications associated with hormonal therapy.
          (a) Orchiectomy—psychological trauma as a result of surgical castration.
          (b) LHRH analogues—initial testosterone "flare" may increase symptoms (bone pain and/or urinary difficulty), subsequent side effects include hot flashes, loss of libido, impotence, gynecomastia.
          (c) Estrogen—breast enlargement (gynecomastia), sodium retention, cardiovascular complications (pulmonary edema, congestive heart failure), and relapse (usually within 2 to 3 years) to hormone-resistant form.
    b. Radiation therapy—for local extension and distant metastases.
       (1) May be primary treatment for stage D lesions if hormonal manipulation is ineffective or contraindicated.
       (2) Used for palliation of pain from bone metastasis.
       (3) Emergency treatment for spinal cord compression.

E. Trends in survival.
  1. Localized—5-year survival rate, 94%.
  2. Metastatic disease—usual prognosis, 1 to 2 year survival.
  3. Survival for all stages combined, 80%.

Assessment

I. Pertinent personal and family history.
  A. Age.
  B. Ethnicity.
  C. Exposure to cadmium (which may accumulate in prostate, and is associated with higher incidence.)

II. Physical examination.
  A. Subjective data.
    1. Early disease—dysuria, hesitancy, straining to start stream; weak urinary stream, nocturia, dribbling, urgency, sensation of incomplete voiding.

    2. Advanced disease—lumbosacral back pain, migratory back pain, lethargy.
  B. Objective data.
    1. Early disease—on DRE, nonraised firm nodule with sharp edge, also may be induration, asymmetry.
    2. Advanced disease—on DRE, hard and stone-like nodule, may be induration, hematuria, weight loss, and secondary disease (e.g., bronchopneumonia).
III. Evaluation of laboratory data.
  A. Elevated serum alkaline phosphatase level.
  B. Elevated serum acid phosphatase level.
  C. Elevated prostatic acid phosphatase level.
  D. Elevated PSA level.

Nursing Diagnoses

  I. Urinary incontinence, functional.
  II. Sexual dysfunction.
  III. Self-care deficit: toileting.
  IV. Urinary elimination, altered.
  V. Altered tissue perfusion: cardiopulmonary.

Outcome Identification

  I. Client lists signs and symptoms of immediate and long-term side effects of treatment—wound infection, fecal incontinence, sexual dysfunction (impotence, decreased libido), urinary bleeding, urinary incontinence, urinary tract infection, side effects of hormonal therapy.
  II. Client demonstrates self-care measures to decrease incidence and severity of symptoms associated with disease and treatment.
    A. Exercises to strengthen perineal muscles and decrease urinary dribbling or incontinence.
    B. Drinks 2 L of fluid daily.
    C. Seeks sexual counseling if problem is present.
  III. Client identifies a follow-up schedule of every 6 months to every year (or as prescribed).
  IV. Client lists signs and symptoms of recurrent disease.
    A. Bone pain.
    B. Further changes in urinary habits.
    C. Abdominal pain.
  V. Client identifies resources to assist with responses to disease and treatment—American Cancer Society, the National Cancer Institute.

Planning and Implementation

  I. Interventions to maximize safety for client.
    A. Maintain closed urinary catheter drainage system and aseptic technique during irrigation to prevent infection.
    B. Maintain patency of urinary and/or bladder irrigation systems; risk of blockage greatest first 3 hours after surgery.
      1. Maintain continuous or intermittent bladder irrigation to remove blood clot and/or mucous plugs.
      2. Avoid kinked tubing by positioning of client and securing of tubes.

C. Apply antiembolic hose; teach client proper application technique.
D. Maintain positioning and patency of urethral catheter (serves as splint for urethral anastomosis and for bladder drainage after radical prostatectomy); usually left in place 2 to 3 weeks.
E. Facilitate healing of perineal wound (with perineal prostatectomy):
   1. Irrigate wound.
   2. Provide sitz baths.
   3. Apply heat lamp to perineum.
   4. Minimize pressure on perineal wound:
      a. Administer low-residue diet and stool softeners to avoid straining at stool.
      b. Avoid and teach client to avoid use of rectal tubes, rectal thermometers, or enemas until healing is complete.
      c. Bed rest may be extended to lessen pressure on suture line.
F. Protect skin integrity (e.g., use of T-binder versus tape to hold dressing in place after perineal prostatectomy.
G. Assess for symptoms of hypercalcemia (polyuria, polydipsia, confusion, weakness), pulmonary edema, congestive heart failure if initiation of hormonal therapy with DES (see Chapters 15, 16, and 17).

II. Interventions to promote comfort.
   A. Administer antispasmodics and/or analgesics for bladder spasms; initiate use of stool softeners with antispasmodics to avoid constipation.
   B. Consult with enterostomal therapist as indicated for perineal wound care, radiation reactions, or management of incontinence.
   C. Administer antidiarrheal medications as ordered for proctitis and teach client to avoid a high-residue diet.

III. Interventions to monitor and decrease incidence or severity of symptoms of prostatic cancer or recurrence.
   A. Teach client to report symptoms of urinary obstruction promptly— diminished stream, abdominal pain and distention, dysuria, retention with dribbling, bladder spasms.
   B. Teach client to report early symptoms of urinary tract infection—fever, dysuria, urgency, hematuria.
   C. Teach client to report symptoms of recurrence—hematuria, urinary obstruction, bone pain, abdominal pain, neuritic pain, weight loss, debilitation, back pain.
   D. Describe follow-up schedule as determined by physician.

IV. Interventions to monitor effects of treatment of prostatic cancer.
   A. Facilitate physician-nurse-client discussion of potential impact of treatment on sexual functioning and interventions to minimize effects.
      1. Give permission before and after treatment to discuss functional and anatomical changes with treatment and resultant sexual concerns (having testicles removed as an adult does not affect masculinity).
      2. Provide information on potential effects of treatment (e.g., impotence after radical prostatectomy; feminization after hormonal therapy).
      3. Provide specific suggestions related to treatment used and alternatives (e.g., penile implants after radical prostatectomy; testicular implants after orchiectomy; or to ask physician if alternative hormonal therapy may be used if estrogens cause severe decrease in libido).
      4. Initiate referral for sexual counseling if indicated.

    B. Record amount and frequency of voiding after removal of urethral catheter.

    C. Inform clients to report lymphedema of legs, scrotum, or penis after lymph node dissection.

    D. Teach clients symptoms of proctitis, which may occur with radiotherapy—diarrhea, cramps, rectal pain.

    E. Teach side effects of hormonal therapy (edema, mood changes) as indicated; possible therapies (fluid restriction, diuretics); and need for continued medical follow-up for laboratory tests (serum sodium and calcium levels) and blood pressure monitoring.

V. Interventions to enhance adaptation and rehabilitation.

    A. Teach care of Foley catheter, three-way irrigation equipment, or other equipment.

    B. Instruct client to drink at least 2 L of fluid per day to alleviate cystitis associated with radiotherapy.

    C. Initiate appropriate referrals for home care (e.g., visiting nurse, enterostomal therapist).

    D. Teach perineal exercises to manage dribbling, urgency, or urinary incontinence (in most cases, problem gradually diminishes).

VI. Interventions to incorporate the client/family in care.

    A. Assess resources and coping strategies of the client/family.

    B. Incorporate personal and cultural values of the client/family in discussing sexual concerns.

        1. Respect reticence in discussing sexual concerns (most clients are elderly and socialized not to discuss sexuality).

        2. Use terminology appropriate to social and cultural level.

        3. Provide written information and anatomic drawings as indicated for clarity and to reinforce teaching.

    C. Identify resources, as needed, for home care, follow-up, reconstructive treatment, or palliation.

Evaluation

The oncology nurse systematically and regularly evaluates the client's and/or family's responses to interventions to determine progress toward the achievement of expected outcomes. Relevant data are collected and actual findings are compared with expected findings. Nursing diagnoses, outcomes, and plans of care are reviewed and revised as necessary.

BIBLIOGRAPHY

Bono, A.V. (1994). Superficial bladder cancer: State of the art. *Cancer Chemother Pharmocol 35*(suppl.), S101–S109.

Chodak, G.W., Thisted, R.A., Gerber, G.S., et al. (1994). Results of conservative management of clinically localized prostate cancer. *N Engl J Med 330*(4), 242–248.

Davis, M. (1993). Renal cell carcinoma. *Semin Oncol Nurs 9*(4), 267–271.

Esrig, D., Freeman, J., Stein, J., & Skinner, E. (1995). Surgery in the management of bladder cancer. *Compr Ther 21*(1), 20–24.

Gnarra, J., Lerman, M., Zbar, B., & Linehan, W.M. (1995). Genetics of renal cell carcinoma and evidence for a critical role for von Hippel-Lindau in renal tumorigenesis. *Semin Oncol 22*(1), 3–8.

Hossan, E., & Striegel, A. (1993). Carcinoma of the bladder. *Semin Oncol Nurs 9*(4), 252–266.

Hostetler, R.M., Mandel, I.G., & Marshburn, J. (1996). Prostate cancer screening. *Med Clin North Am 80*(1), 83–98.

Lind, J., Kravitz, K., & Grieg, B. (1993). Urologic and male genital malignancies. In S.L. Groenwald, M.H. Frogge, M. Goodman, C.H. Yarbro (eds.). *Cancer Nursing Principles and Practice* (3rd ed.). Boston: Jones & Bartlett, pp. 1258–1315.

Long, B.C., Phipps, W.J., & Cassmeyer, V.L. (eds.). (1993). *Medical-surgical Nursing: A Nursing Process Approach* (4th ed.). St. Louis: C.V. Mosby, pp. 1047–1065.

McFarlene, M., deKernion, J., & Figlin, R. (1993). Neoplasms of the bladder. In J.F. Holland, & E. Frei (eds.). *Cancer Medicine* (3rd ed.). Malvern, PA: Lea & Febiger, p. 1546.

McLeod, D.G., & Kolvenbag, G.J. (1996). Defining the role of antiandrogens in the treatment of prostate cancer. *Urology 47*(1A), 95–96.

McLeod, D.G., & Moul, J.W. (1995). Controversies in the treatment of prostate cancer with maximal androgen deprivation. *Surg Oncol Clin North Am 4*(2), 345–359.

Mandelson, M.T., Wager, E.H., & Thompson, R.S. (1995). PSA screening: A public health dilemma. *Annu Rev Public Health 16,* 283–306.

Maxwell, M.B. (1993). Cancer of the prostate. *Semin Oncol Nurs 9*(4), 237–251.

Novick, A.C. (1995). Current surgical approaches, nephron-sparing surgery, and the role of surgery in the integrated immunologic approach to renal cell carcinoma. *Semin Oncol 22*(1), 29–33.

Ofman, U.S. (1993). Psychosocial and sexual implications of genitourinary cancers. *Semin Oncol Nurs 9*(4), 286–292.

Palmer, L.S., Laor, E., & Skinner, W.K., et al. (1995). Prostate cancer screening using fine-needle aspiration cytology prior to open prostatectomy. *Eur Urol 27*(2), 96–98.

Potosky, A.L., Miller, B.A., & Albertsen, P.C., et al. (1995). The role of increasing detection in the rising incidence of prostate cancer. *JAMA 273*(7), 548–552.

Razor, B.R. (1993). Continent urinary reservoirs. *Semin Oncol Nurs 9*(4), 272–285.

Richie, J. (1993). Renal cell carcinoma. In J.F. Holland, & E. Frei (eds.). *Cancer Medicine* (3rd ed.). Malvern, PA: Lea & Febiger, pp. 1529–1545.

Slawin, K.M., Ohori, M., Dillioglugil, O., et al. (1995). Screening for prostate cancer: An analysis of the early experience. *CA Cancer J Clin 45*(3), 134–147.

Taneja, S.S., Pierce, W., Figlin, R., & Belldegrun, A. (1994). Management of disseminated kidney cancer. *Urol Clin North Am 21*(4), 625–637.

Trump, D.L., & Robertson, C.N. (1993). Neoplasms of the prostate. In J.F. Holland, & E. Frei (eds.). *Cancer Medicine* (3rd ed.). Malvern, PA: Lea & Febiger, pp. 1562–1586.

Zietman, A.L., Coen, J.J., Dallow, K.C., et al. (1995). The treatment of prostate cancer by conventional radiation therapy: An analysis of long-term outcome. *Int J Radiat Oncol Biol Phys 32*(2), 287–292.

24

Nursing Care of the Client With Lung Cancer

Julena Lind, RN, MN

Theory

I. Physiology and pathophysiology associated with lung cancer.
   A. Anatomy—see Figure 24–1 for schematic representation of the lungs, locations, and presenting symptoms of various types of tumors.
   B. Primary functions of the lungs are air exchange and filtering of microparticles from the air.
      1. Normal bronchial epithelial cells serve as a lining and have a protective function.
      2. Columnar epithelial cells line the tracheobronchial tree from the trachea to the terminal bronchioles.
      3. Columnar cells consist of ciliated cells that filter particles from the air and mucous-secreting cells that facilitate clearance of particles from the lungs.
   C. Changes associated with cancer.
      1. Long-term exposure to cigarette smoke or irritants such as coal dust damage the ciliated cells and mucus-producing cells and result in replacement by dysplastic cells.
      2. If the irritation continues, the atypia of the epithelial cells progresses to nuclear enlargement, nuclear variability, hyperchromatism, and abnormal mitotic activity.
   D. Histologic types.
      1. Small cell lung cancer (SCLC)—most rapidly growing.
         a. Oat cell.
         b. Intermediate.
         c. Mixed (small cell combined with other cell types of lung carcinoma).
      2. Non-small cell lung cancer (NSCLC)
         a. Epidermoid (squamous cell)—incidence decreasing.
            (1) Spindle cell variant.
         b. Adenocarcinoma—incidence increasing; most common type.
            (1) Acinar.
            (2) Papillary.
            (3) Bronchoalveolar.
            (4) Solid tumor with mucin.
         c. Large cell.
            (1) Giant cell.
            (2) Clear cell.

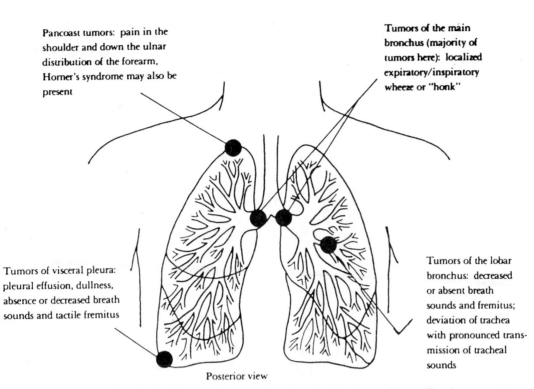

Pancoast tumors: pain in the shoulder and down the ulnar distribution of the forearm, Horner's syndrome may also be present

Tumors of the main bronchus (majority of tumors here): localized expiratory/inspiratory wheeze or "honk"

Tumors of visceral pleura: pleural effusion, dullness, absence or decreased breath sounds and tactile fremitus

Tumors of the lobar bronchus: decreased or absent breath sounds and fremitus; deviation of trachea with pronounced transmission of tracheal sounds

Posterior view

Figure 24–1. Anatomic relationships and tumor locations in the lung. (From Frank-Stromborg, M., & Cohen, R. [1990]. Assessment and interventions for cancer prevention and detection. In S. Groenwald, M.H. Frogge, M. Goodman, & C.H. Yarbro [eds.]. *Cancer Nursing Principles and Practice.* Boston: Jones & Bartlett, p. 128.)

E. Presentation and metastatic patterns (see Figure 24–1).
   1. Squamous cell carcinoma typically arises in segmental bronchi and grows exophytically, causing bronchial obstruction or involvement of the adjacent lymph nodes.
   2. Adenocarcinomas usually are located peripherally and spread more diffusely to brain, bones, other lung, and liver.
   3. Small cell cancer usually occurs endobronchially in a segmental bronchus; however, because of its aggressiveness, hilar and mediastinal nodes are involved in 80% of cases at presentation.
   4. Large cell lung cancer usually presents as bulky peripheral tumors and spreads as peripheral masses before metastasizing to brain, bones, adrenal glands, and liver.
   5. In general, a 3 : 2 ratio of involvement of right versus left lung is reported.
F. Trends in epidemiology.
   1. Lung cancer is the leading cause of cancer incidence and cancer death for both men and women in the U.S.
   2. The incidence rate for men is declining and is currently 80 in 100,000. The incidence rate for women is increasing and is currently 42 in 100,000.
   3. Lung cancer rates started to decline in young white men ages 35 to 44 years in the 1970s and in white men 55 to 64 in the 1980s; incidence and mortality are increasing in all other groups.
   4. Increase in lung cancer deaths in women is attributed to the increase in the number of women smoking.
   5. Tobacco smoking accounts for approximately 90% of lung cancer and is closely associated with all histologic types.

6. In addition to being a carcinogen, tobacco smoke promotes the carcinogenic effect of other carcinogens.
7. Smoking cessation is associated with a gradual decrease in the risk of lung cancer, but 5 or more years must elapse before an appreciable decrease in risk occurs.
8. Environmental and occupational factors.
   a. Asbestos exposure has been linked to the incidence of lung cancer (especially mesothelioma) in shipyard workers, miners, and pipe fitters.
   b. Uranium miners appear to have a particularly high incidence of small cell cancer of the lung (probably caused by radon, which is a radioactive gas that exists in the atmosphere).
   c. Indoor exposure to radon seems to present a risk for lung cancer, but current epidemiologic studies are inconclusive in estimating risks of exposure to radon gas.

II. Principles of medical management.
   A. Screening tests.
      1. No reliable screening or early detection methods exist.
      2. Chest x-ray examinations, lung health questionnaires, and sputum cytology at regular intervals are ineffective in screening.
   B. Diagnostic tests.
      1. Tests to determine the size, histology, and location of the primary tumor.
         a. Chest x-ray examination.
         b. Thoracic computed tomographic (CT) scan (has revolutionized staging) (Table 24–1).
         c. Lung tomography.
         d. Flexible fiberoptic bronchoscopy (with brush or needle biopsy) (Table 24–1).
         e. Transthoracic fine-needle aspiration biopsy.
      2. Tests that aid in determining the lymph node involvement.
         a. Mediastinoscopy generally used for patients for whom CT scan shows mediastinal lymph nodes larger than 1.5 cm (Table 24–1).
         b. Scalene node biopsy.
         c. Hilar tomography.
      3. Tests that aid in detecting distant metastases.
         a. Liver and spleen scans.
         b. Bone scan.
         c. CT scan of the brain.
         d. Thoracentesis (to detect tumor cells in pleural fluid).
   C. Staging methods and procedures.
      1. Stage I, II, III, IV (Table 24–2).
      2. TNM system (Table 24–3).
      3. Performance scales that measure physical status (see Table 19–6).
      4. Procedures as outlined above under Diagnostic Tests.
   D. Treatment options by stage.
      1. Small cell cancer of the lung.
         a. Limited stage.
            (1) Combination chemotherapy and chest irradiation (with or without prophylactic cranial irradiation [PCI] given to clients with complete responses).
            (2) Combination chemotherapy (with or without PCI given to clients with complete responses); especially for clients with impaired pulmonary function or poor performance status.
            (3) Surgical resection of pulmonary tumor in highly selected cases, followed by combination chemotherapy with or without PCI.

TABLE 24–1. **Nursing Care Related to Pulmonary Tests**

Procedure	Physical Alteration	Intervention
Bronchoscopy—to localize and/or perform a biopsy on a lesion		
Local anesthetic (duration 2–8 hr)	Gag reflex	Give client nothing by mouth Maintain flat or semi-Fowler's position
Hyperextended neck	Tension on neck muscles and vertebrae	Apply ice collar first 24 hrs, then heat Provide lozenges and gargles when gag reflex returns Administer analgesics if pain is severe
Insertion of bronchoscope	Laryngeal edema Possible laryngospasms Possible brochospasms	Observe for and report respiratory distress Administer oxygen Administer bronchodilator
Possible biopsy (brush or needle)	Possible bleeding and/or infection Possible pneumothorax	Observe and report: Hemoptysis Symptoms of upper respiratory infection Report dyspnea, decreased breath sounds, cyanosis Administer oxygen
Mediastinoscopy—to evaluate lymph node involvement		
General anesthetic		Give client nothing by mouth before and after procedure
Insertion of scope into intercostal space	Manipulation of trachea Possible air leaks into skin Possible pneumothorax Possible bleeding Possible mediastinitis	Administer analgesics as needed Palpate for crepitus Report dyspnea, decreased breath sounds, cyanosis Administer oxygen Check dressing Report fever, cough
Thoracic Computed Tomographic (CT) Scan—to localize lesion and/or detect node involvement		
Serial x-ray examinations of sectional planes of thorax and computer analysis to provide three-dimensional studies of the tissue	Noninvasive; client to lie still; rotation of large machine, making clicking noises, around client	Instruct client that procedure is painless Tell client what to expect
Possible use of contrast media containing iodides and/or radioactive materials	Intravenous administration Possible adverse reactions to contrast media Possible hypersensitivity to contrast media (rare)	Warn client of immediate sensations of warmth, flushing, bitter or salty taste, nausea/vomiting, and itching and that pain at insertion site may occur Perform cardiopulmonary resuscitation Follow emergency procedures.

TABLE 24–2. **Stage Grouping
of Carcinoma of the Lung**

Defined By the Following TNM Group:
Stage 0
Tis, N0, M0
Stage I
T1, N0, M0
T2, N0, M0
Stage II
T1, N1, M0
T2, N1, M0
Stage III
T1, N2, M0
T2, N2, M0
T3, N0, M0
T3, N1, M0
T3, N2, M0
Stage IIIb
any T, N3, M0
T4, any N, M0
Stage IV
any T, any N, M1

Used with permission of the American Joint Committee on Cancer (AJCC®), Chicago, Illinois. The original source for this material is the AJCC® *Manual for Staging of Cancer,* 4th edition (1992), published by Lippincott-Raven Publishers, Philadelphia.

   b. Extensive stage.
     (1) Combination chemotherapy (with or without PCI).
     (2) Combination chemotherapy and chest irradiation with or without PCI.
     (3) Radiotherapy to sites of metastatic disease that are unlikely to be palliated by chemotherapy (brain, bone, epidural).
2. Non-small cell cancer of the lung.
   a. Stage I.
     (1) Lobectomy or segmental resection.
     (2) Radiotherapy with curative intent for potentially resectable patients who have medical contraindications to surgery.
     (3) Clinical trials of adjuvant chemotherapy following resection.
   b. Stage II.
     (1) Lobectomy, pneumonectomy, or segmental resection.
     (2) Radiotherapy with curative intent for potentially operable tumors in clients who have medical contraindications to surgery.
     (3) Radiotherapy combined with curative surgery.
     (4) Hyperfractionated radiotherapy with or without chemotherapy.
     (5) Adjuvant chemotherapy combined with other modalities.
   c. Stage IIIA.
     (1) Surgery alone in highly selected cases.
     (2) Chemotherapy combined with other modalities.
     (3) Surgery and radiotherapy.
     (4) Radiotherapy alone.
   d. Stage IIIB.
     (1) Radiotherapy alone.
     (2) Chemotherapy combined with radiotherapy.

TABLE 24–3. **TNM Classification Carcinoma of the Lung**

T = Primary Tumor

TX: Primary tumor cannot be assessed or tumor proven by the presence of malignant cells in sputum or bronchial washings but not visualized by imaging or bronchoscopy

T0: No evidence of primary tumor

TIS: Carcinoma in situ

T1: A tumor that is 3.0 cm or less in greatest diameter, surrounded by lung or visceral pleura, and without evidence of invasion more proximal than the lobar bronchus (i.e., not in the main bronchus)*

T2: A tumor with any of the following features of size or extent:
More than 3.0 cm in greatest dimension
Involving the main bronchus, 2.0 cm or more distal to the carina
Invading the visceral pleura
Associated with atelectasis or obstructive pneumonitis that extends to the hilar region but does not involve the entire lung

T3: A tumor of any size with direct extension to the chest wall (including superior sulcus tumors), diaphragm, mediastinal pleura, parietal pericardium; a tumor in the main bronchus less than 2.0 cm distal to the carina but without involvement of the carina; associated atelectasis or obstructive pneumonitis of the entire lung

T4: A tumor of any size that invades any of the following: mediastinum, heart, great vessels, trachea, esophagus, vertebral body, carina; or tumor with a malignant pleural effusion†

N = Nodal Involvement

NX: Regional lymph nodes cannot be assessed

N0: No regional lymph node metastasis

N1: Metastasis in ipsilateral peribronchial and/or ipsilateral hilar lymph nodes, including direct extension

N2: Metastasis in ipsilateral mediastinal and/or subcarinal lymph node(s)

N3: Metastasis in contralateral mediastinal, contralateral hilar, ipsilateral or contralateral scalene, or supraclavicular lymph node(s)

M = Distant Metastasis

MX: Presence of distant metastasis cannot be assessed

M0: No distant metastasis

M1: Distant metastasis (beyond the ipsilateral supraclavicular nodes)

Occult Stage by TNM Group

TX, N0, M0 (Bronchopulmonary secretions contain malignant cells on multiple samples but no other evidence of the primary tumor or evidence of metastasis to the regional lymph nodes or distant metastasis is found.)

*Note: The uncommon superficial tumor of any size with its invasive component limited to the bronchial wall, which may extend proximal to the main bronchus, is also classified as T1.

†Note: In the few patients for whom multiple cytopathologic examinations of pleural fluid are negative for tumor (i.e., fluid is non-bloody and is not an exudate), and clinical judgment dictates that the effusion is not related to the tumor, the effusion should be excluded as a staging element and the patient should be staged as T1, T2, or T3.

Used with permission of the American Joint Committee on Cancer (AJCC®), Chicago, Illinois. The original source for this material is the AJCC® *Manual for Staging of Cancer,* 4th edition (1992), published by Lippincott-Raven Publishers, Philadelphia.

      (3) Chemotherapy and concurrent radiotherapy followed by resection.
      (4) Chemotherapy alone.
  E. Surgery—treatment of choice for cure for non-small cell cancer of the lung.
    1. Lobectomy—removal of a lobe of the lung; associated with lower morbidity and mortality rates than pneumonectomy; generally the preferred treatment for small tumors.
    2. Pneumonectomy—removal of one lung; higher incidence of perfusion and ventilation problems, circulatory overload, and pulmonary hypertension.
    3. Contraindications to curative surgery (thoracotomy).
      a. Metastasis outside the lung.
      b. Scalene node metastasis.
      c. Metastasis to the other lung.
      d. Inadequate pulmonary function.
    4. In the general population only approximately 50% of lung cancer clients are candidates for curative surgery; but about one half of those people do not have a resection after the opening of the chest because of metastasis found during surgery.
  F. Radiotherapy; external beam radiotherapy may be used.
    1. Alone with curative intent for Stage I or II non-small cell lung cancer if lung function is impaired or other conditions preclude surgery.
      a. 5500 to 6000 cGy to midplane of tumor.
    2. As adjuvant to surgery, either preoperatively or postoperatively; the effect on survivorship is controversial.
    3. As prophylactic cranial irradiation (PCI) to prevent or retard the incidence of brain metastases in small cell lung cancer (a retrospective study that revealed the high incidence of central nervous system [CNS] toxicity associated with prophylactic cranial irradiation raises questions about the value of this treatment or therapy). Adding PCI does not improve overall survival.
    4. As palliation for control of symptoms associated with lung cancer (severe cough, hemoptysis, pain, obstructive pneumonitis, superior vena cava syndrome) or to prolong the functional life of the client.
  G. Chemotherapy.
    1. Treatment of choice for small cell lung cancer.
      a. Improves survival rates (12- to 18-month median survival with chemotherapy versus 6 to 8 weeks without).
      b. Has been combined with cranial irradiation to improve survival.
      c. The following combinations produce similar survival.
        (1) Etoposide-cisplatin or carboplatin.
        (2) Cyclophosphamide-doxorubicin-vincristine.
        (3) Cyclophosphamide-doxorubicin-etoposide.
        (4) Ifosfamide-carboplatin-etoposide.
    2. May be used as adjuvant therapy in non-small cell lung cancer.
      a. Not shown to improve survival.
      b. May improve disease-free survival.
      c. May be combined with surgery or radiotherapy.
      d. Cisplatin-based combinations generally used (e.g., cyclophosphamide-doxorubicin-cisplatin).
    3. Commonly used for advanced disease.
      a. Generally yields frequent but brief response rates (up to 40% in some studies).
      b. Cisplatin-based combinations generally used.
  H. Trends in survival.
    1. Overall survival rate at 5 years for lung cancer is only 13% in all clients.
    2. Five-year survival rate is 47% when disease is still localized, but only 15% of cases are detected that early.

    3. Survival depends on the size, location, and extent of metastases at the time of diagnosis.

    4. Survival rates have improved only slightly over the past 10 years.

Assessment

  I. Pertinent personal and environmental history (risk factors).

    A. Tobacco use (number of packs per day multiplied by number of years smoked).

      1. At highest risk are people over 45 who have smoked two or more packs per day for 10 years or more (20 pack years).

      2. Mortality rates for 20-pack-year persons are 15 to 25 times higher than for nonsmokers.

    B. Occupational and environmental exposures (asbestos, uranium, radon).

    C. Onset and duration of symptoms, including client's understanding of disease and treatment.

 II. Physical examination (client may be asymptomatic).

    A. Pulmonary manifestations.

      1. Cough.

      2. Hemoptysis.

      3. Dyspnea.

      4. Pneumonia.

    B. Local manifestations (related to the growth of tumor and compression of adjacent structures).

      1. Shoulder pain.

      2. Arm pain.

      3. Superior vena cava syndrome (distention of arm and neck veins; facial, neck, and arm edema; suffusion of mucous membranes).

III. Evaluation of laboratory data.

    A. Metabolic complications (small cell especially).

      1. Elevated antidiuretic hormone (ADH) level (because of ADH-mimic produced by the tumor).

      2. Elevated adrenocorticotropic hormone (ACTH) level (because of ACTH-mimic produced by the tumor).

    B. Blood gas values.

    C. Pulmonary functions test results.

      1. FEV_1 greater than 70%, lung function normal.

      2. FEV_1 35 to 70%, mild to moderate ventilatory impairment.

      3. FEV_1 less than 35%, severe ventilatory impairment.

Nursing Diagnoses

    I. Knowledge deficit about the disease and its treatment.

   II. Anxiety.

 III. Pain.

 IV. Impaired gas exchange.

  V. Impaired tissue integrity.

 VI. Ineffective airway clearance.

VII. Anticipatory grieving.

VIII. Risk for fluid volume excess.

Outcome Identification

  I. Client verbalizes risks of smoking and the benefits of quitting.

 II. Client experiences pain relief.

   III. Client demonstrates normal respiratory status.

   IV. Client demonstrates optimal gas exchange.

   V. Client explains regimen to follow after discharge, including:

     A. Demonstrates postural drainage techniques.

     B. Demonstrates the use of oxygen or other equipment.

     C. Demonstrates exercise program.

     D. Explains any changes required in lifestyle.

     E. Describes plans for follow-up care.

   VI. Client identifies external and internal factors that increase risk of upper respiratory infection—exposure to crowds; inadequate rest, nutrition, or hydration.

   VII. Client lists signs and symptoms of upper respiratory infection—fever, cough, expectoration (yellow or green in color).

   VIII. Client identifies side effects of radiation therapy and methods to treat side effects.

   IX. Client identifies side effects of chemotherapy and methods to treat side effects.

   X. Client verbalizes indicators of hope (constitutional, psychological, and prognostic).

   XI. Client lists signs and symptoms of metastatic disease.

   XII. Client lists resources available for lung cancer clients.

     A. Local American Cancer Society (e.g., *Facts on Lung Cancer*).

     B. Local American Lung Association.

     C. Local hospice organizations.

     D. Visiting nurse agencies.

     E. National Cancer Institute (e.g., *What You Need to Know About Lung Cancer*).

     F. Cancer Hotline 1-800-4-CANCER.

     G. Internet Cancer Information Web Sites: National Cancer Institute (NCI), other large cancer centers.

     H. Local support groups.

Planning and Implementation

   I. Postoperative interventions to maximize client safety by prevention and detection of hemorrhage, pneumothorax, and/or mediastinal shift.

     A. Check the chest tube drainage system (if present; chest tubes are not necessary for clients post-pneumonectomy) for obstruction every 1 to 2 hours; observe and document:

       1. Absence of fluctuations in the waterseal chamber.

       2. Lack of drainage fluid in the drainage tubing or collection chamber.

     B. Reposition the chest tube drainage tubing as frequently as necessary.

       1. Secure chest tubes with a tight dressing.

       2. Minimize chest tube movement by securing tubes to body.

     C. Examine the drainage tubing and connections for clots and/or debris.

     D. Assess the drainage system for breaks in the system every 8 hours and as needed; document findings; immediately report:

       1. Continuous large amount of bubbling in the waterseal chamber.

       2. "Air leak" noises in the system.

     E. Assess for cause of air leak by checking:

       1. For occlusive seal at the insertion site.

       2. To determine if the chest tube has moved; if so, notify physician.

       3. For an improper fit at the connector site.

       4. For a defect in the equipment.

     F. Auscultate and document breath sounds every 2 to 4 hours.

    G. Monitor and document early signs of respiratory distress—increased respiratory rate, nasal flaring, use of accessory muscles.

    H. Instruct the client to report increase in shortness of breath.

    I. Document client teaching.

    J. Assess and document signs of pneumothorax every 2 to 4 hours—absent breath sounds unilaterally, tracheal deviation, increased shortness of breath.

    K. Obtain chest x-ray examination and blood gas values as ordered and monitor reports.

    L. Monitor position of trachea and report shift from midline.

    M. Avoid deep suctioning that may cause trauma to suture line.

II. Interventions to decrease severity of symptoms associated with the disease and/or treatment.

    A. Interventions related to surgical treatment.

        1. Teach the client and family preoperatively about equipment (may receive mechanical ventilation or supplemental oxygen immediately postoperatively), breathing exercises, and postoperative recovery.

        2. Apply elastic stockings and teach leg exercises to prevent postoperative emboli.

        3. Provide pain relief to promote comfort, early ambulation, and coughing and deep breathing.

        4. Position the client to protect remaining lung tissue:

            a. After lobectomy—promote expansion to fill lung space by avoiding prolonged lying on operative side.

            b. After pneumonectomy—client may lie on back or operated side only.

        5. Promote optimal pulmonary function—coughing and deep breathing, hydrating, changing positions, ambulating.

        6. Teach breathing exercises and the need for cessation of smoking.

    B. Interventions related to radiation therapy of pulmonary and/or cranial fields (see Chapter 35).

    C. Nursing intervention related to chemotherapy (see Chapter 37).

III. Interventions to monitor disease progression.

    A. Schedule follow-up care.

    B. Discuss purpose of brain, bone, and liver scans or other surveillance procedures for metastatic disease.

    C. Teach the client and family signs and symptoms of metastatic disease.

        1. Changes in affect or personality.

        2. Bone pain.

        3. Changes in respiratory status.

        4. Jaundice.

IV. Interventions to enhance adaptation and rehabilitation.

    A. Pulmonary rehabilitation.

    B. Range of motion exercises on side of the thoracotomy.

V. Interventions to incorporate the client/family in care.

    A. Help family to allow the client to maintain roles and activities most important to him or her.

        1. Place emphasis on short-term goals in daily care and priority setting.

        2. Refer to local American Cancer Society or American Lung Association branches for respiratory program, if available.

    B. Teach supportive care skills.

        1. Instruct the client and family in the use of oxygen equipment, postural drainage, self-pacing program.

2. Teach general strengthening exercises.
3. Instruct in relaxation techniques.
4. Assist to maintain realistic hope, yet prepare for changes in lifestyle if prognosis is poor.
5. Assist to resume previous roles and responsibilities if prognostic factors are favorable (small, solitary, isolated lesion).

Evaluation

The oncology nurse systematically and regularly evaluates the client's and/or family's responses to interventions to determine progress toward the achievement of expected outcomes. Relevant data are collected and actual findings are compared with expected findings. Nursing diagnoses, outcomes, and plans of care are reviewed and revised as necessary.

BIBLIOGRAPHY

Brogden, J.M., & Nevidjon, B. (1995). Vinorelbine tartrate (Navelbine): Drug profile and nursing implications of a new vinca alkaloid. *Oncol Nurs Forum 22*(4), 635–646.

Bunn, P.A., & Kelly, K. (1995). New treatment agents for advanced small cell and non-small cell lung cancer. *Semin Oncol 22*(3), 53–63.

Glover, J., & Miaskowski, C. (1994). Small cell lung cancer: Pathophysiologic mechanisms and nursing implications. *Oncol Nurs Forum 21*(1), 87–95.

Greco, F.A., & Hainsworth, J.D. (1994). Practical approaches to the treatment of patients with extensive stage small cell lung cancer. *Semin Oncol 21*(4), 3–6.

Harvey, J.C., Erdman, C., Pisch, J., et al. (1995). Surgical treatment of non-small cell lung cancer in patients older than seventy years. *J Surg Oncol 60*(4), 247–249.

Holmes, E.C., Livingston, R., & Turrisi, A. (1993). Neoplasms of the thorax. In J.F. Holland, & E. Frei (eds.). *Cancer Medicine* (3rd ed.). Malvern, PA: Lea & Febiger, pp. 1285–1372.

Jaklitsch, M.T., Strauss, G.M., Healey, E.A., et al. (1995). An historical perspective of multi-modality treatment for resectable non-small cell lung cancer. *Lung Cancer 12*(2), 17–32.

Kubota, K., Furuse, K., Kawahara, M., et al. (1994). Role of radiotherapy in combined modality treatment of locally advanced non-small cell lung cancer. *J. Clin Oncol 12*(8), 1547–1552.

Long, B.C., Phipps, W.J., & Cassmeyer, V.L. (eds.). (1993). *Medical-surgical Nursing: A Nursing Process Approach* (4th ed.). St. Louis: C.V. Mosby.

Maxwell, M.B. (ed.). (1996). New developments in lung cancer. *Semin Oncol Nurs 12*(4).

Shahidi, H., & Kvale, P.A. (1996). Long-term survival following surgical treatment of solitary brain metastasis in non-small cell lung cancer. *Chest 109*(1), 271–276.

Shaw, E.G., Su, J.Q., Eagan, R.T., et al. (1994). Prophylactic cranial irradiation in complete responders with small cell lung cancer: Analysis of the Mayo Clinic and North Central Cancer Treatment Group databases. *J Clin Oncol 12*(11), 1227–1232.

Shepherd, F.A. (1994). Future directions in the treatment of non-small cell lung cancer. *Semin Oncol 21*(3), 48–62.

Shepherd, F.A. (1994). Treatment of advanced non-small cell lung cancer. *Semin Oncol 21*(4), 7–18.

Shepherd, F.A., Amdemichael, E., Evans, W.K., et al. (1994). Treatment of small cell lung cancer in the elderly. *J Am Geriatr Soc 43*(1), 64–70.

Srensen, J.B., & Hansen, H.H. (1994). Recent advances in diagnosis and treatment of small cell and non-small cell lung cancer. *Curr Opin Oncol 6*(2), 162–170.

25

Nursing Care of the Client With Cancer of the Gastrointestinal Tract

Roberta Anne Strohl, RN, MN, AOCN

ESOPHAGEAL CANCER

Theory

I. Anatomy of organs.
  A. Located between hypopharynx and stomach.
  B. Originates at cricoid cartilage at the sixth cervical vertebra.
  C. Cervical esophagus is more than 5 cm long; thoracic esophagus begins at the thoracic inlet, ends at the gastroesophageal junction, and is 20 to 25 cm long.
  D. Critical adjacent structures.
    1. Trachea.
    2. Aorta.
    3. Lung.
II. Physiology and pathophysiology associated with esophageal cancer.
  A. Primary functions include:
    1. Conducting food from pharynx to stomach.
    2. Primary and secondary peristalsis.
    3. Preventing reflux of stomach contents.
  B. Changes in function associated with esophageal cancer.
    1. Esophagus is a distensible structure.
    2. Symptoms occur late when circumference is less than 13 mm.
    3. Achalasia—benign spasm of lower esophageal sphincter with marked dilation of the esophagus.
    4. Difficulty swallowing.
    5. Painful swallowing of food (odynophagia).
    6. Regurgitation.
    7. Retrosternal or epigastric pain.
    8. Hematemesis.
    9. Melena.
  C. Metastatic patterns.
    1. Local spread.
    2. Visceral metastases.
      a. Liver.
      b. Lung.
      c. Pleura.

       d. Stomach.
       e. Peritoneum.
       f. Kidney.
       g. Adrenal gland.
       h. Bone.
       i. Brain.

III. Trends in epidemiology.
    A. Uncommon cancer in the United States (U.S.).
       1. 2% of US cancer deaths.
       2. Seventh most common cancer worldwide.
       3. Squamous cell cancer most common worldwide, accounts for 90% of esophageal cancer in the U.S.
       4. Higher incidence in African Americans for squamous cell cancer.
       5. Adenocarcinoma of esophagus has a higher incidence in whites, incidence appears to be increasing.
    B. Worldwide incidence.
       1. Mortality highest in China, Puerto Rico, and Singapore.
       2. High rates also in Iran, France, Switzerland.

IV. Principles of medical management.
    A. Screening and diagnostic procedures.
       1. Routine screening has not been reported.
       2. Diagnostic procedures.
         a. Esophagoscopy and biopsy.
         b. Esophagogram.
         c. Computed tomography (CT) of the chest.
         d. Endoscopic ultrasound.
         e. Chest radiography.
         f. Assessment of the head and neck because 20% of patients may present with a second primary lesion.
    B. Staging methods and procedures.
       1. Tumor-node-metastasis (TNM) system used (Table 25–1).
       2. CT of the chest, bone scan, bronchoscopy, pulmonary function studies may add to staging.
       3. Surgical staging with lymph node sampling.
    C. Treatment strategies.
       1. Surgery. Table 25–2 describes surgical procedures in esophageal cancer.
         a. Esophagectomy in local or loco-regional disease.
         b. Disease is often systemic at diagnosis with lymph node involvement and distant metastases.
         c. Surgery may be curative or palliative.
         d. Preoperative pulmonary function values are obtained, forced expiratory volume (FEV) should be at least 70%.
         e. Cardiac assessment.
         f. Nutritional status.
         g. Oral sepsis increases risk of intrathoracic infection, indicating the need for preoperative dental evaluation.
       2. Radiation therapy.
         a. Single modality is used curatively, palliatively.
         b. Combined with surgery preoperatively or postoperatively.
         c. Combined with chemotherapy and surgery.
       3. Chemotherapy.
         a. 5-fluorouracil (5-FU) and mitomycin C and radiation therapy are used in early trials.

TABLE 25–1. **Staging of Esophageal Cancer**

Stage	Description
T = Primary Tumor	
TX	Minimum requirements to assess the primary tumor cannot be seen
T0	No evidence of primary tumor
Tis	Preinvasive carcinoma (carcinoma in situ)
T1	Tumor invades into but not beyond the submucosa
T2	Tumor invades into but not beyond the muscularis propria
T3	Tumor invades into the adventitia
T4	Tumor invades contiguous structures
N = Regional Lymph Nodes	
Cervical esophagus (cervical and supraclavicular lymph nodes)	
NX	Lymph nodes cannot be assessed
N0	No demonstrable metastasis to regional lymph nodes .
N1	Regional lymph nodes contain metastatic tumor
Thoracic esophagus (nodes in the thorax, not those of the cervical, supraclavicular, or abdominal areas)	
N0	No nodal involvement
N1	Nodal involvement
M = Distant Metastasis	
MX	Distant metastasis cannot be assessed
M0	No evidence of distant metastasis
M1	Distant metastasis present

    b. 5-FU and cisplatin, mitomycin C used with radiation therapy in most current trials.

    c. Other agents used include bleomycin, vinblastine, etoposide, doxorubicin.

V. Trends in survival.

  A. Prognosis remains poor because most cancers are diagnosed late. Approximately 7% of patients affected will be alive 5 years after diagnosis.

  B. Risk factors cause many clients to present in poor general condition.

Assessment

I. Pertinent client and family history.

  A. Predisposing conditions.

    1. Tylosis. *formation of a callus*

      a. Hyperkeratosis of the skin of palms and soles. *overgrowth of the horny layer of the epidermis*

      b. Papillomata of the esophagus.

      c. Inherited in an autosomal dominant fashion.

      d. Squamous cell cancer of the esophagus in affected families.

    2. Achalasia—benign spasm of lower esophageal sphincter; a neuromuscular disorder resulting from absent or defective nerves of the myenteric plexus.

      a. Risk of esophageal cancer is 20%.

TABLE 25–2. **Surgical Approaches in Esophageal Cancer**

Location of Lesion	Procedure	Technique	Morbidity Related to *All* Techniques of Esophageal Resection
Lower third of esophagus and cardia	Transthoracoscopy Esophagectomy	Removes distal esophagus and proximal stomach with clear margins of 5–10 cm Resection includes paraesophageal, pericardial, left gastric, and celiac nodes Stomach is mobilized with vascular pedicle, advanced into thorax with end-to-side anastomosis	Atelectasis Pneumonia Postoperative hypoxia (secondary to atelectasis and increased intra-pulmonary shunting) Dehiscence of esophageal anastomosis (7–10 days postop) Early symptoms of leak Low-grade fever, chest pain Late signs: dyspnea, tachycardia, cervical crepitus, pneumo-thoraces, pleural effusion (on operative side with brown fluid) Postoperative bleeding Recurrent laryngeal nerve paralysis (cervical sites)
	En bloc esophagectomy	Dissection includes esophagus surrounding pleura, thoracic duct, lymphatics, and adjacent portions of pericardium and diaphragm	
Upper and middle thirds	Combined right thoracotomy and abdominal approach	Requires anastomosis at or above aortic arch Resection of whole intrathoracic esophagus and dissection of lymph nodes Mobilization of gastric or intestinal conduit for bypass	
Cervical esophagus		Dissection includes head and neck as well as thorax; surgery may require resection of larynx and hypopharynx	

      b. Most common in middle third of the esophagus.
      c. 17 years from diagnosis of achalasia to cancer.
  3. Barrett's esophagus.
      a. Mechanism unclear.
      b. Failure of normal developmental progression from columnar to epi-thelial cells in utero.
      c. May be related to congenitally short esophagus.
      d. Acquired condition related to cephalad migration of gastric columnar epithelium in response to reflux injury of squamous epithelium.

        e. Premalignant in cases when Barrett's lesion extends from proximal to distal 10 cm of the esophagus.

        f. Results in adenocarcinoma.

    4. Caustic injury.

        a. Arise in patients with lye strictures in 1 to 4% of cases.

        b. 40 years after injury.

    5. Esophageal webs.

        a. Plummer-Vinson iron deficiency, anemia, glossitis, cheilosis, koilonychia, brittle fingernails, and splenomegaly.

        b. More common in females.

    6. Secondary primary.

        a. Other cancers associated with risk factors (tobacco, alcohol).

        b. Most arise in upper aerodigestive epithelium.

    7. Age and gender.

        a. Usually in people 55 to 65 years old.

        b. Men.

  B. Dietary factors and lifestyle risk factors.

    1. Tobacco abuse.

    2. Alcohol abuse.

    3. Low-calorie diet.

    4. Low-protein diet.

    5. Pickled vegetables.

II. Physical examination.

  A. Weight loss.

  B. Dysphagia.

  C. Odynophagia.

  D. "Food sticking."

  E. Melena.

  F. Cough (with fistula).

  G. Hematemesis.

  H. Horner's syndrome—miotic pupils and ptosis of the eyelid. Loss of sweating over affected side. Enophthalmos (recession of the eyeball into the orbit) caused by paralysis of the cervical sympathetic trunk.

  I. Exsanguinating hemorrhage with aortic erosion.

III. Laboratory data.

  A. Hemoglobin, hematocrit levels.

  B. Liver enzyme studies.

  C. Electrolyte levels.

Nursing Diagnoses

  I. Anxiety.

 II. Altered nutrition, less than body requirement.

III. Pain.

IV. Risk for injury: aspiration.

Outcome Identification

  I. Client describes personal risk factors for esophageal cancer.

 II. Client discusses rationale, schedule, and personal demands of treatment and follow-up plan.

III. Client lists potential side effects of disease and treatment.

IV. Client describes self-care measures to decrease the severity of complications of treatment.
V. Client demonstrates competence in self-care measures.
VI. Client and family/significant other specify symptoms to report immediately to the health care team.
    A. Bleeding.
    B. Aspiration.
    C. Shortness of breath.

Planning and Implementation

I. Intervention to decrease incidence and severity of complications of treatment unique to esophageal cancer.
    A. Monitor for postoperative complications.
        1. Wound healing.
        2. Anastomotic leak.
        3. Aspiration.
        4. Respiratory complications.
           a. Severe atelectasis.
           b. Pulmonary edema.
           c. Adult respiratory distress syndrome (ARDS).
    B. Monitor for side effects of radiation.
        1. Nausea and vomiting.
        2. Dysphagia.
        3. Fatigue.
        4. Myelosuppression in combined radiation/chemotherapy regimen.
        5. Fistula (in advanced lesions a tracheoesophageal fistula may occur as the tumor regresses).
    C. Monitor for side effects of chemotherapy.
        1. Nausea and vomiting.
        2. Diarrhea.
        3. Myelosuppression.
        4. Neurotoxicity.
II. Interventions to incorporate the client and family in care.
    A. Prevention and early detection.
        1. Instruct family members about predisposing conditions and risk factors for esophageal cancer.
        2. Refer the client and family to substance abuse programs if indicated.
        3. Teach the family to recognize signs and symptoms of esophageal cancer.
    B. Treatment and follow-up demands.
        1. Educate the client and family about self-care measures to reduce complications of disease and treatment.
        2. Inform them about written and service resources (see Chapter 8).
           a. Alcoholics Anonymous or other substance abuse programs.
           b. Smoke cessation programs.
        3. Teach the client and family *signs and symptoms* to report immediately to the health care team, including fever, bleeding, intractable nausea and vomiting, dizziness, and syncope.

Evaluation

The oncology nurse systematically and regularly evaluates the client's and/or family's responses to interventions to determine progress toward the achievement

of expected outcomes. Relevant data are collected and actual findings are compared with expected findings. Nursing diagnoses, outcomes, and plans of care are reviewed and revised as necessary.

GASTRIC CANCER

Theory

I. Anatomy of organs.
  A. Stomach.
    1. Begins at the gastroesophageal junction, ends at the pylorus.
    2. Divided into three major parts.
      a. Fundus.
      b. Corpus or body.
      c. Antrum.
  B. Critical adjacent structures.
    1. Diaphragm.
    2. Liver.
    3. Abdominal wall.
    4. Colon.
    5. Greater omentum.
    6. Spleen.
    7. Pancreas.
    8. Left adrenal gland and kidney.
    9. Duodenum.
II. Physiology and pathophysiology associated with gastric cancer.
  A. Primary functions include:
    1. Storage of food until it can enter the lower portion of gastrointestinal tract.
    2. Mixing of food with gastric secretions until chyme, a semifluid mixture, is formed.
    3. Slow emptying of food into small intestine at rate that accommodates absorption and digestion.
  B. Changes in function associated with gastric cancer.
    1. Nonspecific.
    2. Epigastric discomfort.
    3. Dysphagia.
    4. Early satiety.
    5. Persistent vomiting.
    6. Weight loss.
    7. Pain.
  C. Metastatic patterns.
    1. Penetration of gastric wall.
    2. Invasion of intramural lymphatics.
    3. Local spread to esophagus or duodenum.
    4. Through serosa to omentum, spleen, liver, kidney, pancreas, bowel.
III. Trends in epidemiology.
  A. Decrease in incidence in U.S.
    1. 33 of 100,000 persons affected in 1935, 9 of 100,000 in last decade.
    2. 22,800 new cases occur annually, 14,000 deaths.
    3. 90% of cancers are adenocarcinomas.

4. Other lesions with greater than 1% incidence are gastric lymphoma and leiomyosarcoma.
B. Incidence worldwide.
  1. Leading cause of cancer death in Japan.
  2. High incidence in Eastern Europe and South America, especially Chile and Costa Rica.
IV. Principles of medical management.
  A. Screening and diagnostic procedures.
    1. High-risk areas (Japan) screen with double-contrast barium studies and upper endoscopy.
    2. Results of barium study with biopsy yield diagnosis.
    3. Abdominal and chest radiographs.
    4. Endoscopic ultrasonography (EUS).
  B. Laboratory tests.
    1. Hemoglobin and hematocrit levels because anemia is a common presenting symptom.
    2. Liver enzyme studies to rule out spread.
  C. Staging methods and procedures.
    1. TNM system is used (Table 25–3).
    2. Surgical staging with lymph node sampling.
  D. Treatment strategies.
    1. Surgery.
      a. Curative modality in local disease.
      b. Nutritional assessment is critical preoperatively.
      c. Feeding jejunostomy may be needed in those who are nutritionally compromised.
      d. Surgical techniques presented in Table 25–4.
    2. Chemotherapy.
      a. Postoperative in high-risk patients.
      b. Combination regimens include:
        (1) FAM—5-FU, Adriamycin (doxorubicin), mitomycin C.
        (2) FAP—5-FU, Adriamycin, Platinol.
        (3) FAMTX—5-FU, Adriamycin, methotrexate (with rescue leucovorin).
        (4) EAP—etoposide, Adriamycin, Platinol (cisplatin).
      c. Single agents include:
        (1) 5-FU.
        (2) Doxorubicin.
        (3) Cisplatin.
        (4) Etoposide.
        (5) Mitomycin C.
        (6) Nitrosoureas—bischloroethylnitrosourea (BCNU) and methyl-CCNU.
      d. Delivery systems.
        (1) Intraperitoneal, intraoperative, intra-arterial administration.
        (2) Systemic.
    3. Radiation therapy.
      a. As adjuvant with chemotherapy and/or surgery.
      b. Limited dose without severe acute toxicity.
V. Trends in survival.
  A. Most gastric cancer in the U.S. are diagnosed at an advanced stage.
  B. Survival ranges from 94 to 82% T_1, 82 to 51% T_2, 20% T_3, 5 to 30% T_4 depending on depth of penetration.

TABLE 25–3. **Staging of Gastric Cancer**

Stage	Description
T = Primary Tumor	
TX	Primary tumor cannot be assessed
T0	No evidence of primary tumor
Tis	Carcinoma in situ
T1	Tumor invades lamina propria or submucosa
T2	Tumor invades muscularis propria
T3	Tumor invades adventitia
T4	Tumor invades adjacent structures
N = Regional Lymph Nodes	
NX	Regional lymph node(s) cannot be assessed
N0	No regional lymph node metastasis
N1	Metastasis in perigastric lymph node(s) within 3 cm of edge of primary tumor
N2	Metastasis in perigastric lymph node(s) more than 3 cm from edge of primary tumor, or in lymph nodes along left gastric, common hepatic, splenic, or celiac arteries
M = Distant Metastasis	
MX	Presence of distant metastasis cannot be assessed
M0	No distant metastasis
M1	Distant metastasis

Stage Grouping

Stage 0	Tis	N0	M0
Stage IA	T1	N0	M0
Stage IB	T1	N1	M0
	T2	N0	M0
Stage II	T1	N2	M0
	T2	N1	M0
	T3	N0	M0
Stage IIIA	T2	N2	M0
	T3	N1	M0
	T4	N0	M0
Stage IIIB	T3	N2	M0
	T4	N1	M0
Stage IV	T4	N2	M0
	Any T	Any N	M1

Assessment

I. Pertinent client and family history.
   A. Two variants of gastric cancer have different etiologic factors.
      1. Intestinal.
         a. More common in men.
         b. More common in older individuals.
         c. More common in areas where gastric cancer is epidemic, suggesting environmental etiology.
         d. Preexisting disease—arises from precancerous areas such as gastric atrophy or intestinal metaplasia.

TABLE 25–4. Surgical Approaches to Gastric Cancer

Procedure	Anatomic Site of Lesion	Technique	Advantages/Disadvantages	Continuity of GI Tract
Radical distal subtotal resection	Body or antrum of stomach	Billroth I—removes first portion of duodenum, distal stomach, pylorus	Procedure of choice for elderly or debilitated patients because surgical time is limited; however, scope of resection is also limited	Gastroduodenostomy
		Billroth II—removes 80% of stomach, first portion of duodenum, gastrohepatic and gastrocolic omentum, and nodal tissue adjacent to celiac axis	Preserves a small part of the stomach, which is a better material for anatomosis than esophagus. Limited by tumor extent. If clear margins cannot be obtained, total gastrectomy is needed	Gastrojejunostomy
Total gastrectomy	Extensive or proximal lesions	Entire stomach is removed along with lymph nodes and structures as indicated above. In addition, spleen and distal pancreas may be removed	Increased morbidity/mortality related to anastomotic leaks
Extensive lesions can be treated	Esophagoduodenostomy
Esophagojejunostomy

>>   2. Diffuse.
>>   a. More frequent in women.
>>   b. More frequent in younger individuals.
>>   c. Preexisting disease not a factor.
>>   d. Familial pattern suggesting genetic predisposition.
>   B. Predisposing diet.
>>   1. Low fat and protein.
>>   2. Salted meat and fish.
>>   3. High nitrate.
>>   4. Low vitamin A and C.
>>   5. Smoked foods.
>   C. Environmental factors.
>>   1. Lack of refrigeration.
>>   2. Poor-quality drinking water.
>>   3. Occupation (rubber and coal workers).
>>   4. Smoking.
>   D. Medical factors.
>>   1. Prior gastric surgery.
>>   2. *Helicobacter pylori* infection.
>>   3. Gastric atrophy and gastritis.
> II. Physical examination.
>   A. Epigastric discomfort.
>   B. Dysphagia.
>   C. Weight loss.
>   D. Fatigue.
>   E. Epigastric mass.
>   F. Vomiting.
>   G. Vague symptoms often present.
>   H. Jaundice in advanced disease.
> III. Laboratory data.
>   A. Decreased hemoglobin and hematocrit levels.
>   B. Elevated liver enzyme levels.

Nursing Diagnoses

>   I. Anxiety.
> II. Altered nutrition, less than body requirements.
> III. Pain.

Outcome Identification

>   I. Client describes personal risk factors for gastric cancer.
> II. Client discusses rationale, schedule, and personal demands of the treatment and follow-up plans.
> III. Client lists potential side effects of the disease and treatment.
> IV. Client describes self-care measures to decrease the severity of complications of treatment.
>   V. Client demonstrates competence in self-care measures.
> VI. Client and family/significant other specify symptoms to report immediately to the health care team.
>   A. Vomiting.
>   B. Bleeding.
>   C. Symptoms of obstruction.

Planning and Implementation

I. Interventions to decrease the incidence and severity of complications of treatment unique to gastric cancer.
  A. Monitor for side effects of surgery.
    1. Dumping syndrome.
    2. Wound healing.
    3. Infection.
    4. Anastomotic leak.
    5. Reflux aspiration.
    6. Bezoar formation (food at gastric outlet).
  B. Monitor for side effects of chemotherapy.
    1. Mucositis.
    2. Diarrhea.
    3. Nausea and vomiting.
    4. Myelosuppression.
  C. Monitor for side effects of radiation.
    1. Nausea.
    2. Vomiting.
    3. Fatigue.
II. Interventions to incorporate the client and family in care.
  A. Prevention and early detection.
    1. Instruct family members about familial and dietary risks for gastric cancers.
    2. Discuss recommended screening in high-risk areas.
    3. Teach the family to recognize signs and symptoms of gastric cancer.
  B. Treatment and follow-up demands.
    1. Educate client and family about self-care measures to reduce complications of disease and treatment.
    2. Inform about written and service resources (see Chapter 8).
    3. Signs and symptoms to report immediately to health care team, such as vomiting, fever, pain.

Evaluation

The oncology nurse systematically and regularly evaluates the client's and/or family's responses to interventions to determine progress toward the achievement of expected outcomes. Relevant data are collected and actual findings are compared with expected findings. Nursing diagnoses, outcomes, and plans of care are reviewed and revised as necessary.

COLORECTAL CANCER

Theory

I. Anatomy of organs.
  A. Colon (Fig. 25–1).
    1. Extends from the terminal ileum to the anal canal.
    2. Consists of four parts—ascending or right colon, transverse or middle colon, descending or left colon, and sigmoid colon.
  B. Rectum (see Fig. 25–1).
    1. Is continuous with the sigmoid colon and terminates at the distal anal canal.

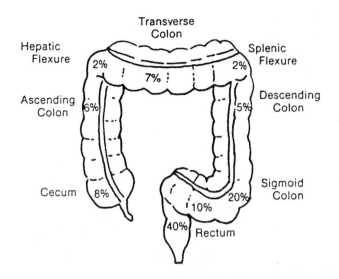

Figure 25–1. Anatomic regions of the colon and associated cancer incidence. Two thirds of all colorectal cancers occur in the rectosigmoid and rectum. Many of these cancers are within reach of the examining finger, and 50% are within the reach of a sigmoidoscope. (From Otte, D.M. [1988]. Nursing management of the patient with colon and rectal cancer. *Semin Oncol Nurs* 4(4), 286.)

    2. Contains a transitional zone between keratinized and nonkeratinized stratified squamous epithelium at the anal verge.

    3. Is covered with peritoneum.

  C. Anus—landmarks of anorectal ring, pectinate line, and anal verge represent transitions in epithelium.

  D. Critical adjacent structures.

    1. Venous drainage from the colon and upper to middle third of the rectum enters the portal system to the liver.

    2. Lower third of the rectum drains to the portal vein and inferior vena cava.

    3. Colon, rectum, and anus lie in proximity to the vagina in females and to the bladder, seminal vesicles, prostate, and urethra in males.

II. Physiology and pathophysiology associated with colorectal cancers.

  A. Primary functions of the colon include:

    1. Processing of ileal contents.

      a. Colon receives 800 to 1000 mL of ileal contents per day.

      b. Absorption of water and electrolytes occurs primarily in the proximal or right colon.

      c. Feces in the right colon are more fluid than in the sigmoid colon.

    2. Movement of ileal contents through bowel.

      a. Innervation of gut responds to both parasympathetic and sympathetic signals.

      b. Secretion, blood flow, and sensory perception are controlled by submucosal structures.

      c. Ileal contents are moved through the colon by a mixture of circular constrictions and longitudinal contractions.

       d. Fecal material is exposed to the bowel wall for absorption of nutritional elements.

       e. Feces are pushed into the rectum.

    3. Storage of feces—in the left colon until defecation.

    4. Defecation.

       a. Rectal wall is distended by feces.

       b. Peristalsis is initiated; the anal sphincter relaxes and defecation occurs.

       c. External anal sphincter is controlled by the conscious mind and can inhibit defecation.

       d. If the impulse for defecation is ignored, the reflex fades.

  B. Changes in function associated with colorectal cancers.

    1. Increase or decrease in consistency of stool.

    2. Changes in color of stool.

    3. Inability to move stool through bowel (obstruction) or pencil-shaped stool because of partial obstruction of bowel.

  C. Metastatic patterns.

    1. Colorectal cancers.

       a. Local extension through penetration of layers of bowel.

       b. Deeper penetration increases chance of spread.

       c. Tumors that have invaded beyond submucosal layer have direct access to vascular and lymphatic systems.

       d. Distant metastases most frequently occur in the liver and lungs and less frequently occur in the brain, bone, and adrenal glands.

    2. Anal cancers.

       a. Local extension to sphincter ani muscles, prostate, urethra, and bladder in males and vagina in females.

       b. Distant metastases occur in lung and liver.

III. Trends in epidemiology.

  A. Colorectal cancer is a common tumor, second only to lung cancer in the number of new cases.

  B. Age-adjusted death rates per 100,000 population compared between 1955 and 1957 and 1985 and 1987 indicate:

    1. Decrease in the death rate related to colon cancer among women.

    2. No change in the death rate related to colon cancer among men.

    3. Decrease in the death rate related to rectal cancer among both men and women.

  C. Over a 30-year period the population-adjusted incidence is unchanged—47 cases per 100,000 persons.

IV. Principles of medical management.

  A. Screening and diagnostic procedures (Table 25–5).

    1. Digital examination detects 10% of anorectal lesions.

    2. Stool for occult blood is controversial with respect to cost-effectiveness as a screening test.

    3. Flexible fiberoptic sigmoidoscopy allows examination of up to 60 cm of colon.

  B. Laboratory tests.

    1. Hemoglobin and hematocrit levels to evaluate anemia commonly found with lesions on the right side.

    2. Carcinoembryonic antigen (CEA)—although not valuable as a diagnostic or screening test, CEA has been used to monitor the response to therapy and follow-up care.

TABLE 25–5. **Diagnostic Tests for Colorectal Cancer**

Description/Purpose	Time Required for Test	Sensations Experienced	Potential Side Effects/ Complications	Self-Care Measures	Critical Symptoms to Report to Health Care Team
Barium Enema					
Identify extent of lesion in colon Identify obstruction	30–45 min	Fullness, abdominal pain, discomfort, urge to defecate	Perforation Bowel obstruction	Preparation includes liquid diet day before, and low-residue diet 1–3 days before test Bowel preparation—laxatives or enema before and after examination Client must hold anal sphincter against tube and breathe slowly to minimize discomfort	Failure to pass barium Signs of gastrointestinal obstruction
Computed Axial Tomographic (CAT) Scan					
Identify lymph node involvement, liver metastases	45–60 min	May be claustrophobic when in scanner Sound of machine going on and off Warm feeling with injection of dye	Allergic reaction to dye Nausea from dye Blood samples for determining blood urea nitrogen (BUN) and creatinine levels are drawn first to assess renal function	May receive nothing by mouth or be instructed to eat lightly before examination because of potential nausea from dye	With contrast, immediately report any discomfort, breathing difficulty, itching
Stool for Occult Blood					
	Preparation— 48–72 hr		False-positive results: Results from meat in diet, hemorrhoids, fissures, peroxidases in	No red meat, poultry, fish, turnips, horseradish for 72 hr before test Withhold iron and aspirin	

Table continued on following page

TABLE 25–5. **Diagnostic Tests for Colorectal Cancer** (*Continued*)

Description/Purpose	Time Required for Test	Sensations Experienced	Potential Side Effects/ Complications	Self-Care Measures	Critical Symptoms to Report to Health Care Team
			skin of vegetables and fruits (cherries, tomatoes), gastritis from aspirin False-negative results: Failure to use high-residue, high-fiber diet 72 hr before test Vitamin C in diet Delay between collection and examination Failure to prepare slides properly Lesion not bleeding at time of examination	Collect three specimens Client urinates first into toilet, uses bedpan to collect stool Send specimen to laboratory or return as instructed	
Colonoscopy, Sigmoidoscopy, Proctoscopy Visualize gastrointestinal tract	15–30 min	Pressure discomfort Intravenous infusion with sedation Lying on left side Scope feels cool Sensation of need to defecate	If tissue removed, bleeding Adverse effects from sedatives	Clear liquid diet for 24 hr, laxative evening before, cleansing enema 3–4 hr before test Deep breathing during examination Expect a large amount of flatus after examination	Pain Bleeding

C. Staging methods and procedures.
   1. Colorectal (Table 25–6).
      a. TNM system is used.
      b. Staging based on clinical data or surgical data.

TABLE 25–6. **Staging of Colorectal Cancer**

Stage	Description
T—Primary Tumor	
TX	Primary tumor cannot be assessed
T0	No evidence of primary tumor
Tis	Carcinoma in situ
T1	Tumor invades submucosa
T2	Tumor invades muscularis propria
T3	Tumor invades through muscularis propria into subserosa or into nonperitonealized pericolic or perirectal tissues
T4	Tumor perforates visceral peritoneum, or directly invades other organs or structures
N—Lymph Node	
NX	Regional lymph nodes cannot be assessed
N0	No regional lymph node metastasis
N1	Metastasis in one to three pericolic or perirectal lymph nodes
N2	Metastasis in four or more pericolic or perirectal lymph nodes
N3	Metastasis in any lymph node along course of a major named vascular trunk
M—Distant Metastasis	
MX	Presence of distant metastasis cannot be assessed
M0	No distant metastasis
M1	Distant metastasis

Stage Grouping

0	Tis	N0	M0
I	T1	N0	M0
	T2	N0	M0
II	T3	N0	M0
	T4	N0	M0
III	Any T	N1	M0
	Any T	N2	M0
	Any T	N3	M0
IV	Any T	Any N	M1

Histopathologic Grade (G)

GX	Grade cannot be assessed
G1	Well differentiated
G2	Moderately well differentiated
G3	Poorly differentiated
G4	Undifferentiated

From American Joint Committee on Cancer (1988). *Manual for Staging of Cancer* (3rd ed.). Philadelphia: J.B. Lippincott.

2. Duke system.
    a. Lesions limited to mucosa—Duke A.
    b. Lesions extending into muscularis propria but not through it—Duke B_1.
    c. Lesions extending through the muscularis propria—Duke B_2.
    d. Lesions of B_1 or B_2 type but with involvement of lymph nodes—Duke C.
D. Treatment strategies.
    1. Surgery.
        a. Surgical resection is the primary treatment for 75% of clients with colorectal cancer.
        b. Surgical procedures for colorectal and anal cancers are presented in Table 25–7.
    2. Radiation therapy.
        a. Preoperative radiation therapy is used to:
            (1) Decrease tumor size and render the tumor resectable.
            (2) Eradicate microscopic disease.
            (3) Decrease the incidence of local recurrence.
        b. Postoperative radiation therapy is used to eradicate remaining disease if:
            (1) Surgical margins are positive for cancer.
            (2) Residual tumor is present.
            (3) A Duke B_2 or C lesion is present.
        c. Combined preoperative and postoperative radiation therapy may be used.
        d. Early rectal cancers in the low- and midrectal regions and anal cancer have been treated with endocavitary radiation (three treatments to a total dose of 8000 to 15,000 cGy).
            (1) High complication rate resulting from superficial effect of high doses of radiation, although they are delivered with low-energy sources.
            (2) Complications—radionecrosis, anal canal ulcers, strictures, bleeding.
    3. Chemotherapy.
        a. Used in combination with surgery and radiation therapy.
        b. Agents used for colorectal cancer—5-FU, levamisole, methotrexate, 5-fluorouracil deoxyribonucleotide (FUDR), and cisplatin.
        c. Agents used for anal cancer—mitomycin C and 5-FU.
V. Trends in survival.
    A. Survival is determined by the stage of disease, grade of tumor, histologic type of tumor, and general health status of the client.
    B. Colon cancer—general 5-year survival rate by stage:
        1. Duke A, 90%.
        2. Duke B, 60 to 80%.
        3. Duke C, 20 to 50%.
    C. Anal cancer overall 5-year survival rate is 48 to 66%.

Assessment

I. Pertinent client and family history.
    A. Age—incidence increases slightly at 40 years; increases sharply at 50 years; doubles each decade thereafter.

TABLE 25–7. Surgical Management of Colorectal Cancer

Site	Procedure	Technique	Physical Alterations	Possible Complications
Rectum	Low anterior resection—for lesions more than 10 cm from anal verge	Resect tumor and 2- to 5-cm margins; staple or suture bowel, conserving sphincter	Sphincter preserved	Anastomotic leak Abscess, infection, irregular bowel function
	Abdominal incision—remove tumor and adjacent involved or potentially involved structures	Performed through abdomen and perineum; perineal wound closed with drain or open to heal by granulation	Colostomy Perineal wound Foley catheter postoperatively Nasogastric tube postoperatively until peristalsis returns	Urinary dysfunction Wound infection Stomal complications Impotence in males Sexual dysfunction related to scarring in females
Anus	Removal of perianal skin, anal canal	Wide excision; anterior-posterior resection may include total pelvic exenteration if lesions involve bladder or urethra	Colostomy Urinary diversion if total pelvic exenteration	As above
Colorectum	Hemicolectomy	Small tumors may be resected with enough margin so that permanent colostomy not needed; may have temporary colostomy	Temporary colostomy possible	Anastomotic leak
	Single-barreled colostomy	Proximal colon brought out and sutured to abdominal wall Defunctionalized colon removed or placed into abdomen (Hartmann pouch)	Permanent colostomy Type of stool depends on location of stoma—*ascending*, fluid; *transverse*, mush, semifluid; *descending*, solid; *rectum*, solid; *anus*, hard solid	Stomal complications Herniation Prolapse Hemorrhage
	Double-barreled colostomy	Two stomas Defunctionalized colon not removed Proximal portion suture to abdominal wall end Stoma Distal mucous fistula		
All sites	Relief of obstruction May be done for palliation of symptoms	Debulking	May have temporary colostomy, nasogastric tube	

    B. Genetic factors.
        1. Familial polyposis, gene leads to successive chromosomal loss.
        2. Gardner syndrome.
        3. Turcot syndrome.
        4. Peutz-Jeghers syndrome.
        5. Juvenile polyposis.
        6. Family cancer syndrome.
        7. Changes in 5q chromosome and ras oncogene lead to deletion in region of chromosome.
        8. Diethyldithiocarbamic acid (DCC) deleted in colon cancer gene.
           a. Role in cell-to-cell contact.
           b. Loss of contact inhibition.
    C. Preexisting bowel disease.
        1. Villous adenoma.
           a. Polyps most likely to become malignant.
           b. Excision of polyps recommended, with annual colonoscopy follow-up examinations.
        2. Ulcerative colitis.
           a. Increased duration of colitis increases risk for malignant change.
           b. The longer the length of involved bowel, the greater the risk for malignancy.
        3. Crohn's disease—risk of malignancy is related to duration and extent of disease.
    D. Other cancers such as breast and gynecologic cancers.
    E. Diet.
        1. High fat intake is proposed as an increased risk for colorectal cancer.
        2. Low-fiber diet increases transit time in the colon; therefore, fecal bile acids and carcinogens in stool have a longer time to interact with mucosa.
    F. Irritation of anal canal related to condylomata, fistula, fissures, abscesses, and hemorrhoids.
 II. Physical examination.
    A. Early signs and symptoms.
        1. Malaise and fatigue.
        2. Signs and symptoms depend on location of cancer (Table 25–8).
        3. Palpation of a mass in the transverse or right colon.
    B. Late signs and symptoms.
        1. Pain.
        2. Weight loss.
        3. Presence of symptoms of metastatic disease.
           a. Pulmonary—cough, chest pain, dyspnea, hemoptysis, wheezing, or dysphagia.
           b. Hepatic—ascites, abdominal distention, nausea, anorexia, increasing abdominal girth, jaundice, changes in color of urine and stool, or pruritus.
III. Laboratory data.
    A. Decreased hemoglobin and hematocrit levels.
    B. Elevated results of liver function tests—lactate dehydrogenase (LDH), serum glutamate pyruvate transaminase (SGPT), or serum glutamic-oxaloacetic transaminase (SGOT).
    C. Elevated CEA.

TABLE 25–8. **Characteristics of Colorectal Cancer**

Site	Pathology	Characteristics	Presentation
Colon	Adenocarcinoma (95%)	Most are relatively slow-growing, poorly differentiated, more aggressive; lymph node involvement common with progression	
Ascending			Anemia, nausea, weight loss, pain (vague and dull); palpable mass uncommon Late symptoms—diarrhea, constipation, anorexia
Transverse			Palpable mass, blood in stool, change in bowel habits, obstruction
Descending			Obstruction, pain (cramps), change in bowel habits
Sigmoid			Blood in stool, constipation, pencil-like stool, obstruction
Rectum	Adenocarcinoma	Same as above	Mucous discharge, bright red rectal bleeding (most common), tenesmus, sense of incomplete evacuation, mucous diarrhea, pain Late symptoms—feeling of rectal fullness, constant ache
Anus	Adenocarcinoma	Higher incidence in fifth through seventh decades; tend to be highly malignant; increasing incidence in male homosexuals	Rectal bleeding, pruritus, mucous discharge, tenesmus, pain or pressure in rectal region
	Squamous cell	May be multifocal; generally well differentiated and slow-growing	
	Basal cell	Local spread only but may be highly malignant; does not behave like basal cell in skin—may metastasize	Sensation of lump, bleeding, pruritus, mucous discharge
	Kaposi's sarcoma (see Chapter 29)		

Nursing Diagnoses

  I. Anxiety.
 II. Altered nutrition, less than body requirements.
III. Risk for sexual dysfunction.
 IV. Risk for impaired skin integrity.
  V. Body image disturbance.

Outcome Identification

  I. Client describes personal risk factors for colorectal cancers.
 II. Client discusses rationale, schedule, and personal demands of treatment and the follow-up plan.

III. Client lists potential side effects of the disease and treatment.
IV. Client describes self-care measures to decrease the incidence, severity, and complications of treatment.
 V. Client demonstrates competence in self-care measures demanded by structural or functional effects of disease or treatment.
VI. Client and family/significant other specify symptoms to report immediately to the health care team.
   A. Changes in structure or function of ostomy.
   B. Symptoms of obstruction.
   C. Blood in stool.
   D. Symptoms of metastatic disease to lung or liver.

Planning and Implementation

 I. Interventions to decrease the incidence and severity of complications of treatment unique to colorectal cancer.
   A. Stoma placement to decrease the incidence of skin reactions.
      1. Mark site at least 2 inches below the waist and away from leg creases.
         a. Avoid stoma placement near scars, bony prominence, skin folds, fistulas, pendulous breasts, or belt line.
         b. Allow for 2 inches of smooth skin around stoma for appliance adherence.
      2. Mark the site while client is lying flat, sitting, standing, and bending.
      3. Mark the site within borders of rectus muscles to minimize risk or herniation and prolapse.
   B. Appliance selection is based on character of stool, contour of skin surrounding stoma, client's manual dexterity, and cost.
   C. Stoma care.
      1. Change appliance every week.
      2. Use skin barriers cut to fit the stoma exactly.
      3. Avoid use of skin products and appliances that contain materials that cause allergic reactions.
      4. Assess the stoma and skin around stoma for complications with each appliance change—erythema, edema, erosion, bleeding, and stomal protrusion, retraction, herniation, or narrowing.
   D. Management of common problems associated with an ostomy (Table 25–9).
      1. Avoid odor-producing foods—legumes, cabbage, onions, carbonated beverages, beer, alcohol, and fatty foods.
      2. Discuss use of odor-absorbing pouches or products such as charcoal.
II. Interventions to monitor for side effects of treatment.
   A. Monitor for postoperative complications related to bowel surgery.
      1. Obstruction or paralytic ileus—pain, diarrhea, nausea, vomiting, or abdominal distention.
      2. Bleeding—pulse rate, respiratory rate, blood pressure, amount and color of drainage from wound and/or stoma.
      3. Infection—fever, pain, redness at incision site, edema, or changes in amount or color of wound drainage.
      4. Stomal complications—retraction, changes in color of stoma, protrusion of stoma onto abdomen, narrowing of stomal opening, herniation, or drainage from fistulous tracts around the stoma.

TABLE 25–9. **Management of Common Colostomy,
Ileostomy, or Urostomy Problems**

Problem	Cause or Sign	Treatment
Odor		
Fecal	Normal intestinal flora	Pouch deodorant
		Air freshener
	Food	Dietary experimentation
	Oral medications	Medications
		Bismuth subgallate, 250 mg four times daily
		Bismuth subcarbonate, 0.6 g four times daily
		Derifil, one tablet, three times daily
Urinary	Poor hygiene	Commercial ostomy deodorant
	Infection	Soak appliance in vinegar-water solution (1:4)
	Concentrated urine	Reassess client/family's technique in care of ostomy
		Treatment of infection
		Increase fluid intake
Skin irritation	Improperly sized stoma opening	Resize stoma opening
		Use skin barrier powder or wafer
	Leakage due to inappropriate appliance	Refer to enterostomal therapist (ET)
		Use skin barrier powder or wafer
	Poor technique	Observe technique and make adjustments as needed
		Use skin barrier powder or wafer
	Allergy	Patch test
		Eliminate offending products
	Flush stoma	Convex appliance and belt
Hyperplasia	Peristomal skin overexposed to urine	Resize stoma opening
		Assess pouching system for pooling on skin
		Refer to ET nurse
Candidiasis	Antibiotic therapy	Nystatin powder applied sparingly with pouch change
	Moist environment	
Folliculitis	Traumatic hair removal	Use of electric razor or scissors to remove hair
Mechanical trauma	Abrasive cleaning technique	Teach client appropriate pouch removal and cleaning techniques
	Traumatic tape removal	
Peristomal malignancy	Disease recurrence	Consider surgical revision of stoma
	Second primary	Use of flexible pouching system
		Refer to ET nurse

Modified from Rowbotham, J.L. (1982). *Managing Colostomies*. Pub No. 3422-PE. Atlanta: American Cancer Society.

    5. Changes in sexual function.
        a. Males—may have erectile and ejaculatory problems with severing of nerves (vertebral segments S2 to S4 and L2 to L4).
        b. Females—enervation not a problem but they may have a decrease in length of the vagina, lack of lubrication, or discomfort with intercourse because of surgical dissection in which the vagina is separated from the rectum.
  B. Monitor for return of bowel function.
    1. Presence of bowel sounds, passage of flatus, and passage of stool.
    2. Tolerance of progressive oral diet.

C. Monitor for complications of radiation therapy to the gastrointestinal tract.
   1. Inflammation of the bowel or bladder.
   2. Blood in stool or urine.
   3. Ulceration of gastrointestinal mucosa—pain.
   4. Necrosis.
   5. Changes in sexual activity related to inflammation of perineal skin.
D. Monitor for complications of chemotherapy for colorectal cancers—5-FU, leucovorin, cisplatin, methotrexate, and semustine (MeCCNU).
   1. Mucositis.
   2. Diarrhea.
   3. Nausea and vomiting.
   4. Myelosuppression.
   5. Decreased libido.
III. Interventions to incorporate the client and family in care.
   A. Prevention and early detection.
      1. Instruct family members about familial risks for colorectal cancers.
      2. Discuss recommended screening guidelines for high-risk individuals.
      3. Suggest dietary modifications to reduce risks of colorectal cancers. (See Chapter 40.)
      4. Teach the family to recognize early signs and symptoms of colorectal cancers.
   B. Treatment and follow-up demands.
      1. Educate the client and family about self-care measures to reduce complications of the disease and treatment.
      2. Inform them about written and service resources available for client and family facing a diagnosis of colorectal cancer. (See Chapter 8.)
         a. American Cancer Society (ACS).
            (1) Services—education and support groups (I Can Cope, Can Surmount, ostomy clubs), Service & Rehabilitation (ACS) direct aid program for ostomy supplies, and publications, including *Sexuality and Cancer.*
         b. United Ostomy Association.
            (1) Address: 36 Executive Park, Suite 120, Irvine, CA 92714, phone number: (714) 660–8624.
            (2) Services—local chapters; *Ostomy Quarterly;* other publications, including *Sex, Courtship, and the Single Ostomate; Sex and the Female Ostomate;* and *Sex and the Male Ostomate.*
         c. International Ostomy Association, c/o Maria Siegel, 73 Widdicombe Hill Boulevard, Suite PH2, Western Ontario, Canada, M9R 4B3.
      3. Teach the client and family signs and symptoms to report immediately to health care team (e.g., bleeding, nausea, and vomiting).

Evaluation

The oncology nurse systematically and regularly evaluates the client's and/or family's responses to interventions to determine progress toward the achievement of expected outcomes. Relevant data are collected and actual findings are compared with expected findings. Nursing diagnoses, outcomes, and plans of care are reviewed and revised as necessary.

BIBLIOGRAPHY

Ahlgren, J. (1992). Colorectal cancer chemotherapy. In J. Ahlgren & J. McDonald (eds.). *Gastrointestinal Oncology*. Philadelphia: J.B. Lippincott, pp. 339–359.

Ahlgren, J. (1992). Esophageal cancer: Chemotherapy and combined modalities. In J. Ahlgren & J. McDonald (eds.). *Gastrointestinal Oncology.* Philadelphia: J.B. Lippincott, pp. 135–151.

Alabaster, O. (1992). Colorectal cancer: Epidemiology, risks, and prevention. In J. Ahlgren & J. McDonald (eds.). *Gastrointestinal Oncology.* Philadelphia: J.B. Lippincott, pp. 243–261.

American Cancer Society. (1996). *Cancer Facts and Figures.* Atlanta: American Cancer Society.

Beart, R. (1995). Colon and rectum. In M. Abeloff, J. Armitage, A. Lichter, & J. Niederhuber (eds.). *Clinical Oncology.* New York: Churchill Livingstone, pp. 1267–1287.

Fisher, S., & Brady, L. (1992). Esophagus. In C. Perez & L. Brady (eds.). *Principles and Practices of Radiation Oncology.* Philadelphia: J.B. Lippincott, pp. 853–871.

Gomes, M. (1992). Esophageal cancer: Surgical approach. In J. Ahlgren & J. McDonald (eds.). *Gastrointestinal Oncology.* Philadelphia: J.B. Lippincott, pp. 89–123.

Gunderson, L., Donohue, J., & Burch, P. (1995). Stomach. In M. Abeloff, J. Armitage, A. Lichter, & J. Niederhuber (eds.). *Clinical Oncology.* New York: Churchill Livingstone, pp. 1267–1287.

Heitmiller, R., & Forastiere, A. (1995). Esophagus. In M. Abeloff, J. Armitage, A. Lichter, & J. Niederhuber (eds.). *Clinical Oncology.* New York: Churchill Livingstone, pp. 1189–1209.

Neugut, A., Hayek, M., & Howe, G. (1996). Epidemiology of gastric cancer. *Semin Oncol 23*(2), 281–292.

Vezeridis, M., & Wanebo, H. (1992). Gastric cancer: Surgical approach. In J. Ahlgren & J. McDonald (eds.). *Gastrointestinal Oncology.* Philadelphia: J.B. Lippincott, pp. 159–171.

26

Nursing Care of the Client With Leukemia

Molly J. Moran, RN, MS, ANP, OCN
Susan A. Ezzone, RN, MS, ANP

Theory

I. Physiology of the hematologic system.
   A. Hematopoiesis is the process of blood cell formation.
      1. Blood-forming organs include bone marrow, liver, and spleen.
         a. Normal bone marrow is essential to develop immunity; maintain hemostasis; and transport hemoglobin, oxygen, and carbon dioxide.
         b. Liver and spleen are primarily blood-forming organs in the fetus, but are capable of blood cell production in response to demand or disease processes in an adult.
      2. Pluripotent progenitor cell (stem cell) originates in the bone marrow and is responsible for production of all hematopoietic cells.
         a. Pluripotent stem cell is capable of self-replication, proliferation, and differentiation into myeloid and lymphoid stem cells.
         b. Myeloid stem cell differentiates into hematopoietic cells including red blood cells; white blood cells (neutrophil, eosinophil, basophil, monocyte, and lymphocyte); and platelets.
         c. Lymphoid stem cell differentiates into B and T lymphocytes, which are responsible for activities of the immune system.
   B. Primary functions of specific hematopoietic cells are described in Table 26–1.
II. Pathophysiology of leukemia.
   A. Leukemia—malignant disorder of blood cells and lymphatic tissue, most commonly involving the white blood cell.
      1. Leukemic or malignant cells excessively proliferate, resulting in overcrowding of bone marrow and inability to produce normal-functioning hematopoietic cells.
      2. Leukemic cells are capable of infiltrating and accumulating in other organs (e.g., central nervous system [CNS], eyes, testes, and skin). Organ involvement is most common in acute leukemia.
      3. Classification of leukemias (Tables 26–2, 26–3, and 26–4) based on predominant cell line affected and level of maturation reached.
      4. Symptoms of leukemia attributed to:
         a. Type of leukemia cell.
         b. Degree of leukemic cell burden.

TABLE 26–1. **Functions of Hematopoietic Cells**

Red blood cell	Transport hemoglobin Transport oxygen from the lungs to the tissues Transport carbon dioxide from the tissues to the lung
Platelet	Formation of hemostatic plug Initiate intrinsic clotting mechanism Maintain capillary integrity
Granulocyte	
Neutrophil	Phagocytosis of bacteria; first line of defense
Basophil	Release of histamine, heparin, and enzymes in acute inflammation
Eosinophil	Phagocytosis and release of enzymes to counteract effects of inflammatory mediators in allergic reactions
Monocyte	
Blood monocyte	Phagocytosis of bacteria, fungus, tumor
Tissue monocyte	Phagocytosis, filtration of particles
Lymphocyte	
B cell	Humoral immunity, antibody production
T cell	Cellular immunity
Helper and suppressor	Regulate function of other lymphocytes
Cytotoxic "killer"	Delayed hypersensitivity reaction, graft-versus-host disease, graft rejection, and attacks tumor cells

Adapted from Haeuber, D., & Spross, J.A. (1994). Protective mechanisms: Bone marrow. In B.L. Johnson & J. Gross (eds.). *Handbook of Oncology Nursing* (2nd ed.). Boston: Jones and Bartlett, pp. 375–379.

TABLE 26–2. **French-American-British (FAB) Classification of Acute Leukemia**

Myeloid		**Lymphocytic**	
M1	Undifferentiated myelocytic	L1	Childhood (pre B- and T-cell)
M2	Myelocytic	L2	Adult (pre B- and T-cell)
M3	Promyelocytic	L3	Burkitt's type (B-cell)
M4	Myelomonocytic		
M5	Monocytic		
M6	Erythroleukemia		
M7	Megakaryocytic		

Reprinted with permission from Wujcik, D. (1993). Leukemia. In S.L. Groenwald, M. Goodman, M.H. Frogge, & C.H. Yarbro (eds.). *Cancer Nursing: Principles and Practice* (3rd ed.). Boston: Jones & Bartlett, pp. 1152. Source: Bennett, J.M., Catovsky, D., Daniel, M.T., et al. (1976). Proposals for the classification of the acute leukemias. *Br J Haemat 33*, 451–458. Bennett, J.M., Catovsky, D., Daniel, M.T., et al. (1985). Criteria for the diagnosis of acute leukemia of megakaryocyte lineage (M7). *Ann Intern Med 103*, 460–462. Bennett, J.M., Catovsky, D., Daniel, M.T., et al. (1985). Proposed revised criteria for the classification of acute myeloid leukemia. *Ann Intern Med 103*, 626–629.

TABLE 26–3. **Rai and Binet Staging Systems for Chronic Lymphocytic Leukemia**

Stage	Lympho-cytosis	Lymph-adenopathy	Hepatomegaly or Splenomegaly	Hemoglobin (g/dL)	Platelets × 10³/μL
Rai System					
0	+	−	−	≥11	≥100
I	+	+	−	≥11	≥100
II	+	±	+	≥11	≥100
III	+	±	±	<11	≥100
IV	+	±	±	Any	<100
Binet System					
A	+	± (<3 lymphatic groups* positive)	±	≥10	≥100
B	+	± (≥3 lymphatic groups* positive)	±	≥10	≥100
C	+	±	±	<10	<100

* Cervical, axillary, inguinal nodes; liver, and spleen are each considered one group whether unilateral or bilateral.
From Deisseroth, A.B., Andreeff, M., Champlin, R., et al. (1993). Chronic leukemias. In V.T. DeVita, Jr., S.S., Hellman, & S.A. Rosenberg (eds.). *Cancer: Principles and Practice of Oncology* (4th ed.). Philadelphia: J.B. Lippincott, p. 1968.

TABLE 26–4. **Phases of Chronic Myelogenous Leukemia**

Chronic phase	Excessive proliferation and accumulation of mature granulocytes Absence of lymphadenopathy Splenomegaly Philadelphia chromosome (Ph¹) present in 90% of persons
Accelerated phase	Progressive leukocytosis Increased myeloid precursors (including blasts); increased basophils Splenomegaly Weight loss Weakness Progressive chromosomal abnormalities
Blast Crisis	Presence of 30–40% blasts or promyelocytes in bone marrow Leukostasis Microvascular occlusion of the CNS or lungs Myeloblastic transformation more common than lymphoblastic Resembles AML

Adapted from Wujcik, D. (1993). Leukemia. In S.L. Groenwald, M. Goodman, M.H. Frogge, & C.H. Yarbro (eds.). *Cancer Nursing: Principles and Practice* (3rd ed.). Boston: Jones & Bartlett, pp. 1161–1163.

       c. Degree of myelosuppression.

       d. Effects of organ involvement (Table 26–5).

  B. Leukemia may occur in any phase of the life cycle and is treated over time, from months to years.

III. Epidemiology (Table 26–6).

  A. Estimated 2% of all new cases of cancer in men and women in the United States (US) in 1997 will be leukemias. Approximately 28,300 cases of leukemia will be diagnosed in 1997 (50% chronic and 50% acute).

  B. Leukemia is expected to occur in more adults than children in 1997.

  C. Acute lymphocytic leukemia is the most common form of leukemia in children.

IV. Etiology and risk factors.

  A. Etiology of leukemia unknown.

  B. Risk factors most often associated with leukemia are exposure to chemicals and drugs (such as alkylating agents), genetic predisposition, exposure to radiation, and viruses.

V. Principles of medical management.

  A. Acute leukemia.

    1. Acute myelogenous leukemia (AML).

      a. Induction—initial treatment with chemotherapy agents given at high doses to eradicate leukemia and achieve complete remission (CR) resulting in bone marrow repopulation with normal cells.

        (1) Induction regimen usually includes cytarabine plus an anthracycline. In children, other agents, such as etoposide and thioguanine, may be added.

        (2) All-trans-retinoic acid (ATRA) is being used as initial treatment in acute promyelocytic leukemia (M3). ATRA induces differentiation of cells, restoring growth of normal blood cells.

        (3) Intrathecal cytarabine or methotrexate, with or without cranial radiation, is given if CNS leukemia is present. In children, cranial irradiation is incorporated into most protocols and is considered a standard part of treatment.

        (4) In a majority of children with M3 leukemia, remission and cure can be accomplished with the use of ATRA and chemotherapy.

        (5) Cytokines—use of granulocyte colony stimulating factors (G-CSF) or granulocyte-macrophage colony stimulating factors (GM-CSF) after completion of induction therapy is being studied to determine efficacy in modifying granulocytopenia in leukemia treatment. Already has been shown to decrease infectious episodes in elderly patients with acute leukemia.

      b. Post-remission therapy given to reduce leukemic cell population and achieve long-term, disease-free survival (DFS). Includes consolidation, intensification, maintenance, and bone marrow transplantation.

        (1) Consolidation therapy—one to two cycles of the same chemotherapy agents used in the induction therapy. Usually given after remission occurs.

        (2) Intensification therapy—high-dose chemotherapy given immediately or within several months of induction therapy. Same chemotherapy agents may be used at higher doses, or different drugs thought to be cross-resistant with induction therapy drugs may be used.

TABLE 26–5. Common Clinical Presentation of Leukemia

Diagnosis	Symptoms	Signs	WBC	Platelet	RBC	Other
AML	Fatigue Malaise Weight loss Fever Recurrent infections Unexplained bleeding Palpitations Dyspnea Anorexia Bone Pain Neurologic complaints: Headache Vomiting Visual changes Seizures	Sudden onset Rapid downhill course Bone marrow failure Anemia Thrombocytopenia Neutropenia Hepatomegaly Organ infiltration Pale skin	Myeloblasts Low Normal High Neutropenia ANC <1000 cells/mm^3	Low	Low	Hyperuricemia Elevated lactate dehydrogenase
ALL	Same as AML	Same as AML Lymphadenopathy Splenomegaly	Lymphoblasts Same as AML	Low	Low	
CML	Malaise Anorexia Weight loss Left upper quadrant pain Abdominal fullness Bone and joint pain Fever Night sweats	Insidious onset Pale skin Hepatomegaly Splenomegaly Bleeding disorders Anemia Peripheral blood leukocytosis	Mature myelocytes >100,000 cells/mm^3	Normal or high	Low	High serum B$_{12}$ level Low leukocyte alkaline phosphatase level (LAP)
CLL	Asymptomatic in early stages Recurrent infections Malaise Anorexia Fatigue Early satiety Abdominal discomfort	Insidious onset Splenomegaly Hepatomegaly Lymphadenopathy Anemia Thrombocytopenia Hypogammaglobinemia Rashes	Small mature or immature lymphocytes B cells >20,000 cells/mm^3 in early disease >100,000 cells/mm^3 in advanced disease	Low	Low	

AML = acute myelogenous leukemia; ALL = acute lymphocytic leukemia; CML = chronic myelogenous leukemia; CLL = chronic lymphocytic leukemia

TABLE 26–6. **Overall Remission and Survival Rates for Leukemia**

Description	Median Age	Initial Remission Rate	Median Survival With Treatment
AML	50–60 years	60–70%	10–15 months
ALL	4 years	Adult—70% Children—90%	Adult—2 years Children—5 years
CML	49 years	90%	3 years
CLL	60 years	90%	4–6 years

Adapted from Wujcik, D. (1993) Leukemia. In Groenwald, S.L., Goodman, M., Frogge, M.H., & Yarbro, C.H. (eds.). *Cancer Nursing: Principles and Practice* (3rd ed.). Boston: Jones & Barlett, p. 1154.

  (3) Maintenance therapy—lower doses of the same drugs used for induction therapy or different drugs given monthly for a prolonged time period to "maintain" a disease-free state. Maintenance therapy not currently recommended in treatment of AML.
    (a) ATRA is not used for maintenance therapy in acute promyelocytic leukemia (M3) because the drug becomes less effective with prolonged therapy.
  (4) Bone marrow transplant (BMT).
    (a) Allogeneic or matched unrelated BMT has become standard therapy for treatment of AML in first remission with long-term DFS rates of 45 to 65%. Transplantation in second or subsequent remissions or relapse decreases DFS to approximately 20% or less. Interest is growing in the use of allogeneic peripheral blood stem cells for transplantation.
    (b) Autologous bone marrow or peripheral blood stem cell transplantation is controversial, and further investigation is underway to evaluate risk of disease recurrence.
 2. Acute lymphocytic leukemia (ALL).
  a. Prognostic factors used to predict outcomes include cell morphology, age, white blood cell (WBC) count at presentation, success of initial induction therapy, and chromosomal abnormalities.
  b. Adults.
   (1) Initial treatment consists of protocol that includes vincristine, prednisone, and anthracycline with or without asparaginase or cyclophosphamide.
   (2) CNS prophylaxis includes intrathecal chemotherapy and/or high-dose systemic chemotherapy and possibly cranial irradiation.
   (3) Post-remission therapy options include short-term, relatively intensive chemotherapy followed by longer-term therapy at lower doses.
   (4) BMT.
    (a) Allogeneic BMT from histocompatible sibling donor should be considered for treatment of clients younger than age 50 years in first CR with high-risk ALL. Effect on DFS of transplantation in first CR remains to be determined.
    (b) Autologous BMT for treatment of ALL is optimally accomplished by collecting marrow during first CR. Various approaches have been used for marrow purging to remove resid-

ual leukemic cells. Wide variation in DFS exists because of differences in timing of transplantation and efforts to decrease residual leukemic cells.

   c. Children.

     (1) Induction chemotherapy regimens consist of prednisone, vincristine, with asparaginase and/or daunorubicin. Usually the four-drug regimen is limited to use in higher risk patients because of toxicities.

       (a) CNS treatment is given if CNS disease present or as prophylaxis. Treatment may consist of intrathecal methotrexate with or without radiation. Intrathecal therapy with methotrexate, cytarabine, and hydrocortisone may be given.

     (2) Postremission therapy continues for 2 to 3 years. Numerous drug combinations and schedules are used for maintenance. Low-risk ALL is treated with methotrexate and mercaptopurine with or without vincristine and prednisone. Additional drugs are used for intermediate and high-risk ALL.

     (3) BMT.

       (a) Allogeneic BMT for treatment of ALL in children should be considered if relapse occurs within 18 months of therapy or during therapy. Estimated DFS for clients transplanted in second CR is 40 to 62%.

       (b) Autologous BMT for children with ALL generally is not a treatment option because most clients have high-risk disease, and transplantation in first CR is not possible.

B. Chronic leukemia.

   1. Chronic myelogenous leukemia (CML).

     a. Chronic phase.

       (1) Two commonly used agents are hydroxyurea and busulfan. These oral agents are used to control leukocytosis but do not eradicate disease or induce cytogenetic remission.

       (2) Several recent studies have shown that alpha-2a interferon has prolonged overall survival and suppressed the growth of Philadelphia chromosome (Ph^1)-positive cells if present.

     b. Accelerated phase of CML is treated with increasing doses of chemotherapy with generally poor results.

     c. Blastic crisis.

       (1) Transformation into lymphoid leukemia—treatment is similar to that for ALL using combinations of vincristine and prednisone.

       (2) Transformation in myeloid leukemia—treatment is similar to that for AML and includes investigational protocols.

       (3) Hydroxyurea may be given for palliation.

       (4) Radiation therapy may be given for lytic bone lesions.

       (5) CNS or meningeal disease may be treated with intrathecal methotrexate, cytarabine, or cranial irradiation.

     d. BMT.

       (1) Allogeneic or syngeneic BMT may be used as effective treatment for CML and may result in long-term DFS. Controversy exists regarding optimal timing of undergoing BMT. According to the International Bone Marrow Transplant Registry (IBMTR) data, patients undergoing BMT in chronic phase have a 50 to 60%

long-term DFS, whereas in accelerated or blastic phase DFS is estimated to be 35 to 40% and 10 to 20%, respectively.

    (2) Autologous bone marrow or peripheral blood stem cell transplantation for treatment of chronic or transformed CML has been used with varying results. Stem cells are collected during the chronic phase of the disease with the intent to reinfuse the cells following myeloablative therapy.

2. Chronic lymphocytic leukemia (CLL).
   a. Treatment is delayed until the client is symptomatic, such as exhibiting signs of hemolytic anemia, cytopenia, lymphadenopathy that is painful and/or disfiguring, or symptomatic organomegaly.
   b. Disease is followed by monitoring lymphocyte count.
   c. Chlorambucil is used to suppress production of well-differentiated, small lymphocytes.
   d. Cyclophosphamide inhibits growth of less mature lymphocytes with limited effect on neutrophils and platelets.
   e. Leukocytosis and immune-mediated cytopenias can be controlled by use of corticosteroids. Splenectomy may be used for symptom relief when steroids are no longer effective.
   f. Radiation therapy is effective treatment for lymphadenopathy and/or splenomegaly that is painful.
   g. Fludarabine has been approved for treatment of B-cell CLL, and its use is being evaluated for first line therapy.
   h. BMT—clinical trials are currently underway to evaluate the use of transplantation for the treatment of CLL.

3. Hairy cell leukemia.
   a. Decision to treat is based on presence of symptomatic cytopenias, massive splenomegaly, or other complications.
   b. 10% of clients will never require treatment.
   c. Treatment options.
      (1) 2-Chlorodoxyadenosine (2-cda).
      (2) Pentostatin.
      (3) Alpha-interferon.
      (4) Splenectomy is rare but indicated when the client has low WBC count, splenomegaly, and minimal bone marrow involvement.

Assessment

I. Patient history.
  A. Exposure to radiation.
    1. Previous treatment with radiation therapy.
    2. Accidental exposure through environmental sources of radiation.
    3. Exposure to radiation in the work setting.
  B. Exposure to chemicals.
    1. Previous treatment with antineoplastic agents (e.g., alkylating agents, etoposide).
    2. Previous treatment with medications such as chloramphenicol, phenylbutazone.
    3. Accidental or work-related exposure to chemicals (e.g., benzene).
  C. Exposure to viruses.
    1. Human immunodeficiency virus (HIV) associated with T-cell lymphocytic leukemia.
    2. Epstein-Barr virus (EBV).

   D. Genetic abnormalities.
     1. Down syndrome.
     2. Turner's syndrome.
     3. Bloom syndrome.
     4. Klinefelter's syndrome.
     5. Fanconi's anemia.
   E. Family history of genetic abnormalities or cancer.
   F. Chief complaint (see Table 26–5, common symptoms).
   G. Psychosocial profile.
II. Physical examination.
   A. Head and neck—pale mucous membranes, bleeding gums, lymphadenopathy.
   B. Abdomen—hepatomegaly, splenomegaly.
   C. Neurologic—headache, papilledema, meningismus, abnormal cranial nerve responses.
   D. Respiratory—abnormal lung sounds if pneumonia is present.
   E. Cardiovascular—tachycardia, murmurs.
   F. Musculoskeletal—joint pain and inflammation.
   G. Integumentary—bruising, ecchymoses, and petechiae.
   H. Lymph nodes—cervical, supraclavicular, axillary, mediastinal, or inguinal lymphadenopathy.
   I. Genitourinary—urinary tract infections, hematuria, testicular mass, menorrhagia.
III. Diagnostic studies.
   A. Complete blood count with WBC differential (see Table 26–5 for values at diagnosis for each type of leukemia).
     1. Thrombocytopenia.
     2. Anemia.
     3. Abnormal differential.
       a. Neutropenia.
       b. Leukocytosis.
       c. Blasts.
   B. Other blood tests.
     1. Liver function tests (e.g., for elevated lactate dehydrogenase [LDH]).
     2. Uric acid (hyperuricemia).
   C. Bone marrow aspirate and biopsy.
     1. Cell morphology.
     2. Immunophenotype.
     3. Cellularity.
     4. Cytogenetic analysis.
   D. Cerebral spinal studies.
     1. Increased protein.
     2. Decreased glucose.
     3. Leukemic cells.

Nursing Diagnoses

   I. Potential for injury.
  II. Risk for infection.
 III. Knowledge deficit.
 IV. Ineffective individual coping.
  V. Ineffective family coping: compromised.

Outcome Identification

  I. Client and family describe the type of leukemia and rationale for treatment.
 II. Client and family list signs and symptoms of immediate and long-term effects of leukemia and treatment.
III. Client lists self-care measures to decrease the incidence and severity of symptoms and complications associated with disease and treatment.
 IV. Client demonstrates skills in self-care necessary because of effects of disease and treatment.
  V. Client and family describe schedule and procedures for routine follow-up care including blood work, bone marrow biopsy, and lumbar puncture.
 VI. Client and family list signs and symptoms of recurrent disease.
VII. Client and family describe potential community resources available to assist with diagnosis, treatment, rehabilitation, and survivorship.

Planning and Implementation

  I. Interventions to decrease the incidence and severity of complications unique to leukemia.
  A. Myelosuppression (see Chapter 12).
  B. Septic shock (see Chapter 17).
  C. Disseminated intravascular coagulation (DIC) (see Chapter 17).
 II. Interventions for management of unique side effects of disease or treatment.
  A. Myelosuppression (see Chapter 12).
  B. Septic shock (see Chapter 17).
  C. DIC (see Chapter 17).
  D. Tumor lysis syndrome (see Chapter 17).
  E. Mucositis (see Chapter 13).
  F. Leukostasis.
   1. Physiologic effect—increase in blood viscosity that may result in obstruction of the microcirculation or formation of thrombi of WBCs in small vessels, resulting in capillary plugging, vessel rupture, bleeding, and organ damage.
   2. Clients at risk—diagnosis of acute or chronic leukemia with a WBC count greater than 50,000 to 100,000/mm^3.
   3. Most common sites.
    a. Brain/CNS.
    b. Lung.
    c. Other organs may be involved.
   4. Most common signs.
    a. Increased intracranial pressure. (See also Chapter 18.)
    b. Respiratory distress.
    c. Other signs depend on organs involved.
   5. Most common complications.
    a. Pulmonary hemorrhage.
    b. Cerebral hemorrhage.
   6. Medical management.
    a. Initiation of chemotherapy to treat the disease process.
    b. Initiation of leukapheresis to temporarily decrease the WBC count.
    c. Administration of intravenous fluids.
    d. Initiation of cranial radiation if appropriate.

7. Nursing interventions.
   a. Frequency of monitoring dependent on individual patient and his/her symptoms. General guidelines are as follows:
      (1) Perform neurologic checks every 2 to 4 hours when the WBC count is greater than 50,000 to 100,000/mm^3.
      (2) Monitor vital signs including blood pressure every 2 to 4 hours.
         (a) Assess respiratory rate, depth, effort, and effectiveness every 2 to 4 hours.
         (b) Auscultate lung sounds.
      (3) Monitor for signs of bleeding every 2 to 4 hours.
      (4) Interventions for management of myelosuppression (see Chapter 12).
      (5) Contact physician with any aberrant findings.
   b. Initiate safety measures as appropriate.
III. Interventions for management of vascular access devices (see Chapter 9).
IV. Interventions for management of alterations in coping.
   A. Psychosocial issues (see Chapter 2).
   B. Altered body image and alopecia (see Chapter 3).
   C. Cultural issues (see Chapter 4).
   D. Survivorship issues (see Chapter 5).
V. Interventions for management of sexuality concerns or abnormalities (see Chapter 6).
VI. Interventions for supportive care related to death and dying issues (see Chapter 7).
VII. Interventions for rehabilitation (see Chapter 8).

Evaluation

The oncology nurse systematically and regularly evaluates the client's and/or family's responses to interventions to determine progress toward the achievement of expected outcomes. Relevant data is collected and actual findings are compared with expected findings. Nursing diagnoses, outcomes, and plans of care are reviewed and revised as necessary.

BIBLIOGRAPHY

Allan, N.C., Richards, S.M., & Shepherd, P.C.A. (1995). UK Medical Research council randomised, multicentre trial of interferon alpha-n1 for chronic myeloid leukaemia: Improved survival irrespective of cytogenetic response. *Lancet 345*(8962), 1392–1397.
American Cancer Society. (1997). *Cancer Facts and Figures–1997*. Atlanta: American Cancer Society.
Carson, C., & Callaghan, M. (1991). Hematopoietic and immunologic cancers. In S.B. Baird, R. McCorkle, & M. Grant (eds.). *Cancer Nursing: A Comprehensive Textbook*. Philadelphia: W.B. Saunders, pp. 536–547.
Campbell, K. (1995). The causes and incidence of haematological malignancies. *Nurs Times 91*(31), 25–28.
Deisseroth, A.B., Andreeff, M., Champlin, R., et al. (1993). Chronic leukemias. In V.T. DeVita, Jr., S. Hellman, & S.A. Rosenberg (eds.). *Cancer: Principles and Practice of Oncology* (4th ed.). Philadelphia: J.B. Lippincott, pp. 1965–1980.
Forman, S.J., Blume, K.G., & Thomas, E.D. (1994). *Bone Marrow Transplantation*. Boston: Blackwell Scientific Publications.
Groenwald, S.L., Frogge, M.H., Goodman, M., & Yarbro, C.G. (eds.). (1995). Leukemia. *Comprehensive Cancer Nursing Review* (2nd ed.). Boston: Jones & Bartlett, pp. 448–464.
Haeuber, D., & Spross, J. (1994). Protective mechanisms: Bone marrow. In B.L. Johnson & J. Gross (eds.). *Handbook of Oncology Nursing* (2nd ed.). Boston: Jones and Bartlett, pp. 373–380.

Italian Cooperative Study Group on Chronic Myeloid Leukemia. (1994). Interferon alfa-2a as compared with conventional chemotherapy for the treatment of chronic myeloid leukemia. *N Engl J Med 330*(12), 820–825.

Keating, M.J., Estey, E., & Kantarjian, H. (1993). Acute leukemia. In V.T. DeVita, Jr., S. Hellman, & S.A. Rosenberg (eds.). *Cancer: Principles and Practice of Oncology* (4th ed.). Philadelphia: J.B. Lippincott, pp. 1938–1959.

Parker, S.L., Tong, T., Bolden, S., & Wingo, P.A. (1996). Cancer statistics 1996. *CA Cancer J Clin 46*(1), 5–27.

Wujcik D. (1993). Leukemia. In S.L. Groenwald, M. Goodman, M.H. Frogge, & C.H. Yarbro (eds.). *Cancer Nursing: Principles and Practice* (3rd ed.). Boston: Jones & Bartlett, pp. 1149–1173.

Wujcik, D., Viele, C.S., & Caudell, K.A. (1996). Leukemia management strategies: The next generation. *Oncol Nurs Forum 23*(3), 477–502.

Yeager, K.A., & Miaskowski, C. (1994). Advances in understanding the mechanisms and management of acute myelogenous leukemia. *Oncol Nurs Forum 21*(3), 541–548.

Nursing Care of the Client With Lymphomas and Multiple Myeloma

Joyce Alexander, RN, MSN, AOCN

Theory

I. Pathophysiology of the lymphoid system.
   A. Primitive or pluripotent stem cell, located in the bone marrow, is ancestor for both myeloid and lymphoid cell lines.
   B. Primary lymphoid tissues are the bone marrow and the thymus.
      1. Lymphocytes develop from committed lymphoid stem cells in the bone marrow.
      2. A portion migrates to the thymus.
         a. Proliferate and mature into T cells.
         b. In adults, T cells continue to proliferate peripherally.
      3. Lymphoid cells maturing in the bone marrow become B cells.
         a. Mature B cells, known as plasma cells, produce immune globulins.
   C. Secondary lymphoid tissues.
      1. Lymph nodes, spleen, Waldeyer's ring (oropharyngeal lymphoid tissue).
      2. Groups of cells in the gut, called Peyer's patches.
      3. Lymphoid cells in the epithelium of the gut and respiratory tract called mucosa-associated lymphoid tissue (MALT).
      4. Distributed in interstitium, in most tissues, except in the central nervous system.
   D. Cells of the lymphoid system include:
      1. T cells and B cells.
      2. Monocytes and macrophages.
      3. Reticular supporting cells, which form the lymph node structure.
      4. Langerhans cells, found in the skin as well as lymph nodes.
      5. See Chapter 20 for information on function of the immune system.
II. Malignancies of the lymphoid system.
   A. Hodgkin's disease.
      1. Malignant cell is Reed-Sternberg cell.
         a. Cells express antigens characteristic of activated B and T cells.
         b. Cells also have characteristics of reticular cells.
         c. Hodgkin's disease may actually be a group of related diseases.
      2. Clinical presentation.
         a. Enlarged lymph nodes with or without systemic symptoms.
            (1) Cervical, supraclavicular, or mediastinal regions most common.
            (2) Tends to spread first to adjacent lymph nodes. Immune suppression before treatment is common.
         b. Systemic symptoms include fever, weight loss, and night sweats.

B. Non-Hodgkin's lymphoma (lymphocytic lymphoma).
   1. Malignancies of T and B lymphocytes.
      a. A collection of diseases rather than a single disease.
      b. Majority are B-cell, some are T-cell neoplasms.
   2. Rarely diagnosed as a single lymph node or region.
      a. Most often presentation is with disseminated disease.
      b. Involvement of bone marrow or liver is common.
   3. Aggressiveness varies among types.
C. Myeloma.
   1. Malignancy of the plasma cell, a B cell differentiated to produce immuno-globulins.
      a. Although a solitary plasmacytoma can occur, multiple myeloma, by definition, is a systemic disease.
      b. Myeloma cells produce abnormally high blood levels of monoclonal immunoglobulins.
         (1) Referred to as M protein.
         (2) Not effective in immune function.
      c. Myeloma cells also produce osteoclast-activating factor (possibly interleukin-1 beta).
         (1) Produces lytic bone lesions, resulting in a "punched out" appearance on radiographs and often in pathologic fractures.
         (2) Increases bone resorption, which can cause hypercalcemia.
   2. Clinical presentation.
      a. Occasionally diagnosed with routine laboratory tests as an elevated blood protein or anemia.
      b. Commonly presents with bone pain resulting from lytic lesions.
      c. Renal insufficiency is common owing to hypercalcemia, hyperviscosity, or deposits of amyloids or immunoglobulins.
III. Diagnostic measures.
   A. Hodgkin's disease.
      1. Excisional lymph node biopsy is required.
      2. Diagnosis requires presence of the Reed-Sternberg cell on pathology examination.
   B. Non-Hodgkin's lymphoma: Excisional lymph node biopsy is required for diagnosis and differentiation of types of non-Hodgkin's lymphoma.
   C. Multiple myeloma is diagnosed by:
      1. Bone marrow biopsy showing the presence of more than 10% plasma cells.
      2. Serum protein electrophoresis showing increased levels of M protein.
      3. Urine immunoelectrophoresis showing increased levels of M protein.
IV. Classification.
   A. Hodgkin's disease.
      1. Pathologic classification and grade: Rye classification.
         a. Lymphocyte predominant.
         b. Mixed cellularity.
         c. Nodular sclerosis.
         d. Lymphocyte-depleted.
      2. Staging.
         a. Hodgkin's disease is staged on the basis of the extent of spread and the presence or absence of systemic symptoms.
         b. Ann Arbor staging system.
            (1) Stage I—single lymph node region or structure.
            (2) Stage II—two or more lymph node regions, same side of diaphragm.

(3) Stage III—lymph nodes on both sides of diaphragm.

(4) Stage IV—extranodal sites.

(5) If the client has fever or night sweats, B is added to stage.

   c. Cotswald modifications to the Ann Arbor system.

     (1) Further subdivided stages based on bulk and location of disease and response to therapy.

   d. Staging workup is done to determine extent of disease.

     (1) History, physical, chest x-ray examination, and complete blood count (CBC).

     (2) Computed tomography (CT) scans of the chest, abdomen, and pelvis.

     (3) Lymphogram is done if the CT scan result is negative.

     (4) Staging laparotomy should be done only if results will alter the initial treatment plan.

  3. Prognosis is related to pathologic classification, stage, age of the client, and response to treatment.

   a. 10-year survival rates for early-stage disease are near 90%.

   b. In treated, advanced disease, 10-year survival is over 50%.

B. Non-Hodgkin's lymphoma.

  1. Pathologic classification and grade.

   a. Working formulation divides lymphomas into grades.

     (1) Low, intermediate, and high.

     (2) Low-grade lymphomas are indolent, higher grades are more aggressive.

   b. Revised European-American Classification of Lymphoid Neoplasms (REAL).

     (1) Categorizes lymphoid malignancies using morphologic, immunologic, and genetic information.

     (2) Lists disease entities with varying aggressiveness and prognosis.

  2. Ann Arbor staging with Cotswald modifications.

   a. Staging workup includes history, physical, chest x-ray examination, blood counts, other blood studies, abdominal-pelvic CT scans.

   b. Lymphangiogram should be performed on most clients.

   c. Bilateral bone marrow biopsy is required.

   d. Staging laparotomy is no longer recommended.

  3. Prognosis depends on grade or aggressiveness of lymphoma and responsiveness to treatment.

   a. Low-grade lymphomas have an indolent course with prolonged survival without aggressive therapy.

   b. Prognosis of aggressive histology lymphomas depends on tumor bulk, responsiveness to therapy, and the client's ability to tolerate treatment.

C. Multiple myeloma.

  1. Multiple myeloma is included in the REAL classification system.

  2. Staging quantifies tumor volume on the basis of hemoglobin level, M protein in urine and blood, serum calcium level, and presence of bone lesions.

  3. Although median survival time from diagnosis is 10 years, most clients with multiple myeloma die of the disease.

V. Treatment (Table 27–1).

A. Hodgkin's disease.

  1. Stage I or IIA—external beam radiation therapy.

  2. Stage II with bulky mediastinal disease—concurrent radiation therapy and chemotherapy.

  3. Advanced disease—combination chemotherapy.

   a. MOPP (mechlorethamine, vincristine, procarbazine, and prednisone).

   b. ABVD (doxorubicin, bleomycin, vinblastine, dacarbazine).

TABLE 27-1. **Treatment of Lymphoid Malignancies**

Disease	Radiation	Chemotherapy	Salvage
Hodgkin's disease	External beam for stages I and IIA. Concurrent with chemotherapy for stage II/bulky disease.	Combination chemotherapy for stages IIB, III, and IV MOPP (mechlorethamine, vincristine, procarbazine, prednisone) or ABVD (doxorubicin, bleomycin, vinblastine, dacarbazine)	Alternative chemotherapy regimen, or Autologous bone marrow transplant, or Peripheral blood stem cell (PBSC) transplant
Non-Hodgkin's lymphoma	Low-grade, stage I or II disease	Combination chemotherapy; regimens including: cyclophosphamide, doxorubicin, prednisone, along with other drugs	Autologous or allogenic bone marrow transplant or PBSC transplant
Multiple myeloma	Palliative	Melphalan and prednisone or VAD (vincristine, doxorubicin, dexamethasone) Autologous bone marrow transplant or PBSC transplant as consolidation for appropriate clients	Allogeneic bone marrow transplant, autologous bone marrow, or PBSC transplant

    4. Salvage therapy for clients who suffer a relapse after chemotherapy.
        a. Alternative chemotherapy (crossover to MOPP or ABVD if not previously used) or, if more than 1 year has passed since treatment, repeat previously used chemotherapy.
        b. Autologous marrow or peripheral blood stem cell (PBSC) transplantation following high-dose chemotherapy has produced complete remission rates of 40 to 70%.

  B. Non-Hodgkin's lymphoma.
    1. Low-grade, stage I or II—radiation therapy.
    2. Aggressive lymphomas are considered systemic disease and treated with combination chemotherapy.
        a. Regimens generally include cyclophosphamide, doxorubicin, and prednisone along with other drugs, given on a complex schedule.
        b. In stage I or II, radiation therapy may be used with chemotherapy.
    3. Preferred treatment for recurrent non-Hodgkin's lymphoma is autologous or allogeneic bone marrow or PBSC transplant.

  C. Multiple myeloma.
    1. Treatment for symptomatic multiple myeloma is chemotherapy.
        a. Melphalan and prednisone or VAD (vincristine, doxorubicin, dexamethasone) have shown excellent response rates.
        b. Interferon alpha inhibits plasma cell growth and may prove useful.
    2. Allogeneic bone marrow transplant has shown benefit but the technique is limited because of age of clients and lack of appropriate donors.
    3. Autologous bone marrow and PBSC transplantation have produced complete response in almost 50% of clients, up to 70 years of age, when used as consolidation.

Assessment

I. During diagnosis and staging.
  A. Personal and family history.
    1. Age.
        a. Hodgkin's disease is more common in young adults with a second peak in older adults.
        b. Non-Hodgkin's lymphoma incidence increases with age.
        c. Peak incidence of multiple myeloma is around 60 years of age.
    2. Family history of Hodgkin's disease in first-degree relatives increases risk.
    3. Personal history of immunosuppression increases risk of lymphoma.
    4. Symptoms prompting client to seek treatment.
        a. Enlarged lymph nodes.
        b. Presence of B symptoms.
            (1) Fever.
            (2) Night sweats.
            (3) Anorexia and/or weight loss.
            (4) Weakness, shortness of breath.
        c. Presence of pain, especially bone pain.
        d. Changes in urinary function.
  B. Physical examination.
    1. Palpation of enlarged lymph nodes.
    2. Palpation of liver and spleen for enlargement.
    3. Neurologic examination for deficits.

  C. Coping skills.
   1. Feelings about staging procedures and possible diagnosis.
   2. Coping strategies used in the past.
   3. Effectiveness of previous coping strategies.
  D. Social situation.
   1. Ability to keep appointments for diagnosis and staging procedures.
    a. Transportation.
    b. Economic issues.
    c. Understanding of need for procedures.
   2. Additional stresses in home and family.
   3. Social support systems.
  E. Knowledge of procedures and potential outcomes.
 II. During treatment.
  A. Side effects of therapy (see Chapters 35 and 37).
   1. Laboratory values, for neutropenia, thrombocytopenia, and electrolyte abnormalities.
   2. Symptoms of infection or bleeding.
   3. Nutritional status, anorexia, nausea and vomiting.
   4. Fatigue.
  B. Symptoms of oncologic emergencies.
   1. Tumor lysis syndrome is common during initial treatment of lymphoma.
   2. Hypercalcemia occurs in clients with multiple myeloma and lymphoma.
   3. Clients with lymphoma or Hodgkin's disease must be observed for superior vena cava syndrome when mediastinal disease is present.
   4. Chapters 17 and 18 give specific assessment parameters for these emergencies.
  C. Presence of bone pain and effectiveness of measures to manage pain.
  D. Mobility and ability to perform activities of daily living.
  E. Body image and adaptation to illness.
 III. Rehabilitation phase.
  A. Sexual or endocrine dysfunction.
  B. Symptoms of second malignancies. (Treatment with alkylating agents or with high-dose combination chemotherapy increases risk of second malignancy.)

Nursing Diagnoses

 I. During diagnosis and staging.
  A. Fear.
  B. Ineffective individual coping.
  C. Ineffective family coping: compromised.
  D. Decisional conflict.
 II. During treatment.
  A. Knowledge deficit.
  B. Fatigue.
  C. Risk for infection.
  D. Altered nutrition, less than body requirements.
  E. Impaired physical mobility.
  F. Chronic pain.
  G. Self-esteem disturbance.
 III. During the rehabilitation phase.
  A. Sexual dysfunction.
  B. Fear.

Outcome Identification

I. During diagnosis and staging, the client and family:
   A. Communicate feelings about a potential diagnosis.
   B. Identify and use effective coping skills.
   C. Arrive on time and prepared for scheduled tests and procedures.
   D. Verbalize information about disease and treatment.
   E. Participate in treatment decisions.
II. During the treatment phase, the client:
   A. Verbalizes knowledge of treatment regimen.
   B. Identifies measures to manage fatigue.
   C. Lists symptoms of infection.
   D. Describes situations requiring professional intervention.
   E. Discusses measures to enhance nutritional intake.
   F. Maintains active or passive motion within mobility limitations.
   G. Uses effective strategies for pain management.
   H. Participates in measures to enhance self-esteem.
III. During the rehabilitation phase, the client:
   A. Identifies potential or actual alterations in sexual function related to disease and treatment.
   B. Demonstrates adaptive behaviors.
      1. Incorporates possibility of disease recurrence into lifestyle without being overwhelmed by threat.
      2. Participates in health maintenance behaviors.

Planning and Implementation

A. A plan of care for the client with a lymphoid malignancy is based on achieving outcomes related to identified nursing diagnoses.
B. The plan of care is developed in cooperation with the client, the client's family, and the multidisciplinary team.
C. Standards of care, care maps, or pathways, when available, provide a blueprint for client care.
D. Appropriate nursing interventions for the client with lymphoid malignancy include, but are not limited to, the following:
   1. Encourage communication of feelings about disease and treatment.
   2. Refer to community resources (support groups, American Cancer Society, I Can Cope).
   3. Explore coping options with the client and family and validate effective mechanisms.
   4. Develop a written schedule and specific instructions for preparation for tests and procedures.
   5. Provide culturally sensitive information in written format at an appropriate reading level or in an alternative format understandable to the client and family.
   6. Clarify and explain information verbally.
   7. Implement measures to assist the client in managing fatigue (see Chapter 1).
   8. Discuss effects of treatment and symptoms requiring professional intervention.
   9. Discuss measures to assist the client in maintaining nutritional intake (see Chapters 9 and 13) and provide nutritional supplements.

10. Encourage active participation in care.
11. Assist the client in maintaining activity. (Inactivity increases the risk of bone resorption.)
12. Provide pharmacologic and nonpharmacologic interventions to manage pain. (See Chapters 1, 10.)
13. Encourage verbalization of feelings about changes in appearance.
14. Provide information on measures to cope with appearance changes (e.g., wigs, scarves, hats for alopecia; Look Good, Feel Better program).
15. Discuss options for sperm banking, when appropriate, before beginning treatment.
16. Refer to appropriate resources for sexual dysfunction including gynecologist, fertility specialist, or sexuality counselor.
17. Review symptoms of endocrine dysfunction that should be reported to the health care team.

Evaluation

The oncology nurse systematically and regularly evaluates the client's and/or family's responses to interventions to determine progress toward the achievement of expected outcomes. Relevant data are collected and actual findings are compared with expected findings. Nursing diagnoses, outcomes, and plans of care are reviewed and revised as necessary.

BIBLIOGRAPHY

Alexanian, R., & Dimopoulos, M. (1995). Management of multiple myeloma. *Semin Hematol 32*(1), 20–30.

Barlogie, B., Jagannath, S., Vesole, D., & Tricot, G. (1995). Autologous and allogeneic transplants for multiple myeloma. *Semin Hematol 32*(1), 31–44.

Clark, J. (1994). Multiple myeloma. In S. Otto (ed.). *Oncology Nursing* (2nd ed.). St. Louis: C.V. Mosby, pp. 356–360.

DeVita, V. Jr., Hellman, S., & Jaffe, E. (1993). Hodgkin's disease. In V. DeVita, Jr., S. Hellman, & S. Rosenberg (eds.). *Cancer: Principles and Practice of Oncology* (4th ed.). Philadelphia: J.B. Lippincott, pp. 1819–1858.

Harris, N.L., Jaffe, E.S., Stein, H., et al. (1994) . A revised European-American classification of lymphoid neoplasms: A proposal from the International Lymphoma Study Group. *Blood 5,* 1361–1392.

Iwamoto, R.R., Rumsey, K.A., & Summers, B.L.Y. (1996). *Statement on the Scope and Standards of Oncology Nursing Practice.* Washington, D.C.: American Nurses Publishing.

Longo, D., DeVita, V. Jr., Jaffe, E., et al. (1993). Lymphocytic lymphomas. In V. DeVita, Jr., S. Hellman, & S. Rosenberg (eds.). *Cancer: Principles and Practice of Oncology* (4th ed.). Philadelphia: J.B. Lippincott, pp. 1859–1927.

Moore, J. Malignant lymphoma. In S. Otto (ed.). *Oncology Nursing* (2nd ed.). St. Louis: C.V. Mosby, pp. 340–355.

Sheridan, C. (1996). Multiple myeloma. *Semin Oncol Nurs 12*(1), 59–69.

Weinshel, E., & Peterson, B. (1993). Hodgkin's disease. *CA Cancer J Clin 43*(6), 327–343.

28

Nursing Care of the Client With Bone and Soft Tissue Cancers

Ellen Carr, RN, MSN, AOCN

Theory

I. Common malignant bone and soft tissue cancers (with cell or tissue of origin).
  A. Osteosarcoma (osseous tissue).
  B. Chondrosarcoma (cartilaginous tissue).
  C. Fibrosarcoma (fibrous tissue).
  D. Ewing's sarcoma (reticuloendothelial tissue).
  E. Miscellaneous soft tissue sarcomas.
    1. Examples.
      a. Liposarcoma (adipose tissue).
      b. Leiomyosarcoma (smooth muscle).
      c. Rhabdomyosarcoma (striated muscle).
      d. Angiosarcoma (vascular tissue).
      e. Malignant fibrous histiocytoma (histiocytic origin).
      f. Kaposi's sarcoma (unknown origin).
II. Epidemiology.
  A. Incidence of primary malignant bone and soft tissue tumors is low.
    1. Bone.
      a. 1997 estimates—2500 new cases; deaths—1410.
      b. Comprise less than 0.2% of all malignant tumors in the US.
    2. Soft tissue.
      a. 1997 estimates—6600 new cases; incidence slightly higher for men. Deaths in 1997—4100.
      b. Comprise less than 5% of all cancers in US adults.
III. Risk factors.
  A. Bone—no definitive risk factors. Factors suggested:
    1. Previous high-dose irradiation.
    2. Chemicals—vinyl chloride gas, arsenic, dioxin, Agent Orange.
    3. Prior treatment with antineoplastic agents—melphalan, procarbazine, nitrosoureas, chlorambucil.
    4. Immunosuppression.
    5. Familial, genetic connections.
    6. Preexisting bone conditions (e.g., Paget's disease).
    7. Skeletal maldevelopment.

B. Soft tissue.
  1. Uncommon and diverse presentations do not suggest common risk factors.
  2. Some suggested factors.
    a. Approximately 5% of sarcomas occur at previous radiation therapy sites (e.g., treated for osteosarcoma).
    b. History of trauma.
    c. Chemical exposure—asbestos, polyvinyl chloride gas, arsenic, Agent Orange.
IV. Pathophysiology and classification.
  A. Bone.
    1. From mesoderm and ectoderm; pseudocapsule contains tumor, then breaks through to surrounding tissue. (This is called *skip metastasis.*)
    2. Staging based on biologic behavior and tumor aggressiveness.
      a. 30% of lesions (stage I) present as intracompartmental.
      b. 70% of lesions (stages II–III) present as extracompartmental.
    3. Osteosarcoma (osteogenic sarcoma)—20% of all primary malignant tumors.
      a. Most often affect adolescents.
      b. Males are affected more frequently than females (1.6:1.0).
      c. Tumor cells are spindle-shaped, from bone-forming mesenchyma in the medullary cavity. Reactive osteoclasts interact with normal bone to destroy it.
      d. Start in metaphysis of long bones (area of highest growth); 50% of cases occur in knee region.
      e. Metastasize to the lung first; at diagnosis, 80% of patients have micro-metastasis.
    4. Chondrosarcoma.
      a. Occurs most often in adults ages 40 to 60 years.
      b. More often in men (2:1).
      c. Origin—malignant cartilaginous tumor cells from medullary canal or outside bone, destroying the bone.
      d. Commonly affect pelvis, femur, and shoulder.
      e. Often slow growing, but it can metastasize distantly.
    5. Fibrosarcoma.
      a. Most often seen in adolescents and young adults.
      b. Commonly affects the femur and tibia.
      c. Arises from the medullary cavity, affects metaphyseal area.
      d. Constitutes approximately 4% of all primary malignant bone cancers.
    6. Ewing's sarcoma.
      a. Constitutes approximately 6% of all primary malignant bone cancers.
      b. Found in children 10 to 15 years old (tall children especially). Rare in African Americans, Chinese.
      c. Highly malignant; origin in nonmesenchymal area of bone marrow; from shaft of long bones.
      d. Most often affects pelvis and lower extremities; femoral diaphysis is the most common site.
      e. Spreads to adjacent tissue via many round cells; indistinct borders, necrotic and hemorrhagic areas are common.
      f. Metastasizes to lungs, lymph nodes, and other bones. At diagnosis, 15 to 35% of patients have metastasis.

g. Associated with retinoblastoma and skeletal anomalies.

h. Disease-free survivors—50% (due to multimodality therapies, precision in surgery [wide resections]).

B. Soft tissue sarcomas.

1. Classified by cell type, origin—connective tissue (fat, muscle, tendons, fibrous tissue).

2. Sarcomas can appear anywhere because of the body's widespread connective tissue; most are found in the lower extremities or trunk.

3. When they metastasize, prognosis is poor.

V. Treatments.

A. Overview.

1. Goals.

a. Rid tumor.

b. Avoid amputation.

c. Preserve functioning.

2. Surgery.

a. Based on size, location, tumor composition.

b. Treatment of choice with osteosarcoma, fibrosarcoma, chondrosarcoma.

c. Amputation versus limb salvage issues:

(1) Acceptable surgical margins.

(2) Blood vessel and nerves involved with the tumor.

(3) Age (in children younger than 10 years old, surgery affects limb growth).

(4) Limb salvage when tumor metastasizes late.

(5) Amputation—when tumor extends to incisional surface or when location necessitates (e.g., tumor extends to vertebral body and pelvis).

(6) At present there is an option for limb salvage surgery; before, amputation was the only choice.

(7) Cryosurgery (insert liquid nitrogen in cavity); sometimes is effective.

d. Reconstruction.

(1) Bone autografts, allografts.

(2) After soft tissue resection, three common methods.

(a) Arthrodesis or fusion (with implants or grafts).

(b) Arthroplasty for joints.

(c) Allografts (since the 1960s)—bone, tendon, ligament, connective tissue.

(3) Tested for match, viral and bacterial contamination.

(4) Method—bone frozen to accept graft.

(5) Intercalary allograft placed between two segments of host bone; used for long bone grafts.

(6) Issues—nonunion, infections, healing.

3. Radiotherapy.

a. Usually added with other modalities.

b. Used when tumor is localized.

c. Used after surgical debulking or tumor removal.

4. Chemotherapy or immunotherapy.

a. Used as an adjuvant or neoadjuvant with surgery.

b. Since the addition of chemotherapy and immunotherapy in a multimodality approach to treatment, disease-free periods for patients have increased remarkably.

   c. Common chemotherapeutic agents—doxorubicin, cisplatin, cyclophosphamide, dacarbazine (DTIC), ifosfamide, methotrexate.

B. Treatment of common malignant bone and soft tissue tumors.

   1. Osteosarcoma.

      a. Surgery.

      b. Multimodality.

         (1) Surgery.

         (2) Radiotherapy.

         (3) Chemotherapy and immunotherapy.

   2. Chondrosarcoma.

      a. Surgery.

   3. Fibrosarcoma.

      a. Surgery.

         (1) Radical surgery.

         (2) Amputation.

      b. Radiotherapy only for inoperable tumors.

   4. Ewing's sarcoma.

      a. Multimodality.

         (1) Surgery.

         (2) Radiotherapy.

         (3) Chemotherapy.

   5. Miscellaneous soft tissue sarcomas (e.g., liposarcoma, leiomyosarcoma, rhabdomyosarcoma, angiosarcoma, malignant fibrous histiocytoma, Kaposi's sarcoma).

      a. Surgery.

         (1) Resection (thoracotomy) when spread to lung, provided that the primary tumor is controlled.

      b. Radiotherapy.

      c. Chemotherapy.

Assessment

I. Osteosarcoma.

   A. Clinical symptoms.

      1. Pain—onset, location, duration, quality; may be radicular; gradual onset, worse at night, increases with tumor burden.

      2. Swelling in affected area.

      3. Bone—rule out injury.

      4. If pathologic fracture, there can be acute, sudden pain.

   B. Physical examination.

      1. Mass visible, palpable; may be firm, nontender, warm.

      2. Size noted, bilateral comparison.

      3. Limited range of motion (ROM).

   C. Diagnostic data.

      1. Laboratory.

         a. Elevated serum alkaline phosphatase level (due to increased osteoblastic activity).

      2. Radiographs (cannot see changes until tumor is advanced); three patterns of tumor (can occur isolated or together).

        a. Geographic (slow-growing) tumor meets nontumor tissue.

        b. Moth-eaten (moderately aggressive).

        c. Permeative (aggressive, infiltrating).

    3. Other tests—computed tomography (CT), fluoroscopy, magnetic resonance imaging (MRI).

    4. Bone scan can show additional skeletal lesions.

II. Chondrosarcoma.

  A. Clinical symptoms.

    1. Dull, aching pain (like arthritis).

  B. Physical examination.

    1. Firm, swollen area; high-grade tumor can appear soft, viscous.

  C. Diagnostic data.

    1. Similar strategies as for osteosarcoma.

III. Fibrosarcoma.

  A. Clinical symptoms.

    1. Pain in affected area.

  B. Physical examination.

    1. Swelling in affected area.

  C. Diagnostic data.

    1. On radiographs, usually seen within the bone; low-grade lesions have well-defined margins, high-grade lesions have poorly defined margins with a more moth-eaten pattern.

    2. Similar strategies as for osteosarcoma.

IV. Ewing's sarcoma.

  A. Clinical symptoms.

    1. Symptom report can be vague; pain progressing, swelling progressing.

    2. Flu-like symptoms, fever, fatigue.

    3. Anemia.

  B. Physical examination.

    1. Swelling, progressing in affected area.

  C. Diagnostic data.

    1. Appear onion-like on radiographs, from multiple layers of subperiosteal new bone reacting to tumor invading the bone cortex.

    2. Diagnosed after rule out other malignant cell possibilities (e.g., rhabdomyosarcoma, lymphoma, neuroblastoma).

    3. Similar diagnostic studies as for osteosarcoma.

V. Soft tissue.

  A. Clinical symptoms.

    1. Painless, swollen mass; unless affecting blood vessels or nerves.

    2. Tumor infiltrates can be distant from the site of origin.

    3. Variety of presenting symptoms—peripheral neuralgias, vascular ischemia, paralysis, bowel obstruction.

  B. Physical examination.

    1. Depending on origin—lung, nerve, mobility affected.

  C. Diagnostic data.

    1. Tissue/cells from incisional, frozen, needle biopsies.

    2. Staging is not standard; grading system is based on mitotic activity.

    3. New technologies that offer more precision—electron microscope examination, immunohistochemical staining, deoxyribonucleic acid (DNA) analysis, ultrasound (for size and density).

    4. Lesions may recur after resection, reappearing deeper and larger, more aggressive with metastasis.

VI. Metastatic disease.
   A. Spread from primary lesions to:
      1. Lung, breast, colon, pancreas, kidney, thyroid, prostate, gastric, testicular.
   B. To evaluate spread—CT of chest and regional lymph nodes.
   C. Sarcomas frequently metastasize to lung.
   D. Other early metastatic sites—spine, ribs, pelvis (90% in axial skeleton).
   E. Presents as dull aching pain, increasing at night.
   F. Risk for pulmonary fractures is high.
   G. Palliative therapies include surgery, radiotherapy, and chemotherapy.
VII. Other issues.
   A. Phantom limb pain or sensation.
      1. One to four weeks postoperative; resolves in a few months.
      2. Patient is aware of itching, pressure, tingling, severe cramping, throbbing, burning pain.
      3. Usually tripped by fatigue, stress, excitement, other stimuli.
      4. Greater when the amputation site is more proximal.

Nursing Diagnoses

   I. Activity intolerance.
   II. Impaired adjustment.
   III. Body image disturbance.
   IV. Ineffective breathing pattern.
   V. Constipation.
   VI. Ineffective individual coping.
   VII. Ineffective denial.
   VIII. Risk for infection.
   IX. Fatigue.
   X. Impaired skin integrity.
   XI. Acute or chronic pain.

Outcome Identification

   I. Client describes symptoms that prompt a physician visit.
   II. Client describes the disease state, plan of care, and actions to maintain health.
   III. Client identifies strategies and resources to cope.
   IV. Client remains free of infection, anemia, and delayed wound healing.
   V. Client communicates pain (e.g., quality, source, intensity) to the health care providers.
   VI. Client identifies means to maintain fluid and nutritional balance.
   VII. Client maintains muscle tone, range of motion (ROM), levels of activity, mobilization, weight-bearing, and incorporates prosthesis if applicable.
   VIII. Client identifies ways to maintain adequate elimination.
   IX. Client describes alterations in sexual function and feelings.
   X. Client identifies and practices ways to conserve energy, optimize ventilatory functioning.
   XI. Client describes signs and symptoms of altered circulation.

Planning and Implementation

   I. The nurse provides information and teaching on prevention and early detection.

II. Preoperative teaching is provided, which may include information on immobilization; wound care; risk for infection; implants; drains; postsurgical or delayed prosthetic fitting (if applicable); issues of endurance, muscle tone; psychosocial issues of depression, anxiety, fear, body image, self-esteem; and physical therapy (e.g., gait training, muscle development, motor function, and lifestyle changes).

III. The nurse provides counseling and teaches strategies to the client/family to assist them to cope with, for example, anxieties, fears, and body image and sexuality issues. Assistance in identifying resources and sources of social support is also provided.

Evaluation

The oncology nurse systematically and regularly evaluates the client's and/or family's responses to interventions to determine progress toward the achievement of expected outcomes. Relevant data are collected and actual findings are compared with expected findings. Nursing diagnoses, outcomes, and plans of care are reviewed and revised as necessary.

BIBLIOGRAPHY

American Cancer Society. (1997). *Cancer Facts and Figures—1997.* Atlanta: American Cancer Society.

Chang, S. (1994). Bone cancers and soft tissue sarcomas. In Otto, S. (ed.). *Oncology Nursing.* St. Louis: C.V. Mosby, pp. 59–73.

Damron, R., & Pritchard, D. (1995). Current combined treatment of high-grade osteosarcomas. *Oncology* 9(4):327–343.

Dorfman, H., & Czerniak, B. (1995). Bone cancers. *Cancer* 75[Suppl. 1], 203–210.

Eiber, F., Morton, D., Eckardt, J., et al. (1994). Limb salvage for skeletal and soft tissue sarcomas. *Cancer* 54:2579–2589.

Inwards, C., & Unni, K. (1995). Classification and grading of bone sarcomas. *Hematol Oncol Clin North Am* 9(4):545–569.

Jaffe, N., Patel, S., & Benjamin, R. (1995). Chemotherapy in osteosarcoma. Basis for application and antagonism to implementation; early controversies surrounding its implementation. *Hematol Oncol Clin North Am* 9(4):825–840.

Malawer, M., Link, M., & Donaldson, S. (1993). Sarcomas of bone. In V. DeVita, Jr., S. Hellman, & S. Rosenberg (eds.). *Cancer: Principles and Practice of Oncology* (4th ed.). Philadelphia: J.B. Lippincott, pp. 1509–1566.

Pizzo, P., Polack, D., Hayes, D., et al. (1993). Solid tumors of childhood. In V. DeVita, Jr., S. Hellman, & S. Rosenberg (eds.). *Cancer: Principles and Practice of Oncology* (4th ed.). Philadelphia: J.B. Lippincott, pp. 1778–1783.

Putnam, J., & Roth, J. (1995). Surgical treatment for pulmonary metastasis from sarcoma. *Hematol Oncol Clin North Am* 9(4):869–887.

Raymond, A., Simms, W., & Ayala, A. (1995). Osteosarcoma. Specimen management following primary chemotherapy. *Hematol Oncol Clin North Am* 9(4):841–867.

Seater, G., Hie, J., Stenwig, A., et al. (1995). Systemic relapse of patients with osteogenic sarcoma. Prognostic factors for long term survival. *Cancer* 75(5):1084–1093.

Yang, J., Glatstein, E., Rosenberg, S., & Antman, K. (1993). Sarcomas of soft tissues. In V. DeVita, Jr., S. Hellman, & S. Rosenberg (eds.). *Cancer: Principles and Practice of Oncology* (4th ed.). Philadelphia: J.B. Lippincott, pp. 1436–1488.

Zalupski, M., & Baker, L. (1995). Systemic adjuvant chemotherapy for soft tissue sarcomas. *Hematol Oncol Clin North Am* 9(4):787–800.

29

Nursing Care of the Client With HIV-Related Cancer

James Halloran, RN, MSN, ANP

Theory

I. Human immunodeficiency virus (HIV) as a predisposing factor to cancer.
   A. Definition of HIV.
      1. Cytopathic retrovirus of lentivirus family.
         a. Causes chronic disease in host.
         b. Long incubation and gradual progression are typical.
      2. Structure.
         a. p24 protein core surrounds the ribonucleic acid (RNA) genome.
         b. Bilayered lipid envelope.
         c. Surface antigens—gp120, gp41.
            (1) gp120—attracted to CD4 surface marker on host cells.
            (2) Human cell with most abundant CD4—T lymphocyte; CD4 also prominent on macrophages and monocytes, microglial cells, Langerhans' cells, dendritic cells.
         d. Reverse transcriptase enzyme, a virus component, mediates transcription of viral ribonucleic acid (RNA) to deoxyribonucleic acid (DNA) in infected cell.
   B. Immunologic structures.
      1. T lymphocyte.
         a. Stem cells from bone marrow mature in thymus, acquire surface markers, seed peripheral lymphoid tissue and circulation; approximately 80% of circulating lymphocytes are T cells.
         b. Pivotal agent in cell-mediated immunity; produces lymphokines, which regulate overall immune response, both promoting and inhibiting proliferation and differentiation of immunoreactive cells and molecules.
         c. Protects against intracellular parasites and tumors; provides immunosurveillance; responsible for graft rejection; displays memory effect.
         d. T4 helper cells are primary HIV targets.
      2. B lymphocyte.
         a. Believed to mature in bone marrow; circulates to and seeds peripheral lymphoid germinal centers; 12 to 15% of circulating lymphocytes are B cells.
         b. Stimulated B cell produces plasma cells, which produce antigen-specific antibody.
         c. Protects against bacterial and viral infections.
         d. B memory cells provide anamnestic effect (stores template of specific antibodies).

3. Lymphoid organs and circulation.
   a. Primary organs—bone marrow and thymus.
   b. Also included—lymphatic vessels, lymph nodes, spleen, and liver.
   c. Nonencapsulated clusters of lymphoid tissue are found around lining of aerodigestive tract.
   d. Lymph nodes are located at junction of lymphatic channels.
      (1) Small and bean shaped; store T and B cells and macrophages.
      (2) Lymphadenopathy (increase in size of lymph nodes) occurs when immune response is invoked by presence of antigen.
4. Natural killer (NK) cells.
   a. Large granular lymphocytes without surface markers of T or B cells.
   b. Primary function is cytotoxicity; target tumor and virally infected cells.
   c. Nonspecific action; no memory function.
C. Physiologic basis of HIV infection and HIV-related cancers.
   1. HIV effect on T4 lymphocytes.
      a. HIV binds to CD4 surface marker on T4 cells.
      b. Fusion and release of viral RNA into host cells.
      c. Viral RNA is transcribed to DNA through action of reverse transcriptase and is integrated into host nuclear DNA; viral particles also are found in host cell cytoplasm.
      d. May remain dormant for variable period, or immediate viral production by infected cell may occur.
      e. Protease enzyme required for assembly of new virus.
      f. Newly produced virion buds from surface of infected cell and infects other cells.
      g. Host cells eventually are depleted.
   2. HIV effect on immune system.
      a. Progressive infection leads to qualitative and quantitative T4 lymphocyte dysfunction, with resultant defect in both cellular and humoral immunity as immunoregulatory function of T4 cells is gradually impaired.
         (1) Progressive destruction of T cells results from viral replication in host.
         (2) HIV may cause polyclonal B-cell activity (also may be due to coinfection with Epstein-Barr virus [EBV]).
         (3) Impaired immune function allows proliferation of malignantly transformed cells.
         (4) No conclusive data exist about quantitative changes in the T4 cell count and stage of disease.
      b. Cofactors in disease progression.
         (1) Definitive role of specific cofactors in disease progression is controversial; may be difficult to distinguish between comorbid infection and true causal relationship.
         (2) Infectious cofactors may include presence of cytomegalovirus (CMV), EBV, and other viruses.
         (3) Lifestyle factors may also influence course of infection; risk for disease progression increases in presence of inadequate nutrition, general poor health, smoking, activities that may result in infection with other strains of HIV.
   3. Clinical staging and classification of HIV infection.
      a. Infection with HIV produces a continuum of changes in health status.
      b. Clinical status may change rapidly in either direction.

    c. Knowledge of disease stage guides selection of therapeutic intervention and psychosocial support.

    d. Two major systems for classifying HIV disease—Centers for Disease Control (CDC) system and Walter Reed system.

      (1) CDC classification system (Table 29–1).

        (a) Considers both laboratory and clinical parameters.

        (b) Provides surveillance definition to guide epidemiologic data collection and serves as framework for stratifying levels of illness (see Table 29–1).

      (2) Walter Reed staging system.

        (a) Based on clinical presentation of individual client.

        (b) Designed to correlate with progressive immune dysfunction.

        (c) Excludes neurologic symptoms (Table 29–2).

  4. Malignant disease as a result of HIV infection.

    a. Impaired immune surveillance function and polyclonal B-cell activity lead to growth of malignantly transformed cells.

    b. Kaposi's sarcoma and B-cell lymphoma—most frequent malignant disease in HIV-infected clients.

    c. Distinguished by abnormal sites of presentation, poor duration of response to therapy, presence of comorbid opportunistic infection.

    d. HIV-infected women are at increased risk for cervical dysplasia and for rapid progression to cervical cancer; diagnosis and staging are same as in non–HIV-positive disease in women with the difference being the aggressiveness of the histology.

II. HIV-related Kaposi's sarcoma (KS).

  A. Definition/pathogenesis—soft-tissue malignancy characterized by malignant growth of reticuloendothelial cell origin in HIV-infected persons.

  B. Cause

    1. Before HIV, pandemic KS occurred primarily in elderly males of Mediterranean origin (classic or non-African KS) and in persons receiving post-organ transplant immunosuppressive agents (transplant-associated KS).

TABLE 29–1. **Centers for Disease Control Classification System for HIV Infection**

	Category A	Category B	Category C
CD4 Count	Asymptomatic; persistent generalized lymphadenopathy; or acute retroviral syndrome	Conditions not usually seen in immunocompetent people (e.g., oral thrush)	AIDS-defining illnesses (e.g., KS, invasive cervical cancer, lymphoma)
>500	A1	B1	**C1**
200–499	A2	B2	**C2**
0–199	**A3**	**B3**	**C3**

CDC 1993 Classification System for HIV Infection: Uses two indices—CD4 count and clinical condition to classify/stage disease in HIV+ persons. By definition, individuals with CD4 count less than 200 qualify for AIDS diagnosis, as well as those diagnosed with category C ("AIDS-defining") conditions (i.e., the categories in bold type).

TABLE 29–2. **Walter Reed Staging System for HIV Infection**

Stage	HIV Antibody Status	Chronic Lymph-adenopathy	CD4 Count	Skin Test	Oral Thrush	Opportunistic Infection
0	Negative	—	>400	WNL	—	—
1	Positive	—	>400	WNL	—	—
2	Positive	Present	>400	WNL	—	—
3	Positive	+/−	<400	WNL	—	—
4	Positive	+/−	<400	Partial anergy	—	—
5	Positive	+/−	<400	Complete anergy	Yes	—
6	Positive	+/−	<400	Partial/complete anergy	+/−	Yes

WNL, *within normal limits*; +/−, may or may not be present.

2. In clients with HIV-related KS (epidemic KS) malignantly transformed cells reproduce unchecked as a result of underlying immune defect.
   a. HIV-associated *tat* gene is thought to promote growth of KS lesions.
   b. Use of nitrite inhalants ("poppers") may be related to development of KS in HIV-infected people.
   c. A herpes-like virus that may be sexually transmitted has been identified and is thought to be associated with HIV-related KS.
C. Appearance and metastasis of HIV-related KS.
   1. Classic presentation includes skin lesions, ranging from pink to purple to brownish, flat or raised, which are usually painless (unless in a sensitive area) and do not blanch with pressure.
   2. HIV-related KS may present as skin lesions or may appear first in any other organ system, including the oral cavity.
   3. Classic KS is typically indolent, whereas HIV-related KS may be very aggressive and progress rapidly.
III. HIV-related lymphoma.
   A. Definition/pathogenesis—majority of clients present with B-cell tumors of high-grade histologic type.
      1. Extranodal involvement is common; primary gastrointestinal (GI) or central nervous system (CNS) lymphoma and bone marrow involvement are common.
      2. Lymphoproliferative conditions seen less frequently in HIV-infected persons include Hodgkin's disease, multiple myeloma, and B-cell acute lymphocytic leukemia.
   B. Cause.
      1. EBV, direct effect of HIV, or activation of *c-myc* oncogene may play causative role.
      2. Lack of effective T-cell mediated immunoregulation allows polyclonal B-cell activity.
   C. Appearance and metastasis—CNS, gastrointestinal (GI) tract, and bone marrow involvement are more frequent in HIV-infected persons; virtually every organ system may be involved.
      1. CNS lesions may cause changes in cognitive function, memory loss, decreased attention span, headaches, personality change, focal neurologic deficits, or generalized seizure activity.
      2. GI tract lesions may cause malabsorption, diarrhea, constipation, or focal

or diffuse abdominal discomfort or may present as an asymptomatic abdominal mass.

3. Blood counts are usually normal despite bone marrow involvement.

IV. Principles of medical management.

A. Diagnostic tests.

1. Diagnosis of HIV infection is usually made on basis of positive antibody test.

a. Enzyme-linked immunosorbent assay (ELISA) test for antibody to HIV is used for screening—high sensitivity and specificity in populations at risk.

b. If ELISA test is positive, test is repeated; if second test is positive, confirmatory Western blot is conducted on same specimen.

c. Other tests to demonstrate infection with HIV—polymerase chain reaction (PCR; a gene amplification technique) or viral culture.

2. Diagnosis of HIV-related KS or lymphoma—similar to testing done for same conditions when not related to HIV infection; because of the wide variance in presenting symptoms, the workup in the HIV-infected person may be more aggressive or comprehensive than in the uninfected person.

a. Once tissue diagnosis of KS lesions has been confirmed, the physician may elect not to biopsy new skin lesions; visceral lesions may be biopsied if the risk-to-benefit ratio permits.

b. Brain biopsy may be performed to establish differential diagnosis between CNS lymphoma and other opportunistic infections; constitutional symptoms such as night sweats may be related to infection with *Mycobacterium avium-intracellulare,* and CNS symptoms may be related to cerebral toxoplasmosis.

c. Because of the risk associated with brain biopsy, a trial of radiotherapy may be undertaken without tissue biopsy.

(1) Response is seen with lymphoma, whereas toxoplasmosis does not respond to radiotherapy.

(2) Alternatively, some physicians may choose to treat for toxoplasmosis (especially if the client has a previous history) and then observe for response.

B. Staging methods and procedures.

1. Staging for HIV-related lymphoma typically follows the same schema for non–HIV-related lymphoma (e.g., the Ann Arbor Staging System) (see Chapter 27).

2. No universally accepted staging system for HIV-related KS has been identified; schema used include parameters of cutaneous, lymph node, and visceral involvement and the occurrence of "B symptoms" (fever, chills, night sweats, diarrhea, unintentional weight loss).

3. Because HIV-related malignancies may present at abnormal sites, diagnostic imaging and/or endoscopic examinations may be more extensive than in HIV-negative persons.

C. Standard therapies.

1. Treatment of HIV-related cancers is based on approaches used for uninfected persons, but the underlying immune deficiency, presence of other opportunistic infections, administration of other medications, and generalized poor health status may require dose reduction, scheduling modifications, and/or selection of alternative approaches.

2. Surgery.

a. May be used to remove KS lesions that interfere with function or appearance such as gingival or upper aerodigestive tract lesions, those obstructing lymphatic flow, or those in cosmetically sensitive areas such as the head and neck; surgical approaches may be limited by the anatomic location of the lesion or client's poor overall health that precludes use of general anesthesia.

  b. Generally not used in clients with HIV-related lymphoma.

 3. Chemotherapy.

  a. May be necessary to adjust dosage based on response, tolerance, comorbidity, contraindication to agents being used to treat other conditions.

  b. HIV-related KS may be treated with single or multiple agents.

   (1) Etoposide may be used as either first-line or salvage therapy.

   (2) Combination approaches include use of vinca alkaloids (especially vinblastine) and bleomycin, vinblastine and methotrexate, vinblastine and doxorubicin, or bleomycin with or without dacarbazine.

   (3) Liposomal doxorubicin or daunorubicin have shown therapeutic response with decreased toxicities.

  c. HIV-related lymphoma is treated with combination chemotherapy, using cyclophosphamide, vincristine, methotrexate, etoposide, cytosine arabinoside, bleomycin, and steroids; use of methotrexate, bleomycin, and doxorubicin, cyclophosphamide, vincristine, and dexamethasone (M-BACOD) is common.

   (1) Primary CNS lymphoma is usually resistant to systemic chemotherapy.

   (2) Intrathecal administration of chemotherapy may be considered.

 4. Radiotherapy.

  a. KS lesions are typically radiosensitive.

   (1) Effective short- to moderate-term local control may be achieved, especially for cosmetic effects or relief of lymphedema caused by lymphatic lesions.

   (2) The aggressive nature of epidemic KS precludes radiotherapy with curative intent.

  b. HIV-related lymphoma may respond to radiotherapy, but control of high-grade tumors is poor; low-grade tumors may be controlled for several months to years.

 5. Biologic response modifiers.

  a. α-Interferon, with or without concomitant zidovudine (AZT), has been approved as treatment for HIV-related KS; the efficacy of other biologic response modifiers is being evaluated.

  b. Other biologic response modifiers are being evaluated as treatment for the underlying HIV infection, but they generally are not used to treat HIV-related lymphomas.

 6. Combined-modality treatment is not well documented as therapy for HIV-related malignancies; synergistic therapeutic and side effects must be weighed carefully.

D. Prognosis.

 1. Survival in persons with HIV-related malignancies depends on multiple factors, including degree of immunosuppression, presence of opportunistic infection(s), nutritional status, location of presenting lesion, lifestyle, and availability and accessibility of adequate care.

 2. HIV-related KS.

  a. In the absence of other major opportunistic infections, clients with HIV-related KS have survived for several years.

  b. In clients with GI tract lesions or B symptoms, survival time is shorter.

  c. Clients with prior or comorbid major opportunistic infection have the worst prognosis, with median survival time of less than 1 year.

3. HIV-related lymphoma.
    a. Most clients present with high-grade, advanced-stage disease, with resultant poor prognosis; high histologic grade, CNS primary tumor, prior persistent generalized lymphadenopathy, and incomplete response to chemotherapy are indicators of poor prognosis.
    b. Median survival time ranges from 4 to 10½ months; shortest survival time is with CNS primary tumor (median, 1 to 2 months); longest survival time is with low-grade lymphomas (12 months to 4 years).

Assessment

I. Clients at risk for HIV-related cancers.
   A. Individuals identified as HIV-positive.
   B. Risks for infection with HIV are highest among people who have:
      1. Been sexually active with more than one partner since 1978.
      2. Shared needles to inject illegal substances or had sex with someone who does.
      3. Received blood or blood products or organ transplant between 1978 and 1985.
      4. Been born to HIV-infected mothers.
      5. Been exposed to HIV in other ways such as through an accidental needle stick.
II. Pertinent history—requires tact and sensitivity on the part of the nurse when inquiring about sensitive topics such as sexuality and illicit drug use.
   A. Inquire about sexual and drug use history.
      1. Unprotected (i.e., without a condom) vaginal or rectal intercourse (highest risk).
      2. Sharing of needles for drug injection, especially in areas of high incidence of HIV infection (major risk); persons with substance abuse disorders may also be at high risk for sexual transmission from engaging in high-risk sex while intoxicated or in "survival sex" (engaging in sex to obtain money, drugs, food, or other needs).
      3. Homosexual or bisexual males may be reluctant to acknowledge sexual activity with other males; use tact and a nonjudgmental approach.
      4. Women may be unaware of bisexual behavior of partner or deny such behavior.
      5. History of one or more sexually transmitted diseases (syphilis, gonorrhea, herpes, chlamydia, hepatitis, genital warts) indicates higher risk.
   B. Inquire about history of blood, blood product, or organ transplantation.
      1. Since 1985 all blood and blood products in United States have been tested for the presence of HIV antibodies; transfusions received in other countries may not have been tested.
      2. Since the early 1980s clotting factors used by hemophiliacs have been treated to kill HIV.
   C. Among children, determine HIV status of mother; children born to mothers infected with HIV have a 30 to 50% chance of being infected if the mother does not receive prenatal antiretroviral therapy.
   D. Inquire about changes in mental status, memory, attention span, or personality; family members or significant others may recognize these changes before the client does; include these findings in data collection.

E. Ask if the person has been tested for the presence of HIV antibody and what the result was.

1. Because of social stigma attached to HIV infection and discrimination against HIV-infected people, the person may be reluctant to acknowledge having been tested or the result.

2. Explain that information about HIV status may be important in determining a diagnosis and treatment plan.

3. Legal restrictions and requirements relative to HIV infection vary among states; the ethical obligation of the nurse to maintain client confidentiality is universal.

III. Physical examination.

A. Signs and symptoms may vary in intensity, may wax and wane over time, but are usually progressive.

B. Inspect the skin.

1. Include gingiva and oral cavity, skin folds, plantar surfaces, scalp, and nares; KS lesions can appear anywhere on the body.

2. Integumentary changes in a client known as infected with HIV may indicate opportunistic infection and should be reported to the attending physician, and/or the client should be referred for further workup.

3. KS lesions may be purple to pink to brown, flat or raised, do not blanch with pressure, and are usually painless unless in a sensitive anatomic area.

4. Despite appearance, KS lesions do not bleed easily.

5. Lymphedema may result from obstruction of lymph flow by neoplastic growth.

C. Assess the thorax and abdomen.

1. Lesions in the lungs can cause rales, wheezes, or cacophonous breath sounds.

2. Cardiac involvement occurs and can cause muffled heart tones or other abnormal heart sounds, palpitations, or chest pain.

3. Evaluate abdomen for tenderness, masses, hyperactive bowel sounds, hepatic or splenic enlargement.

D. Neurologic and mental status examination can reveal changes caused by CNS lesions, opportunistic infections, or HIV-related dementia.

1. Obtain baseline examination for comparison.

2. Assess memory, gait, pupillary response, appearance, behavior, speech, affect, sensorimotor activity, presence of chronic headache, lightheadedness, dizziness, photophobia, syncope, paraesthesias.

3. Findings may vary day to day.

4. Include findings obtained from family, caregiver, and significant others.

E. Other signs and symptoms to assess—unintentional weight loss, diarrhea or constipation, fever, chills, night sweats, lymphadenopathy.

IV. Evaluation of laboratory data.

A. Laboratory studies related to neoplastic processes are the same as those for clients with same pathology who are not infected with HIV.

1. Hematologic values may be skewed in presence of HIV bone marrow invasion: white cell count or platelet count may be elevated or reduced.

2. Schedule of routine testing may differ from that used among non–HIV-infected individuals.

B. Studies to monitor HIV infection.
   1. CD4/T4 lymphocyte count decreases over time at a median rate of 10 cells per month as a result of the progressive destruction of T4 cells by HIV; may be used to quantify the relative immunocompetence of the host, with lower values reflecting decreased immune response.
   2. Virally infected cells produce β_2-microglobulin; increasing serum levels indicate progressive infection.
   3. HIV core antigen p24 serum levels increase with progressive infection.
      a. Levels of β_2-microglobulin and p24 may decrease in end-stage disease.
      b. Decreases may be due to depletion of target cell population rather than to improvement of immune function.
   4. Viral load refers to the amount of HIV RNA detectable in peripheral blood; there are two laboratory methods (polymerase chain reaction or PCR, and branched DNA), which are not interchangeable.
      a. Viral load assays have been demonstrated to be reliable predictors of therapeutic response to antiretroviral therapy.
      b. Viral load assays do not measure virus that may be harbored in anatomic sites other than the peripheral blood (e.g., CNS, lymphatic system).

Nursing Diagnoses

   I. Risk for infection.
  II. Body image disturbance.
 III. Decisional conflict.
  IV. Fatigue.
   V. Altered nutrition: less than body requirements.
  VI. Altered thought process.

Outcome Identification

   I. Client identifies the presence of HIV infection, specific malignancy, and rationale for treatment.
  II. Client and significant other identify immediate and long-term side effects of disease and treatment—exacerbation of immune suppression by myelotoxic therapies, side effects specific to agents used, skin changes caused by radiotherapy.
 III. Client identifies self-care measures to decrease incidence and severity of symptoms associated with disease and treatment—maintenance of adequate rest and nutrition, monitoring body temperature, scheduling of activities to minimize fatigue, use of appropriate skin care techniques, use of prescribed antiemetic agents, or other techniques for symptom management.
  IV. Client demonstrates skills in self-care demanded by structural or functional effects of disease—use of written reminders for routine activities and appointments, use of pillbox with alarm or other means to manage multiple drug administration, use of cosmetic or other means to disguise lesions.
   V. Client describes schedule and procedures for follow-up care, which varies according to condition.
  VI. Client and significant other list signs and symptoms of recurrent disease—growth of old or appearance of new KS lesions, increasing lymphadenopathy or lymphedema, return or exacerbation of sensorimotor changes, increase in

rate of weight loss, change in elimination pattern, exacerbation of prior symptoms.

VII. Client and significant other identify community resources to meet demands of disease, treatment, and survivorship—local acquired immunodeficiency syndromes (AIDS) service organizations, church or civic organizations, American Cancer Society, hospice organizations, self-help groups such as Alcoholics Anonymous or Narcotics Anonymous when appropriate, local credit bureau or other financial services or planning agency, social service program offices such as Social Security.

Planning and Implementation

I. Interventions to maximize safety for client and significant other.
   A. Ensure environmental safety for clients experiencing sensorimotor changes (e.g., provide adequate lighting, especially at night).
   B. Instruct client about avoidance of potential environmental sources of opportunistic infection such as animal waste from pets or uncooked, undercooked, or improperly stored food.
   C. Teach techniques to reduce possibility of HIV transmission.
      1. HIV is transmitted through blood and semen; use a latex condom during every episode of vaginal, rectal, or oral intercourse, with a condom-compatible, water-based lubricant to reduce risk (petroleum-based lubricants or cosmetic creams weaken the condom, increasing the chance of breakage during use).
      2. Do not share toothbrushes, razors, other personal care items.
      3. For cleanup of emesis or other body fluid spills, wear gloves and use a solution of one part household bleach to 10 parts water.
      4. Insist that healthcare workers and volunteer caregivers follow universal precautions as recommended by CDC to reduce the risk of occupational exposure to HIV (Table 29–3).

II. Interventions to decrease incidence and severity of symptoms associated with disease or treatment.
   A. Teach (or refer for teaching) ways to enhance appearance such as use of covering cosmetics to hide KS lesions in cosmetically sensitive areas; use

TABLE 29–3. **Body Fluids in Universal Precautions (CDC)**

Body Fluids to Which Universal Precautions Apply	Body Fluids to Which Universal Precautions DO NOT Apply (unless contaminated by blood)
Blood; any secretion or excretion contaminated with blood	Urine
Cerebrospinal fluid	Feces
Semen; vaginal secretions	Vomitus
Synovial fluid	Perspiration
Amniotic fluid	Nasal secretions
Pericardial fluid	Tears
Pleural fluid	Sputum or saliva (except in dental practice)
Peritoneal fluid	

of scarves or other clothing to cover swollen lymph nodes; use of clothing appropriate to changing body mass with weight loss.

B. Instruct to use acetaminophen or nonsteroidal anti-inflammatory agents rather than aspirin, which may interfere with platelet function, to control fevers, minor aches, and pains (unless otherwise instructed by physician).

C. Encourage to establish routine of regular rest periods and to schedule activities in accordance with energy level.

D. Monitor nutritional status.

1. Teach techniques to increase nutritional intake (e.g., use of supplements, keeping ready-to-eat foods available, eating smaller and more frequent meals).

2. Provide or encourage frequent oral hygiene.

E. Teach appropriate techniques for care of skin in areas being treated with radiotherapy (see Chapter 35).

F. Assess knowledge or use of experimental and/or alternative treatment regimens.

1. Determine and assess client knowledge of any contraindications that may exist between prescribed therapies and those obtained outside usual healthcare channels.

2. Some experimental agents become available before receiving full Food and Drug Administration approval through "parallel track" programs, which allow use of drugs outside the clinical trial setting.

3. Alternative therapies available through various sources (such as "buyers' clubs") may be used by clients.

   a. Ascertain all treatment regimens client is using, regardless of the source.

   b. Monitor interactions between multiple forms of therapy.

   c. Assist client with the process of evaluating alternative therapies in terms of effectiveness, side effects, costs, and safety.

III. Interventions to monitor for sequelae of disease and treatment.

A. Provide teaching about myelotoxic side effects of chemotherapy and signs and symptoms of infection such as acute temperature elevation, appearance of suppurative lesions, bleeding.

B. Assess anorectal skin integrity in clients with diarrhea; teach appropriate skin care.

C. Instruct client to report changes in sense of touch, peripheral tingling, or numbness (may be side effect of vinca alkaloid chemotherapy or due to HIV infection).

IV. Interventions to monitor response to medical management.

A. Assess and document location, appearance, size of KS lesions and/or lymphadenopathy or other tumor effects (abdominal masses, oral lesions).

B. Monitor for changes in size or appearance of lymphomatous lesions.

C. Obtain baseline and ongoing evaluation of mental status, performance status, and self-care ability.

D. Assess nutritional status and document changes.

1. Maintain serial record of body weight, with client wearing approximately same clothing with each recording.

2. Document presence of dysphagia and changes in appetite or taste, which may result from oral lesions or as a side effect of treatment.

V. Interventions to enhance adaptation and rehabilitation.
   A. Use notes, phone calls, or other reminders for appointments and medication administration times (may also use a pillbox with built-in alarm).
      1. Provide written instructions with frequent repetition and reinforcement included.
      2. Provide instruction to caregivers and significant others if client experiences mental status changes.
   B. Refer client and significant others to community agencies, civic organizations, or churches for assistance with social entitlement programs, peer support, and other available services such as home meal delivery.
   C. Refer for physical and/or occupational therapy to assist to learn adaptive techniques to cope with sensorimotor deficits.
   D. Encourage discussion about client's wishes for use of resuscitative measures.
      1. Facilitate decision-making process by establishing atmosphere of trust and acceptance, providing accurate information, respecting client choices.
      2. Ensure that client's wishes are properly documented and communicated to health care providers.
VI. Interventions to incorporate client and significant other in care.
   A. Recognize that the client's family of choice may differ from biologic family of origin.
      1. Determine and follow the client's expressed wishes regarding who is to receive what kind of information, who will be allowed visitation in hospital, and which terms to use to describe relationship (e.g., lover, partner, friend).
      2. Assist or refer for assistance with execution of durable power of attorney, will, and other necessary legal documentation.
   B. Assess resources and coping strategies of client and significant other.
      1. Determine past experience with HIV disease; in areas of high incidence, multiple losses may occur without adequate time for effective grieving.
      2. Consider that the significant other with HIV disease may experience symptoms that limit ability to provide care.
      3. Recognize that a significant other who is not infected with HIV may experience feelings of guilt, uncertainty about own health, concern for the future.
      4. Monitor for indications of maladaptive coping strategies, especially if a history of substance use disorder is present; assist with learning alternative behaviors to manage stress and cope.
      5. Assess knowledge and/or use of alternative therapies.
   C. Include persons identified by the client as significant others in teaching and care decisions when appropriate.

Evaluation

The oncology nurse systematically and regularly evaluates the client's and/or family's response to interventions to determine progress toward the achievement of expected outcomes. Relevant data are collected and actual findings are compared with expected findings. Nursing diagnoses, outcomes, and plans of care are reviewed and revised as necessary.

BIBLIOGRAPHY

Casey, K., Cohen, E., & Hughes, A. (eds.). (1996). *Core Curriculum in HIV/AIDS Nursing.* Philadelphia: Nursecom.

Chang, Y., Cesaman, E., Pessin, M.S., et al. (1994). Identification of a herpes virus-like DNA sequence in AIDS-associated Kaposi's sarcoma. *Science 266,* 1865–1869.

Cohn, J.A. (1989). Virology, immunology and natural history of HIV infection. *J Nurs Midwife 34*(5), 242–252.

Cremer, K.J., Spring, S.B., & Gruber, J. (1990). Role of human immunodeficiency virus type 1 and other viruses in malignancies associated with acquired immune deficiency syndrome. *J Natl Cancer Inst 82*(12), 1016–1024.

Doll, D.C., & Ringenberg, Q.S. (1989). Lymphomas associated with HIV infection. *Semin Oncol Nurs 5*(4), 255–262.

Flaskerud, J.H., & Ungvarski, P.J. (eds.). (1995). HIV/AIDS: A Guide to Nursing Care (3rd ed.). Philadelphia: W.B. Saunders.

Gallo, R.C., & Nerurkar, L.S. (1989). Human retroviruses: Their role in neoplasia and immunodeficiency. *Ann NY Acad Sci 567,* 82–94.

Gallucci, B. (1987). The immune system and cancer. *Oncol Nurs Forum 14*(6, suppl), 3–12.

Gill, P.S., Rarick, M.U., Espina, B., et al: (1990). Advanced acquired immune deficiency syndrome-related Kaposi's sarcoma: Results of pilot studies using combination chemotherapy. *Cancer 65,* 1074–1078.

Glasner, P.D., & Kaslow, R.A. (1990). The epidemiology of human immunodeficiency virus infection. *J Consult Clin Psychol 58*(1), 13–21.

Grady, C. (1988). HIV: Epidemiology, immunopathogenesis, and clinical consequences. *Nurs Clin North Am 23*(4), 683–696.

Grady, C. (1988). Host defense mechanisms: An overview. *Semin Oncol Nurs 4*(2), 86–94.

Halloran, J. (1994). HIV-related malignancies. In D. Grimes & D. Grimes (eds.). *HIV/AIDS Nursing Care.* St. Louis: Mosby-Year Book, pp. 140–152.

Halloran, J.P., & Hughes, A.M. (1991). Knowledge deficit related to prevention and early detection of HIV disease. In J.C. McNally, E.T. Somerville, C. Miaskowski, & M. Rostad (eds.). *Guidelines for Oncology Nursing Practice* (2nd ed.). Philadelphia: W.B. Saunders, pp. 47–54.

Harrison, M., Tomlinson, D., & Stewart, S. (1995). Liposomal-entrapped doxorubicin: An active agent in AIDS-related Kaposi's sarcoma. *J Clin Oncol 13,* 914–920.

Horowitz, M.E., & Pizza, P.A. (1990). Cancer in the child infected with human immunodeficiency virus. *J Pediatr 116*(5), 730–731.

Jacob, J.L., Baird, B.F., Haller, S., & Ostchega, Y. (1989). AIDS-related Kaposi's sarcoma: Concepts of care. *Semin Oncol Nurs 5*(4), 263–275.

Jacobson, L.P., & Armenian, H.K. (1995). An integrated approach to the epidemiology of Kaposi's sarcoma. *Curr Opin Oncol 7,* 450–455.

Kaplan, L.D., Kahn, J.O., Crowe, S., et al. (1991). Clinical and virologic effects of recombinant human granulocyte-macrophage colony stimulating factor in patients receiving chemotherapy for HIV-associated non-Hodgkin's lymphoma: Results of a randomized trial. *J Clin Oncol 9,* 929–940.

Kaplan, L.D., & Northfelt, D.W. (1997). Malignancies associated with AIDS. In M.A. Sande & P.A. Volberding (eds.). *The Medical Management of AIDS.* Philadelphia: W.B. Saunders, pp. 413–439.

Krigel, R.L., & Friedman-Kien, A.E. (1990). Epidemic Kaposi's sarcoma. *Semin Oncol 17*(3), 350–360.

Levine, A.M., Sullivan-Halley, J., Pike, M.C., et al. (1991). HIV-related lymphoma: Prognostic factors predictive of survival. *Cancer 68,* 2466–2472.

Lorenz, H.P., Wilson, W., Leigh, B., et al. (1991). Squamous cell carcinoma of the anus and HIV infection. *Dis Colon Rectum 34,* 336–338.

Lovejoy, N.C. (1988). The pathophysiology of AIDS. *Oncol Nurs Forum 15*(5), 563–571.

Lyter, D.W., Bryant, J., Thackeray, R., et al. (1995). Incidence of HIV-related and non-related malignancies in a large cohort of homosexual men. *J Clin Oncol 13*(10), 2540–2546.

McMahon, K.M., & Coyne, N. (1989). Symptom management in patients with AIDS. *Semin Oncol Nurs 5*(4), 289–301.

Maiman, M., Fruchter, R.G., Guy, L., et al. (1993). HIV infection and invasive cervical carcinoma. *Cancer 71,* 402–406.

Mitsuyasu, R.T., & Groopman, J.E. (1984). Biology and therapy of Kaposi's sarcoma. *Semin Oncol 11,* 53–59.

O'Brien, W.A., Hartigan, P.M., Martin, D., et al. and The Veterans Affairs Cooperative Study Group on AIDS. (1996). Changes in plasma HIV-1 RNA and CD4+ lymphocyte counts and the risk of progression to AIDS. *N Engl J Med 334,* 426–431.

Palefsky, J. (1991). Human papilloma virus infection among HIV-infected individuals. *Hematol Oncol Clin North Am 5,* 357–370.

Presant, C.A., Scolaro, M., Kennedy, P., et al. (1993). Liposomal daunorubicin treatment of HIV-associated Kaposi's sarcoma. *Lancet 341,* 1242–1243.

Selik, R.M., Chu, S.Y., & Ward, J.W. (1995). Trends in infections and cancers among persons dying of HIV infection in the U.S. from 1987–1992. *Ann Intern Med 123,* 933–936.

Vlahov, D. (1989). AIDS: Overview, immunology, virology, and informational needs. *Semin Oncol Nurs 5*(4), 227–235.

Nursing Care of the Client With Genital Cancer

Marie Flannery, RN, MS, AOCN

CERVICAL CANCER

Theory

I. Physiology and pathophysiology associated with cervical cancer.
   A. Anatomy of the cervix (Fig. 30–1).
      1. Consists of the lower portion of the uterus, which is contiguous with the upper portion of the vagina.
      2. Composed of the exocervix and the endocervix.
      3. Surrounded by paracervical tissues rich in lymph nodes.
   B. Changes associated with cancer of the cervix.
      1. Cellular changes exist on a continuum from premalignant changes (mild to moderate to severe cervical intraepithelial neoplasia [CIN]) to carcinoma in situ (CIS) to invasive disease.
      2. The causative agents and risk factors associated with invasive cervical carcinoma (ICC) have been a major focus of research. Human papillomavirus (HPV) is suspected as an initiator with multiple cofactors identified.
      3. The majority of ICC arises in the transformation zone at the squamocolumnar junction (see Fig. 30–1).
         a. Exophytic, fungating, or cauliflower-like lesions protrude from the cervix.
         b. Excavating or ulcerative, necrotic lesions replace the cervix or upper vagina.
         c. Endophytic lesions extend within the cervical canal.
      4. The two main histologic types of cervical cancer are squamous carcinoma and adenocarcinoma.
         a. Squamous carcinoma is most common (75–90%).
         b. Adenocarcinoma occurs in younger women and carries a poorer prognosis; bulky endocervical tumors are aggressive in nature and less responsive to treatment.
   C. Metastatic patterns.
      1. Direct extension within the abdomen to other pelvic structures.
      2. Lymph node metastases.
      3. Metastasis to lung, liver, and bone through the hematologic route.
   D. Trends in epidemiology.
      1. ICC is the sixth most common cancer among women in the United States (US) and the most commonly occurring cancer among women worldwide.

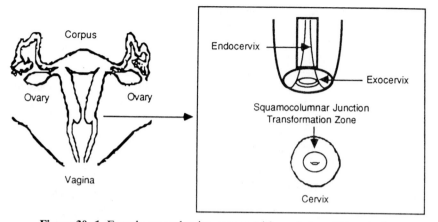

Figure 30–1. Female reproductive organs with anatomy of the cervix.

2. Incidence of ICC has decreased 50% since 1945, with a corresponding increase in the diagnosis of preinvasive disease.
II. Principles of medical management.
  A. Screening and diagnostic procedures.
    1. Screening procedures.
      a. Papanicolaou (Pap) smear with bimanual pelvic examination is recommended as the screening test for premalignant and malignant cervical disease.
        (1) Initial Pap smear at age 18 years or upon initiation of sexual intercourse.
        (2) After three consecutive annual normal Pap smear results, repeat examination every 3 years at discretion of physician.
    2. Diagnostic procedures (Fig. 30–2 for decision-making).
      a. Colposcopy (examination of the cervix under magnification after application of acetic acid) is recommended as a component of evaluation of the cervix after obtaining an abnormal result from a Pap smear.
      b. Cervical biopsy is recommended when abnormalities are identified on the cervix by colposcopy.
      c. Endocervical curettage is recommended when the upper limits of cervical abnormalities are not visualized or the transformation zone within the endocervical canal is not visualized completely.
      d. Cone biopsy (Fig. 30–3) or loop electrosurgical excision procedure (LEEP) may be recommended to obtain a larger wedge of tissue and to rule out invasive cancer.
  B. Staging methods and procedures.
    1. Staging of preinvasive disease (Table 30–1).
    2. For ICC, examination under anesthesia is done to evaluate the extent of the disease.
    3. Evaluation of extension of disease to the bladder or rectum is determined by cystoscopy, intravenous pyelogram (IVP), sigmoidoscopy, proctoscopy, or barium enema examination.
    4. Abdominal or pelvic computed tomographic (CT) scan, ultrasound, or magnetic resonance imaging (MRI) may be done to evaluate the extent of the local lesion and metastasis to regional lymph nodes.
    5. Chest x-ray examination is used to rule out lung metastasis.

Abnormal Pap Smear

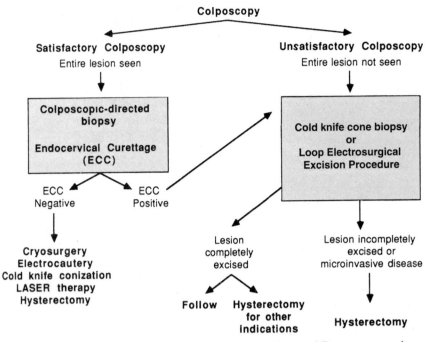

Figure 30–2. Diagnostic decision making after an abnormal Pap smear result.

    6. Although sometimes controversial, ICC is clinically staged and is not altered by subsequent surgical findings (Table 30–2).

C. Treatment strategies.

    1. Preinvasive disease—biopsy, cautery, cryotherapy, laser therapy, conization, LEEP, or hysterectomy; treatment depends on:

       a. Size and location of CIN visualized.

       b. Client desire for preservation of childbearing capacity.

       c. Physician skills and preference.

    2. Invasive disease—surgery and/or radiation.

       a. Treatment choice depends on client age, physical condition, percent

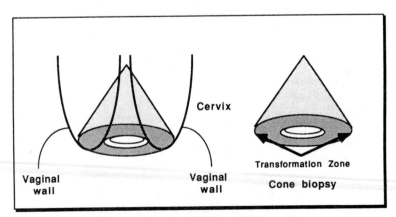

Figure 30–3. Cone biopsy of the cervix.

TABLE 30–1. **Staging for Cervical Cytology**

Pap Smear	WHO System	Bethesda System
Class I	Normal	Within normal limits
Class II	Atypical	Reactive or reparative change
Class III	Dysplasia	Squamous epithelial cell abnormality; atypical squamous cells of undetermined significance; squamous intraepithelial lesion
	Mild dysplasia	Low grade (includes human papilloma virus)
	Moderate dysplasia	High grade
	Severe dysplasia	High grade
Class IV	Carcinoma in situ	High grade
Class V	Invasive squamous cell carcinoma	Squamous cell carcinoma
	Adenocarcinoma	Glandular cell abnormalities: adenocarcinoma or nonepithelial malignant neoplasm

From Wright, T.C., & Richart, R.M. (1992). Pathogenesis and diagnosis of preinvasive lesions of the lower genital tract. In W.J. Hoskins, C.A. Perez, & R.C. Young (eds.). *Principles and Practice of Gynecologic Oncology.* Philadelphia: J.B. Lippincott, p. 528.

TABLE 30–2. **Clinical Staging for Cervical Cancer (FIGO*)**

Stage	Description
0	Carcinoma in situ, intraepithelial carcinoma
I	Carcinoma confined to the cervix (extension to the corpus should be avoided)
IA	Preclinical carcinomas of the cervix (diagnosed only by microscopy)
IA1	Minimal microscopically evident stromal invasion
IA2	Lesions detected microscopically that can be measured, showing no more than a 5-mm depth of invasion when taken from the base of the epithelium and no more than 7 mm of horizontal spread
IB	Lesions of greater dimensions than stage IA2, whether seen clinically or not
II	Involvement of the vagina but not of the lower third or infiltration of the parametria but not out to the side wall
IIA	Involvement of the vagina but no evidence of parametrial involvement
IIB	Infiltration of the parametria but not out to the side wall
III	Involvement of the lower third of the vagina or extension to the pelvic side wall; all cases with hydronephrosis or nonfunctioning kidney unless known to be from another cause
IIIA	Involvement of the lower third of the vagina but not out to the pelvic side wall
IIIB	Involvement of one or both parametria out to the side wall or hydronephrosis or nonfunctioning kidney
IV	Extension beyond the true pelvis
IVA	Involvement of the mucosa of the bladder or rectum
IVB	Distant metastasis

*FIGO: International Federation of Gynecology and Obstetrics.

of ideal body weight, tumor volume, and desire to maintain ovarian function.

  b. Primary surgical treatment—early stage disease:
    (1) Radical hysterectomy with pelvic lymphadenectomy and paraaortic lymph node dissection.
    (2) Bilateral salpingo-oophorectomy included in postmenopausal women or those over age 40 years.
  c. Primary radiation therapy treatment—early or advanced stage disease.
    (1) Combination of external and either high-dose outpatient or conventional inpatient intracavitary brachytherapy implants.
    (2) Intracavitary implants may be given before or after external radiation therapy is completed.
  d. Combination of surgery and radiation therapy for advanced stage disease or early stage disease with positive-testing lymph nodes or positive-testing surgical margins.

3. Recurrent disease presents a treatment challenge.
  a. Recurrent local disease—anterior, posterior, or total pelvic exenteration.
    (1) Extensive preoperative workup done to rule out extrapelvic disease.
    (2) Initial lymph node frozen sections to rule out metastatic disease.
    (3) Anterior pelvic exenteration—radical hysterectomy, pelvic lymph node dissection, removal of bladder, and creation of ileal conduit.
    (4) Posterior pelvic exenteration—radical hysterectomy, pelvic lymph node dissection, removal of rectosigmoid colon, and creation of a colostomy.
  b. Recurrent disseminated disease presents a treatment challenge.
    (1) Chemotherapy is primarily palliative with single agents: cisplatin, paclitaxel, or 5-fluorouracil (5-FU); response rates are low.

D. Trends in survival (Table 30–3).
  1. No overall change in survival rate has occurred for clients with ICC, although mortality rate has decreased because of decreased incidence.
  2. Prognosis is related to stage of disease.
  3. 35% of women have recurrent disease within 3 years of initial therapy.
  4. Cause of death associated most often with uremia, infection, or hemorrhage.

TABLE 30–3. **Five-Year Survival Rates for Clients With Cervical Cancer**

Stage	5-Year Survival Rate (%)
0	95–100
IA	85–90
IB	80
IIA	70–75
IIB	60
III	30
IV	>10

Assessment

I. Pertinent personal and family history.
  A. Bimodal peak of occurrence at 35 to 39 years and 60 to 64 years.
  B. Presence of selected viruses—HPV 16 and 18 and herpes simplex type 2.
  C. Initiation of sexual intercourse during teenage years.
  D. Multiple sexual partners and sexual partners who have had multiple sexual partners.
  E. History of CIN.
  F. Cigarette smoking.
  G. Immunosuppression (e.g., with acquired immunodeficiency disease [AIDS] or after transplantation).
II. Physical examination.
  A. Early signs and symptoms—most women are asymptomatic until disease is advanced. May have a thin, watery vaginal discharge or painless, intermittent, postcoital, intramenstrual, or postmenopausal vaginal bleeding, or an increase in the length and amount of menstrual flow.
  B. Late signs and symptoms—dyspareunia. Urinary symptoms include dysuria, urinary retention, urinary frequency, or hematuria. Bowel symptoms may include rectal bleeding, constipation, or bowel obstruction. Abdominal or pelvic pain referred to the flank or leg. Lower extremity edema.
III. Evaluation of laboratory data.
  A. Elevated blood urea nitrogen (BUN) or creatinine levels.
  B. Decreased hemoglobin or hematocrit levels.
  C. Increased white blood cell count.

Nursing Diagnoses

I. Body image disturbance.
II. Sexual dysfunction.
III. Constipation.
IV. Altered urinary elimination.
V. Ineffective individual coping.
VI. Ineffective family coping: compromised.
VII. Knowledge deficit.

Outcome Identification

I. Client describes personal risk factors for cervical cancer, methods to minimize risks, and plan for screening with Pap smear and pelvic examination.
II. Client discusses rationale, schedule, and personal demands of treatment and follow-up care. Maintains vaginal vault access through regular intercourse or dilation.
III. Client lists potential side effects of disease and treatment.
IV. Client describes self-care measures to decrease the incidence and severity of complications of treatment.
V. Client and family list signs and symptoms of recurrent disease to report to the health care team—pain in hips or lower back, vaginal bleeding, swelling of lower extremities, or unexplained weight loss.
VI. Client and family describe community resources to potentially meet demands of treatment and survivorship (e.g., American Cancer Society and National Coalition for Cancer Survivorship).

Planning and Implementation

I. Interventions to maximize safety for the client.
   A. Teach changes in lifestyle that can modify risks of cervical cancer.
      1. Use of barrier-type contraceptives—diaphragm or condom.
      2. Discontinuation of cigarette smoking.
      3. Screening with a Pap smear as recommended to detect premalignant changes.
   B. See Chapters 34 and 35 for safety concerns with surgery and radiation therapy.

II. Interventions to decrease the severity of symptoms associated with disease and treatment.
   A. Teach the client about possible symptoms associated with treatment modality options.
   B. Primary symptoms related to surgery.
      1. Inability to void—innervation to the bladder can be disrupted during radical hysterectomy and can result in an inability to sense the need to void and an inability to empty the bladder completely; a suprapubic catheter usually will be in place postoperatively. Initiate bladder training by clamping the catheter for 2 to 3 hours. Encourage the client to drink fluids unless contraindicated by physiologic status. Remove the catheter after less than 50 mL residual urine remains after voiding as ordered.
      2. Constipation—bowel is manipulated during radical surgery; peristalsis does not return for several days (see Chapter 14).
      3. Shortened vagina—approximately one third of the upper vagina is excised with hysterectomy; remaining margins are sutured to form a vaginal cuff.
      4. Urinary and stool diversions with pelvic exenteration (see Chapter 14).
   C. Primary symptoms related to radiation therapy (see Chapter 35 for nursing implications of radiation therapy to the ovary, urinary bladder, gastrointestinal tract, and skin).

III. Interventions to monitor for sequelae of disease or treatment.
   A. Surgery.
      1. Assess changes in bowel pattern—constipation, bowel obstruction, and rare fistula formation.
      2. Evaluate changes in bladder pattern—recurrent urinary tract infection and fistula formation.
   B. Radiation therapy.
      1. Assess changes in bowel pattern—diarrhea, bowel obstruction, rectal ulcers, and rectovaginal fistulas.
      2. Assess changes in bladder pattern—urinary retention, cystitis, and vesicovaginal fistulas.
      3. Evaluate changes in vaginal tissues—atrophy, stenosis, and dryness.
   C. Recurrent disease.
      1. Assess for history of vaginal bleeding.
      2. Evaluate occurrence of new pain, particularly in hips or lower back.
      3. Evaluate lower extremities for edema.
      4. Assess for changes in appetite with weight loss.

IV. Interventions to incorporate the client and family in care.
   A. Encourage open communication about the impact of disease and treatment on the client and significant others.

B. Teach the client and significant other new self-care skills required during or after treatment.

C. Identify concerns the client and sexual partner may have about resuming intercourse after treatment.

Evaluation

The oncology nurse systematically and regularly evaluates the client's and/or family's responses to interventions to determine progress toward the achievement of expected outcomes. Relevant data are collected and actual findings are compared with expected findings. Nursing diagnoses, outcomes, and plans of care are reviewed and revised as necessary.

ENDOMETRIAL CANCER

Theory

I. Physiology and pathophysiology associated with endometrial cancer.
  A. Anatomy of the endometrium.
    1. Inner layer of three layers of the uterus (endometrium, myometrium, and parietal peritoneum).
    2. Highly vascular mucous membrane lining.
  B. Primary functions of the endometrium—provides vascular and nutrient supply for developing fetus and responds to variations in estrogen and progesterone levels in a cyclic fashion.
  C. Changes associated with cancer of the endometrium.
    1. Underlying cause of endometrial cancer is believed to be abnormal production and metabolism of endogenous estrogen.
    2. Hyperplasia that may progress to invasive cancer.
    3. Histology is 90% adenocarcinoma; rarer types include clear cell, papillary serous, adenosquamous, and sarcoma.
  D. Metastatic patterns.
    1. Invades inner one third of the endometrium and progresses to the full thickness of the endometrium.
    2. Metastasis occurs through local extension to adjacent structures such as the cervix and vagina.
    3. Metastasis occurs in femoral, iliac, and hypogastric lymph nodes.
    4. Hematologic metastasis is uncommon except in rarely occurring sarcoma.
  E. Trends in epidemiology.
    1. Most common gynecologic malignancy among women in the US. Fourth most common cancer in women in the US.
    2. Incidence has increased over the past several decades and has been associated with increased use of estrogen replacement therapy (without progestins).
II. Principles of medical management.
  A. Screening procedures.
    1. Endometrial aspiration or biopsy. (Pap smear detects less than 50% of cases.)
    2. Bimanual pelvic examination to palpate the size and shape of the uterus.
  B. Diagnostic procedures.
    1. Endocervical curettage to rule out cervical cancer.
    2. Fractional dilation and curettage (D and C) if previous endometrial biopsy results have been negative and abnormal bleeding persists.

C. Staging methods and procedures (Table 30–4).
   1. Procedures.
      a. Bladder involvement—cystoscopy or intravenous pyelogram (IVP).
      b. Bowel involvement—barium enema examination, proctoscopy, or sig-moidoscopy.
      c. Chest x-ray examination to rule out metastasis.
      d. Hysterography, hysteroscopy, lymphangiography, ultrasound, CT scan, or MRI to evaluate size of tumor and extension to lymph nodes.
   2. Surgical staging based on findings from exploratory laparotomy, total abdominal hysterectomy–bilateral salpingo-oophorectomy (TAH-BSO), and peritoneal washing.
   3. Results of staging reported as anatomic stage, histopathologic grade, depth of myometrial invasion, and evaluation of peritoneal cytology (see Table 30–4).
D. Treatment strategies.
   1. Treatment decisions are based on stage of disease, grade, depth of myometrial invasion, and client characteristics.
   2. Preinvasive disease—administration of progesterone or simple hysterectomy.
   3. Invasive disease—surgery and/or radiation therapy; optimal dose and sequencing remains under investigation.
      a. Surgery.
         (1) Surgical staging procedure (TAH-BSO) serves as primary treatment for early stage disease.
         (2) Pelvic and paraaortic lymphadenectomy included for grade 2 and 3 lesions.
      b. Radiation therapy (RT).
         (1) Primary treatment for high-risk surgical candidates. (Because of risk factors and comorbidities, many clients are not surgical candidates and receive primary RT.)
      c. Adjuvant radiation therapy.
         (1) Preoperative therapy for clients with extensive lesions involving the cervix or high-grade lesions.

TABLE 30–4. **Staging for Endometrial Carcinoma (FIGO*)**

Stage	Description
0	Atypical hyperplasia or carcinoma in situ
IA	Tumor limited to the endometrium
IB	Invasion to less than one half of myometrium
IC	Invasion to more than one half of myometrium
IIA	Endocervical glandular involvement only
IIB	Cervical stromal invasion
IIIA	Invasion of serosa and adnexa and/or positive peritoneal cytology
IIIB	Vaginal metastases
IIIC	Metastases to pelvic and/or para-aortic lymph nodes
IVA	Invasion of bladder and/or bowel mucosa
IVB	Distant metastasis, including intra-abdominal and/or inguinal lymph nodes

*FIGO: International Federation of Gynecology and Obstetrics.

(2) Postoperative therapy for clients with risk factors for recurrent disease; high-grade lesions, deep myometrial invasion; or cervical involvement.

(3) Techniques include intracavitary brachytherapy and teletherapy.

d. Hormonal therapy for disseminated disease.

(1) Synthetic progestational agents—megestrol acetate or medroxy-progesterone acetate.

e. Chemotherapy for recurrent disease—single-agent cyclophosphamide, doxorubicin, or cisplatin remains an area for further investigation for optimal therapy.

f. Recurrent disease—surgery or radiation therapy to previously untreated areas.

E. Trends in survival (Table 30–5).

1. Most curable gynecologic malignancy.

2. Prognostic factors include stage, grade, and depth of myometrial invasion.

3. 25 to 35% of clients have recurrent disease.

Assessment

I. Pertinent personal and family history.

A. Age—peak incidence, 50 to 64 years.

B. Menopausal status—80% of clients are postmenopausal.

C. Socioeconomic status—higher status places women at increased risk.

D. History of changes in hormone levels—obesity, nulliparity, late menopause, infertility, irregular menstrual history, Stein-Leventhal syndrome, and estrogen replacement therapy without progestational agents.

E. Personal history of endometrial hyperplasia; breast, ovarian, or colorectal cancers.

F. Family history of multiple endocrine-related cancer.

G. Triad of obesity, diabetes, and hypertension greatly increases risk.

II. Physical examination.

A. Early signs and symptoms—bleeding in postmenopausal women, irregular or heavy menstrual flow in premenopausal women, vaginal discharge, lumbosacral pain.

B. Late signs and symptoms—hemorrhage, ascites, jaundice, bowel obstruction, respiratory distress.

TABLE 30–5. **Five-Year Survival Rates for Clients With Endometrial Cancer**

Stage	5-Year Survival Rate (%)
I Overall	76
Grade 1	92
Grade 2	74
Grade 3	48
II	50
III	30
IV	9

III. Evaluation of laboratory data.
   A. Decreased hemoglobin or hematocrit level.
   B. Abnormal liver enzyme levels.
   C. Abnormal chemistry profile results.

Nursing Diagnoses

   I. Body image disturbance.
   II. Sexual dysfunction.
   III. Ineffective individual coping.
   IV. Ineffective family coping: compromised.
   V. Fear.
   VI. Knowledge deficit.

Outcome Identification

   I. Client describes personal risk factors for endometrial cancer.
   II. Client discusses rationale, schedule, and personal demands of treatment and follow-up care.
   III. Client and family list potential side effects of disease and treatment.
   IV. Client describes self-care measures to decrease the incidence and severity of complications of treatment.
   V. Client and family list signs and symptoms of recurrent disease to report to the health care team, such as vaginal bleeding, constipation, and pelvic pain.
   VI. Client and family describe potential community resources to meet demands of treatment and survivorship.

Planning and Implementation

   I. Interventions to maximize safety for the client.
      A. Teach changes in lifestyle that can modify risks of endometrial cancer.
         1. Encourage the client to maintain ideal body weight.
         2. Suggest a combination of estrogen and progesterone hormone replacement postmenopausally if the uterus is present.
      B. See Chapters 34 and 35 for safety concerns about surgery and radiation therapy.
   II. Interventions to decrease the severity of symptoms associated with disease and treatment from surgery and radiation therapy such as altered urinary and bowel function and pain.
      A. Venous stasis.
         1. Encourage turning in bed and ambulating as soon as possible.
         2. Teach isometric leg exercises to do while in bed.
         3. Apply antiembolic stockings.
         4. Monitor for discomfort in legs and thighs.
         5. Avoid use of a knee gatch in the bed.
      B. Urinary retention.
         1. Monitor urinary output.
         2. Assess for bladder distention above the symphysis pubis.
         3. Assess for lower abdominal discomfort.
   III. Interventions to monitor for sequelae of disease and treatment.
      A. See Chapters 13 and 14 for issues related to nutrition and elimination, and Chapter 1 for comfort issues.

B. See Chapters 2, 3, and 6 for coping, body image, and sexuality issues.
C. Assess for signs of recurrent disease.
  1. Vaginal bleeding.
  2. Change in bowel habits—constipation.
  3. Pelvic pain.

Evaluation

The oncology nurse systematically and regularly evaluates the client's and/or family's responses to interventions to determine progress toward the achievement of expected outcomes. Relevant data are collected and actual findings are compared with expected findings. Nursing diagnoses, outcomes, and plans of care are reviewed and revised as necessary.

OVARIAN CANCER

Theory

 I. Physiology and pathophysiology of ovarian cancer.
  A. Anatomy of the ovary.
    1. Ovaries are located on each side of the uterus behind the fallopian tubes.
    2. Ovarian lymphatics drain into the iliac and periaortic lymph nodes.
  B. Primary functions of the ovary—production and release of ova and production of hormones to meet needs of female for development, growth, and function (estrogen, progesterone, and testosterone).
  C. Metastatic patterns.
    1. Local extension to adjacent organs.
    2. Exfoliation of the ovarian capsule.
    3. Serosal seeding by tumor nests throughout the peritoneal cavity.
    4. Hematologic spread to the lungs and liver.
  D. Trends in epidemiology.
    1. Steady increase in the incidence of ovarian cancer.
 II. Principles of medical management.
  A. Screening procedures.
    1. Bimanual pelvic examination.
      a. Increase in size or irregularity of the ovary.
      b. Palpable ovary in a postmenopausal woman.
    2. Serial CA-125 determinations in high-risk women, supplemented by transvaginal ultrasound remain controversial but are sometimes used for high-risk women.
  B. Diagnostic procedures.
    1. Laparoscopy or exploratory laparotomy to obtain tissue for diagnosis.
    2. Paracentesis of ascitic fluid.
  C. Staging (Table 30–6) procedures and methods.
    1. Bowel involvement—barium enema examination, proctosigmoidoscopy, and upper gastrointestinal series.
    2. Bladder involvement—cystoscopy and IVP.
    3. Pulmonary involvement—chest x-ray examination.
    4. Liver involvement—liver enzyme values.
    5. Surgical staging laparotomy is mandatory to evaluate pelvic and abdominal contents—TAH-BSO; peritoneal cytology; omentectomy; lymph node biopsies or removal; multiple biopsies of bladder, bowel, liver, and

TABLE 30–6. **Staging for Ovarian Cancer (FIGO*)**

Stage	Description
I	Growth limited to the ovaries
IA	Growth limited to one ovary; no ascites; no tumor on the external surface; capsule intact
IB	Growth limited to both ovaries; no ascites; no tumor on the external surfaces; capsules intact
IC	Either stage IA or IB tumor but with tumor on surface of one or both ovaries, with capsule ruptured, with ascites present containing malignant cells, or with positive peritoneal washings
II	Growth involving one or both ovaries with pelvic extension
IIA	Extension and/or metastases to the uterus and/or tubes
IIB	Extension to other pelvic tissues
IIC	Either stage IIA or IIB tumor but with tumor on the surface of one or both ovaries, with capsule(s) ruptured, with ascites present and containing malignant cells, or with positive peritoneal washings
III	Tumor involving one or both ovaries, with peritoneal implants outside the pelvis and/or positive retroperitoneal or inguinal nodes; superficial liver metastasis equals stage III
IIIA	Tumor grossly limited to the true pelvis, with negative nodes but histologically confirmed microscopic seeding of abdominal peritoneal surfaces
IIIB	Tumor of one or both ovaries, with histologically confirmed implants of abdominal peritoneal surfaces, with none exceeding 2 cm in diameter; nodes are negative.
IIIC	Abdominal implants greater than 2 cm in diameter and/or positive retroperitoneal or inguinal nodes
IV	Growth involving one or both ovaries with distant metastases; if pleural effusion is present, cytology must be positive to allot a case to stage IV; parenchymal liver metastasis equals stage IV

*FIGO: International Federation of Gynecology and Obstetrics.

diaphragm surfaces; appendectomy; and debulking cytoreduction of all visible tumor.
   6. Majority of clients with ovarian cancer are diagnosed with late-stage disease.
   D. Treatment strategies.
      1. Primary surgical treatment.
         a. Cytoreduction, with removal of all tumor or tumors greater than 3 cm in size so that minimal residual disease remains.
         b. Surgery may be used alone to treat early stage disease or borderline tumors with "low malignant potential."
         c. Surgery may be used to evaluate the response to chemotherapy treatment ("second-look" procedures), for secondary cytoreduction, and for palliation of recurrent bowel obstruction.
            (1) Goals are to detect residual tumor, debulk remaining tumor, and determine further treatment.
            (2) Second-look procedures are done only in the presence of a complete response clinically.
            (3) One fourth to one third of clients with a complete response clinically have evidence of disease on second look.

2. Adjuvant chemotherapy.
    a. Treatment of clients with late-stage disease.
    b. Combination chemotherapy with paclitaxel and cisplatin/carboplatin is now first-line therapy. Recurrent progressive disease may be treated with cisplatin, cyclophosphamide, paclitaxel, hexamethylmelamine, hydroxyurea.
    c. Chemotherapy may be administered intravenously and intraperitoneally; advantages of intraperitoneal method include:
        (1) Higher concentrations of drug to the surface of the tumor.
        (2) Decreased systemic side effects.
        (3) Systemic tolerance of higher doses of drug.
    d. Hormonal therapy may be used for salvage therapy (e.g., megestrol acetate and tamoxifen citrate).
    e. Adjuvant radiation therapy.
        (1) Pelvic or whole abdominal extended fields may be used for treatment of metastatic disease to the pelvis or abdomen.
        (2) Acute and chronic gastrointestinal complications are common.
        (3) Radioactive isotopes, such as ^{32}P, may also be given intraperitoneally to treat abdominal metastases.
    f. Biologic response modifiers are used as single agents and in combination with chemotherapy as adjuvant therapy.
        (1) Biologic response modifiers can be administered intravenously or intraperitoneally.
        (2) Interferon, interleukin-2, and monoclonal antibodies are under investigation.
E. Trends in survival (Table 30–7).
    1. Overall 5-year survival rate ranges from 30 to 35%.
    2. Stage and grade are important prognostic factors.
    3. Abdominal carcinomatosis commonly occurs and results in intestinal obstruction, malabsorption, and fluid and electrolyte imbalances.

Assessment

I. Pertinent personal and family history.
    A. Age—occurs commonly in premenopausal women ages 40 to 65 years old. Peak incidence is at age 55 to 59 years. Germ cell tumors are more common in children and adolescents.
    B. Infertility.

TABLE 30–7. Five-Year Survival Rates for Clients With Ovarian Cancer

Stage	5-Year Survival Rate (%)
I	80
II	60
IIIa	60
IIIb	30
IIIc	5–10
IV	5

   C. Nulliparity.
   D. Personal history of breast, endometrial, or colon cancers.
   E. Family history of breast, endometrial, or colon cancers.
   F. 10% of ovarian cancers are familial, receiving great investigative attention including genetic investigation.
II. Physical examination.
   A. Early signs and symptoms are vague and diffuse—gastrointestinal distress, dyspepsia, abdominal discomfort, flatulence, eructation, increased pelvic pressure.
   B. Late signs and symptoms—palpable abdominal or pelvic mass, increased abdominal girth, ascites, pleural effusions, intestinal obstruction, weight loss.
III. Evaluation of laboratory data.
   A. CA-125 may be used to monitor treatment response or disease recurrence.
   B. Beta-human chorionic gonadotropin (β-hCG) levels may be used to detect and monitor germ cell tumors.

Nursing Diagnoses

   I. Body image disturbance.
   II. Constipation.
   III. Altered nutrition, less than body requirements.
   IV. Ineffective individual coping.
   V. Ineffective family coping: compromised.
   VI. Anticipatory grieving.
   VII. Sexual dysfunction.
   VIII. Knowledge deficit.

Outcome Identification

   I. Client describes personal risk factors for ovarian cancer.
   II. Client and family discuss rationale, schedule, and personal demands of treatment and follow-up care.
   III. Client lists potential side effects of disease and treatment.
   IV. Client describes self-care measures to decrease the incidence and severity of complications of treatment.
   V. Client and family identify signs and symptoms of recurrent disease to report to the health care team.
   VI. Client and family describe community resources to meet potential demands of treatment and survivorship.

Planning and Implementation

   I. Interventions for management of symptoms related to disease and treatment modalities, that is, surgery and chemotherapy.
   A. See Chapters 13 and 14 for issues related to nutrition and elimination and Chapter 1 for comfort issues.
   B. See Chapters 2, 3, 6, and 7 for coping, body image, sexuality, and death and dying issues.
   II. Aggressive symptom management is necessary while women receive complex chemotherapy regimens (e.g., antiemetic control, prevention of neuropathies, maintenance of fluid and electrolyte balance).

III. Coping issues need to be addressed because diagnosis is often delayed, therapy may be prolonged, and prognosis is poor.

Evaluation

The oncology nurse systematically and regularly evaluates the client's and/or family's responses to interventions to determine progress toward the achievement of expected outcomes. Relevant data are collected and actual findings are compared with expected findings. Nursing diagnoses, outcomes, and plans of care are reviewed and revised as necessary.

GESTATIONAL TROPHOBLASTIC NEOPLASIA

Theory

I. Physiology and pathophysiology associated with gestational trophoblastic neoplasia (GTN).
  A. A continuum exists from an abnormal pregnancy to molar pregnancy to invasive mole to choriocarcinoma to placental tumor.
  B. Chromosomal abnormalities that correspond to the disease are under investigation.
  C. Metastatic patterns.
      1. Hematologic spread to lung, liver, and brain usually with choriocarcinoma.
  D. Trends in epidemiology.
      1. Varies geographically and ethnically; in US 1 per 1700 pregnancies; African Americans have higher incidence.
II. Principles of medical management.
  A. Screening and diagnostic procedures—ultrasound to evaluate suspected pregnancy if fetal abnormality or absence, hCG laboratory evaluation and metastatic workup if necessary.
  B. Staging methods and procedures include ultrasound, D and C, metastatic evaluation of chest and brain if appropriate. (Table 30–8).
  C. Treatment strategies.
      1. Depend on classification and desired fertility.
          a. Suction evacuation of uterine contents eliminates mole and preserves childbearing.
          b. Hysterectomy may be done if childbearing is not desired.
      2. Invasive disease—removal of uterine contents with suction.
      3. Chemotherapy is extremely effective in management of GTN.
          a. Single-agent therapy with methotrexate, actinomycin D, etoposide for low-risk and nonmetastatic disease.
          b. Combination chemotherapy for high-risk disease.

TABLE 30–8. **FIGO* Staging for Gestational Trophoblastic Tumors**

Stage I	Confined to uterine corpus
Stage II	Metastasis to pelvis
Stage III	Metastasis to lungs
Stage IV	Distant metastasis

* FIGO: International Federation of Gynecology and Obstetrics.

      4. Surgical removal of isolated chemotherapy-resistant metastasis.

      5. Radiation therapy of resistant metastatic sites.

   C. Trends in survival—80% of clients with metastatic disease are cured.

Assessment

    I. Pertinent personal and family history.

      A. Age—highest risk for women over 40 years of age becoming pregnant. Some increased risk for women under 20 years.

      B. Previous molar pregnancy greatest risk factor.

   II. Physical examination.

      A. Early signs and symptoms include abnormal uterine bleeding while presumed pregnant; abdominal pain; absence of fetal heartbeat.

  III. Evaluation of laboratory data.

      A. hCG extremely sensitive; weekly serial tests until results are normal and then monthly for 1 year. Used to monitor presence of disease, response to treatment, and recurrence.

Nursing Diagnoses

    I. Body image disturbance.

   II. Sexual dysfunction.

 III. Grieving.

 IV. Ineffective individual coping.

  V. Ineffective family coping: compromised.

 VI. Knowledge deficit.

Outcome Identification

    I. Client describes personal risk factors for GTN, methods for screening.

   II. Client discusses rationale, schedule, and personal demands of treatment and follow-up care, especially obtaining routine hCG.

  III. Client and family list potential side effects of disease and treatment.

 IV. Client identifies self-care measures to decrease the incidence and severity of complications of treatment.

  V. Client and family address issues of loss related to pregnancy and/or future fertility.

 VI. Client and family describe community resources to meet potential demands of treatment and survivorship, such as the American Cancer Society and National Coalition for Cancer Survivorship.

Planning and Implementation

    I. Interventions to decrease the severity of symptoms associated with disease and treatment.

      A. See Chapters 13 and 14 for issues related to nutrition and elimination and Chapter 1 for comfort issues.

      B. See Chapters 2, 3, and 6 for coping, body image and sexuality issues.

   II. Interventions to incorporate the client and family in care.

      A. Encourage open communication about the impact of disease and treatment on the client and significant others.

      B. Teach the client and significant other new self-care skills required during or after treatment.

   C. Identify concerns the client and her sexual partner may have about future fertility.

Evaluation

The oncology nurse systematically and regularly evaluates the client's and/or family's responses to interventions to determine progress toward the achievement of expected outcomes. Relevant data are collected and actual findings are compared with expected findings. Nursing diagnoses, outcomes, and plans of care are reviewed and revised as necessary.

VULVAR CANCER

Theory

   I. Physiology and pathophysiology associated with vulvar cancer.
      A. Anatomy of the vulva—lies beneath the labia majora, labia minora, and clitoris.
      B. Changes associated with cancer of the vulva.
         1. Cellular changes exist on a continuum from premalignant changes to invasive carcinoma.
         2. Histology—85% squamous; rare—melanoma, leiomyosarcoma, basal cell.
      C. Metastatic patterns.
         1. Direct extension to other pelvic structures.
         2. Lymph node metastases common.
      D. Trends in epidemiology—very rare cancer, comprise only 5% of all female cancers.
  II. Principles of medical management.
      A. Screening and diagnostic procedures.
         1. Screening procedures—careful pelvic inspection and examination; acetic acid staining and colposcopy may be used to evaluate any suspicious lesions.
         2. Diagnostic procedure—biopsy.
      B. Staging methods and procedures include biopsy of suspected area and evaluation of lymph node involvement with CT. The International Federation of Gynecology and Obstetrics (FIGO) system is used.
      C. Treatment strategies.
         1. Preinvasive disease—surgical management with wide local excision or vulvectomy.
         2. Invasive disease—surgery has been the major modality (i.e., vulvectomy and nodal dissection).
         3. Radiation therapy as an adjunct pre- or postoperatively.
      D. Trends in survival are difficult to identify accurately because of low incidence (Table 30–9).

Assessment

   I. Pertinent personal and family history.
      A. Age—postmenopausal women at ages ranging from the 60s to 70s have peak incidence.
      B. History of vulvar inflammation and other genitourinary (GU) cancers increases risk.

TABLE 30–9. **Five-Year Survival Rates for Clients With Vulvar Cancer**

Stage	5-Year Survival Rate (%)
I	98
II	85
III	74
IV	31

II. Physical examination.
    A. Early signs and symptoms—vaginal lump or itching.
    B. Late signs and symptoms—bleeding, discharge, dysuria.

Nursing Diagnoses

  I. Body image disturbance.
 II. Sexual dysfunction.
III. Ineffective individual coping.
IV. Ineffective family coping: compromised.
 V. Knowledge deficit.

Outcome Identification

   I. Client describes personal risk factors to minimize risks and plan for screening.
  II. Client discusses rationale, schedule, and personal demands of treatment and follow-up care.
III. Client and family list potential side effects of disease and treatment.
IV. Client and family address concerns of altered sexual functioning and perception.
 V. Client and family describe community resources to meet potential demands of treatment and survivorship.

Planning and Implementation

   I. Interventions to decrease the severity of symptoms associated with disease and treatment.
    A. Teach client about possible symptoms associated with treatment modality options (e.g., attention to skin care and promotion of healing without infection or pain is important after surgery). (See Chapter 34.)
  II. Monitor for the development of leg edema if lymph node dissection completed.
III. Identify concerns the client and her sexual partner may have about resuming sexual functioning after treatment.

Evaluation

The oncology nurse systematically and regularly evaluates the client's and/or family's responses to interventions to determine progress toward the achievement of expected outcomes. Relevant data are collected and actual findings are compared with expected findings. Nursing diagnoses, outcomes, and plans of care are reviewed and revised as necessary.

VAGINAL CANCER

Theory

I. Physiology and pathophysiology associated with vaginal cancer.
   A. Anatomy of the vagina—the mucous membrane tube forming the passageway between the uterus and the vulva.
   B. Changes associated can be premalignant to invasive.
   C. Role of HPV under investigation as causative agent.
   D. Pathology—squamous cell carcinoma 85%; rarely melanoma, adenocarcinoma, clear cell cancers.
   E. Metastatic patterns.
      1. Local extension and lymph node involvement.
      2. More commonly a metastatic site for cervical cancer.
   F. Incidence—extremely rare cancer; comprises 1 to 2% of female genitourinary cancer.
II. Principles of medical management.
   A. Screening procedures.
      1. Careful pelvic inspection and examination.
      2. Cytologic washings, even after hysterectomy.
   B. Diagnostic procedures.
      1. Biopsy of lesion, usually an outpatient procedure.
      2. Examination under anesthesia—cystoscopy, proctoscopy
      3. Chest x-ray examination, CT of abdomen and pelvis.
   C. The FIGO staging system is used.
   D. Treatment strategies.
      1. Preinvasive disease—vaginal intraepithelial neoplasia: 5-FU local application, laser vaporization, brachytherapy, or surgical excision.
      2. Invasive disease—surgery and/or radiation therapy.
         a. Surgery—vaginectomy and hysterectomy for early stage disease.
         b. Radiation therapy—main treatment for all stages, implant may be added to teletherapy, lymph node fields depend on staging.
      3. Recurrent disease—surgery or radiation therapy to previously untreated areas.
   E. Trends in survival are poor (Table 30–10).

Assessment

I. Pertinent personal and family history.
   A. Age—primarily a disease of the elderly, over age 60 years.
   B. Personal history of maternal diethylstilbestrol use during pregnancy; should be screened for rare clear cell pathology.
   C. Prior history of ICC increases risk.

TABLE 30–10. **Five-Year Survival Rates for Clients With Vaginal Cancer**

Stage	5-Year Survival Rate (%)
I	53
II	43
III	28
IV	12

II. Physical examination.
  A. Early signs and symptoms—vaginal bleeding or discharge.
  B. Late signs and symptoms—gastrointestinal or genitourinary changes.

Nursing Diagnoses

  I. Body image disturbance.
  II. Sexual dysfunction.
  III. Ineffective individual coping.
  IV. Ineffective family coping: compromised.
  V. Knowledge deficit.

Outcome Identification

  I. Client describes personal risk factors for vaginal cancer.
  II. Client discusses rationale, schedule, and personal demands of treatment and follow-up care.
  III. Client and family list potential side effects of disease and treatment.
  IV. Client identifies self-care measures to decrease the incidence and severity of complications of treatment.
  V. Client lists signs and symptoms of recurrent disease to report to the health care team.
  VI. Client and family describe community resources to meet potential demands of treatment and survivorship.

Planning and Implementation

  I. Interventions to monitor for sequelae of disease and treatment.
  A. See Chapters 13 and 14 for issues related to nutrition and elimination and Chapter 1 for comfort issues.
  B. See Chapters 2, 3, and 6 for coping, body image, and sexuality issues.
  II. Interventions to incorporate the client and family in care.
  A. Identify concerns the client and her sexual partner may have about resuming sexual functioning after treatment.

Evaluation

The oncology nurse systematically and regularly evaluates the client's and/or family's responses to interventions to determine progress toward the achievement of expected outcomes. Relevant data are collected and actual findings are compared with expected findings. Nursing diagnoses, outcomes, and plans of care are reviewed and revised as necessary.

TESTICULAR CANCER

Theory

  I. Physiology and pathophysiology associated with testicular cancer.
  A. Anatomy of the testes—testes are ovoid glands located in the scrotal sac that descend from the abdomen through the inguinal canal during the seventh month of fetal life.
  B. Primary functions of the testes include spermatogenesis and production of a hormone (testosterone) for male development, growth, and function.

   C. Changes associated with cancer of the testes.
     1. Testicular cancers arise from germinal epithelium.
     2. Usually occur in only one testis.
     3. Etiology is unknown. Risk factors include: cryptorchidism, chromosomal abnormalities (e.g., Klinefelter's syndrome), and abnormalities in reproductive tract development in utero.
     4. Behavior of testicular cancer varies with histologic subtype.
       a. Seminomas.
         (1) Occur in approximately 45% of cases.
         (2) Spread slowly, primarily through the lymphatics.
         (3) Are responsive to radiation therapy.
       b. Nonseminoma germ cell testicular tumors (NSGCTT)—embryonal tumor (20%), teratoma, choriocarcinoma; yolk sac, interstitial cell, and gonadal stromal tumors.
         (1) More aggressive than pure seminomas; 60 to 70% have lymph node spread at diagnosis.
         (2) Embryonal tumors invade the spermatic cord and metastasize to lung.
         (3) Embryonal tumors are not responsive to radiation therapy.
       c. Mixed cell types are fairly common.
   D. Metastatic patterns.
     1. Direct extension to adjacent structures.
     2. Lymphatic spread.
     3. Hematologic metastasis to the lung, brain, bone, and liver.
   E. Trends in epidemiology.
     1. Very rare cancer, incidence approximately 1% in American males.
     2. Most commonly occurring cancer among men ages 15 to 35 years.
     3. Incidence is higher and is increasing among white males.
II. Principles of medical management.
   A. Screening and diagnostic procedures.
     1. Screening procedures.
       a. Monthly testicular self-examination.
       b. Annual bimanual palpation and examination of the testes by the health care provider.
     2. Diagnostic procedure—tissue biopsy by high inguinal orchiectomy.
   B. Staging methods and procedures.
     1. Chest x-ray examination, CT scan, and/or tomography to evaluate lung metastasis.
     2. Abdominal CT scan and ultrasound to evaluate lymph node involvement.
     3. IVP to evaluate displacement of the ureter or kidney.
     4. Multiple staging systems are used (Table 30–11).
   C. Treatment strategies (vary by histology).
     1. Surgery.
       a. Transinguinal orchiectomy is the primary treatment for seminomas and nonseminomas.
       b. Retroperitoneal lymph node dissection may be done on the affected side.
       c. Surgery may be used to resect residual disease and isolated metastatic lesions of lung, liver, and retroperitoneum.
     2. Radiation therapy.
       a. Primary or adjuvant treatment for early stage seminomas.
       b. Fields may include iliac, retroperitoneal, and paraaortic lymph nodes or whole abdomen.
       c. Use of RT to lung fields limits use of bleomycin for recurrent disease because the risk of pulmonary fibrosis increases.

TABLE 30–11. **Comparison of Some Staging Systems for Testis Cancer**

Stage	Walter Reed Hospital	AJC/TNM Classification	Stage Grouping
I	Tumor confined to one testis No clinical or radiographic evidence of spread beyond	T_1 Limited to body of the testis, incl rete T_2 >Tunica albuginea/epididymis T_3 Invasion of spermatic cord T_4 Invasion of scrotal wall	I I II II
IIA	As in stage I but minimal metastases to iliac or para-aortic lymph nodes	N_1 Single homolateral ≥2 cm	III
IIB	Clinical or radiographic evidence of metastases to femoral, inguinal, iliac, or para-aortic lymph nodes. No metastases above diaphragm or visceral organs	N_2 2-5 cm or multiple regional lymph nodes, if inguinal, mobile N_3 >5 cm or fixed	IV IV
III	Clinical or radiographic evidence of metastases above the diaphragm or other distant metastases to body organs	M_1 Distant metastasis present	IV

T = tumor; N = node; M = metastasis.
AJC (1)/UICC(2)
From Keller, J.W., Sahasrabudhe, D.M., & McCune, C.S. (1993). Urologic and male genital cancers. In P. Rubin (ed.). *Clinical Oncology: A Multidisciplinary Approach for Physicians and Students* (7th ed.). Philadelphia: W.B. Saunders (p. 444).

    3. Chemotherapy.
        a. Treatment for NSGCTT and high-risk seminoma; clients with elevated tumor markers, advanced stage disease, or recurrent disease.
        b. Aggressive combination chemotherapy regimens (agents commonly used include cisplatin, vinblastine, bleomycin, etoposide, ifosfamide, vincristine, and doxorubicin). Response rates are excellent—complete response (70%) and partial response (30%).
    4. Recurrent disease also responds to chemotherapy. Surgical resection of recurrent disease or isolated resistant metastasis may be done.
  D. Trends in survival (Table 30–12).
    1. Survival from testicular cancer has increased dramatically over the past 10 years.
    2. Testicular cancer is considered curable, and the prognosis for clients is excellent.

TABLE 30–12. **Five-Year Survival Rates for Clients With Testicular Cancer**

Seminomas		Nonseminomas	
Stage	5-Year Survival Rate (%)	Stage	5-Year Survival Rate (%)
A	98	A	90–100
B1-B2	75–94	B	90
B3-C	71	C	80–85

3. Prognosis depends on bulk of disease at diagnosis.
4. Recurrences usually occur within 2 years; however, recurrences beyond 5 years have been reported, and recurrent disease is also responsive to treatment.

Assessment

I. Pertinent personal and family history.
  A. Age.
    1. Most commonly occurs in men age 20 to 40 years.
    2. Incidence decreases for men age 40 to 60 years and increases again after age 60 years.
  B. Cryptorchidism (undescended testicle) increases risk twenty-fold to forty-fold; if orchipexy is done after 6 years of age, protection is lost.
  C. Polythelia (multiple nipples) is associated with increased risk.
II. Physical examination.
  A. Early signs and symptoms are usually absent. Patients may have an asymptomatic mass; gynecomastia; infertility; or testicular fullness, heaviness, swelling, or pain.
  B. Late signs and symptoms are back pain, bone pain, or respiratory distress.
III. Evaluation of laboratory data.
  A. Serum tumor markers—α-fetoprotein (AFP) and β-hCG to establish a differential diagnosis, assess response to treatment, and monitor long-term responses.
  B. NSGCTT more commonly has elevated levels of markers—AFP (70%) and β-hCG (50%). AFP is not elevated in pure seminomas.

Nursing Diagnoses

I. Body image disturbance.
II. Sexual dysfunction.
III. Ineffective individual coping.
IV. Ineffective family coping: compromised.
V. Knowledge deficit.
VI. Anticipatory grieving.

Outcome Identification

I. Client describes personal risk factors for testicular cancer and a plan for testicular self-examination.
II. Client discusses rationale, schedule, and personal demands of treatment and follow-up care.
III. Client and family list potential side effects of disease and treatment.
IV. Client identifies self-care measures to decrease the incidence and severity of complications of treatment.
V. Client and family list signs and symptoms of recurrent disease to report.
VI. Client and family describe community resources to meet potential demands of treatment and survivorship.

Planning and Implementation

I. Teach adolescent men to perform monthly testicular self-examination (TSE).
II. See Chapters 34 and 37 for interventions related to surgical needs and chemotherapy.

A. Chemotherapy regimens are aggressive and require intensive nursing support and symptom management for fluid and electrolyte maintenance, monitoring renal function, antiemetic control, and prevention of constipation and neuropathies.

III. Interventions to decrease the severity of symptoms associated with disease and treatment.
   A. Edema.
      1. Apply ice bags to scrotal area for first 12 hours after surgery.
      2. Apply compression dressing to surgical site.
      3. Teach the client to avoid standing for long periods of time.
      4. Advise the client to take 20-minute tub baths three times a day for 1 week.
      5. Instruct the client to avoid heavy lifting for 4 to 6 weeks after surgery.
   B. Comfort.
      1. Encourage bed rest for 24 to 48 hours after surgery.
      2. Encourage use of an athletic supporter when ambulating.
   C. Body image, sexuality, and fertility.
      1. Discuss the potential of sperm banking as an option before treatment begins.
      2. Encourage open discussion about changes in body image between the client and his sexual partner.

IV. Interventions to incorporate the client and family in care.
   A. Identify concerns the client and his sexual partner may have about resuming sexual functioning after treatment.

Evaluation

The oncology nurse systematically and regularly evaluates the client's and/or family's responses to interventions to determine progress toward the achievement of expected outcomes. Relevant data are collected and actual findings are compared with expected findings. Nursing diagnoses, outcomes, and plans of care are reviewed and revised as necessary.

PENILE CANCER

Theory

I. Physiology and pathophysiology associated with penile cancer.
   A. Anatomy of the penis (Fig. 30–4).

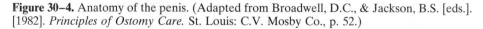

Figure 30–4. Anatomy of the penis. (Adapted from Broadwell, D.C., & Jackson, B.S. [eds.]. [1982]. *Principles of Ostomy Care.* St. Louis: C.V. Mosby Co., p. 52.)

1. Composed of the shaft and the glans.
2. Shaft has three cylindrical layers—bilateral corpus spongiosum, corpora cavernosa, and erectile tissues.
   B. Primary functions of the penis are urination and copulation.
   C. Causative factors unknown; HPV investigated; poor penile hygiene and no circumcision increase risk.
   D. Metastatic patterns.
   1. Direct extension to adjacent tissues.
   2. Metastasis to regional lymphatics—inguinal and iliac nodes.
II. Principles of medical management.
   A. Diagnostic procedures include biopsy of the penile lesion.
   B. Staging methods and procedures.
   1. Abdominal CT scan and x-ray examination to evaluate regional lymph nodes; intravenous urography, lymphangiography, chest x-ray examination, liver and bone scans.
   2. Staging is done clinically.
   C. Treatment strategies.
   1. Premalignant lesions—local excision, topical fluorouracil, or laser therapy.
   2. Invasive cancer.
      a. Surgery.
         (1) Partial or total penectomy with groin node dissection is controversial.
         (2) Total penectomy requires creation of a perineal urostomy for urination.
         (3) Radical lymphadenectomy or lymph node sampling may be done, depending on the stage of disease.
      b. Radiation therapy.
         (1) Interstitial, surface mold, or external beam therapy may be used for small penile lesions.
         (2) RT may also be used for palliative treatment.
      c. Chemotherapy.
         (1) May be used as palliative treatment for clients with stage III and IV disease.
         (2) Chemotherapy agents—cisplatin, methotrexate, and bleomycin are used.
   D. Trends in survival—because the disease is extremely rare, accurate trends in survival are not available (Table 30–13).

TABLE 30–13. **Five-Year Survival Rates for Clients With Penile Cancer**

Stage	5-Year Survival Rate (%)
I	80
II	60
III	25
IV	0

Assessment

   I. Pertinent personal and family history.
     A. Age—60 years or older.
     B. Penile hygiene practices—poor hygiene increases risk.
     C. Circumcision status—no circumcision increases risk.
  II. Physical examination.
     A. Early signs and symptoms—mass, nodule, or ulceration of the penis; foul-smelling penile discharge; inguinal lymphadenopathy; bleeding on the surface of the penis.
     B. Late signs and symptoms—fungating lesion of the penis, bone pain, respiratory distress.
 III. Evaluation of laboratory data—none specific to penile cancer.

Nursing Diagnoses

   I. Body image disturbance.
  II. Sexual dysfunction.
 III. Ineffective individual coping.
  IV. Ineffective family coping: compromised.
   V. Knowledge deficit.

Outcome Identification

   I. Client describes personal risk factors for penile cancer.
  II. Client discusses rationale, schedule, and personal demands of treatment and follow-up care.
 III. Client and family list potential side effects of disease and treatment.
  IV. Client identifies self-care measures to decrease the incidence and severity of complications of treatment.
   V. Client and family list signs and symptoms of recurrent disease to report.
  VI. Client and family describe community resources to meet potential demands of treatment and survivorship.

Planning and Implementation

   I. Interventions to maximize safety for the client.
     A. Discuss the option of circumcision before puberty for protective effect.
     B. Instruct high-risk clients in penile self-examination.
     C. Teach penile hygiene practices.
       1. Retraction of foreskin for cleansing.
       2. Washing penis with mild soap and water.
  II. For patients requiring assistance with urinary continence and maintenance, see Chapter 14.
 III. Interventions to enhance adaptation and rehabilitation.
     A. Encourage open discussion of sexual concerns.
       1. Reinforce information that clients with partial penectomy maintain sexual desire and the ability to penetrate, reach orgasm, and ejaculate.
       2. Discuss prosthetic options with clients who have had a total penectomy.
     B. Discuss alternate forms of sexual expression with the client and his sexual partner.

Evaluation

The oncology nurse systematically and regularly evaluates the client's and/or family's responses to interventions to determine progress toward the achievement of expected outcomes. Relevant data are collected and actual findings are compared with expected findings. Nursing diagnoses, outcomes, and plans of care are reviewed and revised as necessary.

BIBLIOGRAPHY

Berek, J.S., & Hacker, N.F. (1994). *Practical Gynecologic Oncology* (2nd ed.). Baltimore: Williams & Wilkins.

Broadwell, D.C., & Jackson, B.S. (eds.). (1982). *Principles of Ostomy Care.* St. Louis: C.V. Mosby Co.

DeVita, V.T., Jr., Hellman, S., & Rosenberg, S.A. (eds.). (1993). *Cancer: Principles and Practice of Oncology* (4th ed.). Philadelphia: J.B. Lippincott.

DiSaia, P.J., & Creasman, W.T. (1993). *Clinical Gynecologic Oncology* (4th ed.). St. Louis: Mosby-Year Book.

Hawkins, C., & Miaskowski, C. (1996). Testicular cancer: A review. *Oncol Nurs Forum 23,* 1203–1211.

Ibbotson, T., & Wyke, S. (1995). A review of cervical cancer and cervical screening: Implications for nursing practice. *J Adv Nurs 22,* 745–752.

Lovejoy, N.C. (1994). Precancerous and cancerous cervical lesions: The multicultural "male" risk factor. *Oncol Nurs Forum 21,* 497–504.

McCorkle, R., Grant, M., Frank-Stromborg, M., & Baird, S. (eds.). (1996). *Cancer Nursing: A Comprehensive Textbook* (2nd ed.). Philadelphia: W.B. Saunders.

NIH Consensus Development Panel on Ovarian Cancer. (1995). Ovarian cancer: Screening, treatment, and follow-up. *JAMA 273*(6)491–497.

Ozols, R. (1995). Current status of chemotherapy for ovarian cancer. *Semin Oncol 22*(5[suppl. 2]), 61–66.

Rubin, P. (ed.). (1993). *Clinical Oncology: A Multidisciplinary Approach for Physicians and Students* (7th ed.). Philadelphia: W.B. Saunders.

Wright, Jr., T.C., & Richart, R.M. (1992). Pathogenesis and diagnosis of preinvasive lesion of the lower genital tract. In W.J. Hoskins, C.A. Perez, & R.C. Young (eds.). *Principles and Practice of Gynecologic Oncology.* Philadelphia: J.B. Lippincott, pp. 509–536.

Zacharias, D.R., Gilg, C.A., & Foxall, M.J. (1994). Quality of life and coping in patients with gynecologic cancer and their spouses. *Oncol Nurs Forum 21,* 1699–1706.

Nursing Care of the Client With Skin Cancer

Alice J. Longman, RN, EdD, FAAN

Theory

I. Physiology and pathophysiology associated with skin cancers.
   A. Anatomy of the skin.
      1. Epidermis is the uppermost layer—composed of keratinocytes, flat, scale-like stratified squamous epithelial cells and sphere-shaped basal cells.
      2. Dermis, or cornium, is the underlying layer—contains collagen-producing fibroblasts, giving skin strength.
      3. Melanocytes, cells that produce melanin, are in the epidermis between the basal cells.
   B. Primary organ functions.
      1. Protects body from mechanical, thermal, and chemical injuries and from infection-causing microorganisms.
      2. Helps maintain homeostasis and temperature regulatory functions.
      3. Carries the cutaneous and autonomic nerves, produces vitamin D, and stores water and fat.
   C. Changes in function associated with skin cancers.
      1. Ultraviolet portion of the solar spectrum affects incidence of skin cancers.
      2. Aging skin.
         a. Epidermis flattens and thins with age.
         b. Melanin production decreases with changes in skin and hair color.
   D. Metastatic pattern.
      1. Basal cell carcinoma.
         a. Recurrence rates vary, depending on the size of the tumor and length of follow-up.
         b. Rarely metastasizes but has the possibility of creating extensive damage.
         c. Predisposing factors are the size of the primary tumor and the resistance of the tumor to surgery and radiotherapy.
      2. Squamous cell carcinoma.
         a. Recurrence rates vary, but most recurrences develop within 2 years of diagnosis.
         b. Metastasizes almost exclusively via lymphatics.
         c. Degree of metastasis varies according to causative factors, morphologic characteristics, and size and depth of the tumor.

3. Malignant melanoma.
    a. Most important prognostic features are the size and depth of the tumor at the time of removal.
    b. Metastasizes to regional lymph nodes and then to other distant sites.
    c. Difficult and unpredictable problem of hematogenous dissemination has not been solved.
E. Trends in epidemiology.
    1. Nonmelanoma skin cancers (basal cell and squamous cell carcinoma).
        a. Most common malignant neoplasm in the United States (US) Caucasian population.
        b. Incidence has been increasing for several decades.
        c. Estimated 900,000 new cases in 1997 in the US.
    2. Cutaneous malignant melanoma.
        a. Accounts for 3% of all skin cancers.
        b. Estimated 40,300 cases in 1997 in the US.
        c. Accounts for an estimated 7300 deaths annually.
        d. Highest rates are found in southern Arizona.
F. Characteristics of skin cancers.
    1. Nonmelanoma skin cancers (basal cell carcinoma and squamous cell carcinoma) (Table 31–1).
        a. Nodular basal cell carcinoma.
            (1) Bulky nodular growth caused by lack of keratinization in the epidermis.
            (2) Semitransparent surface producing a shiny, translucent, pearly hue.
            (3) Ulcerated center with elevated margins.
        b. Superficial basal cell carcinoma.
            (1) Develops in multiple sites growing peripherally across the skin surface.
            (2) Well-demarcated, erythematous, scaly patch.
            (3) Raised pearly border.
        c. Pigmented basal cell carcinoma.
            (1) Melanin in the epidermis and dermis, and in the tumor itself.
            (2) Blue, black, or brown appearance.
            (3) Contains telangiectases and has a raised pearly border.
        d. Morpheaform or sclerotic basal cell carcinoma.
            (1) Flat or depressed scar-like plaque that is pale yellow or white.
            (2) Nodularity, ulceration, and bleeding may occur.
            (3) Finger-like projections of fibroepitheliomatous strands of tumor.
        e. Squamous cell carcinoma.
            (1) Arises from the keratinizing cells of the epidermis.
            (2) Round to irregular shape with a plaque-like or nodular character.
            (3) Varies from an ulcerated infiltrating mass to an elevated, erythematous nodular mass.
            (4) Potential for metastasis to regional and distant sites.

TABLE 31–1. **Common Sites of Nonmelanoma Skin Cancers**

Type of Skin Cancer	Common Sites
Nodular basal cell carcinoma	Face, head, neck
Superficial basal cell carcinoma	Trunk, extremities
Pigmented basal cell carcinoma	Face, head, neck
Morpheaform basal cell carcinoma	Head, neck
Squamous cell carcinoma	Head, nose, border of lips, hands

    2. Malignant melanoma (Table 31–2).
      a. Major features.
        (1) Arises from melanocytes, which are cells specializing in the biosynthesis and transport of melanin.
        (2) Characterized by radial and vertical growth phases.
        (3) Precursor lesions.
          (a) Dysplastic nevi that may be familial (B-K moles) or nonfamilial (sporadic dysplastic nevi).
          (b) Congenital melanocytic nevi covering large areas of the body.
      b. Classification of malignant melanoma.
        (1) Lentigo maligna melanoma (LMN).
          (a) Found in chronically sun-exposed skin.
          (b) Large, freckle-like lesion, tan to black in color.
          (c) Raised nodule with notched border.
        (2) Superficial spreading melanoma (SSM).
          (a) Commonly arises in preexisting nevus.
          (b) Variety of colors, ranging from tan, brown, or black to a characteristic red, white, blue, and gray.
          (c) Irregular plaque, scaly, crusty, surface-notched border.
        (3) Nodular melanoma (NM).
          (a) Raised, dome-shaped, blue-black lesion.
          (b) Elevated lesion with well-demarcated borders.
          (c) Rapid vertical growth phase.
        (4) Acral-lentiginous melanoma (ALM).
          (a) Flat and irregular in shape.
          (b) Variegated colors in shades of tan, blue, and black.
          (c) Smooth or ulcerated lesion that may be raised or flat.
      c. Features of early malignant melanoma (Table 31–3).
        (1) Asymmetry.
        (2) Border irregularity.
        (3) Color variegation.
        (4) Diameter greater than 6 mm.
II. Principles of medical management.
    A. Diagnostic procedures.
      1. General procedures.
        a. Nonmelanoma skin cancers.
          (1) Electrosurgery and histology examination with 0.5- to 1-cm margins are recommended if the lesion is small.
          (2) Incisional biopsy, including 1-cm margin, is justified for larger lesions.
        b. Malignant melanoma.
          (1) Most important characteristic is the vertical depth of melanotic penetration through the skin.

TABLE 31–2. **Common Sites of Malignant Melanoma**

Type of Melanoma	Common Sites
Lentigo maligna melanoma	Face, neck, trunk, dorsum of hands
Superficial spreading melanoma	Backs of men; legs of women
Nodular melanoma	Trunk, head, neck
Acral-lentiginous melanoma	Palms of hands, soles of feet, nail beds, mucous membranes

TABLE 31–3. **Danger Signs
of Malignant Melanoma**

Change in color

Change in size

Change in shape

Change in elevation

Change in surface

Change in surrounding skin

Change in sensation

Change in consistency

From Friedman, R.J., Rigel, D.D., Silverman, M.K., et al. (1991). Malignant melanoma in the 1990s: The continued importance of early detection and the role of physician examination and self-examination of the skin. *CA Cancer J Clin 41,* 210.

    (2) Refinement of classification relates the prognosis of melanoma to the actual measured depth or thickness of invasion.

  2. Specific procedures.

    a. Accurate histologic diagnosis.

      (1) Excisional biopsy, yielding a specimen with a few millimeters of normal tissue.

      (2) Step sections of biopsy specimen at 3 mm or closer.

    b. Microstaging describes the level of invasion of malignant melanoma and maximal tumor thickness.

B. Staging methods and procedures—parameters assessing the depth of invasion of malignant melanoma (Table 31–4).

  1. Anatomic level of invasion of Clark grading level (five histologic levels).

  2. Maximal vertical tumor thickness or Breslow measurement (five measures in millimeters).

  3. New staging system for melanoma (American Joint Committee on Cancer).

TABLE 31–4. **New Staging System for Melanoma**

Stage	Criteria
IA	Localized melanoma <0.75 mm or level II* (T1N0M0)
IB	Localized melanoma 0.76–1.5 mm or level III* (T2N0M0)
IIA	Localized melanoma 1.5–4 mm or level IV* (T3N0M0)
IIB	Localized melanoma >4 mm or level V* (T4N0M0)
III	Limited nodal metastases involving only one regional lymph node basin, or less than 5 in-transit metastases but without nodal metastases (AnyTN1M0)
IV	Advanced regional metastases (AnyTN2M0) or any patient with distant metastases (AnyT, anyN, M1 or M2)

*When the thickness and level of invasion criteria do not coincide within a T classification, thickness should take precedence.

Adapted by the American Joint Committee on Cancer. (1992). In Balch, C.M. Cutaneous melanoma: Prognosis and treatment results worldwide. *Semin Surg Oncol 8*(6), 406.

C. Treatment strategies.
1. Nonmelanoma skin cancers—definitive treatment depends on location and size of the tumor, exact histologic type, possible extension into nearby structures, metastases, previous treatment, anticipated cosmetic results, age, and general condition of the client.
   a. Surgery.
      (1) Excision of the lesion.
      (2) Curettage and electrodesiccation for small, superficial, or recurrent lesions.
      (3) Mohs micrographic surgery—surgically removes tissue in multiple, progressively thin layers.
   b. Radiotherapy.
      (1) Recommended for lesions that are inoperable and larger than 1 cm but smaller than 10 cm.
      (2) Administered in fractional doses.
   c. Cryotherapy.
      (1) Tumor destruction by use of liquid nitrogen to freeze and thaw tumor tissue.
      (2) Lesions with well-defined margins benefit from treatment.
   d. Chemotherapy.
      (1) Topical 5-fluorouracil (5-FU) for premalignant keratosis.
      (2) For recurrent skin cancers, particularly squamous cell carcinoma no longer manageable by surgery or radiotherapy, cisplatin and doxorubicin have been used.
2. Malignant melanoma.
   a. Surgery.
      (1) Local excision, leaving a 2- to 3-cm margin if anatomically possible.
      (2) Split-thickness skin grafting may be required for cosmetic reasons.
      (3) Regional lymph node dissection may be indicated but is controversial.
      (4) Used for palliative management in relief of symptoms or solitary lesions.
   b. Radiotherapy.
      (1) Most effective when tumor volume is low.
      (2) Used for palliative management when subcutaneous, cutaneous, and nodal metastases are inaccessible for surgical removal.
   c. Chemotherapy agents with consistent activity include dacarbazine (DTIC) and the nitrosoureas (carmustine [BCNU], lomustine [CCNU], semustine [Me-CCNU], and chlorozotocin).
   d. Hormonal therapy and biotherapy.
      (1) Trials with hormonal therapy such as tamoxifen and diethylstilbestrol remain inconclusive.
      (2) Agents such as interferon, interleukin, tumor necrosis factor, monoclonal antibodies, and retinoids are being studied.
3. Special considerations.
   a. Primary melanoma of the eye.
      (1) Melanoma primarily in the iris responds well to local resection.
      (2) Ciliary body and choroidal melanoma require enucleation.
      (3) Success of treatment for metastatic disease from eye melanoma is uniformly poor.
   b. Local advanced disease.
      (1) Development of massive, local disease, frequently in the neck and in axillary or inguinal nodal areas.
      (2) Combination of radiotherapy and hyperthermia offers palliation.

Assessment

I. Pertinent personal and family history.
   A. Risk factors (basal cell and squamous cell carcinoma) (Table 31–5).
      1. Exogenous factors.
         a. Ultraviolet radiation from sunlight over a long period of time.
         b. Exposure to ionizing radiation, arsenic, or petroleum.
         c. Scars following injury.
      2. Endogenous factors.
         a. Fair or freckled complexion.
         b. Red, blond, or light brown hair.
         c. Light-colored eyes.
         d. Xeroderma pigmentosum, basal cell nevus syndrome, albinism, and epidermodysplasia verruciformis.
      3. Premalignant states or lesions.
         a. Actinic, or senile, keratoses.
         b. Seborrheic keratoses.
         c. Bowen's disease.
   B. Risk factors (malignant melanoma) (see Table 31–5).
      1. Exogenous factors.
         a. Ultraviolet radiation from sunlight.
         b. Poor tolerance of ultraviolet radiation from sunlight.
         c. Intense, intermittent exposure to sunlight.
      2. Endogenous factors.
         a. Atypical moles (dysplastic nevi).
         b. Familial atypical mole and melanoma syndrome (FAM-M).
   C. Pertinent history.
      1. Skin exposure to sunlight.
         a. Time of day during exposure.
         b. Geographical area of residences or recreation.
         c. Altitude or overcast weather conditions.
         d. Time of year exposed to the sun.
         e. Length of exposures.
      2. Skin type (Table 31–6).
         a. Pigmentation or erythema type.
         b. Genetic history.

TABLE 31–5. **Major Risk Factors for Skin Cancers**

Risk Factor	Skin Cancer Risk
Personal factors	Excessive exposure to sunlight Easily burned Increasing age Premalignant states
Lifestyle	Outdoor work Outdoor recreational activities Chronic exposure to chemical agents
Drugs	Treatment for psoriasis (psoralen ultraviolet A [PUVA])
Immunologic factor	Organ transplant recipients

TABLE 31–6. **Skin Types and Skin Reactions**

Skin Type	Skin Reactions
1	Burns easily and severely; tans little or not at all
2	Burns easily and severely; tans minimally or lightly
3	Burns moderately; tans approximately average
4	Burns minimally; tans easily
5	Burns rarely; tans easily and substantially
6	Never burns; tans profusely

II. Physical examination.
  A. Skin assessment.
    1. Inspection and palpation of all accessible skin surfaces.
    2. Assessment of preexisting lesions.
    3. Inspection of the scalp and entire hairline.
    4. Inspection of the face, lips, and neck.
    5. Inspection and palpation of all surfaces of upper extremities.
    6. Inspection and palpation of the skin of the back, buttocks, and back of the legs.
  B. Signs and symptoms—changes in existing moles.
    1. Size.
    2. Shape.
    3. Color.
    4. History of itching in existing moles.
    5. History of burning in existing moles.

Nursing Diagnoses

  I. Knowledge deficit.
  II. Ineffective individual coping.
  III. Ineffective family coping: compromised.

Outcome Identification

  I. Prevention and early detection of skin cancers.
    A. Client identifies factors that place an individual at risk for skin cancers.
    B. Client describes specific health-promoting activities such as minimal skin exposure to ultraviolet radiation during specific hours of the day.
  II. Skin self-assessment.
    A. Client describes systematic assessment of skin for suspicious lesions.
    B. Client identifies resources that provide information.
  III. Warning signs of early malignant melanoma.
    A. Client describes importance of assessing for early signs of changes in nevi.
    B. Client and/or nurse conducts a family pedigree to determine family history of skin cancers.
  IV. Coping related to diagnosis of malignant melanoma.
    A. Client participates in care and ongoing decision-making.
    B. Client sets realistic goals.

V. Changes in recreational activities or work because of skin cancers.
   A. Client uses appropriate personal and community resources in managing changes.
   B. Client identifies alternative resources when present strategies do not meet needs.
VI. Changes in lifestyle as a result of the diagnosis of malignant melanoma.
   A. Client and family participate in the decision-making process pertaining to the plan of care and life activities.
   B. Client and family identify community resources that assist coping.

Planning and Implementation

I. Nonmelanoma skin cancers (basal cell carcinoma and squamous cell carcinoma).
   A. Preventive measures.
      1. Minimize exposure to sunlight between the hours of 10 AM and 3 PM.
      2. Use protective clothing such as a hat, long-sleeved shirt, and long pants during prolonged exposure to the sun.
      3. Use sunglasses that meet ultraviolet (UV) requirements.
      4. Use sunscreens (absorbers) and sunblocks (reflectors).
         a. Use commercial sunscreens with a sun protection factor (SPF) of 15 or more.
         b. Reapply sunscreen every 2 to 3 hours during prolonged exposure to the sun; reapply sunscreen after swimming.
      5. Use sunscreen with benzophenones because of photosensitivity if taking thiazides, sulfonamides, and antineoplastic agents.
      6. Avoid tanning salons and sunbeds.
      7. Keep infants out of the sun.
   B. Screening and early detection measures.
      1. Obtain a history of any recent changes in lesions.
      2. Teach systematic assessment of skin lesions for changes.
      3. Use educational resources.
         a. American Academy of Dermatology—*The Sun and Your Skin.*
         b. American Cancer Society—*Cancer of the Skin.*
         c. Skin Cancer Foundation—*Sun and Skin News.*
   C. Therapeutic measures.
      1. Prepare the client and family for surgical intervention and other treatment.
      2. Stress importance of early treatment.
   D. Rehabilitative measures.
      1. Assess impact of treatment for skin cancer.
      2. Stress importance of evaluation at regular intervals for potential recurrence.
II. Malignant melanoma.
   A. Preventive measures.
      1. Teach high-risk clients to do monthly skin self-examination.
      2. Stress importance of monthly skin self-examination.
   B. Screening and early detection.
      1. Do a family pedigree to determine family history of malignant melanoma.
      2. Use educational resources.
         a. American Academy of Dermatology—*Melanoma Skin Cancer.*
         b. National Cancer Institute—*What You Need to Know About Melanoma.*
         c. Skin Cancer Foundation—*The Melanoma Letter.*

C. Therapeutic measures.
   1. Prepare the client and family for extensive intervention and treatment.
   2. Use an open, optimistic approach in discussing feelings and attitudes about the diagnosis and treatment.
D. Rehabilitative measures.
   1. Stress importance of evaluation at regular intervals for potential recurrence.
   2. Stress importance of changes in lifestyle in relation to sun exposure for high-risk individuals and families to decrease chances of further development of malignant melanoma.

Evaluation

The oncology nurse systematically and regularly evaluates the client's and/or family's responses to interventions to determine progress toward the achievement of expected outcomes. Relevant data are collected and actual findings are compared with expected findings. Nursing diagnoses, outcomes, and plans of care are reviewed and revised as necessary.

BIBLIOGRAPHY

American Cancer Society. (1997). *Cancer Facts and Figures–1997.* Atlanta: American Cancer Society.

Bargoil, S.C., & Erdman, L.K. (1993). Safe tan: An oxymoron. *Cancer Nurs 16,* 139–144.

Entrekin, N.M., & McMillan, S.C. (1993). Nurses' knowledge, beliefs, and practices related to cancer prevention and detection. *Cancer Nurs 16,* 431–439.

Friedman, R.J., Rigel, D.D., Silverman, M.K., et al. (1991). Malignant melanoma in the 1990s: The continued importance of early detection and the role of physician examination and self-examination of the skin. *CA Cancer J Clin 41,* 201–226.

Holmstrom, H. (1992). Surgical management of primary melanoma. *Semin Surg Oncol 8,* 366–369.

Ketcham, A.S., & Balch, C.M. (1985). Classification and staging systems. In C.M. Balch, G.W. Milton, H.M. Shaw, & S.J. Soong (eds.). *Cutaneous Melanoma.* Philadelphia: J.B. Lippincott, pp. 55–62.

Loescher, L.J. (1993). Skin cancer prevention and screening update. *Semin Oncol Nurs 9,* 184–187.

Loescher, L.J., & Meyskens, F.L. (1991). Chemoprevention of human skin cancer. *Semin Oncol Nurs 7,* 45–52.

Longman, A. (1992). Skin cancer. In J.C. Clark & R.F. McGee (eds.). *Core Curriculum for Oncology Nursing* (2nd ed.). Philadelphia: W.B. Saunders, pp. 488–498.

Longman, A.J. (1996). Malignant melanoma. In M. Liebman & D. Camp-Sorrell (eds.). *Multimodal Therapy in Oncology Nursing.* St. Louis: Mosby-Year Book, pp. 271–280.

Longman, A.J. (1996). Skin cancers. In R. McCorkle, M. Grant, M. Frank-Stromborg, & S.B. Baird (eds.). *Cancer Nursing: A Comprehensive Textbook* (2nd ed.). Philadelphia: W.B. Saunders, pp. 860–869.

Marks, R. (1996). Prevention and control of melanoma: The public health approach. *CA Cancer J Clin 46,* 199–216.

Olsen, S.J., & Frank-Stromborg, M. (1993). Cancer prevention and early detection in ethnically diverse populations. *Semin Oncol Nurs 9,* 198–209.

Parker, S.L., Tong, T., Bolden, S., & Wingo, P.A. (1996). Cancer statistics, 1996. *CA Cancer J Clin 46,* 5–27.

Tokar, I.P., Fraser, M.C., & Bale, S.J. (1992). Genodermatoses with profound malignant potential. *Semin Oncol Nurs 8,* 272–280.

Urist, M.M. (1996). Surgical management of primary cutaneous melanoma. *CA Cancer J Clin 46,* 217–224.

Vargo, N.L. (1991). Basal and squamous cell carcinoma: An overview. *Semin Oncol Nurs 7,* 13–25.

Nursing Care of the Client With Cancer of the Neurologic System

Marva Bohen, RN, MS

BRAIN TUMORS

Theory

I. Physiology and pathophysiology associated with brain tumors.
  A. Anatomy.
    1. Primary structures (Figs. 32–1 and 32–2).
      a. Cerebrum—two hemispheres consisting of pairs of lobes: frontal, temporal, parietal, occipital.
      b. Thalamus and hypothalamus located at the base of the cerebrum.
      c. Cerebellum—located in the posterior fossa at the back of the head below the occipital lobes.
      d. Brainstem—located at the base of the brain, and the top of the spinal cord; consists of midbrain, pons, and medulla oblongata.
    2. Critical adjacent structures.
      a. Meninges—membranes that cover brain and spinal cord; outermost layer is the dura, a thick, whitish, inelastic covering.
      b. Ventricles—four connected cavities in the brain through which cerebrospinal fluid (CSF) flows (Fig. 32–3).
        (1) CSF is a clear, colorless, odorless fluid that bathes the brain and spinal cord within the dural covering.
        (2) Blockage of CSF flow due to tumor growth can cause hydrocephalus.
      c. Cerebral blood vessels.
        (1) Two vertebral arteries and two internal carotid arteries supply blood to the brain.
        (2) Circle of Willis connects the anterior and posterior arteries to provide alternative routes if blood flow to a single vessel is blocked.
        (3) Venous drainage is accomplished via dural sinuses, vascular channels between the two layers of the dura.
      d. Blood-brain barrier.
        (1) Tighter junctions between the cells of the brain capillaries that selectively allow substances to cross neuronal membranes.
        (2) Movement across the barrier is dependent on particle size, lipid solubility, chemical dissociation, and protein-binding potential of the substance.

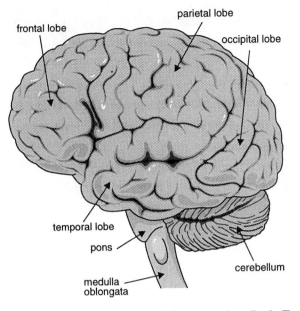

Figure 32–1. Lobes of the cerebral hemispheres. (From American Brain Tumor Association [1996]. *A Primer of Brain Tumors* [6th ed.]. Chicago: American Brain Tumor Association, p. 5.)

    e. Skull.
      (1) Normally acts as a protective framework.
      (2) With malignant tumors, its rigidity forces an increase in intracranial pressure as the tumor grows and cerebral edema increases.
    f. Cranial nerves.
      (1) Twelve pairs—10 arise from the brainstem and two arise from the cerebrum.
      (2) Peripheral nerves of the brain.
      (3) Tumors near the brainstem produce cranial nerve deficits.
  3. The most common primary malignant tumors tend to arise from support (glial) cells in the brain.
    a. Astrocytes—connective tissue cells.
    b. Oligodendrocytes—cells that produce myelin.
    c. Ependyma—lining of the ventricles.
  4. Some tumors, more common in children, arise from primitive neuroectodermal cells. These are called primitive neuroectodermal cell tumors (PNETs).
    a. Medulloblastomas.
    b. Ependymoblastomas.
    c. Pinealblastomas.
  5. All of these tumors occur within the structures of the brain.
B. Functions of the brain (Fig. 32–4).
  1. Frontal lobes.
    a. Personality.
    b. Intellect.
    c. Judgment.
    d. Abstract thinking.
    e. Mood and affect.

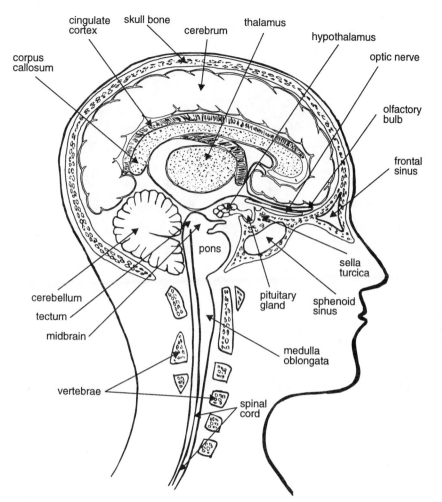

Figure 32–2. Cross-section of the brain. (From American Brain Tumor Association [1996]. *A Primer of Brain Tumors* [6th ed.]. Chicago: American Brain Tumor Association, p. 8.)

    f. Memory.

    g. Speech (in the left frontal lobe for most right-handed people).

  2. Motor strip—at the conjunction of the frontal lobe with the parietal lobe.

    a. Right motor strip area controls motor function on the left side.

    b. Left motor strip area controls motor function on the right side.

  3. Parietal lobes—sensory input.

    a. Pain.

    b. Temperature.

    c. Pinprick.

    d. Light touch.

    e. Proprioception.

    f. Two-point discrimination.

    g. Double simultaneous discrimination.

    h. Stereognosis.

    i. Graphesthesia.

  4. Occipital lobes.

    a. Sight.

    b. Visual identification of objects.

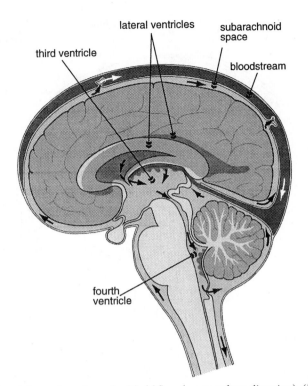

Figure 32–3. Ventricles and cerebrospinal fluid flow (*arrows show direction*). (From American Brain Tumor Association [1996]. *A Primer of Brain Tumors* [6th ed.]. Chicago: American Brain Tumor Association, p. 17.)

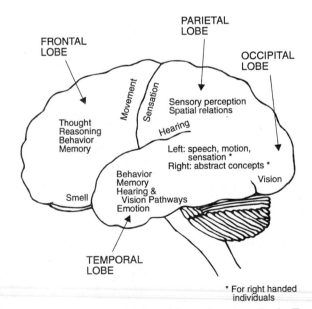

Figure 32–4. Functions of the cerebral lobes. (From American Brain Tumor Association [1996]. *A Primer of Brain Tumors* [6th ed.]. Chicago: American Brain Tumor Association, p. 18.)

  5. Temporal lobes.
     a. Hearing.
     b. Memory.
     c. Receptive speech.
  6. Cerebellum.
     a. Coordination.
     b. Balance.
  7. Thalamus.
     a. Monitors sensory input.
     b. Acts as a relay station for sensory information.
  8. Hypothalamus controls:
     a. Water balance.
     b. Sleep.
     c. Temperature.
     d. Appetite.
     e. Blood pressure.
     f. Coordinates overall patterns of activity.
  9. Brainstem (pons, midbrain, medulla) controls:
     a. Blood pressure.
     b. Heartbeat.
     c. Respirations.
C. Changes associated with cancer.
  1. Direct injury to brain tissue.
     a. Focal neurologic deficits specific to tumor location (see list of functions).
     b. Abnormal firing of neurons resulting in seizure activity.
  2. Cerebral edema.
     a. Compression of normal tissues from swelling around the tumor.
     b. Symptoms are more diffuse than focal.
        (1) Increased sleepiness.
        (2) Headaches, usually unilateral and worse in the morning.
        (3) Confusion.
        (4) Herniation.
            (a) Decreased level of consciousness.
            (b) Pupillary abnormalities or other cranial nerve dysfunctions.
            (c) Decorticate or decerebrate posturing.
            (d) Coma.
            (e) Irregular breathing.
            (f) Death.
  3. Hydrocephalus—resulting from blockage of CSF pathways due to tumor growth and/or edema. Symptoms include:
     a. Headache.
     b. Loss of balance.
     c. Memory loss.
     d. Confusion.
     e. Urinary incontinence.
  4. Increased intracranial pressure (ICP) related to tumor growth, edema, or hydrocephalus. See earlier descriptions for symptoms.
D. Histology.
  1. Astrocytomas—most common brain tumors.
     a. Grade I: pilocytic astrocytoma. Usually found in children. Also referred to as juvenile pilocytic astrocytoma (JPA).

  b. Grade II: astrocytoma—low-grade tumors with little evidence of malignant behavior.
  c. Grade III: anaplastic astrocytoma—tumors that exhibit nuclear pleomorphism, mitosis, or increased cellularity, which indicate a tendency for rapid growth.
  d. Grade IV: glioblastoma multiforme—a tumor with all the features of rapid growth plus necrosis. This is the most malignant of brain tumors and also the most common, accounting for about 30% of all brain tumors.
2. Oligodendrogliomas: comprise about 5% of all brain tumors.
  a. Grades I and II are called oligodendrogliomas and are quite indolent.
  b. Grades III and IV are called anaplastic oligodendrogliomas and feature the more aggressive features of a malignant tumor.
3. Medulloblastomas.
  a. Occur primarily in children (70%).
  b. Start in the cerebellum.
  c. Metastasize to other areas of the central nervous system (CNS) through the CSF.
4. Ependymomas.
  a. Arise from the lining of the ventricles.
  b. May be malignant or benign, but are usually benign.
  c. Account for 10% of childhood brain tumors, but only 5% of adult brain tumors.
5. Primary CNS lymphoma.
  a. Until 1974, only comprised about 1% of all brain tumors. Since then, a three-fold increase has been noted.
  b. More likely to occur in immunosuppressed individuals (transplant recipients and those who test human immunodeficiency virus [HIV]-positive).
  c. Brain has no lymph tissue. Mechanism for development of central nervous system lymphomas is not understood.
6. Mixed tumors.
  a. More than one cell type.
  b. Usually astrocytes and oligodendrocytes.
  c. May be astrocytes and ependymal cells.
7. Tumors of neuronal origin are quite rare and tend to be benign.
E. Presentation.
  1. Seizure (30%).
  2. Headache.
    a. Usually unilateral.
    b. Usually more severe when the person first awakens.
  3. Hemiparesis.
  4. Aphasias.
  5. Visual field cuts.
  6. Confusion.
F. Metastatic patterns.
  1. Recurrence is usually restricted to the CNS.
  2. Distant metastases rarely occur; when present, they occur in lung or bone.
G. Epidemiology.
  1. Approximately 17,500 new primary brain tumors every year in the United States (US).

2. Brain tumor is the most common solid tumor in children.
3. Incidence is increasing for unknown reasons. The following have been postulated:
   a. Better diagnostic procedures.
   b. Lengthening of the lifespan allows for a greater chance to develop brain tumors.
   c. Unknown environmental factors.
   d. Men are more likely than women to develop a malignant brain tumor (ratio of 1.5 : 1).

II. Principles of medical management.
   A. Screening and diagnostic procedures.
      1. Currently no screening tests to identify clients with brain tumors.
      2. Computerized tomography (CT).
         a. Often used as initial study for clients suspected of having a brain tumor.
         b. Less expensive than magnetic resonance imaging (MRI).
         c. Malignant tumors are best visualized with contrast enhanced scans.
      3. MRI.
         a. Provides the best imaging of brain tumors.
            (1) Contrast is used to enhance the area of tumor.
            (2) Shows the tumor on different planes: sagittal, axial, coronal.
            (3) Easier for the surgeon to identify critical structures.
            (4) Can see patterns of cerebral edema more clearly.
         b. Normally used:
            (1) Preoperatively.
            (2) Postoperatively within 24 hours to assess residual tumor volume. Postoperative scan provides the baseline value to measure treatment effect.
            (3) For follow-up examination about every 3 months while undergoing treatment.
      4. Stereotactic biopsy.
         a. Done when tumor cannot be surgically resected.
         b. Requires a special frame that can only be used on the head (Fig. 32–5).
         c. Provides a small sample of tissue with which to make a diagnosis.

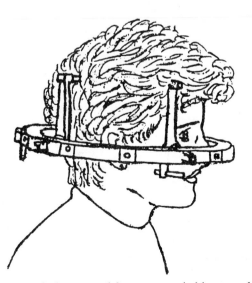

Figure 32–5. Stereotactic frame used for stereotactic biopsy and radiosurgery.

d. Sampling error is possible, so that the tumor may be read out as less malignant than it actually is.

5. Surgical resection.

    a. Subtotal—removal of a portion of the tumor for diagnostic purposes and to reduce mass effect.

    b. Gross total—removal of all visible tumor.

        (1) Diagnostic tissue sample.

        (2) Reduction of mass effect.

        (3) Theoretically improves response to treatment (smaller tumor burden).

        (4) Done only when surgery will not create a worsening of neurologic deficits.

B. Staging methods.

1. Size of tumor, location, and degree of malignancy are the best indicators of prognosis.

2. TNM classification (Table 32–1).

    a. TNM classification is limited because two of three indicators are usually not applicable to brain tumors.

    b. Tumor size: applicable.

    c. Node involvement: does not apply to brain tumors.

    d. Metastases outside the brain and spinal cord are extremely rare.

C. Standard therapies.

1. Surgery: See descriptions in diagnostic section later.

    a. Clients may receive surgery two or three times to:

        (1) Decrease tumor burden.

        (2) Differentiate tumor from treatment effects.

        (3) Restage tumor—lower-grade tumors may become more malignant over time.

    b. A biopsy may be indicated to restage tumor if a resection would:

        (1) Increase or create neurologic deficit.

        (2) Be risky for the client because of other health concerns.

2. Radiotherapy—currently considered the most effective therapy for most malignant brain tumors.

    a. Standard (conventional) radiation.

        (1) Given over 6 to 7 weeks.

        (2) Total dose ranges from 5500 to 6200 cGy—varies depending on tumor type.

        (3) Higher dose can result in severe long-term side effects (dementia, cognitive problems, radiation necrosis).

        (4) Radiate the tumor plus a 2- to 3-cm margin.

        (5) Whole-brain radiation is seldom used except for metastatic tumors.

    b. Stereotactic radiosurgery.

        (1) Uses the same type of head frame used for stereotactic biopsy (see Fig. 32–5).

        (2) The frame allows the radiation to be focused on the tumor.

        (3) Radiation is delivered in several arcs so that the tumor receives the full dose, but normal tissues are spared.

        (4) The dose is calculated depending on the tumor type, size of tumor, proximity to critical structures (e.g., the optic nerve) that can be easily damaged by high-dose radiation.

        (5) The dose is delivered in a single high-dose fraction.

        (6) Usually used in conjunction with or following standard radiation.

    c. Fractionated stereotactic radiotherapy.

        (1) Uses a relocatable stereotactic frame so that several focused fractions can be delivered over several days (Fig. 32–6).

TABLE 32–1. **TNM Classification of Brain Tumors**

Primary Tumor (T)

TX	Primary tumor cannot be assessed
T0	No evidence of primary tumor

Supratentorial Tumor

T1	Tumor 5 cm or less in greatest dimension; limited to one side
T2	Tumor more than 5 cm in greatest dimension; limited to one side
T3	Tumor invades or encroaches on the ventricular system
T4	Tumor crosses the midline, invades the opposite hemisphere, or invades infratentorially

Infratentorial Tumor

T1	Tumor 3 cm or less in greatest dimension; limited to one side
T2	Tumor more than 3 cm in greatest dimension; limited to one side
T3	Tumor invades or encroaches on the ventricular system
T4	Tumor crosses the midline, invades the opposite hemisphere, or invades supratentorially

Regional Lymph Nodes (N)

This category does not apply to this site.

Distant Metastasis (M)

MX	Presence of distant metastasis cannot be assessed
M0	No distant metastasis
M1	Distant metastasis

Histopathological Grade (G)

GX	Grade cannot be assessed
G1	Well differentiated
G2	Moderately well differentiated
G3	Poorly differentiated
G4	Undifferentiated

Stage Grouping

Stage IA	G1	T1	M0
Stage IB	G1	T2	M0
	G1	T3	M0
Stage IIA	G2	T1	M0
Stage IIB	G2	T2	M0
	G2	T3	M0
Stage IIIA	G3	T1	M0
Stage IIIB	G3	T2	M0
	G3	T3	M0
Stage IV	G1, G2, G3	T4	M0
	G4	Any T	M0
	Any G	Any T	M1

From Beahrs, O.H., Henson, D.E., Hutter, R., et al. (1992). *Manual for Staging of Cancer* (ed. 4). Philadelphia: J.B. Lippincott Co., pp. 247–252.

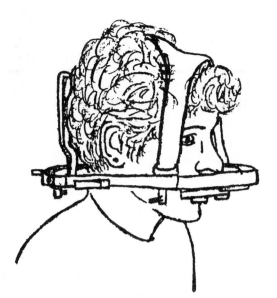

Figure 32–6. Relocatable stereotactic frame used for fractionated stereotactic radiotherapy.

   (2) Provides doses equivalent to the amount delivered by conventional radiation.
   (3) Spares normal tissue—reduction in side effects (hair loss, dementia, cognitive dysfunction).
   (4) May replace or augment conventional radiotherapy.
   d. Brachytherapy.
   (1) Implantation of radioactive seeds into the tumor bed.
   (2) Seeds are left in place for 3 to 4 days.
   (3) Approximately 35% of patients who receive brachytherapy develop severe radiation side effects.
   (4) Rarely used because of side effects.
3. Chemotherapy.
   a. Usually reserved as an adjunct to radiation.
   b. Median survival increases only by 1 to 2 months with addition of standard chemotherapy for treatment of malignant astrocytomas.
   c. Number of long-term survivors increases with the use of chemotherapy in high-grade tumors.
   d. Anaplastic oligodendrogliomas are more sensitive to chemotherapy than other tumors. Complete responses may occur.
   e. Commonly used drugs.
   (1) Carmustine (BCNU).
      (a) Used since the 1970s for brain tumors.
      (b) Lipid solubility allows it to pass the blood-brain barrier.
   (2) PCV3—regimen using three drugs: procarbazine, lomustine (CCNU), and vincristine.
      (a) The regimen of choice for treating anaplastic oligodendrogliomas.
      (b) Also used as the standard regimen for treating other malignant gliomas by some cancer treatment centers.
4. Investigational modalities.
   a. Blood-brain barrier disruption.
   (1) Requires intra-arterial infusion of mannitol or RMP-7 to open the barrier, then infusion of chemotherapy.

          (2) Initial results very promising for treatment of CNS lymphoma in clients who are not HIV-positive.

          (3) Appears to double median survival time for clients with malignant gliomas.

    b. Bone marrow transplant/stem cell rescue.

          (1) Pediatric protocols.

          (2) Patients with recurrent anaplastic oligodendrogliomas.

    c. Gene therapy—used primarily for malignant gliomas.

          (1) Herpesvirus.

          (2) Diphtheria toxin.

    d. Immunotherapy—animal studies using a brain tumor vaccine have been completed at a few centers. Cells are taken from the client, grown in a laboratory, killed with radiation, and reinjected into the client, along with other drugs to stimulate the immune response.

  D. Trends in survival.

    1. Dependent on location, size, and accessibility of tumor.

    2. Use of multimodality therapy has increased the number of long-term survivors.

    3. Chemotherapy has been useful particularly with:

      a. Anaplastic oligodendroglioma—median survival has doubled from 2 years to about 4 years using PCV3 chemotherapy.

      b. Primary CNS lymphoma median survival.

          (1) No treatment—1 to 3 months.

          (2) Surgery—not indicated.

          (3) Radiation therapy—12 to 18 months.

          (4) Chemotherapy—varies with regimen; best is 44.5 months using blood-brain barrier disruption.

Assessment

  I. Pertinent personal and family history.

    A. Risk factors are not known.

    B. Exposure to some environmental factors has been explored but not confirmed, for example:

      1. Vinyl chloride.

      2. Radiation.

      3. Petrochemical products.

      4. Inks and solvents.

      5. Hair dyes.

      6. Cellular telephones.

      7. High-power lines.

    C. Most common solid tumor of childhood.

    D. Incidence slightly higher in males.

    E. Although no hereditary pattern has been established for malignant tumors, they are more likely to occur in people with:

      1. Neurofibromatosis.

      2. Tuberous sclerosis.

      3. von Hippel-Lindau disease.

    F. Immunocompromised patients are at higher risk for primary CNS lymphoma.

 II. Pertinent medical history.

    A. Sudden onset of seizure activity.

    B. Headaches.

      1. Recent onset or more severe than usual.

      2. Usually unilateral.
      3. May be worse in the morning or awaken the client.
    C. Describes focal neurologic deficits.
    D. Family reports change in personality.
    E. Family reports episodes of memory loss or confusion.
  III. Physical examination.
    A. Neurologic examination.
    B. Look for focal neurologic deficit.
  IV. Diagnostic evaluation.
    A. CT with and without contrast medium, or
    B. MRI with and without contrast medium.

Nursing Diagnoses

    I. Knowledge deficit.
   II. Decreased intracranial adaptive capacity.
  III. Risk for activity intolerance.
  IV. Body image disturbance.
   V. Risk for caregiver role strain.
  VI. Altered family processes.
 VII. Risk for injury.
VIII. Sexual dysfunction.

Outcome Identification

    I. Client identifies the tumor type.
   II. Client and caregivers describe treatment options.
  III. Client and caregivers identify resources for support and learning, such as:
    A. Members of the health care team.
    B. Brain tumor support groups.
    C. Other cancer support groups.
    D. American Brain Tumor Association.
    E. American Cancer Society.
    F. National Brain Tumor Foundation.
  IV. Client's caregivers recognize signs and symptoms of increased intracranial pressure and seek assistance.
   V. Client and/or caregivers identify medications, know the correct doses, and describe possible side effects.
  VI. Client and caregivers identify reasons for decreased activity tolerance.
    A. Radiation.
    B. Chemotherapy.
    C. Cerebral edema.
    D. Hemiparesis.
    E. Steroid myopathy (due to dexamethasone used to control cerebral edema).
    F. Poor balance.
 VII. Client and caregivers identify strategies to conserve energy and increase activity tolerance.
    A. Frequent rest periods.
    B. Gradual increase to normal activities.
    C. Physical therapy to improve muscular tone and develop balance-compensation techniques.

VIII. Client identifies methods for coping with body image disturbances.
   A. Hair loss from radiation, which will most likely be permanent.
      1. Wigs.
      2. Hats or scarves.
      3. Shaving the head.
   B. Neurologic deficits.
      1. Use of appliances and aids.
      2. Speech therapy, physical therapy (PT), occupational therapy (OT) sessions to enhance function.
   IX. Caregivers identify resources for respite and self-care.
   X. Family identifies changes in its structure and processes.
   XI. Family identifies resources to assist in coping with changes, such as:
      A. Social services.
      B. Psychologists and family counselors.
      C. Attorney to assist with estate planning and power of attorney issues if the client becomes unable to competently manage affairs.
      D. Child support group dealing with chronically ill parent, loss of parent.
   XII. If the client has seizures, the caregivers demonstrate first aid procedures for a person having seizures.
   XIII. Client and/or caregivers recognize the potential for injury when neurologic deficits interfere with balance, ambulation, driving, and ability to perform activities of daily living (ADLs).
   XIV. Client and caregivers identify resources for assisting with safety issues.
      A. Physical therapy: balance compensation, strengthening.
      B. Occupational therapy: assistive devices and safety assessments.
   XV. Client and his or her sexual partner identify issues that may affect sexual function.
      A. Radiation in which the field includes the pituitary region.
      B. Need for birth control with chemotherapy regimens.
      C. Potential for sterility with certain chemotherapy agents.
      D. Fatigue.
      E. Neurologic deficits.

Planning and Implementation

   I. Identify knowledge deficits related to brain tumor.
      A. Provide information in written and oral forms.
      B. Be available to answer questions.
      C. Provide information about other resources.
         1. American Brain Tumor Association
            2720 River Road
            Des Plaines, IL 60018-4110
            Patient Line: 1-800-886-2282
         2. National Brain Tumor Foundation
            323 Geary Street, Suite 510
            San Francisco, CA 94102
            415-296-0404
   II. Assess neurologic status for evidence of:
      A. Increasing intracranial pressure or cerebral edema.
      B. Progression of the tumor.
      C. Effectiveness of antiseizure medication.

D. Effectiveness of steroid treatment.

E. Side effects of medications.

III. Assess the client for evidence of activity intolerance.

A. Counsel the client and family on available resources.

B. Discuss methods for conserving energy.

IV. Identify resources for clients with body image disturbance.

V. Identify resources for a caregiver experiencing stress.

VI. Assess family processes.

A. Identify altered processes.

B. Provide information regarding resources and support.

VII. Assess the client for risk of injury.

A. Poor balance.

B. Seizures.

C. Poor insight or judgment.

VIII. Counsel caregivers and client when safety concerns arise.

IX. Provide information regarding possibility of sexual dysfunction.

A. Discuss effects of brain tumor and treatment.

B. Provide information specific to the individual's situation.

1. Use of birth control.

2. Possibility of sterility.

3. Banking of sperm or fertilized ova.

4. Loss of menstrual cycling in women who lose pituitary function due to radiation.

5. Alternative sexual positions.

6. Loss of libido.

Evaluation

The oncology nurse systematically and regularly evaluates the client's and/or family's responses to interventions to determine progress toward the achievement of expected outcomes. Relevant data are collected and actual findings are compared with expected findings. Nursing diagnoses, outcomes, and plans of care are reviewed and revised as necessary.

SPINAL CORD TUMORS

Theory

I. Physiology and pathophysiology associated with spinal cord tumors.

A. Anatomy.

1. The spinal cord is an extension of the brain.

a. Cord body begins at the brainstem and extends through the spinal foramina of vertebrae to the L1 to L2 vertebral level.

b. Consists of 31 pairs of spinal nerves.

2. Critical adjacent structures.

a. Vertebral column.

(1) 33 vertebrae joined by ligaments.

(2) Bony structure encasing and protecting cord.

(3) Divisions—7 cervical, 12 thoracic, 5 lumbar, 5 sacral (fused), 4 coccygeal (fused).

b. Intravertebral discs—cartilage pads separating vertebrae, allowing flexion of the cord.

c. Meninges—layers of tissue that surround the spinal cord and brain.

    d. Cerebrospinal fluid (CSF)—fluid that bathes and cushions the spinal
       cord; contained within the meninges.

    e. Vertebral blood vessels—supply from vertebral and spinal arteries.

3. Consists of same cell types as brain.

4. Malignant primary tumors tend to arise from intramedullary (within the
   spinal cord) support cells.

    a. Astrocytes.

    b. Ependymal cells. (Fig. 32–7)

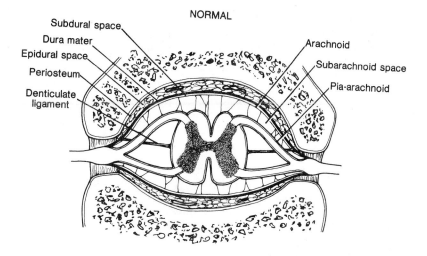

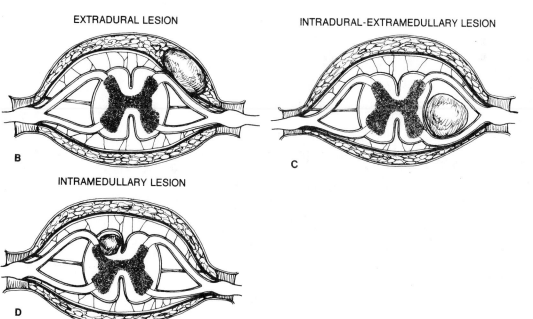

Figure 32–7. The location of intraspinal tumors. *A,* Normal anatomy. *B,* Extradural lesion
(metastases). *C,* Intradural-extramedullary lesion (neurofibroma). *D,* Intramedullary lesion
(glioma). (From Borenstein, D.G., Wiesel, S.W., & Boden, S.D. (1995). Low Back Pain:
Medical Diagnosis and Comprehensive Management (2nd ed.). Philadelphia, W.B. Saunders,
p. 412.

5. Metastatic tumors are more likely to occur outside the dura (extradural), such as in the:
    a. Lung.
    b. Breast.
    c. Prostate.
6. Benign tumors are more likely to occur inside the dura, but outside the spinal cord (extramedullary), such as:
    a. Meningiomas.
    b. Neurofibromas.
    c. Neurilemmomas.
B. Functions of the spinal cord.
    1. Motor function of the body from neck to toes.
    2. Sensory function of the body from the back of the head to the toes.
    3. Loss of function dependent on:
        a. Site of tumor.
            (1) Cervical—neck, arms and hands.
            (2) Thoracic—chest to umbilicus.
            (3) Lumbar—hips to toes.
        b. Size of tumor.
C. Changes in function with spinal tumors.
    1. Growth of tumor creates cord compression as it enlarges.
    2. Can also compress spinal nerves and occlude blood vessels.
D. Histologic types (see Theory, I.A.4–6).
E. Presentation.
    1. Pain.
        a. Along spine.
        b. Radicular.
    2. Sensory impairment.
        a. Numbness or tingling.
        b. Usually unilateral and progressive.
    3. Motor impairment.
        a. Develops in conjunction with sensory impairment.
        b. Paresis, usually unilateral.
        c. Spasticity.
        d. Bladder and bowel dysfunction.
        e. Motor impairment is a late sign and may not be reversible with surgery.
F. Metastatic patterns—primary spinal tumors tend not to metastasize distantly. They may invade dura and adjacent structures.
G. Trends in epidemiology—no trends noted.
II. Principles of medical management.
    A. Screening and diagnostic procedures.
        1. Spine films.
        2. CT—best for bony structures.
        3. MRI—best for defining soft tissues.
        4. Myelogram—aids in seeking source of spinal compression.
        5. Electromyography—detects muscular innervation dysfunctions peripherally.
    B. Staging methods.
        1. Clinical neurologic status.
        2. Degree of malignancy of tumor.

3. Invasion into adjacent structures.
4. Status of systemic disease, if tumor is metastatic.
C. Treatment strategies.
  1. Extradural tumors.
     a. High-dose corticosteroids to reduce edema (e.g., dexamethasone).
     b. Radiation, if primary tumor is known and is radiosensitive.
     c. Surgery if tumor is not radiosensitive, neurologic status is deteriorating, or tumor type is not known, and if surgery will not put the patient at risk for more severe neurologic deficit or other life-threatening complications.
  2. Intradural/extramedullary—surgical resection.
  3. Intradural/intramedullary.
     a. Surgical resection if possible.
     b. Malignant gliomas may require radiation and chemotherapy.
D. Trends in survival.
  1. Life expectancy is normal for patients with benign tumors that can be completely resected.
  2. Treatment for patients with malignant primary spinal cord tumors or metastatic tumors is palliative, and life expectancy is 1 to 2 years.

Assessment

I. Pertinent personal and family history.
   A. History of neurofibromatosis.
   B. History of lung, breast, or prostate cancer.
   C. Describes localized or radicular neck or back pain.
   D. Describes sensory changes.
      1. Numbness and tingling.
      2. Unable to differentiate hot and cold.
      3. Loss of sensation of touch and/or pain.
   E. Describes decreased motor function.
   F. Describes loss of bowel or bladder control.
II. Physical examination.
   A. Neurologic assessment.
      1. Sensation.
      2. Movement and strength.
   B. Assess abdomen for:
      1. Signs of urinary retention.
      2. Bowel sounds.
      3. Hardness and distention.
   C. Attempt to elicit pain at site along spine.

Nursing Diagnoses

I. Acute pain.
II. Altered urinary elimination.
III. Bowel incontinence.
IV. Impaired physical mobility.
V. Tactile sensory alterations.
VI. Sexual dysfunction.

Outcome Identification

I. Client identifies methods for pain control.

II. Client describes signs and symptoms of bladder dysfunction.

III. Client implements a bladder and/or bowel control program.

IV. Client lists safety hazards related to decreased sensation and mobility.

V. Client identifies resources for learning to compensate for loss of motor and sensory functions.

VI. Client has access to information about sexual issues.

Planning and Implementation

I. Pain management.

A. Develop pain control plan in conjunction with the client and family based on:

1. Degree of pain.

2. Degree of control with medications in use.

3. Available alternatives.

4. Expectation that surgery or radiation will help alleviate pain.

B. Implement the plan and assess.

II. Urinary elimination.

A. Assess the status of urinary elimination based on:

1. Urinary retention.

2. Potential for infection.

3. Urinary incontinence with skin irritation.

B. Develop a plan in conjunction with the client and family.

III. Bowel elimination.

A. Assess the status of bowel function.

B. Develop a plan in conjunction with the client and family to:

1. Provide a routine for bowel elimination.

2. Provide back-up strategies if incontinence occurs unexpectedly.

IV. Provide the client and family with information about rehabilitation for sensory and motor loss.

V. Counsel the client and family on safety hazards related to motor and sensory loss.

VI. Provide information on sexuality issues as needed.

Evaluation

The oncology nurse systematically and regularly evaluates the client's and/or family's responses to interventions to determine progress toward the achievement of expected outcomes. Relevant data are collected and actual findings are compared with expected findings. Nursing diagnoses, outcomes, and plans of care are reviewed and revised as necessary.

BIBLIOGRAPHY

Chandler, K.L., Prados, M.D., Maler, M., & Wilson, C.B. (1993). Long-term survival in patients with glioblastoma multiforme. *Neurosurgery 32*(5), 716–720.

Dahlborg, S.A., Henner, D.W., Crossen, J.R., et al. (1996). Non-AIDS primary CNS lymphoma: The first example of a durable response in a primary brain tumor using enhanced chemotherapy delivery without cognitive loss and without radiotherapy. *Cancer J Sci Am 2*(3), 1–9.

Fine, H.A., Dear, K.B.G., Loeffler, J.S., et al. (1993). Meta-analysis of radiation therapy with and without adjuvant chemotherapy for malignant glioma in adults. *Cancer 71*(8), 2585–2597.

Levin, V.C. (ed.). (1996). *Cancer in the Nervous System.* New York: Churchill Livingstone.

Segal, G. (1996). *A Primer of Brain Tumors* (6th ed.). Chicago: American Brain Tumor Association.

Wen, P.Y., & Black, P.M. (eds.). (1995). Brain tumors in adults [entire issue]. *Neurol Clin 13*(4).

Williams, P.C., Henner, D., Roman-Goldstein, S., et al. (1995). Toxicity and efficacy of carboplatin and etoposide in conjunction with disruption of the blood-brain tumor barrier in the treatment of intracranial neoplasms. *Neurosurgery 37,* 17–28.

33

Nursing Care of the Client With Head and Neck Cancer

Ryan R. Iwamoto, ARNP, MN, AOCN

Theory

I. Introduction.
   A. Head and neck cancers include cancers of the oral cavity, oropharynx, nasal cavity, paranasal sinuses, nasopharynx, larynx, hypopharynx, and salivary glands.
   B. Although the incidence of cancer occurring in this area is relatively small in number (5% of all cancers), the devastation of this disease in terms of dysfunction and body image changes calls for intensive nursing interventions to promote adaptation.
   C. Trends in epidemiology.
      1. Usually occurs in the 50- to 70-year age group.
      2. More men than women are affected by cancers of the head and neck.
      3. Risk factors for head and neck cancer are listed in Table 33–1.
      4. Incidence, staging, and treatment of cancer in this area are dependent on the specific location of the tumor.
   D. Use of prosthetic devices and surgical flaps (myocutaneous and free) has resulted in improved cosmetic effects and reduced deformities.
   E. Histology and incidence.
      1. Histology of head and neck tumors—90%, squamous cell; 10% adenocarcinoma (salivary glands), melanoma, sarcoma, or lymphoma.
      2. Majority of head and neck tumors occur in the oral cavity (48%), larynx (25%), and oropharynx (10%).
   F. Metastatic patterns.
      1. Head and neck cancer is a locally aggressive disease that spreads regionally to the lymphatics of the neck (Fig. 33–1).
      2. Most clients present with stage III or IV disease, which indicates tumor spread to the lymphatics and/or a very large invasive primary tumor.
      3. The incidence of local regional failure is as high as 60%, with clinically detected distant metastasis occurring at a rate of 20%.
      4. Autopsy studies indicate that the incidence of distant metastasis is 50%; however, 90% of these clients die with uncontrolled primary tumors or neck disease (i.e., regional disease).
      5. Most common sites of distant metastasis—lung, liver, and bone.
   G. Trends in survival rates.
      1. No appreciable increase in 5-year survival rates has been achieved over the last 30 years, but advances made since the early 1970s include more

TABLE 33–1. **Risk Factors for Head and Neck Cancers**

Personal/environmental	Tobacco use—all forms Cigarettes, cigars, pipe, smokeless tobacco Alcohol Poor oral hygiene Long-term sun exposure
Occupational	Asbestos, coal products, nickel, textiles, wood dust, organic compounds exposure; leather workers and machinists
Ethnicity	Southern Chinese population: nasopharyngeal cancers
Viruses	Epstein-Barr: nasopharyngeal cancers Herpes simplex and human papilloma viruses: oral cancers

conservative surgical techniques and reconstruction, increasing quality of life and decreasing airway, communication, and swallowing dysfunctions.

2. Five-year relative survival rate for all head and neck tumors approximates 50%.
   a. For early stage I and II cancers—40 to 95%.
   b. For stage III and IV lesions—0 to 50%.
3. Five-year survival (all stages) varies by site: oral cavity (40–70%), oropharynx (35–50%), larynx (50–80%), nasopharynx (26%), and nose and sinuses (15–40%).
4. Eliminating aggravating lifestyle factors (smoking and alcohol) decreases the chance of developing recurrent disease.

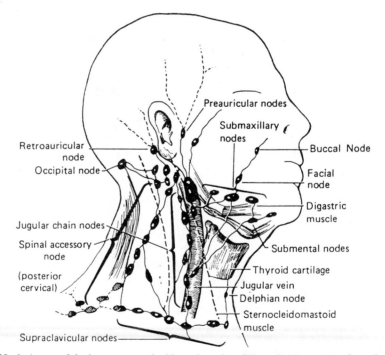

Figure 33–1. Areas of drainage to cervical lymph nodes. (From Schleper, J.R. [1989]. Prevention, detection, and diagnosis of head and neck cancers. *Semin Oncol Nurs* 5[3], 146. Drawing by Greg Patterson.)

II. Anatomy of the head and neck (Fig. 33–2).
    A. Oral cavity—extends from the lips to the hard palate above and the circum-vallate papillae below; structures include lips, buccal mucosa, floor of mouth, upper and lower alveoli, retromolar trigone, hard palate, and anterior two thirds of the tongue.
    B. Oropharynx—extends from the circumvallate papillae below and hard palate above to the level of the hyoid bone; structures include the base of tongue (posterior one third), soft palate, tonsils, and posterior pharyngeal wall.
    C. Nasal cavity and paranasal sinuses—include nasal vestibule; paired maxillary, ethmoid, and frontal sinuses, and a single sphenoid sinus.
    D. Nasopharynx—located below the base of skull and behind the nasal cavity; continuous with the posterior pharyngeal wall.
    E. Larynx—extends from the epiglottis to the cricoid cartilage; protected by the thyroid cartilage, which encases it; subdivided into three anatomic areas.
       1. Supraglottis—located below the base of tongue, extending to but not including the true vocal cord; structures include epiglottis, aryepiglottic folds, arytenoid cartilages, and false vocal cords.
       2. Glottis—area of the true vocal cord.
       3. Subglottis—area below the true vocal cord, extending to the cricoid cartilage.

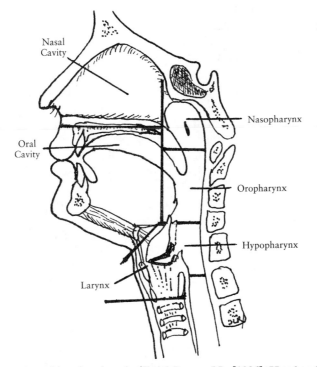

Figure 33–2. Anatomy of head and neck. (From Reese, J.L. [1996]. Head and neck cancers. In R. McCorkle, M. Grant, M. Frank-Stromborg, & S.B. Baird (Eds.), *Cancer Nursing: A Comprehensive Textbook* [2nd ed.]. Philadelphia: W.B. Saunders, p. 775.)

F. Hypopharynx—extends from the hyoid bone to the lower border of the cricoid cartilage; structures include pyriform sinuses, postcricoid region, and the lower posterior pharyngeal wall.

G. Critical adjacent structures.

1. Regional lymph nodes of the neck drain the anatomic structures of the head and neck; area includes submental submaxillary, upper and lower jugular, posterior triangle (spinal accessory), and preauricular nodes (see Fig. 33–1).

2. Head and neck structures are contiguous with the lower aerodigestive tract—trachea, lungs, and esophagus.

3. The nasopharynx and paranasal sinuses are in close approximation to the brain.

III. Primary functions of the head and neck.

A. Respiration—the upper respiratory tract serves as the passageway for transporting air into the lungs by the following process:

1. The diaphragm descends, increasing the intrathoracic pressure.

2. Negative pressure results in air entering the mouth and nose where it is warmed, filtered, and humidified.

3. Air enters the upper air passageways of the pharynx, larynx, and trachea, then enters the lung.

4. The olfactory membrane lies along the superior part of each nostril as well as along the septum and superior turbinates. The olfactory cells within the membrane serve as receptors for the sense of smell.

B. Speech—is formed from sound waves created as air is expelled from the lungs, passes through the vocal cords. Speech is mechanically perfected through the processes of:

1. Phonation—achieved by the larynx.

2. Articulation—achieved by the lips, tongue, and soft palate.

3. Resonation—resonators (pharynx, mouth, nose, and nasal sinuses) create the tone and quality of speech.

C. Swallowing—complex process wherein 26 muscles and six cranial nerves orchestrate the transport of food from the mouth to the stomach in four phases of swallowing.

1. Oral preparatory—bolus of food is prepared for initiating the swallow by mastication of the food into small particles and secretion of saliva into the oral cavity to lubricate the bolus.

a. Taste receptors are located on the tongue, soft palate, glossopalatine arch, and posterior wall of the pharynx.

2. Oral—bolus is propelled into the pharynx by the front-to-back movement of the tongue.

3. Pharyngeal—bolus moves through the pharynx and is propelled toward the esophagus; the vocal cords close and the larynx moves upward and forward, preventing aspiration.

4. Esophageal—bolus moves through the esophagus and enters the stomach.

IV. Changes in function associated with cancers of the head and neck.

A. Respiration.

1. Head and neck cancer affects primarily the structures of the upper airway, which serve to transport warmed, filtered, and humidified air into the lungs.

2. Disease and treatment in this area may result in bypassing the natural

air-conditioning function of the upper air passageways, causing a cooling, drying effect on the trachea and lungs that can lead to infection.

3. The sense of smell may be affected with the inability to sniff due to alterations in the upper airway.

B. Speech.

1. Removing part or all of the *larynx* results in loss of the vibrating component for speech; thus sound waves cannot be produced (total laryngectomy) or are diminished (partial).

2. Surgery to the *mouth, tongue,* or *palate* causes changes in the person's ability to articulate clear, understandable speech.

3. Cancer or treatment of the *nose* or *sinuses* influences the tone and quality of the speech.

C. Swallowing.

1. S*upraglottic laryngectomy* affects the pharyngeal phase of swallowing, resulting in decreased protection of the glottis; aspiration is a danger until swallowing techniques are learned.

2. Extensive resections of structures in the *oral cavity* and *oropharynx* requiring flap reconstruction affect the oral preparatory and oral phase of swallowing and may result in drooling of saliva, decreased mastication, aspiration, pooling of food and fluids; radiation therapy to this area causes decreased saliva production (xerostomia), with loss of lubrication of the food bolus and taste changes.

V. Principles of medical management.

A. Screening and diagnostic procedures.

1. No definitive screening examination or test is recommended for early detection; however, a thorough oral examination should be included in a cancer-related checkup conducted every 3 years for those 20 to 40 years of age and every year for those 40 years of age and older.

2. Clients with head and neck cancer are at an increased risk for synchronous primary tumors as a result of prolonged exposure of the mucosal surface to carcinogens; therefore, the initial workup includes evaluation to rule out multiple primary tumors.

3. Evaluation of suspected head and neck tumors includes a thorough history and examination of all structures of the upper aerodigestive tract.

   a. History of risk factors (see Table 33–1).

   b. Signs and symptoms of disease (Table 33–2).

   c. Physical examination.

      (1) Visualization.

      (2) Mirror examination of the pharynx and larynx.

      (3) Palpation via a bimanual examination to assess the oral cavity and upper neck.

4. Radiologic studies.

   a. Computed tomographic (CT) scan—to assist in determining the extent of the primary tumor and in identifying metastasis to the cervical lymph nodes.

   b. Chest x-ray examination—to identify disease in the lung, a second primary tumor, or distant metastasis.

   c. Panorex—panoramic views to evaluate mandibular invasion from oral cavity and oropharyngeal lesions (Table 33–3).

   d. Magnetic resonance imaging (MRI) scan—superior to the CT scan in staging nasopharyngeal primaries.

TABLE 33–2. **Signs and Symptoms of Head and Neck Cancers**

Early	**Late**
Oral Cavity and Oropharynx	
Leukoplakia	Dysphagia
Erythroplakia	Aspiration (oropharyngeal)
Pain or ulcer that fails to heal	Speech difficulties
Painless, persistent mass	Trismus (lockjaw)
Difficulty with dentures	Referred otalgia (ear pain)
	Weight loss
	Cervical adenopathy
Larynx and Hypopharynx	
Persistent hoarseness	Pain
Throat pain	Dysphagia
	Dyspnea and stridor
	Hemoptysis
	Referred otalgia (supraglottic)
	Aspiration (supraglottic)
	Cervical adenopathy
Nose and Paranasal Sinuses	
Nasal stuffiness	Bloody nasal discharge
Headache	Pain in teeth
	Asymmetry, pain, and/or numbness over involved sinus
	Trismus
	Proptosis (eyes protrude)
	Diplopia (cranial nerves III, IV, VI)
Nasopharynx	
No early symptoms	Bloody nasal discharge
	Unilateral nasal obstruction
	Unilateral serous otitis media
	Unilateral hearing loss
	Poorly localized headaches
	Cranial nerve compression
	Presence of an enlarged posterior high-cervical lymph node (most common presenting symptom)

    e. Cine-esophagography/barium swallow—to identify the extent of lesions in the oropharynx that may extend into the hypopharynx (see Table 33–3).

    f. Bone and liver scans—to evaluate distant metastasis among high-risk clients (bone pain or elevated liver enzyme levels).

  5. Laboratory studies—complete blood count, chemistry studies, liver function tests.

  6. Histologic diagnosis obtained by:

    a. Fine-needle aspiration—performed on suspicious neck nodes and accessible lesions in the oral cavity.

    b. Excisional biopsy of the entire lesion—for diagnostic or curative purposes.

      (1) Performed on small oral cavity, lip, or skin lesions.

      (2) As a rule, an open or excisional biopsy of suspicious neck nodes is contraindicated (to avoid seeding of the tumor) except when all other examinations fail to identify a primary site or when lymphoma is suspected.

TABLE 33–3. **Specific Diagnostic Procedures in Evaluation of Head and Neck Tumors**

Description	Time Required	Sensations Experienced	Potential Side Effects/ Complications	Self-Care Measures	Symptoms to Report to Health Care Team
Panoramic X-ray Examination (*Panorex*)					
Examination of an entire dental arch viewed on one film To evaluate mandibular invasion	10 min	None	None	None	N/A
Cine-esophagography					
Video x-ray examination of oral and pharyngeal stages of swallowing To identify extension of lesions into hypopharynx	30 min	Vary, depending on degree of dysphagia	Aspiration	None	Temperature elevation Productive cough
Barium Swallow and X-ray Examination of Upper Gastrointestinal Tract					
To evaluate tumor invasion of hypopharynx and cervical esophagus	15 min	Chalky taste	Constipation secondary to use of barium	Assess bowel function Take laxative as needed Force fluids	No bowel movement within 3 days Abdominal distention
Panendoscopy					
Surgical procedure in which a lighted scope is passed along the upper aerodigestive tract to inspect and obtain biopsy specimens from areas of the entire mucosa (includes bronchoscopy, esophagoscopy, nasopharyngoscopy, and laryngoscopy) To detect metastasis or second primary tumor	1 hr	Related to general anesthesia	Reactions to general anesthesia Airway obstruction Tracheoesophageal fistula Sore throat Aspiration Hemorrhage from biopsy site Pneumothorax	Deep breathe, turn, ambulate	Difficulty breathing Excessive bleeding Inability to swallow (nurse should check for return of gag reflex) Increased temperature, cough, or sputum production

c. Incisional biopsy—taking a small sample of tumor along with adjoining normal tissue.

d. Panendoscopy (passing an endoscope along the entire mucosa of the upper aerodigestive tract)—to examine and perform a biopsy on suspicious areas, determine the full extent of disease, and identify synchronous primary tumors (see Table 33–3).

B. Staging methods and procedures—TNM classification system, defined by the American Joint Committee on Cancer (AJCC) in 1992, is used for staging head and neck tumors (Table 33–4).

C. Treatment strategies—surgery and radiation are the primary treatment modalities for managing malignant head and neck tumors; chemotherapy is used for recurrent and metastatic disease.

1. Treatment is based on the T and N classification:
   a. T1 and T2 lesions of the oral cavity, larynx, nose, and paranasal sinuses are treated with primary surgery or radiation, whereas T3 and T4 tumors are treated with combination therapy (Table 33–5).
   b. Treatment of N1, N2, and N3 disease is outlined in Table 33–6.
   c. Clinically negative neck nodes and a large primary lesion (T2, N0) of the oral cavity, oropharynx, hypopharynx, or larynx is generally treated with either lymphadenectomy or radiation because of the propensity to spread.

2. Surgery.
   a. Table 33–7 identifies the common surgical procedures used in treating head and neck malignancies, the physical alterations expected, and nursing implications.

3. Radiation therapy.
   a. As primary treatment to control the primary tumor and adjacent lymph nodes yet maintain structure and function; dose range is 6000 to 7000 cGy.
   b. Adjuvant treatment for stages III and IV disease and tumors that have a tendency to spread toward the midline (e.g., oropharyngeal lesions); dose is approximately 5000 cGy.
   c. External beam radiation therapy is used approximately 4 to 6 weeks after surgery, but preoperative radiation or permanently placed iodine-125 seeds may be used to debulk large or unresectable lesions.
      (1) Advantage of postoperative radiation is fewer wound complications.
      (2) Preoperative dental evaluations, removal of diseased teeth, and prophylactic fluoride treatment are indicated.
      (3) Postoperative radiation is initiated after the wounds heal (3 to 6 weeks) and is administered over a 6- to 7-week period.
   d. Cancers of the nasopharynx are treated primarily with radiation.
      (1) Close proximity to vital structures of the brain precludes surgery.
      (2) Carefully selected clients who fail after radiation therapy may be treated with base of skull resection of tumor.
   e. Brachytherapy (implanted iridium-192 or cesium-137) may be used to treat lesions of the anterior and posterior tongue, floor of mouth, and nasal vestibule to maximize dose to the tumor bed and minimize exposure to surrounding tissue.
   f. Table 33–8 describes the side effects associated with radiation therapy to the head and neck region.

4. Chemotherapy.
   a. Chemotherapy alone is not curative; it is used to reduce tumor volume or eradicate clinically detectable squamous cell carcinomas; chemotherapy is also used for recurrent or metastatic disease.
   b. Single agent or combination (cisplatin, bleomycin, 5-fluorouracil [5-FU], paclitaxel, and methotrexate) chemotherapy regimens may be given as adjuvant and neoadjuvant therapy; may be used as palliative therapy for recurrent or unresectable lesions.
   c. Chemotherapy is sometimes given with radiation therapy for its sensitizing effect.

TABLE 33–4. **TNM Staging of Cancers of the Head and Neck**

Classification

T = Primary Tumor

  General: for all sites
  TX   Primary tumor cannot be assessed
  TO   No evidence of primary tumor
  TIS   Carcinoma in situ

Oral Cavity, Oropharynx
  T1   greatest diameter of primary tumor ≤ 2 cm
  T2   >2 cm or ≤ 4 cm
  T3   >4 cm
  T4   Massive tumor, with deep invasion into maxilla, mandible, pterygoid muscles,
            deep tongue muscle, skin, soft tissues of neck

Hypopharynx
  T1   Tumor confined to one subsite of hypopharynx
  T2   Tumor invades more than one subsite of hypopharynx or an adjacent site,
            without fixation of hemilarynx
  T3   Tumor invades more than one subsite of hypopharynx or an adjacent site,
            with fixation of hemilarynx
  T4   Tumor involves adjacent structures (e.g. cartilage or soft tissues of neck)

Nasopharynx
  T1   Tumor confined to one subsite
  T2   Involvement of two subsites within nasopharynx
  T3   Extension into nasal cavity or oropharynx
  T4   Invasion into skull and/or cranial nerve(s)

Larynx
  Glottic
  T1   Limited to true vocal cords; normal vocal cord mobility; may include anterior
            or posterior commissure
  T2   Supra- or subglottic extension; normal or impaired mobility
  T3   Confined to larynx proper; vocal cord fixation
  T4   Cartilage destruction and/or extension out of larynx to other tissues

  Supraglottic
  T1   Limited to subsite of supraglottis; normal vocal cord mobility
  T2   Extension to glottis or adjacent supraglottic subsite; normal vocal cord
            mobility
  T3   Confined to larynx proper; cord fixation and/or extension into hypopharynx
            or preepiglottic space
  T4   Massive tumor, cartilage destruction and/or extension out of larynx

  Subglottic
  T1   Limited to subglottic region
  T2   Extension to vocal cord(s)
  T3   Limited to larynx; vocal cord fixation
  T4   Massive tumor; cartilage destruction and/or extension out of larynx

N = Nodal Metastasis
  NX   Nodes cannot be assessed
  N0   No regional lymph node metastasis
  N1   Single, ipsilateral node: ≤ 3 cm
  N2A   Single, ipsilateral node: > 3 cm or ≤ 6 cm
  N2B   Multiple, ipsilateral nodes: all ≤ 6 cm
  N3A   Ipsilateral node(s): one > 6 cm
  N3B   Bilateral nodes (each side subclassed)
  N3C   Contralateral node(s), only

M = Distant Metastasis
  MX   Presence of distant metastasis cannot be assessed
  M0   No distant metastasis
  M1   Distant metastasis present

Table continued on following page

TABLE 33–4. **TNM Staging of Cancers of the Head and Neck** (*Continued*)

Stage Groupings

Stage I	T1, N0, M0
Stage II	T2, N0, M0
Stage III	T3, N0, M0; T1, T2, or T3 with N1, M0
Stage IV	T4, N0 or N1, M0
	Any T, N2 or N3, M0
	Any T, Any N, M1

From Beahrs, O.H., Henson, D.E., Hutter, R.V.P., & Kennedy, B.J. (1992). *Manual for Staging Cancer* (4th ed.). Philadelphia: J.B. Lippincott, pp. 27–56.

 5. Palliative therapy.
    a. Surgery, radiation, and/or chemotherapy are used for unresectable lesions or recurrent tumors, or for clients who carry a high surgical risk.
    b. Short courses of radiation (3000 cGy over 2 to 3 weeks) may be used to relieve pain, bleeding, or obstruction.

TABLE 33–5. **Treatment Strategies for Head and Neck Cancer by Tumor Classification and Site**

	T0	**T1 and T2**	**T3 and T4**
Oral cavity and oropharynx	Laser excision	Radiation (4500–5500 cGy), with 500–2500 cGy boost to primary site *or* Simple excision with primary closure	Composite resection, with primary closure and adjuvant radiation (5000 cGy) *or* Myocutaneous flap closure and adjuvant radiation (5000 cGy)
Larynx	Laser excision	Glottic lesions—radiation (5500–6500 cGy) Supraglottic lesion—supraglottic laryngectomy Lesions confined to one side of glottis, with posterior extension—hemilaryngectomy	Total laryngectomy and adjuvant radiation (5000 cGy)
Nose and paranasal sinuses	——	Maxillectomy Excision of nasal vault and lesion *or* Radiation therapy	Maxillectomy (may include orbital exenteration) and radiation Excision of nasal vault lesions and radiation
Nasopharynx	——	Excision and/or radiation therapy	Radiation to nasopharynx, retropharyngeal nodes, lymph nodes in both sides of neck Skull base surgery in selected cases that fail with radiation therapy

TABLE 33–6. **Treatment Strategies for Nodal Involvement in Head and Neck Cancer**

N0	N1	N2 and N3
No treatment *or* Lymphadenectomy *or* Modified neck dissection *or* Radiation therapy	Modified neck dissection if tumor has not compromised cranial nerve XI with radiation therapy *or* Radiation therapy (if node <2 cm) *or* Radical neck dissection without radiation therapy	Radical neck dissection with radiation therapy

Assessment

I. Pertinent personal and family history (risk factors).
  A. Assess risk factors (see Table 33–1).
  B. Assess the client for signs and symptoms of the disease (see Table 33–2).
  C. Assess the health history and previous history of carcinoma and/or treatment of the head and neck.
II. Physical examination (see Theory).
III. Laboratory and diagnostic data.
  A. Monitor complete blood count, electrolyte values, liver and renal function test results.
  B. Radiologic studies (see Theory).
IV. Client undergoing treatment.
  A. Surgery.
    1. Adequacy of airway: cleanliness of tracheostomy.
    2. Ability to communicate—use of paper and pen, Magic Slate, electronic communication device, picture board, or nonverbal cues.
    3. Ability to swallow.
    4. Range of motion of head, neck, and shoulders.
    5. Coping with anticipated and actual physical changes associated with surgical procedure.
    6. Skin and suture lines for areas of erythema, induration, and tenderness, which may be signs of impending fistula formation.
    7. Understanding about surgical procedure, preoperative preparation, and postoperative care and rehabilitation.
  B. Radiation therapy.
    1. Skin integrity—color, tenderness, dryness, breakdown, pruritus.
    2. Level of fatigue, activities that exacerbate fatigue, activities that minimize or relieve fatigue. When fatigue occurs and how long it lasts.
    3. Level of appetite.
    4. Oral cavity inspection, assessing for presence of stomatitis, infection, xerostomia, taste changes.
    5. Pharyngitis, globus, dysphagia.
    6. Level of anxiety.
    7. Coping ability with body image changes.
    8. Understanding about radiation therapy and ability to perform self-care measures.

TABLE 33-7. **Surgical Procedures for Head and Neck Cancer**

Procedure	Physical Alteration	Nursing Implications
Laser	Little to none	Minimal bleeding
Composite resection	Resection of oral cavity/ oropharyngeal lesion in continuity with neck dissection Portion of mandible is resected Reconstruction with myocutaneous flaps is usually required, with resections of large amounts of tissue	May experience problems with speech (decreased articulation with tongue involvement), swallowing (impaired mastication, salivary drooling, aspiration), altered facial contour
Supraglottic laryngectomy	Resection of structures above the false vocal cords, including the epiglottis (preserves the true vocal cords)	Aspiration until swallowing techniques are learned Maintains a relatively normal voice
Hemilaryngectomy	Vertical excision of one true and one false cord and underlying cartilage	Hoarse voice Minimal or no swallowing problems
Total laryngectomy	Excision of entire larynx from the hyoid bone to the second tracheal ring	Permanent tracheostomy Aphonia Decreased sense of smell Unable to perform Valsalva maneuver
Maxillectomy	Partial or total en bloc resection of the cavity May include the ethmoid sinus, lateral nasal wall, palate, and floor of orbit	Preoperatively, orthodontist makes dental obturator to fill the large surgical defect and to facilitate swallowing Requires daily care to cavity and placement of obturator
Orbital exenteration	Resection of orbit secondary to extension of maxillary sinus tumor or recurrent disease	Facial defect Unilateral vision loss Requires daily care and cleansing of cavity
Craniofacial/skull base dissection	Surgical approach to inaccessible midfacial and extensive paranasal sinus and nasopharyngeal lesions	May have facial defect and cranial nerve (III, IV, V) deficits
Radical neck dissection	Resection of sternocleidomastoid muscle, jugular vein, spinal accessory nerve, and cervical lymph nodes	Shoulder droop Concave contour of neck
Modified neck dissection	Radical neck dissection with preservation of either the sternocleidomastoid muscle, jugular vein, or spinal accessory nerve	Shoulder droop if spinal accessory nerve resected Concave contour of neck
Lymphadenectomy	Resection of lymph nodes in neck	Surgical scars

TABLE 33–8. **Side Effects from Radiation Therapy for Head and Neck Cancers**

Physical Alterations
Skin reactions
Fatigue
Anorexia
Oral stomatitis
Xerostomia
Taste changes
Pharyngitis

C. Chemotherapy.
  1. Occurrence of nausea and vomiting, use and efficacy of antiemetics.
  2. Intake and output of fluids, daily weight, electrolyte levels including creatinine for renal function.
  3. Oral cavity inspection, assessing for presence of stomatitis and infection.
  4. Vital signs—monitor.
  5. Monitoring of blood counts, assess for infections, fever and myalgias from neutropenia.
  6. Assessing for bleeding from thrombocytopenia; fatigue from anemia.
  7. Understanding about chemotherapy and ability to perform self-care measures.

Nursing Diagnoses

  I. Surgery.
    A. Ineffective airway clearance.
    B. Impaired verbal communication.
    C. Altered nutrition, less than body requirements.
    D. Impaired physical mobility.
    E. Body image disturbance.
    F. Risk for impaired skin integrity.
    G. Knowledge deficit.
 II. Radiation therapy (Table 33–9).
III. Chemotherapy (Table 33–10).

Outcome Identification

The client:
  I. Identifies type of cancer, rationale for treatment, alteration in anatomy and physiology that will result from treatment, and the specific side effects of treatment.
 II. Lists signs and symptoms and treatment of immediate and long-term side effects of disease and treatment.
III. Discusses self-care measures to decrease incidence and severity of symptoms associated with disease and treatment.
    A. Refrain from further tobacco use and drinking of alcoholic beverages.
    B. Maintain prophylactic oral care during and after radiation treatment (removal of diseased teeth, daily fluoride treatments).

Nursing Diagnoses	Nursing Implications
Impaired skin integrity	1. Assess skin reactions 2. Instruct patient and family to keep skin clean. 3. Instruct patient to avoid shaving within area of treatment 4. Apply moisturizing lotion as directed for skin dryness 5. If pruritus occurs, apply thin layer of hydrocortisone cream 6. If moist desquamation occurs, use Burow compresses three to four times a day
Activity intolerance	1. Assess level of fatigue 2. Advise patient to plan rest periods throughout the day 3. Maintain nutritional intake 4. Utilize resources to conserve energy 5. Obtain assistance for chores and transportation as needed
Altered nutrition, less than body requirements related to anorexia	1. Assess appetite 2. Monitor weight 3. Recommend frequent small meals 4. Advise on use of nutrient-dense foods such as nutritional supplements

Altered oral mucous membrane	1. Assess oral cavity: note presence of erythema, xerostomia, ulcerations, infections
	2. Advise on mouth care:
	  a. Brush teeth after each meal.
	  b. Floss teeth at bedtime (if client normally practices flossing teeth)
	  c. Rinse mouth with normal saline every 2 hours or as needed throughout the day
	  d. Use saliva substitutes as needed
	3. Utilize topical anesthetics or systemic analgesics as prescribed before meals and as needed
	4. Recommend soft, nonspicy, nonacidic diet
	5. Maintain hydration status

Sensory/perceptual alterations: gustatory	1. Assess presence of taste changes 2. Recommend experimenting with different food tastes 3. Advise performing mouth care before meals 4. Recommend chewing foods longer, to allow longer contact of food with taste receptors in the mouth
Impaired swallowing	1. Assess for pharyngitis 2. Monitor for infections 3. Monitor weight 4. Use topical anesthetics or systemic analgesics as prescribed for pain 5. Recommend soft, nonspicy, nonacidic diet 6. Maintain hydration
Psychosocial Issues	
Anxiety	1. Assess level of anxixety 2. Allow client and family to verbalize issues and concerns 3. Provide education about illness and treatment
Body image disturbance	1. Assess client understanding about body image changes 2. Provide education about changes and rehabilitative measures available 3. Allow client and family to discuss issues and concerns about body image changes
Knowledge deficit related to radiation therapy and self-care measures	1. Assess client's and family's understanding about radiation therapy and self-care measures 2. Provide education about radiation therapy and self-care measures; utilize available multimedia patient education tools: booklets, videos, audiotapes 3. Evaluate comprehension of patient education materials

TABLE 33–10. **Chemotherapy for Cancers of the
Head and Neck—Nursing Diagnoses and Implications**

Nursing Diagnoses	Nursing Implications
Risk for fluid volume deficit related to nausea and vomiting	1. Assess for nausea and vomiting 2. Instruct client to use antiemetics before chemotherapy and as needed 3. Monitor hydration status 4. Encourage fluids 5. Utilize nonpharmacologic measures to manage nausea and vomiting: relaxation exercises, distraction 6. Encourage small frequent meals 7. Provide diet that is low fat and nonsweet; encourage fluids 8. Provide mouth care frequently during the day
Risk for injury related to nephrotoxicity of cisplatin	1. Monitor laboratory values, electrolytes, especially creatinine and blood urea nitrogen levels 2. Provide hydrating intravenous fluids and medications as ordered 3. Monitor intake and output 4. Encourage fluids 5. Control nausea and vomiting
Altered oral mucous membrane	1. Assess oral cavity: tenderness, ulceration, bleeding, infections 2. Instruct client about mouth care: Brush teeth after each meal Floss teeth at bedtime, if client normally practices flossing Perform frequent oral rinses with warm normal saline 3. Advise on diet consisting of nonspicy, nonacidic, room-temperature or cool foods 4. Maintain hydration
Risk for infection related to neutropenia	1. Monitor blood counts: white blood count, neutrophils; assess for neutropenia 2. Institute neutropenia precautions when white blood cell count is decreased: Monitor temperature: be alert for fever, chills, sweats, myalgias; report these occurrences Avoid crowds Avoid persons with colds or other respiratory infections Avoid sharing eating utensils, beverage containers Avoid handling animal excreta (i.e., litter box, bird cage) Preserve and protect skin integrity
Risk for injury related to thrombocytopenia	1. Monitor platelet count 2. Institute bleeding precautions when platelet count is decreased: Assess skin, mucous membranes, bowel movements, urine, emesis, and secretions for signs of bleeding Assess signs of hemorrhage: hypotension, changes in consciousness, headache, vomiting, and tachycardia Protect skin integrity: avoid venipuncture, intramuscular injections Perform mouth care, avoid traumatizing oral mucosa Institute bowel program to prevent constipation Avoid trauma to rectal tissues: avoid rectal medication, rectal thermometer, enemas Use electric razor Provide safe environment that eliminates hazards for injury

Table continued on following page

TABLE 33–10. **Chemotherapy for Cancers of the
Head and Neck—Nursing Diagnoses and Implications** (*Continued*)

Nursing Diagnoses	Nursing Implications

Risk for activity intolerance related to anemia	1. Assess for fatigue
	2. Monitor blood counts: red blood cells, hematocrit
	3. Recommend measures to minimize fatigue:
	   Pace activities
	   Plan rest periods during the day
	4. Administer blood products as ordered
	5. Ensure adequate nutritional intake

Knowledge deficit related to chemotherapy and self-care measures	1. Assess level of understanding about chemotherapy 2. Provide information about chemotherapy: effects, side effects, and self-care measures as well as symptoms to report 3. Provide educational booklets, videotapes, and audiotapes as they are available 4. Evaluate comprehension of patient education

    C. Maintain high-residue diet and high fluid intake to prevent constipation that may result from absence of Valsalva maneuver (after total laryngectomy).

  IV. Demonstrates skill in self-care demanded by structural or functional effects of disease and treatment by return demonstration of the following:
    A. Wound care.
    B. Airway management.
      1. Perform tracheostomy care.
      2. Perform stoma care.
      3. Perform suctioning.
      4. Provide humidification via stoma.
    C. Nutritional care.
    D. Self-monitoring for disease progression or recurrence:
      1. Demonstrate self-examination of the head and neck area.
      2. List symptoms to report—red areas (erythroplakia), white areas (leukoplakia), ulcers that do not heal in 2 weeks, lymph node enlargement or changes.

   V. Discusses coping strategies.
    A. Independence in activities of daily living and new skills (tracheostomy care, esophageal speech).
    B. Socialization with family and friends.
    C. Return to previous work or activities or occupational training for alternative work and leisure activities.
    D. Participation in support groups and informational systems to assist in problem solving, lifestyle changes, and adjustment (Lost Chord Club, I Quit Clinics, I Can Cope educational programs).

  VI. Describes plan for follow-up care.
    A. To monitor rehabilitation and detect recurrence or a second primary tumor.
      1. Cite schedule for clinical evaluation (e.g., every month for the first year; every 2 months the second year; every 3 months the third year; every 4 months the fourth year; every 5 months the fifth year; and every year thereafter).

    2. List signs and symptoms of recurrence—pain, dysphagia, neck nodes enlargement, ulceration, bleeding, hemoptysis, airway obstruction, bone pain.

  B. To promote physical and psychosocial adjustment—use of physical therapist, occupational therapist, speech therapist, CanSurmount or Laryngectomy Club.

  C. To change lifestyles—stop smoking and/or alcohol cessation programs.

VII. Discusses community resources for clients with cancers of the head and neck.

  A. Support groups and organizations: Lost Chord Club, I Can Cope, CanSurmount, International Association of Laryngectomees (contact the American Cancer Society: 1-800-227-2345).

  B. Booklets:

    1. *Self-Help for the Laryngectomee*
    Edmund Lauder
    11115 Whisper Hollow
    San Antonio, TX 78230
    512-492-1984

    2. *Looking Forward: A Guidebook for the Larynegectomee* (2nd ed.)
    Keith, R.L. (1991)
    New York: Thieme Medical Publishers
    Available from publisher:
    Thieme Medical Publishers
    381 Park Ave., S.
    New York, NY 10061
    or from the author:
    Robert L. Keith, M.D.
    Mayo Comprehensive Cancer Center
    Speech Pathology, E-8A
    Rochester, MN 55905
    507-284-3112

  C. Medical Supply Providers for information about stoma bibs, shower shields, medications, other equipment.

  D. Medic-Alert Foundation International
    2323 Colorado Ave.
    Turlock, CA 95381-1009
    1-800-ID-ALERT (1-800-432-5378)

Planning and Implementation

Overall

I. Interventions to ensure that collaborative, multidisciplinary (including the client), and systematic monitoring and evaluation of the client's condition is ongoing.

  A. Involve members from the various disciplines in care of the client with head and neck cancer: surgery, radiation oncology, medical oncology, nursing, social work, physical medicine, rehabilitation, speech and language pathology, nutrition, others.

  B. Arrange regularly scheduled multidisciplinary patient care conferences.

  C. Determine client goals and time frames for accomplishment of these goals.

Surgery for Head and Neck Cancers

I. Preoperative preparation.

  A. Initiate client and family preoperative teaching at the time of diagnosis and discuss information about the disease, treatment, side effects, and anticipated postoperative changes.

B. Give instructions and demonstrate the use of various types of equipment (tracheostomy tube, drains, nasogastric tube, tonsil-tip suction catheter, others).

C. Counsel and support the client and family as needed.

D. Discuss economic and rehabilitation resources.

E. Arrange a preoperative and a postoperative visit with a Lost Chord or Laryngectomy Club member if indicated (call American Cancer Society [ACS] or local agencies).

F. Determine client's reading ability preoperatively and choose communication mechanisms to be used postoperatively:
   1. Paper and pencil.
   2. Magic Slate.
   3. Picture board.
   4. Nonverbal cues.
   5. Electronic communication board or device.

II. Postoperative interventions to maximize safety for the client.

A. Maintain close proximity to the nurses' station to monitor clients with altered airway.

B. Keep an extra tracheostomy tube of the same size (inner and outer cannula and obturator), scissors, and a tracheal dilator at the bedside of all tracheostomy clients.

C. Keep the call bell within reach at all times.

D. Identify method of communication if the client has a tracheostomy in place.

E. Observe for signs and symptoms of delirium tremens in clients with recent history of alcohol abuse.

F. Observe for signs and symptoms of aspiration in clients who have had a supraglottic laryngectomy, resection of structures in the oropharynx, or cranial nerve (IX, X, XII) deficits.

G. Implement carotid precautions for clients at risk for carotid rupture.

III. Postoperative interventions to decrease the severity of symptoms associated with surgery for cancers of the head and neck.

A. Airway management related to tracheostomy.
   1. Permanent tracheostomy (total laryngectomy) (Fig. 33–3).
      a. Airway.
         (1) A cuffed tracheostomy tube is used while the client requires mechanical ventilation; may be removed by postoperative day 2 or 3.
         (2) Laryngectomy tube may be used if the stoma begins to narrow.
      b. Humidity.
         (1) Provide humidified air or oxygen via a tracheostomy collar to prevent drying of the mucosa and crusting of secretions.
         (2) Apply moistened 4 × 4 gauze pads to cover the stoma to provide humidity.
         (3) Advise that a stoma bib worn over the stoma helps lessen drying of mucosa.
         (4) Teach symptoms of inadequate humidity—thick, tenacious secretions that are difficult to expectorate.
      c. Stoma care.
         (1) Cleanse stoma with half-and-half peroxide and normal saline solution.

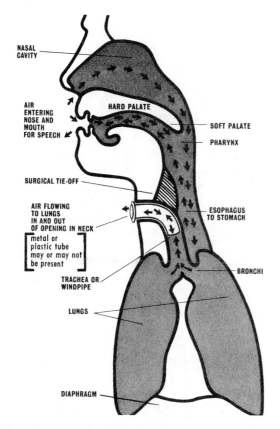

NASAL
CAVITY

AIR
ENTERING
NOSE AND
MOUTH
FOR SPEECH

HARD PALATE

SOFT PALATE

PHARYNX

SURGICAL TIE-OFF

AIR FLOWING
TO LUNGS
IN AND OUT
OF OPENING IN NECK

metal or
plastic tube
may or may not
be present

ESOPHAGUS
TO STOMACH

BRONCHI

TRACHEA OR
WINDPIPE

LUNGS

DIAPHRAGM

Figure 33–3. Physiology of head and neck after total laryngectomy (From *First Aid for [neck breathers] Laryngectomees.* Atlanta: American Cancer Society, p. 3 [1-800-ACS-2345].)

    (2) Remove all mucous crusting, twice each day and as needed.

    (3) Remove visible mucous plugs with a Kelly clamp.

    (4) Apply a thin layer of prescribed ointment around the stoma twice each day.

2. Temporary tracheostomy (Fig. 33–4).

  a. A cuffed tube (generally placed in the operating room and maintained for 5 days) is kept inflated if mechanical ventilation is needed or if the client is at risk for aspiration.

  b. Initial tracheostomy tube is changed by the physician to a noncuffed tube. (If the client is aspirating, the cuffed tube is maintained.)

  c. As edema decreases, the client may be able to breathe without the tracheostomy tube.

    (1) Tube is downsized to a number 4 or 5, or a fenestrated tube is placed.

    (2) Tube is plugged for 24 hours.

    (3) If the client is able to breathe with the tube plugged for prolonged time periods and is able to expectorate secretions through the mouth, the cannula may be removed.

    (4) Dressing over the stoma is changed every day and as needed.

    (5) Client is instructed to place a finger over stoma dressing when coughing or speaking until the wound has sealed.

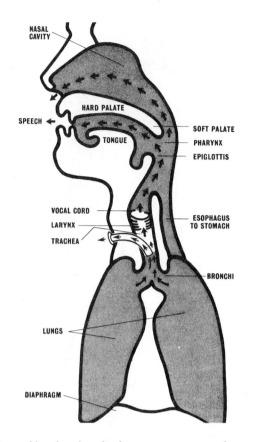

Figure 33–4. Physiology of head and neck after a temporary tracheostomy. (From *First Aid for [neck breathers] Laryngectomees.* Atlanta: American Cancer Society, p. 4.)

    d. Suctioning (all tracheostomies) is based on the need for airway clearance.
      (1) Hyperoxygenate and/or hyperinflate the lungs before and after suctioning to prevent hypoxemia and arrhythmia.
      (2) Instill 2 to 5 mL of normal saline solution into the tracheostomy to lavage and stimulate the trachea and bronchi if needed to precipitate coughing and mobilize secretions.
      (3) Use an incentive spirometer attached via a female adapter to a plastic tracheostomy tube and/or use chest physical therapy, as indicated, to mobilize secretions and prevent atelectasis.
      (4) Record the color, amount, and odor of sputum produced, and how frequently suctioning is required.
  B. Tracheostomy care.
    1. Remove the inner cannula and cleanse off all mucus and crusts with a half-and-half solution of peroxide and normal saline every 4 to 8 hours initially, then twice daily and as needed.
    2. Replace soiled tracheostomy ties as needed; allow one fingerbreadth ease underneath ties when determining tightness.
  C. Wound care.
    1. Assess the surgical wounds every 3 to 4 hours, noting color (pink versus cyanotic), temperature, and capillary refill (immediately after blanching) of skin and muscle flaps.

    2. Avoid excessive pressure that interferes with flap perfusion (tight tracheostomy ties, oxygen collars, hyperextension of the neck, and the client lying on the flap), to ensure flap viability.

    3. Assess integrity of suture lines, both external and intraoral (if applicable); breakdown may be the first sign of wound infection or fistula formation.

    4. Clean external suture lines with a half-and-half solution of peroxide and normal saline; then apply prescribed ointment every 4 to 8 hours.

    5. If client has nasal surgery, a maxillectomy, and/or an orbital exenteration, gently cleanse the cavities to remove accumulated crusts as ordered by the physician; a half-and-half solution of normal saline and sodium bicarbonate or normal saline solution alone can be used.

    6. Assess wound drains for color, amount, and odor of drainage; clotting and air leaks can lead to wound infections if not prevented or treated early.

D. Oral care.

    1. Use or instruct the client, if able, to use a tonsil-tip suction catheter to remove excess secretions from the oral cavity.

    2. Perform oral care with half-and-half peroxide and normal saline solution at least every 4 hours as ordered by the physician.

    3. A gravity gavage or jet-spray dental cleansing system may be used for gentle cleansing of the cavity.

    4. A Kelly clamp or a toothette may be used to remove mucous crusts that develop on immobile suture lines and flaps.

    5. Avoid the use of lemon glycerin swabs and commercially prepared mouthwashes that contain alcohol to minimize drying of the mucosa.

E. Nutrition.

    1. Assess nutritional status before surgery; 60% of head and neck clients initially present with malnutrition.

    2. Identify clients with nutritional deficiencies that necessitate oral, enteral, or parenteral nutritional supplements.

      a. Greater than 10% body weight loss during any treatment phase.

      b. More than 20% below ideal body weight.

    3. Confer with physician regarding methods of nutritional support—enteral tube feedings, other methods.

    4. Assess surgically treated clients after head and neck surgery for swallowing dysfunction.

F. Mobility.

    1. If a neck dissection is performed, the spinal accessory nerve and the sternocleidomastoid muscles are often resected, resulting in shoulder droop, atrophy of the trapezius muscle, forward curvature of the spine, and limited range of motion (approximately 90 degrees) of the shoulder.

    2. Passive and active range of motion exercises of the shoulder are initiated after the wound drains are removed, and clients are progressed to resistive exercises, with the ultimate goal of a functional range of 150 degrees.

G. Body image changes.

    1. Provide and teach wound, oral, and tracheostomy care techniques to promote control of secretion and odors.

    2. Encourage self-care activities (tracheostomy care, tube feeding, suctioning) and activities of daily living (grooming, hair combing, shaving, applying makeup).

    3. Encourage resocialization though progressive ambulation, interaction with others, and support group participation (e.g., Voice Masters, Lost Chord Club, I Can Cope, CanSurmount).

    4. Involve the social worker to assist with counseling and financial, vocational, and adjustment issues.

5. Inform the client of resources for the purchase of tracheostomy covers, scarves, makeup, or other cosmetic assistance; consult ACS Look Good, Feel Better program for further suggestions (e.g., hair care, scarves).

6. Support clients and family through the normal grieving process; allow them to voice concerns, fears, and anxieties.

H. Observe and advise about other possible alterations in functioning related to disease and treatment.
1. Loss of sense of smell and/or taste.
2. Loss of ability to blow nose (may need suctioning with nasal congestion or a cold).
3. Loss of ability to perform Valsalva maneuver may predispose to constipation; stool softeners are often required.
4. Loss of normal airway.
   a. Advise to wear Medic Alert bracelet identifying client as a neck breather and to carry cards and/or windshield stickers for emergency use (Fig. 33–5).
   b. Establish emergency plans with local emergency system (tape recorder at phone with prerecorded call for help).
   c. Teach the client, family, public, and professionals first aid for individuals with a laryngectomy (Fig. 33–6).
5. Loss of ability to blow air from their mouth (cannot extinguish candles on a birthday cake).

IV. Interventions to monitor for unique side effects of treatment for head and neck cancers.
A. Fistula formation.
1. Fistula formation is more common if client has received preoperative radiation.
2. Breakdown of suture lines (pharyngeal, tracheoesophageal) allows secretions to leak into the wounds or under skin flaps.
3. Formation usually occurs 3 to 5 days after surgery.
4. Observe for signs and symptoms—erythema, drainage, tenderness of the suture line, low-grade temperature of 100 to 101°F, fluctuance below the neck skin, local edema.
5. Maintain nothing by mouth (NPO) status to allow healing
6. Perform dressing changes and wound packing every 4 to 8 hours or as needed to promote granulation of wound.

B. Carotid artery rupture.
1. Rupture of the carotid artery occurs in 3.5% of head and neck clients treated with radical surgery.
2. Radiation therapy effects or fistula formation increases risks of carotid artery rupture.
3. Place clients with an exposed carotid artery on "carotid precautions"; supplies placed at the bedside include:
   Three bath towels
   Six packs of 4 × 4 sponges
   Six 5 × 9 combine dressing pads
   One cuffed tracheostomy tube
   10-mL syringe
   Alcohol swabs
   Four packs of 4-inch rolled gauze (e.g., Kling)
   Intravenous solutions (normal saline, lactated Ringer's)
   Type and crossmatch—stamped requisitions for 2 units of blood

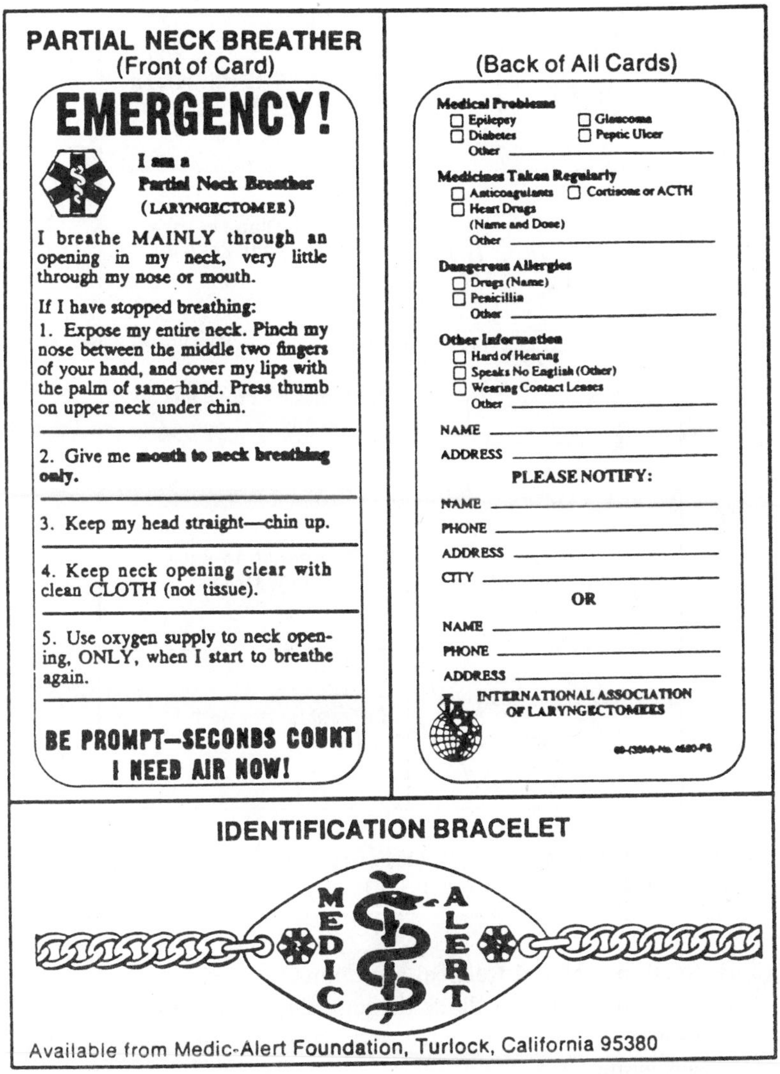

PARTIAL NECK BREATHER
(Front of Card)

EMERGENCY!

I am a
Partial Neck Breather
(LARYNGECTOMEE)

I breathe MAINLY through an opening in my neck, very little through my nose or mouth.

If I have stopped breathing:

1. Expose my entire neck. Pinch my nose between the middle two fingers of your hand, and cover my lips with the palm of same hand. Press thumb on upper neck under chin.

2. Give me **mouth to neck breathing only.**

3. Keep my head straight—chin up.

4. Keep neck opening clear with clean CLOTH (not tissue).

5. Use oxygen supply to neck opening, ONLY, when I start to breathe again.

**BE PROMPT—SECONDS COUNT
I NEED AIR NOW!**

(Back of All Cards)

Medical Problems
☐ Epilepsy ☐ Glaucoma
☐ Diabetes ☐ Peptic Ulcer
Other

Medicines Taken Regularly
☐ Anticoagulants ☐ Cortisone or ACTH
☐ Heart Drugs
(Name and Dose)
Other

Dangerous Allergies
☐ Drugs (Name)
☐ Penicillin
Other

Other Information
☐ Hard of Hearing
☐ Speaks No English (Other)
☐ Wearing Contact Lenses
Other

NAME
ADDRESS
PLEASE NOTIFY:
NAME
PHONE
ADDRESS
CITY
OR
NAME
PHONE
ADDRESS

**INTERNATIONAL ASSOCIATION
OF LARYNGECTOMEES**

IDENTIFICATION BRACELET

MEDIC ALERT

Available from Medic-Alert Foundation, Turlock, California 95380

Figure 33–5. Medic Alert information. (From *First Aid for [neck breathers] Laryngectomees.* Atlanta: American Cancer Society, p. 4.)

    Suction apparatus and setup
    Arterial blood gases kit
    Blood drawing equipment
    Latex gloves, disposable gowns, goggles.
4. Keep an intact heparin/saline lock in place.
5. Place clients on stool softeners to avoid straining.
6. Use wet-to-wet dressing changes to avoid debriding the artery.
7. In the event of a rupture:
    a. Apply pressure if bleeding externally or pack gauze in mouth if bleeding internally and *call for assistance.*
    b. Establish an airway.
    c. Inflate the cuff on the tracheostomy tube to prevent aspiration and to apply internal pressure on the artery.

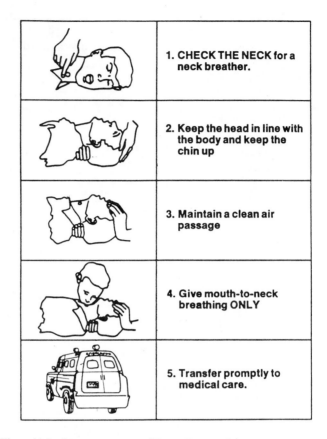

Figure 33–6. First aid for laryngectomees. (From *First Aid for [neck breathers] Laryngectomees.* Atlanta: American Cancer Society, p. 13.)

    d. Suction oral and tracheal secretions.

    e. Infuse intravenous fluids through the heparin lock.

    f. Obtain blood from the blood bank and determine arterial blood gas values.

    g. Call operating room personnel to alert them about the emergency.

    h. Prepare the client and transfer to the operating room.

    i. Initiate universal precautions (as quickly as possible).

    j. If the client is alert, provide supportive and explanatory information throughout the situation.

IV. Interventions to enhance adaptation and rehabilitation.

    A. Communication.

        1. Cancers in the oral cavity affect the function of *articulation;* therapy includes:

            a. Exercises to increase strength, range of motion, coordination, and accuracy of tongue movement.

            b. Use of oral prostheses to compensate for tissue loss and allow for greater contact of the tongue with the palate, creating more intelligible speech.

        2. Cancers in the larynx affect *phonation;* therapy includes:

            a. After a partial laryngectomy, exercises to improve voice quality, pitch, and loudness.

   b. After a total laryngectomy:
      (1) Use of artificial larynx that transmits sound into the vocal tract.
      (2) Use of esophageal speech—air is swallowed and trapped in the esophagus, then released, allowing air to vibrate against the walls of the esophagus.
      (3) Use of tracheoesophageal prosthesis—placement of a prosthesis in a surgically created tracheoesophageal fistula; sound is formed by air from the lungs, creating a better quality of esophageal speech.
B. Swallowing.
   1. Surgeries in the head and neck region can affect swallowing.
   2. A thorough clinical evaluation of the oral preparatory and pharyngeal stages of swallowing is conducted.
   3. A barium swallow and x-ray examination or cine-esophagography are performed to assess the oral and pharyngeal stages of the swallow.
   4. An individual swallowing plan is developed and includes:
      a. Compensatory strategies—postural changes that facilitate passage of food into the oral cavity and pharynx (head elevated); changes in food consistency (i.e., thin versus thick fluids, semisolid versus pureed foods).
      b. Indirect swallowing therapy—jaw and tongue range of motion exercises; adduction of tongue exercises to improve laryngeal closure.
      c. Direct swallowing therapy using supraglottic swallow.
         (1) Prepare the bolus of food in the oral preparatory phase.
         (2) Before initiating the swallow, hold breath to close vocal cords.
         (3) Swallow while still holding breath.
         (4) Cough while exhaling after the swallow to expectorate remaining food or fluids on top of vocal cords.
         (5) Repeat steps three and four (swallow/cough).
   5. The cuff on the tracheostomy tube is partially or totally inflated during meals and 30 minutes afterward to avoid aspiration.
   6. For some clients, removal of the tracheostomy tube improves swallowing by allowing the larynx to elevate.
   7. Until the client can take adequate amounts by mouth, enteral tube feeding is used to maintain nutritional requirements.
C. Patient education and support.
   1. Begin discharge teaching before surgery and reinforce this teaching immediately after surgery; teaching includes care of the tracheostomy tube, stoma care, suctioning techniques, enteral/supplemental feeding, alternative methods of providing humidity (bedside humidifier at bedtime and as needed), swallowing techniques, and speech, occupational, and physical therapy.
   2. Teach self-examination of lips, mouth, and oral cavity and palpation of adjacent nodes (see Fig. 33–1) to monitor disease progression or recurrence.
   3. Include discharge teaching about alleviation of risk factors to minimize risk of recurrence (e.g., use of smoking cessation programs, Alcoholics Anonymous).
   4. Recommend a head and neck cancer support group to discuss fears and help clients and families cope with the disease and treatment.
   5. Provide literature to reinforce or augment teaching; call the American Cancer Society (1-800-227-2345), the International Association of

Laryngectomees (1-800-227-2345) and the National Cancer Institute (1-800-422-6237) for current publications.

Radiation Therapy for Head and Neck Cancer

Table 33–9 lists nursing diagnoses and implications related to radiation therapy for cancers of the head and neck.

Chemotherapy for Head and Neck Cancer

Table 33–10 lists nursing diagnoses and implications related to chemotherapy for cancers of the head and neck.

Evaluation

The oncology nurse systematically and regularly evaluates the client's and/or family's responses to interventions to determine progress toward the achievement of expected outcomes. Relevant data are collected and actual findings are compared with expected findings. Nursing diagnoses, outcomes, and plans of care are reviewed and revised as necessary.

BIBLIOGRAPHY

Aisner, J., Hiponia, D., Conley, B., et al. (1995). Combined modalities in the treatment of head and neck cancers. *Semin Oncol 22*(3[suppl 6]), 28–4.

al-Sarraf, M. (1994). Cisplatin combinations in the treatment of head and neck cancer. *Semin Oncol 21*(5[suppl 12]), 28–34.

Baker, C.A. (1992). Factors associated with rehabilitation in head and neck cancer. *Cancer Nurs 15*(6), 395–400.

Beahrs, O.H., Henson, D.E., Hutter, R.V.P., & Kennedy, B.J. (1992). *Manual for Staging Cancer* (4th ed.). Philadelphia: J.B. Lippincott.

Dimery, I.W., & Hong, W.K. (1993). Overview of combined modality therapies for head and neck cancer. *J Natl Cancer Inst 85*(2), 95–111.

Dropkin, M.J. (1989). Coping with disfigurement and dysfunction after head and neck cancer surgery: A conceptual framework. *Semin Oncol Nurs 5*(3), 213–219.

Grant, M., Rhiner, M., & Padilla, G.V. (1989). Nutritional management in the head and neck cancer patient. *Semin Oncol Nurs 5*(3), 195–204.

Logemann, J.A. (1989). Swallowing and communication rehabilitation. *Semin Oncol Nurs 5*(3), 205–212.

Madeya, M.L. (1996). Oral complications from cancer therapy: Pathophysiology and secondary complications (part 1). *Oncol Nurs Forum 23*(5), 801–807.

Madeya, M.L. (1996). Oral complications from cancer therapy: Nursing implications for assessment and treatment (part 2). *Oncol Nurs Forum 23*(5), 808–819.

Martin, L.K. (1989). Management of the altered airway in the head and neck cancer patient. *Semin Oncol Nurs 5*(3), 182–190.

Mashberg, A., & Samit, A. (1995). Early diagnosis of asymptomatic oral and oropharyngeal squamous cancers. *CA Cancer J Clin 45*(6), 328–351.

Mathog, R.H. (1991). Rehabilitation of head and neck cancer patients: Consensus of recommendations from the International Conference on Rehabilitation of the Head and Neck Cancer Patient. *Head Neck 13*(1), 1–2.

National Institutes of Health. (1989). Oral complications of cancer therapies: Diagnosis, prevention, and treatment. *Consensus Development Conference Statement 7*(7), 1–11.

Norris, C.M., & Blake, C. (1991). Head, neck, and thyroid cancer. In A.I. Holleb, D.J. Fink, & G.P. Murphy (eds.), *American Cancer Society Textbook of Clinical Oncology*. Atlanta: American Cancer Society, pp. 306–328.

Reese, J.L. (1996). Head and neck cancers. In R. McCorkle, M. Grant, M. Frank-Stromborg, & S.B. Baird (eds.). *Cancer Nursing: A Comprehensive Textbook* (2nd ed.). Philadelphia: W.B. Saunders, pp. 773–795.

Schwartz, S.S., & Yuska, C.M. (1989). Common patient care issues following surgery for head and neck cancer. *Semin Oncol Nurs 5*(3), 191–194.

Shah, J.P., & Lydiatt, W. (1995). Treatment of cancer of the head and neck. *CA Cancer J Clin 45*(6), 352–368.

Spitz, M.R. (1994). Epidemiology and risk factors for head and neck cancer. *Semin Oncol 21*(3), 281–288.

Strohl, R.A. (1989). Radiation therapy for head and neck cancers. *Semin Oncol Nurs 5*(3), 166–173.

Tobias, J.S. (1992). Current role of chemotherapy in head and neck cancer. *Drugs 43*(3), 333–345.

Nursing Implications of Surgical Treatment

Thomas J. Szopa, RN, MS, AOCN, CETN

Theory

I. Principles of surgery.
  A. Surgery is the treatment of choice for malignant tumors that:
    1. Have low growth fractions and long cell-cycle times.
    2. Are confined locally and/or regionally.
  B. Surgery is planned to:
    1. Remove the malignant tumor and a margin of adjacent normal tissue.
    2. Remove the malignant tumor with attention to resulting structural, functional, and cosmetic changes.
  C. Surgical procedures include strategies to decrease the local and systemic spread of cancer.
    1. Ligation of local blood vessels and local and regional draining lymphatics.
    2. Irrigation of wounds with cytotoxic agents.
    3. Changing surgical gloves frequently.
    4. Cleaning surgical instruments with cytotoxic solutions.
    5. Using a "no-touch" technique with tumor tissue.
II. Role of surgery in cancer care.
  A. Establish a tissue diagnosis.
    1. Incisional biopsy (Table 34–1).
    2. Excisional biopsy (see Table 34–1).
    3. Needle biopsy (see Table 34–1).
  B. Determine the stage of disease.
    1. Obtain multiple biopsies to identify and determine the extent of disease.
    2. Remove tumor along with affected organs or tissues.
    3. Mark residual tumor on affected organs to assist in subsequent cancer treatment planning and delivery.
  C. Treat disease.
    1. Primary treatment—removal of the malignant tumor and a margin of adjacent normal tissue.
    2. Adjuvant treatment—removal of tissues to decrease the risk of cancer incidence, progression, or recurrence.
      a. Cytoreductive surgery—reduction of the tumor volume to improve the effect of other cancer treatment modalities.
      b. Prophylactic surgery—removal of nonvital organs that have an extremely high risk of subsequent cancer (Table 34–2).

TABLE 34–1. Surgical Procedures

Type of Procedure	Uses in Cancer Care	Advantages	Disadvantages
Incisional biopsy	Obtain tissue for pathology examination	Simple method to obtain diagnosis	Additional, more extensive surgical procedure generally performed to remove tumor
Excisional biopsy	Establish tissue diagnosis and tumor removal	Quick, simple removal of tumor at biopsy time; may not require hospitalization: decreased cost; minimal cosmetic effects	Tumor cells may be implanted along surgical path and incision, resulting in local recurrence
Needle biopsy	Obtain tissue for pathology examination	Simple to perform, reliable, inexpensive, performed with client under local anesthesia on outpatient basis	Risk of injury to adjacent structures; risk of tumor cell implantation along needle track and recurrence
Diagnostic laparotomy	Determine stage and extent of disease	Provides more accurate diagnostic information for treatment planning	Major surgical procedure with risk for postoperative complications; requires hospital stay, costly, multiple lifestyle disruptions.
Local excision	Primary treatment Cytoreductive surgery Removal of solitary metastasis Palliative treatment	Minimal tissue removal with little effect on functional status and appearance; may not require hospital stay or short hospital stay	Risk of microscopic residual disease left in tissue, resulting in local recurrence
Wide excision	Primary treatment Cytoreductive surgery Prophylactic surgery	Eliminates visible and microscopic disease locally and in adjacent tissue that has increased risk for disease spread	Longer, more involved rehabilitation required; may cause major changes in functional ability and appearance; may require reconstructive procedures
Laser	Primary treatment Cytoreductive surgery Palliation	Can be used in all body systems; decreased blood loss and need for blood products; decreased local recurrence rates; minimal side effects, including minimal pain during and after surgery; decreased wound drainage,	None noted

	Uses	Advantages	Limitations/Considerations
(continued)		earlier return of functional ability, reduced incidence of functional disabilities; minimal preparation time and easy to deliver treatment; decreased procedure time; decreased or eliminated hospital stay; may be repeated on recurrent tumor; may perform immediate graft; may be performed when traditional surgery is contraindicated (e.g., because of location of tumor; client is a poor surgical risk as a result of health status)	
Photodynamic therapy	Primary treatment	More precise in locating cancer cells, particularly when all sites of disease are unknown; decreased risks and variety of side effects as compared with traditional surgery	Photosensitivity for 4–6 weeks, causing possible lifestyle disruptions
Stereotaxis	Obtain biopsy Primary treatment Cytoreductive surgery Implantation of radioactive sources, hyperthermia, or chemotherapeutic agents Perform thalamotomy for intractable cancer pain or tremor	Minimize tissue exposed and affected; less trauma to brain tissue than traditional approaches with decreased neurologic deficits; shorter hospital stay and reduced hospitalization costs; lower mortality and morbidity	Use dependent on size and location of tumor, and current expertise and technology in imaging modalities and computer technology Neurologic side effects dependent on size and location of tumor
Laparoscopic surgery	Primary treatment	Decreased postoperative pain and procedure-related complications; earlier recovery and return to activities of daily living Shorter hospital stay with decreased treatment costs	Use dependent on size and location of primary tumor and existence of regional disease; anatomic defects may limit access and use; data inconclusive on long-term effect on prognosis

TABLE 34–2. **Surgery That Can Prevent Cancer**

Underlying Condition	Associated Cancer	Prophylactic Surgery
Cryptorchidism	Testicular	Orchiopexy
Polyposis coli	Colon	Colectomy
Familial colon cancer	Colon	Colectomy
Ulcerative colitis	Colon	Colectomy
Multiple endocrine neoplasia types II and III	Medullary cancer of the thyroid	Thyroidectomy
Familial breast cancer	Breast	Mastectomy
Familial ovarian cancer	Ovary	Oophorectomy

From DeVita, V.T., Jr., Hellman, S., & Rosenberg, S.A. (eds.). (1993). *Cancer: Principles & Practice of Oncology* (4th ed.). Philadelphia: J.B. Lippincott, p. 243.

3. Salvage treatment—use of an extensive surgical approach to treat local disease recurrence after the use of a less extensive primary approach (Table 34–3).
4. Palliative treatment—use of procedures to promote client comfort and quality of life without the goal of cure of disease.
   a. Examples—bone stabilization, relief of obstruction, removal of solitary metastasis, therapy for oncologic emergencies, ablative surgery, and management of cancer pain.
   b. Benefit of palliative treatment depends on the biologic pace of the cancer, projected life expectancy, and expected primary treatment outcome.
5. Combination treatment—use of surgery with other treatment modalities to improve tumor resectability; decrease the extent of tissue removed; limit the change in physical appearance and functional ability; and improve treatment outcomes.
   a. Examples—preoperative chemotherapy, radiation therapy, or immunotherapy; intraoperative chemotherapy or radiation therapy; and postoperative chemotherapy, radiation therapy, or immunotherapy.
   b. Risk of type and severity of side effects experienced increases with each additional treatment modality used.
      (1) Chemotherapy may affect wound healing (methotrexate); renal function (cisplatin); cardiac function (doxorubicin); or pulmonary function (bleomycin).
      (2) Radiation therapy may affect wound healing in the treatment field or function of organs within the treatment field (pulmonary fibrosis).

TABLE 34–3. **Examples of Salvage Therapy**

Cancer Site	Primary Conservative Approach	Salvage Approach
Breast	Lumpectomy and radiation therapy	Mastectomy
Bladder	Primary radiation therapy	Radical cystectomy
Early glottic carcinoma	Primary radiation therapy	Hemilaryngectomy
Prostate	Primary radiation therapy	Radical prostatectomy

   c. Current research issues.
      (1) Timing of combination therapies.
      (2) Sequencing of combination therapies.
      (3) Identifying combination therapies most effective in controlling cancer with minimal untoward effects.
   D. Place therapeutic and supportive hardware such as a gastrostomy tube; hyperalimentation lines; ventricular reservoir; external or implantable vascular access catheters, ports, and pumps; and radioactive implants.
   E. Assess response to treatment by "second-look" procedures.
      1. Procedure performed within a predetermined time frame after initial therapy.
      2. Sites and volume of residual tumor are identified and resected if possible.
   F. Reconstruct affected body parts.
      1. Repair or reduce anatomic defects from cancer surgery to improve function and/or cosmetic appearance.
      2. Examples—fecal or urinary diversion, breast reconstruction, fistula excision, skin flap development, and prosthesis placement.
III. Types and classifications of surgery (see Table 34–1).
   A. Surgical extent.
      1. Local excision—removal of cancer with a small margin of normal tissue.
      2. Wide excision—removal of cancer, tissue containing primary lymph nodes, contiguous structures involved, and contiguous structures at high risk for tumor spread.
   B. Electrosurgery—use of electric current for cell destruction.
   C. Cryosurgery—use of liquid nitrogen to freeze tissue to result in cell destruction.
   D. Chemosurgery—use of combined topical chemotherapy and layer-by-layer surgical removal of abnormal tissue.
   E. Laser (*l*ight *a*mplification by *s*timulated *e*mission of *r*adiation) surgery (see Table 34–1).
      1. Contact tip or "laser scalpel" provides a focused form of energy within a precise location and depth of tissue.
      2. Photodynamic therapy—intravenous injection of a light-sensitizing agent (hematoporphyrin derivative [HPD]) with uptake by cancer cells, followed by exposure to laser light within 24 to 48 hours of injection (see Table 34–1).
         a. Results in fluorescence of cancer cells and cell death.
         b. Used for determining extent of disease and response to treatment.
   F. Stereotactic surgery—method of precisely locating specific sites within brain tissue (see Table 34–1).
      1. Treatment planning and intervention incorporate the use of:
         a. A head frame that provides for rigid skull fixation.
         b. An arc-quadrant that attaches to the head frame providing direction to treatment instrumentation to the localized intracranial target.
         c. Stereotactic data acquisition and processing system that includes the use of various imaging modalities and computer technology to process information regarding the geometric configuration, volume, and extent of the tumor.
         d. A surgical tool to be used to treat the tumor.
   G. Laparoscopic resection—the use of a laparoscope to visualize, reach, and remove tumor through several small incisions (see Table 34–1). Currently under experimental use for localized abdominal tumors.

IV. Safety measures in the delivery of surgery.
   A. Aseptic techniques are used to reduce the risks of infection.
      1. Skin preparation to specific surgical site.
      2. Sterile techniques during procedures.
      3. Wound dressings.
   B. Type of anesthesia is selected based on client preference, previous response to anesthesia, physical and mental history, type and duration of procedure, surgical site, and positioning during the surgical procedure.
   C. Electrical hazards are prevented by proper grounding plate placement within the operating room and by checking electrical cords, plugs, and outlets.
   D. Client is prepared for the surgery.
      1. Delivery of specific operative site or system preparations such as bowel preparations, medications, or nutritional interventions.
      2. Positioning during the surgical procedure to prevent joint damage, muscle stretch or strain, and pressure ulcers.
   E. Informed consent is obtained.
      1. The nature of and reason for surgery is explained.
      2. All available options and risks associated with each option are discussed.
      3. Risks of the surgical procedure and administration of anesthesia are described.
      4. Potential benefits and outcomes of the treatment are explained.

Assessment

I. Pertinent personal history.
   A. Factors that may increase the incidence of complications of surgery.
      1. Presence of preexisting cardiovascular, pulmonary, renal, neurologic, musculoskeletal, gastrointestinal, or liver disease.
      2. Previous surgical history—type of surgery; experience with anesthetic agents, blood transfusions, and surgical complications.
      3. Lifestyle activities such as tobacco use, alcohol ingestion, illegal medications use, or abuse of over-the-counter medications.
      4. Previous cancer therapy and the length of time since therapy was completed.
      5. Present medications.
      6. Allergies.
      7. Physiologic changes of aging (Table 34–4).
   B. Factors that may influence discharge planning.
      1. Home environment.
      2. Financial status.
      3. Self-care capabilities.
      4. Anticipated changes in self-care capabilities resulting from surgery.
      5. Support personnel or services available and patterns of use.
      6. Employment status and type of work.
II. Physical examination.
   A. Cardiovascular—heart rate and rhythm, blood pressure, presence and quality of regional pulses, color and temperature of regional extremities.
   B. Pulmonary—respiratory rate, depth, and rhythm; lung expansion; posture.
   C. Renal—color and odor of urine; urinary elimination patterns; previous urinary output.

TABLE 34–4. **Physiologic Changes Related to the Aging Process That Can Affect Surgery**

Physiologic Changes	Effects	Potential Postoperative Complications
Cardiovascular		
↓Elasticity of blood vessels	↓Circulation to vital organs Slower blood flow	Shock (hypotension), thrombosis with pulmonary emboli, delayed wound healing, postoperative confusion, hypervolemia, decreased response to stress
↓Cardiac output		
↓Peripheral circulation		
Respiratory		
↓Elasticity of lungs and chest wall	↓Vital capacity	Atelectasis, pneumonia, postoperative confusion
↓Residual lung volume	↓Alveolar volume	
↓Forced expiratory volume	↓Gas exchange	
↓Ciliary action	↓Cough reflex	
Fewer alveolar capillaries		
Urinary		
↓Glomerular filtration rate	↓Kidney function Stasis of urine in bladder Loss of urinary control	Prolonged response to anesthesia and drugs, overhydration with intravenous fluids, hyperkalemia, urinary tract infection, urinary incontinence
↓Bladder muscle tone		
Weakened perineal muscles		
Musculoskeletal		
↓Muscle strength	↓Activity	Atelectasis, pneumonia, thrombophlebitis, constipation, or fecal impaction
Limitation of motion		
Gastrointestinal		
↓Intestinal motility	Retention of feces	Constipation or fecal impaction
Metabolic		
↓Gamma globulin level	↓Inflammatory response	Delayed wound healing, wound dehiscence or evisceration
↓Plasma proteins		
Immune System		
Fewer killer T cells	↓Ability to protect against invasion by pathogenic microorganisms	Wound infection, wound dehiscence, pneumonia, urinary tract infection
↓Response to foreign antigens		

From Keeling, A.W., Muro, G.A., & Long, B.C. (1995). Preoperative nursing. In W.J. Phipps, V.I. Cassmeyer, J.K. Sands, & M.K. Lehman (eds.). *Medical-Surgical Nursing: Concepts and Clinical Practice* (5th ed.). St. Louis: Mosby-Year Book, p. 595.

D. Gastrointestinal—color, consistency, and caliber of stool; bowel elimination patterns.
E. Mobility—muscle strength and endurance, range of motion; gait; activity level.
F. Nutrition—weight; skin turgor; amount, content, and patterns of nutritional intake.
G. Comfort level.
III. Psychosocial examination.
A. Explore client and family concerns.
1. Meaning attached to the loss of body part and/or functioning.
2. Expectations related to the procedure, such as pain, disability, or survival.
3. Perceived impact of surgery on lifestyle and relationships.
B. Assess the client's and family's current level of coping.
1. Coping strategies used in previous illnesses or times of stress.
2. Support systems available and patterns of use.
3. Community resources available and patterns of use.
IV. Critical laboratory and diagnostic data unique to surgery.
A. Cardiovascular—electrocardiogram (ECG).
B. Hematologic—complete blood count, prothrombin time, and partial thromboplastin time.
C. Hepatic—liver function studies.
D. Renal—urinalysis, blood urea nitrogen, creatinine, and electrolytes.
E. Pulmonary—chest x-ray examination.
F. Nutritional—serum albumin.

Nursing Diagnoses

I. Pain.
II. Impaired skin integrity.
III. Ineffective airway clearance.
IV. Altered nutrition, less than body requirements.
V. Knowledge deficit.
VI. Anxiety.

Outcome Identification

I. Client and family describe the type of and rationale for surgery.
II. Client and family list potential immediate and long-term complications of the surgery.
III. Client describes self-care measures to decrease the incidence and severity of complications of surgery.
IV. Client demonstrates new self-care skills demanded by structural or functional effects of surgery.
V. Client and family describe schedule and procedures for routine follow-up care.
VI. Client and family list changes in condition that should be reported to the health care team.
A. Signs and symptoms of infection.
B. Persistent nausea, vomiting, or a decrease in appetite.
C. Poor wound healing.
D. Changes in bowel or bladder patterns.
E. Changes in location or increased severity of pain or intolerance to discomfort.
F. Inability to resume functional ability within anticipated time frame.

VII. Client and family identify potential community resources to meet unique demands of therapy and rehabilitation.

Planning and Implementation

I. Interventions to maximize safety for the client and family.
  A. Implement the preoperative medical preparation regimen as ordered.
    1. Dietary restrictions.
    2. Bowel preparation.
    3. Skin preparation.
  B. Use aseptic or clean technique, as indicated, for invasive procedures such as insertion of tubes, drains, or intravenous lines.
II. Interventions to decrease incidence and severity of complications unique to surgery.
  A. Ineffective airway clearance.
    1. Teach turning, coughing, and deep breathing (TCDB) techniques to the client and family and schedule activities postoperatively.
    2. Demonstrate use of incentive spirometry.
    3. Use suction devices to assist the client to remove mucus or sputum.
  B. Impaired skin integrity.
    1. Assist the client to turn and shift positions in bed every 2 hours.
    2. Massage uninjured areas gently.
    3. Use mattress overlays such as therapeutic foam mattress, alternating air mattress, or water mattress or specialty beds such as low-airflow, air-fluidized, or kinetic therapy for high-risk clients.
    4. Establish a schedule for changing the surgical dressing.
    5. Use protective film, hydrocolloid barriers, and/or collection devices around drains or tubes with copious drainage.
    6. Encourage early ambulation.
  C. Pain (acute).
    1. Teach splinting of incision during TCBD or with movement.
    2. Use nonpharmacologic methods for pain control:
      a. Progressive muscle relaxation.
      b. Guided imagery.
      c. Music.
      d. Massage.
      e. Diversional activities.
    3. Administer analgesic and antiemetic medications as ordered by the physician.
  D. Anxiety.
    1. Allow the client and family to discuss feelings, fears, and concerns.
    2. Provide client and family teaching.
      a. Plan of care and rationale for procedures.
      b. Anticipated care settings, equipment, and experiences related to surgery.
      c. Self-care strategies to prevent or minimize complications of surgery.
    3. Encourage use of coping strategies that have been effective in the past during times of stress.
    4. Allow for adequate rest periods between care activities.
III. Interventions to monitor for unique complications of surgery.
  A. Ineffective airway clearance.
    1. Assess the client on a routine basis for changes in respiratory effort, rate, rhythm, and for subjective responses to breathing.

    2. Inspect chest wall for symmetrical movement, use of accessory muscles, diaphragmatic breathing, and sternal retraction.

    3. Auscultate lungs for adventitious or absent breath sounds.

  B. Impaired skin integrity.

    1. Assess incision site for redness, swelling, increased drainage, discomfort, and approximation of surgical margins.

    2. Assess bony prominences for areas remaining red 30 minutes or longer after pressure is relieved.

  C. Altered nutrition, less than body requirements.

    1. Assess for return of bowel sounds.

    2. Assess for physical signs of dehydration—color and moisture of mucous membranes; skin turgor.

    3. Assess fluid loss via incisional or fistular wounds, urinary output, and tube drainage or drain output.

    4. Assess intake and output ratio.

    5. Weigh the client daily.

    6. Evaluate tolerance to progressive diet—appetite, amount and type of foods eaten, and responses to eating.

    7. Monitor laboratory parameters of nutritional status.

IV. Interventions to enhance adaptation and rehabilitation.

  A. Implement postoperative teaching plan that includes changes in self-care activities and activities resulting from surgery, progressive return to maximal level of activity, anticipated discharge medications, wound management, proper use of assistive or prosthetic devices, community resources available for home care, plans for follow-up care, contact person if questions arise, and changes in condition to report to the health care team.

  B. Involve the client and family in assessment, planning, and evaluation of care through transition periods.

  C. Instruct the client and family about rehabilitation programs available such as physical and occupational therapy, speech therapy, ostomy outpatient clinics, and prosthetic fitting services.

  D. Refer the client and family to support programs available such as Reach to Recovery, ReCon Group, Voicemasters, Make Today Count, International Association of Laryngectomees, and United Ostomy Association chapters.

  E. Refer the client and family to professional counselors as indicated.

Evaluation

The oncology nurse systematically and regularly evaluates the client's and/or family's responses to interventions to determine progress toward the achievement of expected outcomes. Relevant data are collected and actual findings are compared with expected findings. Nursing diagnoses, outcomes, and plans of care are reviewed and revised as necessary.

BIBLIOGRAPHY

Bertsch, D., Burak, W.E., Jr., Young, D.C. et al. (1995). Radioimmunoguided surgery system improves survival for patients with recurrent colorectal cancer. *Surgery 118*(4), 634–638.

DeVita, V., Jr., Hellman, S., & Rosenberg, S. (eds.). (1993). *Cancer: Principles and Practice of Oncology* (4th ed.). Philadelphia: J.B. Lippincott.

Drake, D.B., & Oishi, S.N. (1995). Wound healing considerations in chemotherapy and radiation therapy. *Clin Plast Surg 22*(1), 31–37.

Exelby, P. (1993). Pediatric surgical oncology. Introduction. *Semin Surg Oncol 9*(6), 459–460.

Greene, F. (1993). Laparoscopic surgery in cancer treatment. *Important Adv Oncol* 157–166.

Groenwald, S.L., Frogge, M.H., Goodman, M., & Yarbro, C.H. (eds.). (1993). *Cancer Nursing: Principles and Practice* (2nd ed.). Boston: Jones & Bartlett.

Hagle, M., Mioduszewski-McDonagh, J., & Rapp, C. (1994). Patients with long-term vascular access devices: Care and complications. *Orthop Nurs 13*(5), 41–52.

Hammerhofer-Jereb, K. (1996). Laparoscopic bowel resection? *RN 59*(3), 22–25.

Harlow, S.P., Rodriguez-Bigas, M., Mang, T., & Petrelli, N.J. (1995). Intraoperative photodynamic therapy as an adjunct to surgery for recurrent rectal cancer. *Ann Surg Oncol 2*(3), 228–232.

Hassenbusch, S. (1995). Surgical management of cancer pain. *Neurosurg Clin North Am 6*(1), 127–134.

Jako, G. (1987). The road toward 21st century surgery: New strategies and initiatives in cancer treatment. *Lasers Surg Med 7*(3), 217–228.

Keeling, A.W., Muro, G.A., & Long, B.C. (1995). Preoperative nursing. In W.J. Phipps, V.I. Cassmeyer, J.K. Sands, & M.K. Lehman (eds.). *Medical-Surgical Nursing: Concepts and Clinical Practice* (5th ed.). St. Louis: Mosby-Year Book, pp. 589–605.

Markman, M. (1995). Surgery for support and palliation in patients with malignant disease. *Semin Oncol 22*(2[suppl 3]), 91–94.

Nag, S., Petty, L.R. & Parrott, S. (1994). Comprehensive surgical radiation oncology. *AORN J 60*(1), 27–37.

Otto, S. (1994). *Oncology Nursing* (2nd ed.). St. Louis: Mosby-Year Book.

Polomano, R., Weintraub, F.N., & Wurster, A. (1994). Surgical critical care for cancer patients. *Semin Oncol Nurs 10*(3), 165–176.

Sliney, D., & Trokel, S. (1993). *Medical Lasers and Their Safe Use.* New York: Springer-Verlag.

Springfield, D. (1993). Surgical wound healing. *Cancer Treat Res 67,* 81–98.

Weintraub, F., & Neumark, D. (1996). Surgical oncology. In R. McCorkle, M. Grant, M. Frank-Stromborg, & S. Baird (eds.). *Cancer Nursing: A Comprehensive Textbook* (2nd ed.). Philadelphia: W.B. Saunders, pp. 315–330.

Nursing Implications of Radiation Therapy

Ellen Sitton, RN, MSN, OCN, RT(T)

Theory

I. Principles of radiation.
  A. Radiation is energy emitted and transferred through matter or space. Not all radiations are harmful to the tissues.
    1. Examples of radiation: heat, radiowaves, light, x-rays, gamma rays.
    2. Ionizing radiation has sufficient energy to eject one or more orbital electrons from an atom or molecule, changing a stable atom to an ionized, unstable atom. Ionizing radiation interacts with tissues → physical changes → chemical changes → biologic changes.
    3. X-rays and gamma rays and cosmic radiation are ionizing radiations.
    4. Forms of ionizing radiation.
      a. Electromagnetic: radiation in the form of energy waves. Includes photons (x-rays and gamma rays).
      b. Particulate: radiation in the form of subatomic particles. Includes electrons, protons, neutrons, alpha particles, beta particles.
    5. Radiation therapy (RT) is the treatment of disease with ionizing radiation.
  B. Radiobiology is the study of events that occur after ionizing radiation is absorbed by a living organism or cell.
    1. Biologic effects of ionizing radiation.
      a. Cellular targets—the target, or most critical site for radiation damage, is believed to be the deoxyribonucleic acid (DNA). Damage to DNA may lead to cell alteration and/or death.
      b. Cells can successfully repair some radiation damage.
    2. Somatic changes—alterations that occur in the irradiated tissues.
    3. Hereditary changes—potential damage resulting from changes in the individual's reproductive cells (ova and sperm). Hereditary change is associated with the offspring of irradiated individuals.
    4. Normal tissue and tumor are affected by ionizing radiation. Time in which biologic changes appear and the nature and severity of effects depend on the amount of radiation absorbed, fractionation, and rate at which it is administered. Acute- and late-responding tissues are affected differently by these factors.
      a. Possible response of a cell exposed to ionizing radiation.
        (1) Unaffected—no damage in the critical site or target.

(2) Repair—damage is not sufficient to be lethal and recovery is possible with sufficient time, energy, and nutrients.

(3) Cell death—sufficient damage in critical target to be lethal; death occurs when the cell attempts to divide (reproductive death) or immediately during interphase (e.g., lymphocytes, serous acini of parotid glands, lacrimal glands).

b. Radiosensitivity—all normal and cancer cells are vulnerable to effects of radiation and may be injured or destroyed by RT. Cells vary in sensitivity to radiation. Generally, rapidly dividing cells, both normal and cancer cells, are most sensitive (e.g., mucosa) and are referred to as *radiosensitive*. Nondividing or slowly dividing cells are generally less radiosensitive, or *radioresistant* (e.g., muscle cells, neurons) (Table 35–1).

c. Normal tissue response.

(1) Tissue tolerance—normal tissues can tolerate a limited amount of radiation. Dose of radiation to a tumor is limited by the tolerance of the normal tissues in the volume of tissue irradiated. Doses of radiation above the tolerance dose result in permanent injury or death of tissue.

(2) A course of RT is planned to deliver a dose high enough to destroy the tumor in the primary site and surrounding lymph nodes at risk for cancer while not exceeding the tolerance of the normal tissues in the radiation field (or portal).

(3) Side effects and sequelae of RT are generally the result of the effect of radiation on normal tissues.

(4) Early and late tissue responses—all normal tissues do not respond to irradiation the same way (Table 35–2).

(a) Early side effects occur during RT or weeks or months after RT and generally heal after the RT course. They are usually exhibited first by tissues with rapidly proliferating cells (e.g., gastrointestinal mucosa, bone marrow). These tissues are considered acutely responding tissues and generally demonstrate early side effects. The severity of this early response to irradiation is not a predictor of severity of late response.

TABLE 35–1. **Relative Radiosensitivity of Various Tumors and Tissues**

Tumors/Tissues	Relative Radiosensitivity
Lymphoma Leukemia Seminoma Dysgerminoma	High
Squamous cell cancer of the oropharyngeal, glottic, bladder, skin, and cervical epithelia; adenocarcinomas of the alimentary tract	Fairly high
Vascular and connective tissue elements of all tumors; secondary neurovascularization, astrocytomas	Medium
Salivary gland tumors, hepatoma, renal cancer, pancreatic cancer, chondrosarcoma, osteogenic sarcoma	Fairly low
Rhabdomyosarcoma, leiomyosarcoma, and ganglioneurofibrosarcoma	Low

From Rubin, P. (ed.). (1983). Principles of radiation oncology and cancer radiotherapy. In *Clinical Oncology for Medical Students and Physicians.* New York: American Cancer Society.

TABLE 35–2. **Response to Radiation: Acute/Late Responding**

Acute-responding Tissues	Subacute-responding Tissues	Late-responding Tissues
Bone marrow, ovary, testis, lymph node, salivary gland, small bowel, stomach, colon, oral mucosa, larynx, esophagus, arterioles, skin, bladder, capillaries, vagina	Lung, liver, kidney, heart, spinal cord, brain	Lymph vessels, thyroid, pituitary, breast, bone cartilage, pancreas, uterus, bile ducts

Data from Hall, E.J., & Cox, J.D. (1994). Physical and biologic basis of radiation therapy. In J.D. Cox (ed.). *Moss' Radiation Oncology: Rationale, Technique, Results* (7th ed.). St. Louis: Mosby-Year Book, pp. 3–65.

  (b) Late effects occur months to years after RT and are permanent. Tissues composed of slowly proliferating cells develop injury slowly (e.g., central and peripheral nervous system, kidney, dermis, cartilage, bone).

  (c) Subacute-responding tissues show few, if any, early effects but demonstrate damage in weeks to a few months after RT.

  (d) Late-responding tissues (e.g., spinal cord, peripheral nerves, kidney, dermis, cartilage, bone) generally demonstrate little evidence of early effects and show late effects months to years after RT.

 (5) Cancer cells originating from rapidly growing normal cells are generally relatively radiosensitive and can be destroyed with lower doses than cancer cells originating from radioresistant cells.

 d. Tissue response to fractionation.

  (1) External beam irradiation—a total dose tolerated by the tissues in the irradiated field is prescribed and is fractionated, or divided, into daily doses (usually 180–200 cGy/day). High dose per fraction and large total doses have been shown to be related to increased severity of late effects.

  (2) Radioactive source therapy—a total dose tolerated by the tissues in the irradiated area is prescribed. This dose may be given over several days as a continuous application (low-dose rate) or in a single or several doses over several minutes (high-dose rate).

  (3) Excessive prolongation of treatment allows surviving tumor cells to proliferate during treatment.

  (4) Well oxygenated tissues are generally more sensitive to radiation than hypoxic cells.

  (5) Mitosis is the most sensitive phase of the cell cycle followed by G_2.

II. RT fundamentals.

 A. Approximately 50% of clients treated for cancer are treated with RT during the course of the disease.

 B. Goals of RT include delivering a precise dose of ionizing radiation to a defined volume of tissue and minimizing the dose to normal tissue in the treated volume.

 C. Aims of radiation treatments.

  1. Cure. Purpose—kill all cells in a malignant tumor capable of cell division while limiting the dose to the normal tissues. The client is expected to have a normal life span and systematic follow-up evaluation for late effects of RT.

2. Control. Purpose—limit the growth and spread of disease. The client is expected to have a period of symptom-free time.
3. Palliation. Purpose—improve quality of life by reducing or relieving symptoms or impending complications (e.g., relief of pain from bony metastasis, treatment of impending cord compression, relief of superior vena cava syndrome, decreasing obstruction, reduction/relief of symptoms from brain metastasis). Life span is not expected to be extended.
D. Methods of delivery of RT.
  1. Local treatment.
    a. External beam treatment machines in radiation oncology (teletherapy).
      (1) Linear accelerator (may treat with x-rays and/or electrons).
        (a) X-rays: intermediate to deep treatment (depth of penetration varies with energy).
        (b) Electron beam: shallow treatment (spares deeper tissues; depth of penetration varies with energy; high skin doses).
      (2) Cobalt-60.
        (a) Radioactive source: emission of gamma rays.
    b. Radioactive source therapy: brachytherapy.
      (1) Beta particles and gamma rays from sealed radioactive sources.
  2. Systemic treatment.
    a. Radioactive source therapy: radiopharmaceutical therapy.
      (1) Beta particles and gamma rays from unsealed radioactive sources.
E. Progress and innovations in radiation oncology.
  1. Combined modality treatment.
    a. RT and chemotherapy (pre-RT, concurrent, post-RT).
    b. Intraoperative RT.
    c. Radioimmunotherapy (RIT).
    d. Hyperthermia and RT.
  2. 3D-conformal RT (e.g., 6-field conformal prostate RT).
  3. Arc RT (e.g., stereotactic radiosurgery).
  4. Gamma knife.
  5. Altered fractionation (e.g., twice daily [BID] fractionation, high dose rate).
  6. Total body irradiation.
  7. Total skin electron irradiation.
  8. Particle beam therapy (e.g., neutron therapy, proton therapy).
  9. Chemical modification (radiosensitizers and radioprotectors).
III. Teletherapy (external beam RT).
  A. Precise dose delivered to the client from outside the body.
  B. Treatment process.
    1. Client consultation.
    2. Simulation—x-ray examination made to simulate treatment volume. Immobilization devices prn. Treatment marks placed on skin or immobilization device (e.g., mask). Computed tomography (CT), magnetic resonance imaging (MRI), and other modalities are used for tumor localization to plan fields.
    3. CT planning—may be used to precisely locate treatment fields.
    4. Treatment planning—computerized treatment plan developed. Based on pathology of tumor, location, number of fields, radiosensitivity of tumor and normal tissue in treatment volume, goal.
    5. Client education.
    6. Client treatment and follow-up.

RADIOACTIVE ATOM

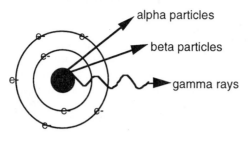

Figure 35–1. Radioactive atom.

IV. Radioactive source therapy.
   A. Radioactivity.
      1. Definition—radioactivity, or radioactive decay, is the spontaneous emission of highly energetic particles (alpha and/or beta) or rays (gamma) from the nuclei of an element (radioisotope) (Fig. 35–1).
      2. Alpha particles—large particles; not used in brachytherapy.
         Beta particles (β)—characteristics similar to electrons; less penetrating than gamma rays.
         Gamma rays (γ)—same as x-rays; penetrating.
      3. Energy—each radioactive element radiates energy as particles and/or rays that are characteristic for that element. Some elements emit particles and/or rays with energies that are more penetrating than others and therefore require more shielding to absorb the radiation. Shielding is measured in centimeters of lead (Pb). Half-value layer (HVL) blocks half of the radiation (Table 35–3).
      4. Half-life—proportion of atoms that disintegrate in a given time is predictable. The time required for one half of the atoms of a given quantity of radioactive material to decay is the physical half-life. Important in unsealed source RT.
      5. Units of measurement (Table 35–4).
         a. Radiation therapy—radiation absorbed dose; gray (Gy), rad.
         b. Radiation protection—dose equivalent; Sievert measure or roentgen-equivalent–man (REM).
         c. Radioactive material—activity; Becquerel, Curie.
   B. Treatment with radioactive sources (Fig. 35–2).
      1. Selection of type and method depends on client and disease factors.
         a. Sealed sources (brachytherapy).

TABLE 35–3. **Characteristics of Radioactive Elements**

Radioactive Elements			
Element	**Half-life**	**Energy**	**HVL (cm Pb)**
Cesium 137 (^{137}Cs)	30.0 years	0.66 MeV (γ)	0.65 cm
Iridium 192 (^{192}Ir)	74.2 days	0.35 MeV (γ)	0.3 cm
Iodine 131 (^{131}I)	8.0 days	0.36 MeV (γ)	0.3 cm
Iodine 125 (^{125}I)	60.2 days	0.03 MeV (γ)	0.4 cm
Strontium 89 (^{89}Sr)	50.5 days	1.46 MeV (β)	(1 mm of lead blocks 100% of ^{89}Sr)

MeV = million electron volts; HVL = half-value layer

TABLE 35–4. **Units of Measurement**

Absorbed Dose (gray, rad)
1 Gy = 100 rad   100 cGy = 100 rad
Therapeutic doses are prescribed in Gy or cGy

Dose Equivalent (Sievert, rem)
(1 Sv = 100 rem)
Badge readings are in mrem (millirem)

Activity (Becquerel, Curie)
1 Bq = 2.7×10^{-11} Ci = 1 dps   1 Ci = 3.7×10^{10} dps

    (1) Dose rate—low dose rate (LDR), high dose rate (HDR).
    (2) Type—intracavitary, interstitial, intraluminal.
  b. Unsealed sources (radiopharmaceutical therapy).
    (1) Dose—therapeutic dose (tracer dose for diagnostic tests).
2. Sealed sources (brachytherapy)—treatment of tumors with radioactive sources placed either temporarily or permanently adjacent to the tumor (intracavitary or surface application), into the tumor (interstitial application), or into a lumen (intraluminal).
  a. Primary advantage is ability to deliver a high dose of radiation to a small volume of tumor while delivering limited dose to adjacent normal tissues. Can be delivered over a period of several days (e.g., LDR) or in a few minutes (e.g., HDR).
  b. Radioactive material is sealed in a container and never comes in direct contact with the client. Energy of the radiation penetrates through the container to treat the client. When the sealed source is removed from the client, the client no longer requires radiation precautions. Sealed sources are used for LDR and HDR brachytherapy.
  c. An LDR remote afterloading device uses computer-controlled loading and unloading of sources from the client from outside the client's

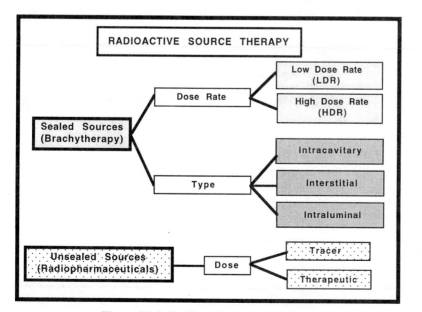

Figure 35–2. Radioactive source therapy.

room to reduce the exposure to the staff to a negligible amount near 0. Physician prescribes treatment in number of hours that the sources are loaded in the client. Each treatment generally lasts several days.

   d. HDR machines are remote afterloading devices and generally use one highly radioactive computer-controlled source to treat clients. They may only be used where adequate shielding is available. Each treatment lasts only a few minutes. Client is not radioactive after the source is removed.

   e. Principles of time, distance, and shielding are utilized to minimize exposure to the staff and visitors.

3. Unsealed sources (radiopharmaceutical therapy)—radioactive materials are administered intravenously (IV), orally, or into a body cavity and result in uptake of the radioactive element into various parts of the body, depending upon the element and the form in which it is administered. Radioactivity may be distributed fairly uniformly over the body or may concentrate in specific organs.

   a. Therapeutic dose—a dose of radiation high enough to treat the tumor. Aim is to deliver a predetermined dose to an organ or area of the body to treat the area with radiation.

   b. Tracer dose—used for diagnostic tests (e.g., bone, liver, and thyroid scans). Dose is very low and client is generally released from the hospital after the test.

IV. Radiation safety and protection.

  A. Dose limitation—radiation protection.

    1. Dose limits are applied to all individuals. Different limits are applied to occupationally exposed radiation workers.

      a. ALARA (as low as reasonably achievable)—the best radiation protection guide is to keep radiation exposure as low as reasonably achievable. Radiation should be continually monitored and controlled.

      b. EDE (effective dose equivalent)—exposure to ionizing radiation from artificial sources is controlled by law (Table 35–5).

  B. Radiation monitoring.

    1. Personnel monitoring—individuals working in a restricted area should wear a personal monitor to measure radiation dose (e.g., film badge). The badge contains a small photographic film and is worn on the trunk of the body. Badges are read and exchanged monthly. Workers should never wear a badge belonging to someone else because doing so does not allow determination of how much exposure each person received. Dosimeters are available to measure radiation exposure; they can be read at the time of exposure.

TABLE 35–5. **Total Effective Dose Equivalent (TEDE)**

Radiation worker (occupational exposure)
   5000 mrem/yr = 5 rem/yr = 50 mSv/yr
Declared pregnant woman worker
   <0.5 rem TEDE to the embryo or fetus over the entire pregnancy.
   (If a pregnant woman does not declare her pregnancy in writing, the limit does not apply.)
Nonradiation worker (general public)
   100 mrem/yr = 0.1 rem/yr = 1 mSv/yr

mrem = millirem; mSV = milliSievert

2. Survey meters (e.g., Geiger counter)—used for surveying the client, room, trash, linen, other after brachytherapy or radiopharmaceutical therapy.
   C. Radiation safety.
   1. Essential considerations in minimizing exposure to radiation—time, distance, and shielding.
      a. Time—minimize the amount of time spent near radioactive sources. Work quickly and efficiently. Rotate staff responsibilities.
      b. Distance—intensity of radiation decreases rapidly as the distance increases. Doubling the distance decreases exposure to one fourth of the exposure received at the original distance (e.g., exposure of 40 mrem/hr at 1 meter is 10 mrem/hr at 2 meters). Staff should work as far away from the source as possible and never touch a source (use long-handled forceps for dislodged sources).
      c. Shielding—the type of shielding and its thickness depend on the type and energy of radioactive source.

Assessment

I. Effective communication.
   A. Barriers to learning (e.g., language, hearing deficit, visual problems).
   B. Cultural issues.
   C. Developmental stage.
II. History and physical assessment.
   A. Cancer history (personal and family).
   B. Previous and current cancer treatment.
   C. Intercurrent disease especially any condition involving tissues included in the radiation treatment volume.
   D. Relevant laboratory data (e.g., white blood count [WBC], hemoglobin, hematocrit levels) and diagnostic data (e.g., results of CT scans, pathology examination, staging).
   E. Current symptoms and other medical conditions (e.g., pregnancy, restricted range of motion [ROM]).
   F. Weight.
III. Psychosocial assessment.
   A. Coping patterns.
   B. Support systems and client's ability to meet transportation and care needs during treatment and follow-up care.
   C. Knowledge and perceptions regarding treatment.
IV. Factors influencing side effects of RT.
   A. Site of radiation field (tissues to be irradiated).
   B. Time-dose-volume relationship (length of treatment, fractionation, volume of tissue irradiated).
   C. Radiosensitivity of tissues in treatment volume and potential early and late side effects.
   D. Radiation type and energy including depth of treatment prescribed.
   E. Nutritional status.
   F. Client adherence to recommended care during RT.
   G. Individual differences between clients.

Nursing Diagnoses

I. Table 35–6 lists common, potential nursing diagnoses for specific sites of irradiation.

TABLE 35–6. **Potential Nursing Diagnoses for Specific Sites**

Site of Irradiation	Potential Nursing Diagnoses
Skin	Risk for impaired skin integrity related to radiation-induced changes
	Body image disturbance related to treatment lines, radiation-induced changes, tattoos
Head and neck	Altered oral mucous membranes related to radiation-induced changes
	Altered nutrition, less than body requirements, related to mucositis, xerostomia, altered taste sensation, and radiation caries
	Impaired physical mobility (temporomandibular joint) related to trismus
	Impaired verbal communication related to vocal cord irradiation, mucositis, and xerostomia
Central nervous system	Risk for injury related to radiation-induced increased intracranial edema
	Body image disturbance related to alopecia
Chest	Altered nutrition, less than body requirements, related to esophagitis
	Risk for infection related to leukopenia
	Risk for injury related to thrombocytopenia
	Ineffective breathing pattern related to radiation pneumonitis and/or fibrosis
	Decreased cardiac output related to cardiotoxicity
	Impaired physical mobility (shoulder joint) related to radiation fibrosis
Abdomen	Altered nutrition, less than body requirements, related to gastritis, nausea, and vomiting
	Diarrhea
	Risk for infection related to leukopenia
	Risk for injury related to thrombocytopenia
	Acute pain related to radiation hepatitis
	Risk for fluid volume deficit related to radiation nephritis
Pelvis	Diarrhea
	Risk for infection related to leukopenia
	Risk for injury related to thrombocytopenia
	Altered urinary elimination related to radiation cystitis
	Sexual dysfunction
	Altered sexuality patterns

II. Commonly used nursing diagnoses include:
  A. Fear.
  B. Knowledge deficit.
  C. Altered nutrition, less than body requirements.
  D. Fatigue.
  E. Pain (acute).
  F. Altered role performance.
  G. Altered growth and development.

Outcome Identification

  I. Client and family describe state of the disease, therapy, and potential side effects of RT.

II. Client and family participate in decision-making process regarding the plan of care and life activities as appropriate.
III. Client participates in self-care measures to minimize occurrence, severity, and complications of side effects of RT.
IV. Client and family participate in measures to minimize fear and anxiety associated with treatment.
V. Client and family report signs and symptoms of early and late side effects of RT to a member of the health care team.
VI. Client and family identify appropriate community and personal resources for information and services.
VII. Client and family describe follow-up plan.

Planning and Implementation

I. Client education and interventions to incorporate client and family in care.
II. Interventions to minimize side effects of RT.
   A. Note incidence and severity of side effects.
   B. Perform nursing assessments and interventions related to area treated (Table 35–7).
III. Interventions to maximize radiation protection and safety with sealed and unsealed source RT.
   A. Exposure—utilize principles of time, distance, and shielding to minimize exposure. Remote afterloading—sources automatically withdrawn from the client and kept in a safe in the machine while staff and visitors are present. Negligible radiation exposure to staff and visitors.
   B. Unsealed sources—blood and body fluids become radioactive. Inpatient rooms are specially prepared by radiation safety staff; plastic covers and absorbent floor coverings. Client may use the toilet and flush it three times after each use to dilute radioactive urine, stool, or vomitus. Client uses disposable dishes. Everything exposed to the client's body fluids is potentially contaminated with radiation. Linens and wastes kept in containers in the room and monitored for radiation before removed. Staff wear gowns and gloves. Before leaving room, staff wash hands with the gloves on and then again after they are removed.
   C. Sealed sources—accountability for all sources must be maintained. Shielded container is placed in room in the event of a dislodged source. Long forceps are used to place sources in the lead container. Dressings at implant site are changed by the physician only. Linens and wastes are kept in containers in the room and surveyed for radiation before being removed. Client and room are surveyed upon removal of the sources.
   D. Shielding—room designation for brachytherapy and radiopharmaceutical therapy depends on the facility and radioactive material being used. Many institutions have specially shielded rooms. Clients generally are in a private room.
   E. Shielding (portable)—portable shields may be placed by the radiation safety officer (RSO) or designee at the bedside. Staff should stand behind the shield if possible when radioactive sources are in the client.
   F. Exposure rate—measurements of exposure rate are generally done at 1 m from the client, on the nonclient side of a portable shield, and at the door of the room by the RSO or designee. Measurement of exposure rates in uncontrolled areas (e.g., room next door) may also be done.

TABLE 35–7. **Side Effects of Radiation Therapy**

Site	Potential Early Effects	Potential Intermediate/Late Effects	Nursing Considerations
Skin	Erythema, pigmentation, dry desquamation, moist desquamation, alopecia	Fibrosis, atrophy, telangiectasis, altered pigmentation, slow healing of trauma, carcinogenesis	*Early effects:* Nonmoist reaction: wash with mild soap and water and use nonirritating moisturizing skin cream or cornstarch in dry areas. Moist desquamation: wash with ¼–½ strength peroxide or wound cleanser and use hydrogel dressing or silver sulfadiazine. Observe for increased reaction in skin folds and with electrons. Observe for increased expected reaction if client has had chemotherapy that enhances skin reaction (e.g., doxorubicin, actinomycin D). *Early and late effects:* Protect skin from chemical, mechanical, thermal irritants/injury, and from sun. (See also Chapter 11.)
Bone marrow	Myelosuppression (especially leukopenia, thrombocytopenia)		Large treatment areas covering significant amounts of bone marrow → increased myelosuppression (see Chapter 12)
Spine		Lhermitte sign; significantly damages growth in axial spine in children	*Late:* Radiation to growing bone decreases growth; monitor growth and development patterns after RT in children. Assess neurologic and sensory functions
Brain	Alopecia, somnolence	Hypothyroidism (if pituitary gland is in field)	*Early:* Use mild shampoo. Moisturizing skin creams as needed. Plan for alopecia (generally temporary) (see Chapter 3). *Late:* Assess neurologic and sensory function
Head and neck Mucosa	Mucositis	Pale mucosa, telangiectasia	Pretreatment dental evaluation. Avoid chemical, thermal, and mechanical irritants to mucosa
Salivary glands	Xerostomia	Xerostomia, dental caries	Dental prophylaxis and fluoride program. Assess for signs/symptoms of hypothyroidism (See Chapter 33 for mucositis, xerostomia, and taste alterations interventions)
Teeth		Radiation dental caries	
Tongue, taste buds	Changes in taste		
Larynx	Laryngitis		
Thyroid		Hypothyroidism	
Bone (mandible)		Osteoradionecrosis	

	Acute effects	Late effects	Nursing interventions
Chest			
Lung	Radiation pneumonitis	Radiation pneumonitis, pulmonary fibrosis	Assess breathing. Assess nutritional status (see Chapter 15, pulmonary toxicity)
Heart		Pericarditis, pancarditis, myocardial infarction	See Chapter 16, cardiovascular toxicity
Esophagus	Esophagitis, dysphagia	Stricture, fistula	See Chapter 13 for dysphagia
Abdomen			
Small bowel	Diarrhea, fat malabsorption, nausea and vomiting	Small bowel obstruction, stricture	Antidiarrheal and antiemetic use; Assess nutritional status; Low-residue diet; Adequate fluids (See Chapter 14 for diarrhea, bowel obstruction)
Stomach	Gastritis, nausea and vomiting 1–2 hours posttreatment		(See Chapter 13 for nausea and vomiting)
Pelvis			
Bladder	Radiation cystitis	Fibrosis	Assess bladder function, bladder analgesic use
Large bowel, rectum	Diarrhea, nausea and vomiting, inflammation of hemorrhoids, tenesmus	Bowel ulceration, inflammation	Antidiarrheal use (see Chapter 14)
Ovaries	Premature menopause	Ovarian failure especially if greater than 25 years; altered sexuality	Before treatment, assess ovarian function. Discuss sperm banking before treatment if azoospermia anticipated. Evaluate impact on client (see Chapter 6)
Testes		Azoospermia	
Vagina	Inflammation, dryness, dyspareunia	Dryness, stenosis, vaginal shortening, dyspareunia	Water-based lubricants (women); Vaginal dilator after treatment
Penis	Inflammation	Erectile dysfunction, urethral stenosis	Assess potency prior to RT (men)
All sites	Fatigue	Carcinogenesis	Fatigue reduction strategies. Follow-up assessment (see Chapter 1 for fatigue interventions)

G. Exposure—client movement within the room may be restricted during the procedure. Unless specifically ordered by the physician, the client is to remain in room. Some clients may be out of bed but may be instructed to stay behind the shields unless using the bathroom. Clients remain in bed when visitors are present.

H. Radiation signs and instructions—radiation warning signs are posted on the door, chart, and client's armband. Information regarding source, exposure rate, specific instructions to nurses and visitors is generally placed in the chart.

I. Contamination or lost sealed source—in the event of possible contamination or loss of a source, the RSO and radiation oncology or nuclear medicine physician are notified immediately.

J. Time—minimize amount of time personnel are in room. Personnel are also rotated when radioactive sources cannot be remote afterloaded. Visitors are restricted in amount of time spent in room.

K. Distance—visitors and personnel (when possible) remain 6 feet from client and behind the shield.

L. Children (under the age of 18) and pregnant visitors and staff are not to enter the room when radioactivity is present.

M. Discharge—release of clients containing radioactive elements is very carefully controlled. Limitations on the quantity of radioactivity and exposure at 1 m. Instructions must be given to the client and significant others.

IV. Interventions to monitor for late effects of RT.

V. Communication of the client's responses with the health care team.

VI. Documentation of interventions and the client's responses.

EVALUATION

The oncology nurse systematically and regularly evaluates the client's and/or family's responses to interventions to determine progress toward the achievement of expected outcomes. Relevant data are collected and actual findings are compared with expected findings. Nursing diagnoses, outcomes, and plans of care are reviewed and revised as necessary.

BIBLIOGRAPHY

Alcarese, F. (1995). Addressing sexual dysfunction following radiation therapy for a gynecologic malignancy. *Oncol Nurs Forum 22*(8), 1227–1232.

Bucholtz, J.D. (1994). Comforting children during radiotherapy. *Oncol Nurs Forum 21*(6), 987–994.

Dow, K.H., Harris, J.R., & Roy, C. (1994). Pregnancy after breast-conserving surgery and radiation therapy for breast cancer. *Monogr Natl Cancer Inst 16*, 131–137.

Dow, K.H., Bucholtz, J.D., Iwamoto, R., et al. (eds.). (1997). *Nursing Care in Radiation Oncology* (2nd ed.). Philadelphia: W.B. Saunders.

Dunne-Daly, C.F. (1994). Brachytherapy. *Cancer Nurs 17*(4), 355–362.

Dunne-Daly, C.F. (1994). Education and nursing care of brachytherapy clients. *Cancer Nurs 17*(5), 434–444.

Dunne-Daly, C.F. (1994). External radiation therapy self-learning module. *Cancer Nurs 17*(2), 156–168.

Dunne-Daly, C.F. (1994). Nursing care and adverse reactions of external radiation therapy: A self-learning module. *Cancer Nurs 17*(3), 236–256.

Dunne-Daly, C.F. (1995). Potential long-term and late effects from radiation therapy. *Cancer Nurs 18*(1), 67–79.

Flanguis, A., Bjorvell, H., & Lind, M.G. (1993). Oral- and pharyngeal-cancer clients' perceived symptoms and health. *Cancer Nurs 16*(3), 214–221.

Forester, B., Kornfeld, D.S., Fleiss, J.L., & Thompson, S. (1993). Group psychotherapy during radiotherapy: Effects on emotional and physical distress. *Am J Psychiatry, 150*, 1700–1706.

Hilderley, L., & Dow, K. (1996). Radiation oncology. In R. McCorkle, M. Grant, M. Frank-Stromborg, & S. Baird (eds.). *Cancer Nursing: A Comprehensive Textbook* (2nd ed.). Philadelphia: W.B. Saunders, pp. 331–358.

Kan, M.K. (1995). Palliation of bone pain in patients with metastatic cancer using strontium-89 (Metastron). *Cancer Nurs 18*(4), 286–291.

Lindsey, A.M., Larson, P.J., Dodd, M.J., et al. (1994). Comorbidity, nutritional intake, social support, weight, and functional status over time in older cancer patients receiving radiotherapy. *Cancer Nurs 17*(2), 113–124.

Poroch, D. (1995). The effect of preparatory patient education on the anxiety and satisfaction of cancer patients receiving radiation therapy. *Cancer Nurs 18*(3), 206–214.

Servodidio, C.A., & Abramson, D.H. (1993). Acute and long-term effects of radiation therapy to the eye in children. *Cancer Nurs 16*(5), 371–381.

Sitton, E.T. (1992). Early and late radiation-induced skin alterations. Part I: Mechanisms of skin changes. *Oncol Nurs Forum 19*(5), 801–808.

Sitton, E.T. (1992). Early and late radiation-induced skin alterations. Part II: Nursing care of irradiated skin. *Oncol Nurs Forum 19*(6), 907–912.

Stewart, F.A., & Van Der Kogel, A.J. (1994). Retreatment tolerance of normal tissues. *Semin Radiat Oncol 4*(2), 103–111.

36

Nursing Implications of Biotherapy

Paula Trahan Rieger, RN, MSN, ANP, CS, OCN

Theory

I. Definition.
  A. Biotherapy—treatment with agents derived from biologic sources and/or those agents able to affect biologic responses.
  B. Biologic response modifiers—agents or approaches that change the relationship between the tumor and host by modifying the biologic response of the host to tumor cells with a resultant therapeutic effect.

II. Goals and approaches.
  A. Diagnosis of cancer.
    1. Monoclonal antibodies (MAbs) are used in the differential diagnosis of cancer.
      a. Classification of leukemias/lymphomas (recognition of cell surface markers).
      b. Identification of tumors with light microscopy.
    2. Radiolabeled monoclonal antibodies (low-dose radioisotopes tagged to MAbs) are used to detect tumors using special scans.
  B. Treatment of cancer.
    1. Cure.
      a. Primary treatment.
        (1) Interferon-alpha for the treatment of chronic myelogenous leukemia.
      b. Adjuvant therapy.
        (1) After surgery to maintain the disease-free interval (e.g., interferon-alpha after surgery in patients with melanoma).
    2. Control or stabilization of disease.
    3. Maintenance therapy.
      a. After chemotherapy to maintain remissions and/or decrease the recurrence of disease (e.g., interferon-alpha after chemotherapy in a patient with multiple myeloma or lymphoma).
    4. Combination therapy.
      a. Other biologic agents.
      b. Chemotherapy.
      c. After surgery.
      d. Radiotherapy.

C. Supportive therapy.
  1. Hematopoietic growth factors after antineoplastic therapy to decrease the incidence and severity of neutropenia, anemia, and thrombocytopenia.
D. Investigational.
  1. The use of biotherapy in many cancers and clinical situations remains under investigation. Many applications currently supported in the literature have not received regulatory (Food and Drug Administration [FDA]) approval.
III. Types of agents and indications. Table 36–1 lists complete information on mechanism of action, indications, side effects, and key nursing considerations for specific agents.
  A. Cytokines—generic term for proteins released by cells that affect the function of other cells.
    1. Interferons (IFNs).
      a. Family of glycoprotein hormones with immunomodulatory, antiproliferative, and antiviral effects.
      b. Regulatory approval for the treatment of hairy-cell leukemia, chronic myelogenous leukemia, acquired immunodeficiency syndrome (AIDS)-related Kaposi's sarcoma, and as adjuvant therapy for patients with melanoma at a high risk for recurrence.
    2. Interleukins (ILs).
      a. "Between leukocytes," protein molecules responsible for the signaling and communication between cells of the immune system.
      b. Regulatory approval—interleukin-2 (IL-2) for the treatment of renal cell cancer.
    3. Hematopoietic growth factors (HGFs).
      a. Family of glycoprotein molecules that regulate the reproduction, maturation, and functional activity of blood cells (see Chapter 10).
      b. Approved by the FDA for use after autologous bone marrow transplantation to enhance marrow engraftment and decrease the incidence of neutropenic fever, for the mobilization of peripheral blood stem cells, and after antineoplastic therapy to decrease the incidence of neutropenic fever and hospitalization and reduce the use of antibiotics.
    4. Tumor necrosis factor (TNF).
      a. Monokine (protein produced by activated monocytes) that causes the hemorrhagic necrosis of cancer cells; mediator of septic shock.
      b. Regulatory approval: remains investigational.
  B. Monoclonal antibodies (MAbs).
    1. Highly specific antibodies produced from a single clone of cells.
    2. Regulatory approval—for use in radiolabeled scans for the detection of disease in patients with colon or ovarian cancer.
  C. Effector cells.
    1. Immune cells (e.g., lymphocytes) removed from the patient by pheresis or from the tumor during surgery, grown outside the body, and readministered as an intravenous infusion.
      a. Lymphokine-activated killer (LAK) cells.
      b. Tumor-derived activated cells (TDAC).
    2. Regulatory approval—remain investigational.
  D. Immunomodulators.
    1. Agents that nonspecifically stimulate the immune system (e.g., bacillus Calmette-Guérin [BCG], levamisole).

TABLE 36–1. **Biologic Agents**

Actions	Clinical Uses	Common Side Effects	Key Nursing Considerations
Alpha (α)-interferon (IFN) *Beta (β)-interferon* *Gamma (γ)-interferon*		*Acute*	
Antiviral activity Antiproliferative activities Immunomodulatory activities	Interferon-alpha 2a (Roferon-A,) is FDA-approved for hairy-cell leukemia, acquired immunodeficiency syndrome (AIDS)-related Kaposi's sarcoma, the treatment of chronic myelogenous leukemia, and chronic hepatitis C Interferon-alpha 2b (Intron-A) is FDA-approved for hairy-cell leukemia, AIDS-related Kaposi's sarcoma, condyloma acuminatum, chronic hepatitis B and C, and as adjuvant therapy for patients with melanoma at high risk for recurrence The use of interferon alpha has shown efficacy in other diseases such as renal cell cancer, melanoma and other hematologic malignancies but it remains investigational	Flu-like syndrome (headaches, fever, chills, arthralgia and myalgia) Nausea and vomiting *Chronic* Fatigue Neurologic Decreased short-term memory Decreased concentration/ attention span Decreased ability to perform mathematical calculations Gastrointestinal Taste changes Anorexia Weight loss Integumentary Dry skin Pruritus Partial alopecia Hematologic Neutropenia Thrombocytopenia	Fatigue, anorexia and malaise may be dose-limiting. Neurotoxicity may necessitate discontinuance of drug Chills usually occur 3–6 hr after administration Premedicate with acetaminophen before IFN administration to prevent flu-like symptoms and every 4 hr as needed after IFN dosing Fever occurs 30–90 min after onset of chills and may peak at 104°F (40°C) for as long as 24 hr Fever and chills may decrease or vary in severity and incidence as treatment cycle progresses Maintain fluid balance Institute fatigue management strategies Institute measures to maintain nutritional status Monitor for mental status changes and institute measures as appropriate
Interleukin-2 (IL-2)			
Supports growth and maturation of subpopulations of T cells Stimulates activity of natural killer (NK) and cytotoxic T cells Induces production of other lymphokines	IL-2 (aldesleukin, Prokine) is FDA-approved for the treatment of renal cell cancer It has also shown clinical efficacy in the treatment of melanoma; however, it remains investigational for this purpose	Constitutional symptoms Fatigue Capillary leak syndrome Nausea and vomiting Anorexia Diarrhea Central nervous system (CNS) changes Skin changes Erythema Dry desquamation Pruritus Rash Altered laboratory test values Hepatic Hematologic Hypocalcemia Hypomagnesemia	Medicate with acetaminophen and nonsteroidal anti-inflammatory drugs (NSAIDs) to control temperature Obtain and monitor: Orthostatic blood pressure/ pulse Daily weights Input and output Perform skin care (see Chapters 1 and 11) Institute measures to manage fatigue Institute measures to maintain nutritional status Institute measures to maintain fluid balance
Interleukin-1 (IL-1)			
Induces release of lymphokines from activated T cells, fibroblasts Mediates inflammatory response Hematologic effects	Investigational Clinical trials have evaluated its myeloprotective effects post-chemotherapy and effects as an antitumor agent	Constitutional symptoms Hypotension Phlebitis with peripheral administration	Monitor orthostatic blood pressure Dilute with human serum albumin (HSA) after initial reconstitution Medicate with acetaminophen to control flu-like symptoms
Interleukin-4 (IL-4)			
Stimulates growth of resting B cells Stimulates mast cells Regulates growth and differentiation of hematopoietic bone marrow stem cells	Investigational (antitumor effects)	Constitutional symptoms Nasal congestion *High Doses* Capillary leak-type syndrome Rare—skin rashes	Premedicate for chills and fever Monitor vital signs and orthostatic blood pressure Obtain daily weights
Interleukin-6 (IL-6)			
Differation effects on both T and B cells Effects on hematopoiesis Increases production of acute-phase proteins	Investigational status for hematopoietic effects, antitumor effects	Constitutional symptoms Hyperglycemia Transient anemia	Premedicate with acetaminophen and indomethacin to control flu-like symptoms May require blood glucose monitoring

TABLE 36–1. **Biologic Agents** *Continued*

Actions	Clinical Uses	Common Side Effects	Key Nursing Considerations
Retinoids			

Isotretinoin
13-*cis*-retinoic acid
Tretinoin
all-*trans*-retinoic acid
Vitamin A derivatives with biologic effects in vision, growth, reproduction, epithelial cell differentiation, and immune function
	Tretinoin FDA-approved for the treatment of acute promyelocytic leukemia
	Investigational use as chemopreventive agent in the treatment of oral premalignancies, prevention of secondary squamous cell cancers (head, neck, and lung)
		Teratogenesis
		Headache
		Irritability
		Skin changes
		  Desquamation
		  Dryness
		  Dry and cracked lips
		  Sun sensitivity
		  Alopecia
		Joint pain
		Fatigue
		Dryness of the eyes and mucous membranes
			Should not be used during pregnancy
			Women of childbearing age should be counseled to practice effective contraception
			Protective measures should be used when out in the sun
			Liberal use of skin and lip emollients
			Acetaminophen or NSAIDs for arthralgias

Tumor Necrosis Factor (TNF)			

Causes cell death by arrest at G_2 phase
Damages vascular epithelium in tumor capillaries, resulting in hemorrhage and necrosis of tumor cells
Enhances coagulation and depresses anticoagulation
Mediates septic shock reaction
	TNF remains under clinical investigation	Flu-like syndrome
		Chills occur 1–6 hr after administration of agent; can progress to rigors
		Fever occurs 30–60 min after onset of chills and usually peaks 1–2 hr after administration
		Cardiopulmonary
		  Orthostatic hypotension
		Gastrointestinal
		  Nausea
		  Vomiting
		  Anorexia
		Hepatic (doses $>50~\mu g/m^2$)
		  Elevated transaminases
		  Hypertriglyceridemia
		  Transient increases in coagulation factors
		  Decreased cholesterol
		  Hyperbilirubinemia
		Hematologic (doses $>100~\mu g/m^2$)
		  Reversible neutropenia
		  Reversible thrombocytopenia
		  Reversible monocytosis
		Other
		  Pain at tumor site
		  Erythema at SQ injection site
		  Weight loss
		
		Rare
		Neurologic
		  Seizures
		  Confusion
		  Aphasia
		  Dyspnea
			Treat chills immediately, at onset, with meperidine hydrochloride intravenously as ordered by physician
			Offer meperdine or morphine as a premedication with ensuing doses of TNF (if allergic or refractory to meperidine, use diphenhydramine or morphine sulfate as an alternative as ordered by physician)
			Administer acetaminophen as a premedication and every 4 hr as needed
			Monitor vital signs frequently in clients receiving doses greater than 100 $\mu g/m^2$
			Treat significant decreases in systolic blood pressure with normal saline solution (250-mL boluses) as ordered by physician
			Monitor changes in coagulation parameters and signs of bleeding
			Monitor blood gases as ordered by physician
			Apply warm soaks or dry heat to TNF injection sites

Monoclonal Antibodies
Cause cell death through interaction with immune responses or by delivery of cytotoxic substances to the cell (e.g., toxins, chemotherapy, radiotherapy)
Recognize tumor-associated antigens
	Differential diagnosis of tumors by pathologist
	Satumomab (Oncoscint CR-OV) FDA-approved for use as a radiolabeled infusion for the detection of colon and ovarian cancer
	Investigational
	  Treatment of cancer
	  Bone marrow transplant
		Potential allergic reactions
		Constitutional symptoms
			Keep emergency drugs at bedside
			Monitor vital signs frequently during first hour of infusion
			Administer drug by infusion pumps

Effector Cells Example: lymphokine-activated killer [LAK] cells or tumor-derived activated (TDAC) cells Target tumor cells	Investigational Primarily in combination with IL-2	Chills Fever	Medicate client for chills with intravenous meperidine Administer acetaminophen for fevers Do not filter cell preparations during administration Agitate drug gently and at intervals to reduce clumping

2. Regulatory agencies have given approval for levamisole used as adjuvant therapy in combination with 5-fluorouracil for the treatment of colon cancer (Dukes' C classification) and BCG administered as an intravesical infusion for the treatment of bladder cancer.
   E. Retinoids.
      1. Vitamin A derivatives that have a significant role in vision, growth, reproduction, epithelial cell differentiation, and immune function.
      2. Regulatory approval has been granted for tretinoin (Vesanoid) for the treatment of patients with acute promyelocytic leukemia (APL).
IV. Production of biologic agents.
   A. Recombinant deoxyribonucleic acid (DNA) technology.
      1. Technique for the production of large amounts of pure protein through insertion of the genetic sequence coding for that protein into an expression system (e.g., bacteria, yeast, mammalian cells).
   B. Hybridoma technology.
      1. Technique for the production of large amounts of pure immunoglobulin (e.g., MAbs). Classic technique fused murine myeloma cells with murine lymphocytes to produce *hybridomas*.
   C. Gene therapy.
      1. Technique in which a functioning gene is inserted into a patient's cells to reverse an acquired genetic defect or to add a new function to the cell.
   D. Growth of effector cells ex vivo.
      1. LAK cells.
      2. TDAC.
V. Rationale for biotherapy.
   A. Theory of immune surveillance.
      1. An intact immune system is able to recognize cancer cells as different from normal cells and can destroy the cancer cells.
      2. Cancer cells are constantly produced by the body and destroyed by the functioning immune system.
      3. Cancer develops when the immune system does not function properly or is unable to recognize cancer cells as foreign.
VI. Mechanisms of action.
   A. Biologic effects are mediated through attachment to cell surface receptors.
   B. Biologic agents are pleiotropic (possessing more than one biologic effect).
   C. Administration of one biologic agent often stimulates or suppresses the production of other biologic agents in vivo.
   D. Mechanisms of action for a biologic agent in a given disease are not generally well understood and most likely differ for use of the same agent (e.g., IFN) in different diseases.
   E. Classification.
      1. Agents that augment, modulate, or restore the immune response of the host.
      2. Agents that have direct antitumor activity (cytotoxic or antiproliferative mechanisms of action).
      3. Agents that have other biologic effects such as affecting the differentiation or maturation of cells or the ability of the tumor cell to metastasize or survive.
VII. Safety measures in the delivery of biotherapy.
   A. Aseptic techniques should be used when preparing and administering biologic agents.

B. Most biologic agents are natural body proteins; however, there are few published studies on the mutagenicity and carcinogenicity of these agents.
  1. Universal precautions are recommended.
  2. Generation of aerosols and direct skin contact with agents fused to chemotherapeutic agents should be avoided (see Chapter 38).
  3. Use isotope-specific guidelines for radioisotopes attached to MAbs (see Chapter 35).
C. Consult pharmacy resource personnel and product literature for specific information regarding preparation, storage, administration guidelines and special precautions, and disposal.
D. Institutional guidelines pertaining to investigational protocols should be consulted when biologic agents are given as part of a clinical research protocol.

Assessment

I. Pertinent personal history.
  A. Assess current medications, especially those that may be contraindicated with biologic agents.
    1. Aspirin.
    2. Steroids. Contraindicated with interleukin-2.
    3. Nonsteroidal anti-inflammatory drugs (NSAIDs).
    4. Medications that may alter mentation or coagulation.
    5. Immunosuppressants.
  B. Disease status—type and stage of cancer.
  C. Assess for chronic illnesses that may be exacerbated by side effects associated with biologic therapy—heart disease, diabetes, neurologic or psychiatric disorders, pulmonary disease, hypertension, and psoriasis.
  D. Assess history of and response to prior cancer therapies.
  E. Allergies.
II. Physical examination.
  A. Before initiation of therapy (to serve as a baseline for comparison), and at regular intervals during the course of therapy to evaluate tolerance to therapy, the patient should have a thorough physical assessment by body system:
    1. Cardiovascular—heart rate and rhythm, abnormal heart sounds, blood pressure, and orthostatic blood pressure (with agents known to cause hypotension).
    2. Pulmonary—respiratory rate, breath sounds, shortness of breath, cyanosis, and clubbing.
    3. Gastrointestinal/nutritional—weight, eating patterns, abdominal girth, mucositis, and xerostomia.
    4. Musculoskeletal—range of motion, functional status, and presence and patterns of arthralgias.
    5. Neurologic—affect, orientation, memory, attention span, social engagement, and sensory perception.
    6. Integumentary—erythema, rash, lesions, injection site reactions, dryness, decreased turgor, and alopecia.
    7. General—presence of fever and flulike symptoms, fatigue.
III. Psychosocial examination.
  A. Assess baseline mental status.
  B. Assess current social structure, including support systems, primary caretaker, housing and living arrangements, and work status.

C. Assess type, number, and effectiveness of previous coping strategies used by client and family.
D. Determine response to illness and emotional state.
E. Assess ability to perform self-care activities (especially important if therapy is to be administered in the ambulatory setting).
F. Consider financial status—need for referral to social worker or access to pharmaceutical company reimbursement assistance programs.
G. Assess cultural factors and health-related beliefs.
IV. Evaluation of laboratory data.
A. Hematologic—white blood count, differential, hemoglobin, and hematocrit levels, and platelet count.
B. Renal function—blood urea nitrogen (BUN) and creatinine levels.
C. Liver function—lactate dehydrogenase (LDH), alkaline phosphatase, serum glutamic-oxaloacetic transaminase (SGOT), serum glutamate pyruvic transaminase (SGPT), and bilirubin levels.
D. Nutritional parameters—electrolytes, protein, and albumin levels.
E. Diagnostic and staging results.
V. Client and family perceptions of treatment goals and demands.
A. Treatment goals (e.g., diagnostic, therapeutic, supportive or investigational).
B. Obligations of treatment such as length of hospitalization, follow-up clinic visits, laboratory and diagnostic test requirements, and financial obligations.
C. Expected side effects of biotherapy.
D. Self-care skills required.

Nursing Diagnoses

I. Table 36–2 lists potential nursing diagnoses seen with the administration of biotherapy.
II. Commonly used nursing diagnoses include:
A. Risk for altered body temperature.
B. Fatigue.
C. Knowledge deficit.
D. Impaired memory.
E. Risk for impaired skin integrity.
F. Altered nutrition, less than body requirements.

Outcome Identification

I. Client and family describe the type of and rationale for treatment with biologic therapy.
II. Client and family receive culturally competent care.
III. Client and family list potential immediate and long-term complications of biotherapy—constitutional symptoms, bone pain, fatigue, anorexia, weight loss or gain, somnolence, confusion, psychosis, chest pain, hypotension, irregular heartbeats, shortness of breath, decreased urinary output, and allergic reaction.
IV. Client and family describe self-care measures to decrease incidence and severity of side effects associated with biologic therapy.
V. Client and family demonstrate self-care skills required to administer biotherapy (e.g., medication self-administration, use of ambulatory infusion pumps, care of venous access devices).

TABLE 36–2. **Potential Nursing Diagnoses for Patients Receiving Biotherapy**

Prevention and Detection
  Health-seeking behaviors (specify)

Information and education
  Knowledge deficit (specify)
  Therapeutic regimen: individual, ineffective
    management

Coping
  Anxiety
  Coping, individual ineffective
  Spiritual distress
  Caregiver role strain, risk for

  Body image disturbance
  Social interaction, impaired
  Role performance, altered

Discomfort
  Pain

Nutrition
  Nutrition, altered: less than body
    requirements

Protective mechanisms
  Infection, high risk for
  Oral mucous membrane, altered
  Sensory/perceptual alterations
  Skin integrity, impaired
  Skin integrity, impaired, high risk for

  Thought processes, altered
  Protection, altered
  Sleep pattern disturbance
  Body temperature, altered, high
    risk for

Mobility and activity
  Fatigue
  Activity intolerance

Elimination
  Diarrhea
  Urinary elimination, altered

Sexuality
  Sexuality patterns, altered

Ventilation
  Gas exchange, impaired

Circulation
  Fluid volume deficit, high risk for
  Tissue perfusion, altered (specify)

From Rieger, P.T. Patient management. In P.T. Rieger (ed.). *Biotherapy: A Comprehensive Overview.*
© 1995 Boston: Jones & Bartlett Publishers, p. 198. Reprinted with permission.

  VI. Client and family verbalize changes in condition that should be reported to
     the health care team:
     A. Fever uncontrolled with acetaminophen or unrelated to normal response
       to therapy.
     B. Weight gain greater than 10 pounds in 1 week.
     C. Weight loss of more than 10% of body weight over several months.
     D. Shortness of breath at rest or extreme shortness of breath with exertion.
     E. Dizziness, chest pain, or irregular heartbeats.
     F. Marked changes in volume of urinary output.
     G. Overwhelming fatigue.
     H. Significant changes in mental status (e.g., depression, confusion, or psycho-
       sis); allergic reactions or intense inflammatory reactions at the injection site.

VII. Client and family identify potential community resources to meet unique demands of therapy and rehabilitation.

Planning and Implementation

I. Dosing and administration of biologic agents.
  A. Use aseptic procedures for mixing and administering biologic agents.
  B. Identify the location of emergency equipment and supplies (with administration of MAbs, these should be located at the bedside).
  C. Obtain baseline pulse, respirations, blood pressure, and temperature values before administration of biotherapy.
  D. Administer premedications (e.g., acetaminophen and diphenhydramine) as ordered by the physician.
  E. Perform dosage calculation.
    1. Standardized total dose.
    2. Per body surface area or per kilogram of body weight.
    3. Adjustments in dose based on:
      a. Organ function (e.g., renal, hematologic).
      b. Toxicity grading (e.g., for fatigue, mental status changes, hematologic values).
  F. Identify issues related to stability, compatibility with other drugs, and filterability that are unique to biologic agents.
    1. Most biologic agents are stored refrigerated, not frozen.
    2. Some are administered with albumin to ensure stability.
    3. Agents should not be shaken during reconstitution to avoid denaturing the biologic protein.
  G. Consider common routes of administration.
    1. Subcutaneous.
    2. Intramuscular.
    3. Intravenous (e.g., bolus infusion, continuous infusion).
    4. Additional routes of administration may include intralesional, intravesicular, intraarterial, intraperitoneal, intracavitary, intrathecal, topical, intralymphatic, and oral.
II. Interventions to monitor for unique complications of biologic therapy.
  A. Monitor orthostatic blood pressure and pulse rate with agents known to cause hypotension.
  B. Monitor fever patterns to differentiate normal responses to treatment from septic spikes.
  C. Evaluate symptoms for frequency, severity, duration, and effects on activities of daily living. Most biotherapy-related side effects are more severe with higher doses, and they tend to affect the quality of life.
    1. Excessive fatigue.
    2. Weight loss or gain of 10 pounds or more in 1 week.
    3. Marked mental status changes such as excessive somnolence, psychosis, or confusion.
    4. Cardiac symptoms such as chest pain, arrhythmias, and symptomatic hypotension.
    5. Other symptoms—increased dyspnea, oliguria, edema, and severe allergic or local inflammatory reaction.
  D. Follow client for adherence to outpatient regimen.
  E. Monitor critical changes in laboratory test values as ordered by the physician.

III. Interventions to decrease the incidence and severity of complications unique to biologic therapy.
   A. Impaired skin integrity.
      1. Bathe in shower or bath with tepid water and avoid scrubbing skin.
      2. Apply lubricants (water-based lotions or creams) to skin after bathing and at regular intervals during the day.
      3. Encourage measures to maintain skin integrity such as position changes, weight shifts, getting out of bed, and ambulation.
   B. Mental status changes.
      1. Assess, at regular intervals, mental status and potential for injury (e.g., risk of falling).
      2. Teach family to monitor for subtle behavioral changes and report to a member of the health care team.
      3. Maintain a safe physical environment.
      4. Evaluate the impact of mental status changes on functional status, judgment, and independence in activities of daily living.
   C. Capillary leak syndrome—movement of fluid from the vascular bed into tissues—end results are edema, weight gain, hypotension, and decreased urinary output; seen with IL-2 and sargramostim at high doses.
      1. Administer supportive medical therapy such as albumin, diuretics, fluids, and vasopressors as ordered by the physician.
      2. Instruct the client to change positions from lying to sitting to standing slowly to avoid dizziness.
      3. Report significant changes to physician.
         a. Urinary output less than 30 mL/hour.
         b. Symptomatic hypotension.
         c. Dyspnea.
         d. Weight gain greater than 10 pounds over 1 week.
   D. Fatigue (see Chapter 1).
   E. Flulike symptoms.
      1. Monitor temperature and fever patterns.
      2. Use comfort measures to control fever and chills (e.g., warm blankets or clothing, warm beverages).
      3. Preadminister medications such as acetaminophen to control symptoms.
      4. Monitor at regular intervals and adjust as needed based on client status (e.g., elderly, those with underlying cardiac or pulmonary problems).
   F. Allergic reactions.
      1. Seen primarily with MAbs.
      2. Stop administration of MAbs.
      3. Administer fluids and emergency medications (e.g., diphenhydramine, epinephrine, methylprednisolone) as ordered.
      4. Monitor vital signs.
IV. Client and family education.
   A. Teach strategies to manage chronic side effects of therapy—fatigue, anorexia, and mental status changes (see Chapters 1, 11, 13).
   B. Teach the client and family needed self-care skills for receiving biologic therapy in the ambulatory setting.
   C. Provide literature available for commercially available biologic agents.
   D. Discuss changes in lifestyle resulting from side effects of therapy and continued need for follow-up care.
   E. Teach client and family signs and symptoms of untoward reactions related to biotherapy administration that should be reported to a member of the health care team.

F. Use client logs to document the incidence and severity of side effects and the type and effectiveness of self-care strategies used.

Evaluation

The oncology nurse systematically and regularly evaluates the client's and/or family's responses to interventions to determine progress toward the achievement of expected outcomes. Relevant data are collected and actual findings are compared with expected findings. Nursing diagnoses, outcomes, and plans of care are reviewed and revised as necessary.

BIBLIOGRAPHY

American Society of Clinical Oncology. (1996). Update of recommendations for the use of hematopoietic colony-stimulating factors: Evidence-based clinical practice guidelines. *J Clin Oncol 14,* 1957–1960.

Atkins, M.B., Mier, J.W., & Trehu, E.G. (1995). Combination cytokine therapy. In V.T. DeVita, Jr., S. Hellman, S.A. Rosenberg (eds.). *Biologic Therapy of Cancer* (2nd ed.). Philadelphia: J.B. Lippincott, pp. 443–466.

Bockheim, C.M., & Jassak, P.F. (1993). The expanding world of colony-stimulating factors. *Cancer Pract 1*(3), 205–216.

Conrad, K.J., & Horrell, C.J. (eds.). (1995). *Biotherapy: Recommendations for Nursing Course Content and Clinical Practicum.* Pittsburgh: Oncology Nursing Press.

DeVita, V.T., Jr., Hellman, S., & Rosenberg, S.A. (eds.). (1995). *Biologic Therapy of Cancer* (2nd ed.). Philadelphia: J.B. Lippincott.

Engleking, C., & Wujcik, D. (1994). Biologic response modifiers (BRMs). In L. Tenenbaum (ed.). *Cancer Chemotherapy and Biotherapy: A Reference Guide* (2nd ed.). Philadelphia: W.B. Saunders, pp. 151–179.

Estrov, Z., Kurzrock, R., & Talpaz, M. (eds.). (1993). *Interferons: Basic Principles and Clinical Application.* Austin: R.G. Landes.

Fisher, R. (ed.). (1993). Interleukin-2: Advances in clinical research and treatment. *Semin Oncol 20*(6[suppl 9]), 1–59.

Goldenberg, D. (1994). New developments in monoclonal antibodies for cancer detection and therapy. *CA Cancer J Clin 44*(1), 43–64.

Graydon, J.E., Bubela, N., Irvine, D., & Vincent, L. (1995). Fatigue-reducing strategies used by patients receiving treatment for cancer. *Cancer Nurs 18,* 23–28.

Jenkins, J., Wheeler, V., & Albright, L. (1994). Gene therapy for cancer. *Cancer Nurs 17,* 447–456.

Lippman, S.M., Benner, S.E., & Hong, W.K. (1994). Cancer chemoprevention. *J Clin Oncol 12,* 851–873.

Mertelsmann, R., & Herrmann, F. (eds.). (1995). *Hematopoietic Growth Factors in Clinical Applications* (2nd ed.). New York: Marcel Dekker.

Miller, L. (ed.). (1994). American Society of Clinical Oncology recommendations for the use of hematopoietic colony-stimulating factors: Evidence-based, clinical practice guidelines. *J Clin Oncol 12,* 2471–2508.

Post-White, J. (1996). The immune system. *Semin Oncol Nurs 12*(2), 89–96.

Rieger, P.T. (ed.). (1995). *Biotherapy: A Comprehensive Overview.* Boston: Jones & Bartlett.

Rieger, P.T. (1995). Interferon-alpha: A clinical update. *Cancer Pract 3*(6), 356–365.

Rieger, P.T. (ed.). (1996). Biotherapy: Present accomplishments and future projections. *Semin Oncol Nurs 12*(2), 81–171.

Rieger, P.T., & Haeuber, D. (1995). A new approach to managing chemotherapy-related anemia: Nursing implications of epoetin alfa. *Oncol Nurs Forum 22,* 71–81.

Rieger, P.T., & Rumsey, K.A. (1992). Responding to the educational needs of patients receiving biotherapy. In R.M. Carroll-Johnson (ed.). *The Biotherapy of Cancer V* (monograph). Pittsburgh: Oncology Nursing Press, pp. 10–15.

Straw, L.J., & Conrad, K.J. (1994). Patient education resources related to biotherapy and the immune system. *Oncol Nurs Forum 212,* 1223–1228.

Vose, J.M., & Armitage, J.O. (1995). Clinical applications of hematopoietic growth factors. *J Clin Oncol 4,* 1023–1035.

Wheeler, V.S. (1997). Biotherapy. In S.L. Groenwald, M.H. Frogge, M. Goodman & C.H. Yarbro (eds.). *Cancer Nursing: Principles and Practice* (4th ed.). Boston: Jones & Bartlett, pp. 426–458.

Nursing Implications of Antineoplastic Therapy

Catherine Bender, RN, PhD

Theory

I. Principles of cancer chemotherapy.
  A. Cancer chemotherapy is the treatment of choice for malignancies of the hematopoietic system and for solid tumors, including solid tumors that have metastasized regionally or distally.
  B. The application of antineoplastic agents to the treatment of cancer is based on concepts of cellular kinetics, which include the cell life cycle, cell cycle time, growth fraction, and tumor burden.
    1. Cell life cycle—a five-stage process of reproduction that occurs in both normal and malignant cells (Fig. 37–1).
      a. Gap 0 (G_0) or resting phase.
        (1) Cells are not dividing and are temporarily out of the cell cycle.
        (2) Duration of time in G_0 phase is highly variable.
      b. Gap 1 (G_1): post-mitotic phase or interphase.
        (1) As cells are activated they enter the cell cycle at the G_1 phase.
        (2) Enzymes necessary for deoxyribonucleic acid (DNA) synthesis are produced.
        (3) Protein and ribonucleic acid (RNA) synthesis also occur.
        (4) Duration of time in G_1 is variable, lasting from hours to days.
      c. Synthesis (S).
        (1) Cellular DNA is duplicated in preparation for DNA division.
        (2) Duration of time in the S phase is approximately 10 to 20 hours.
      d. Gap 2 (G_2) or premitotic phase.
        (1) Further protein and RNA synthesis occurs.
        (2) Precursors of the mitotic spindle apparatus are produced.
        (3) Duration of time in G_2 is short, ranging from 2 to 10 hours.
      e. M (mitosis).
        (1) Cellular division occurs in four phases—prophase, metaphase, anaphase, and telophase.
          (a) Prophase—nuclear membrane breaks down and chromosomes clump.
          (b) Metaphase—chromosomes align in the middle of the cell.
          (c) Anaphase—chromosomes segregate to the centriole.
          (d) Telophase—cellular division occurs with the production of two daughter cells.

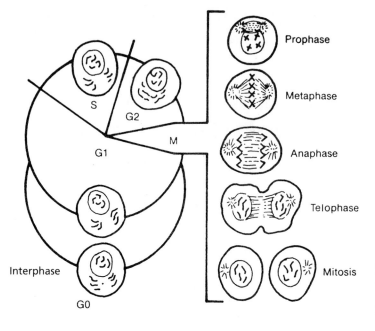

Prophase

Metaphase

Anaphase

Telophase

Mitosis

S

G2

M

G1

Interphase

G0

Figure 37–1. Cell life cycle. (Redrawn from Marino, L. [1981]. *Cancer Nursing.* St. Louis: C.V. Mosby.)

   (2) Duration of time in M phase is approximately 30 minutes to 1 hour.

 2. Cell cycle time—the amount of time required for a cell to move from one mitosis to another mitosis.

  a. The length of the total cell cycle varies with the specific type of cell; the length of the G_0 phase is the major determinant of the cell cycle time.

  b. A shorter cell cycle time results in higher cell kill with exposure to cell cycle–specific agents.

  c. Continuous infusion of cell cycle–specific agents results in exposure of a greater number of cells and in a higher cell kill in tumors with short cell cycle times.

 3. Growth fraction of tumor—the percentage of cells actively dividing at a given point of time.

  a. A higher growth fraction results in a higher cell kill with exposure to cell cycle–specific agents.

  b. Tumors with a greater fraction of cells in G_0 are more sensitive to cell cycle–nonspecific agents.

 4. Tumor burden—the number of cells present in the tumor.

  a. Cancers with a small tumor burden are usually more sensitive to antineoplastic therapy.

  b. As the tumor burden increases, the growth rate slows, and the number of cells actively dividing decreases.

  c. The higher the tumor cell burden, the higher the probability of drug-resistant sublines.

C. Approaches to chemotherapy.

 1. Combination chemotherapy—the use of two or more antineoplastic agents to produce additive or synergistic results against tumor cells.

  a. Combining agents with actions in different phases of the cell cycle increases the number of cells exposed to cytotoxic effects during a given treatment cycle.

    b. Combining agents, in which one agent is an antidote and serves to rescue the host from the toxic effects of the other agent.

    c. Combining agents decreases the incidence and severity of side effects of therapy.

    d. Effective in patients with large tumors containing a small number of proliferating cells. Agent kills a high proportion of tumor cells and stimulates remaining tumor cells to enter the proliferative phase. Additional agents kill newly proliferating cells.

    e. Combining agents decreases the possibility of drug resistance.

    f. Criteria for selection of antineoplastic agents for combination therapy.

       (1) Demonstrate cytotoxic activity when used alone to treat a specific cancer.

       (2) Possess different dose-limiting toxicities.

       (3) Exhibit toxicities that occur at different points of time from the treatment.

       (4) Exhibit biologic effects that result in enhanced cytotoxicity.

  2. Regional chemotherapy—method of delivering higher doses of chemotherapy to the specific site of the tumor, such as the liver, while reducing the intensity of systemic toxicity.

  3. High-dose chemotherapy administered with supportive therapy (e.g., granulocyte/granulocyte-macrophage colony stimulating factors for neutropenia) or with an antidote to diminish toxicity (e.g., high-dose methotrexate with leucovorin rescue).

  D. Factors influencing the response to antineoplastic agents.

    1. Characteristics of the tumor—location, size, growth rate, presence of resistant cells, and ratio of sensitivity of malignant cells and normal target cells.

    2. Availability of combination antineoplastic regimens.

    3. Hormone receptor status.

    4. Administration schedule—bolus, infusion, or combined modality therapy (combination of chemotherapy with other forms of anticancer therapy such as radiation therapy or surgery).

    5. Physical status of the client.

    6. Psychosocial status of the client.

II. Roles of chemotherapy in cancer care.

  A. Cure—complete response.

    1. Single treatment modality—for example, acute lymphocytic leukemia in children, Hodgkin's disease, lymphosarcoma, Burkitt lymphoma, testicular carcinoma, gestational trophoblastic tumors, non-Hodgkin's lymphoma (in children), diffuse large cell lymphoma, and Ewing's sarcoma.

    2. Combined treatment modality (e.g., Wilms' tumor, osteogenic sarcoma, rhabdomyosarcoma).

  B. Control.

    1. Goal is to extend the length and quality of life when hope of cure is not realistic.

    2. Examples—breast cancer, chronic lymphocytic leukemia, chronic and acute myelogenous leukemia, small cell carcinoma of the lung, prostatic cancer, multiple myeloma, gastric carcinoma, endometrial carcinoma, non-Hodgkin's lymphoma (indolent), hairy-cell leukemia, ovarian carci-

noma, neuroblastoma, colorectal cancer, liver cancer, and soft tissue sarcomas.

   C. Palliation.
1. Goal is to improve comfort when neither cure nor control is possible.
2. Relief of pressure on nerves, lymphatics, and vasculature, and reduction of organ obstruction.

III. Types and classifications of chemotherapy.

Antineoplastic agents are classified according to the phase of action during the cell cycle, mechanism of action, biochemical structure, or physiologic action.

   A. Phase of action during the cell cycle.
1. Cell cycle–specific agents.
   a. Major cytotoxic effects are exerted on cells actively dividing at specific phases throughout the cell cycle.
   b. Agents are not active against cells in the resting phase (G_0).
   c. Agents are most effective if administered in divided doses or by continuous infusion.
   d. Cytotoxic effects occur during the cell cycle and are expressed when cell repair or division is attempted.
2. Cell cycle–nonspecific agents.
   a. Major cytotoxic effects are exerted on cells at any phase, including G_0, in the cell cycle.
   b. Agents are most effective if administered by bolus doses because the number of cells affected is proportional to the amount of drug given.
   c. Cytotoxic effects occur during the cell cycle and are expressed when cell division is attempted.

   B. Biochemical structure, mechanism of action, or derivation (Table 37–1).
1. Alkylating agents.
   a. Mechanisms of action—interfere with DNA replication through cross-linking of DNA strands, DNA strand breaking, and abnormal base pairing of proteins.
   b. Most agents are cell cycle–nonspecific.
   c. Major toxicities occur in the hematopoietic, gastrointestinal, and reproductive systems (Table 37–2).
2. Nitrosoureas.
   a. Mechanisms of action—interfere with DNA replication and repair.
   b. Nitrosoureas are noncross-resistant to alkylating agents.
   c. Most agents are cell cycle–nonspecific.
   d. Most agents cross the blood-brain barrier.
   e. Major toxicities occur in the hematopoietic and gastrointestinal systems.
3. Antimetabolites.
   a. Mechanisms of action—inhibit protein synthesis, substitute erroneous metabolites or structural analogues during DNA synthesis, and inhibit DNA synthesis.
   b. Most agents are cell cycle–specific, S phase.
   c. Major toxicities occur in the hematopoietic and gastrointestinal systems.
4. Antitumor antibiotics.
   a. Mechanisms of action—interfere with nucleic acid synthesis and function, inhibit ribonucleic acid (RNA) synthesis, and inhibit DNA synthesis.

TABLE 37–1. **Classifications of Antineoplastic Agents**

Antimetabolites

5-azacytidine	Fludarabine
5-fluorouracil	Gemcitabine
6-thioguanine	Hydroxyurea
6-mercaptopurine	Methotrexate
Cladribine (2-CdA) (Leustatin)	Pentostatin
Cytosine arabinoside	Vidarabine
Floxuridine	

Alkylating Agents

Altretamine (Hexalen)	Ifosfamide
Busulfan	Mechlorethamine
Carboplatin	Melphalan
Chlorambucil	Procarbazine
Cisplatin	Thiophosphoramide
Cyclophosphamide	Triethylenethiophosphoramide (thiotepa)
Dacarbazine	

Antitumor Antibiotics

Bleomycin	Epirubicin
Dactinomycin (actinomycin D)	Idarubicin
Daunorubicin	Mitomycin-C
Doxorubicin	Mitoxantrone

Nitrosoureas

Carmustine	Semustine
Chlorozotozin	Streptozotocin
Lomustine	

Plant Alkaloids

Etoposide (VP-16)	Vinblastine
Paclitaxel (Taxol)	Vincristine
Taxotere	Vindesine
Teniposide (VM-26)	Vinorelbine (Navelbine)

Topoisomerase I Inhibitors

Irinotecan
Topotecan hydrochloride

Hormones

Aminoglutethimide	Leuprolide
Anastrozole	Medroxyprogesterone acetate (Provera)
Diethylstilbestrol	Megestrol acetate (Megace)
Fluoxymesterone (Halotestin)	Nilutamide (Nicandron)
Flutamide	Octreotide
Goserelin (Zoladex)	Tamoxifen citrate (Nolvadex)
Hydroxyprogesterone caproate (Delalutin)	Testosterone

Miscellaneous Agents

Amsacrine
L-asparaginase
Tretinoin

    b. Most agents are cell cycle–nonspecific.
    c. Major toxicities occur in the hematopoietic, gastrointestinal, reproductive, and cardiac systems (cumulative doses) (see Table 37–2).
  5. Plant alkaloids.
    a. Mechanisms of action—arrest or inhibit mitosis.
    b. Most agents are cell cycle–specific, M phase.

TABLE 37–2. **Potential Side Effects of Chemotherapy**

System	Side Effects
Hematopoietic	Anemia Leukopenia Thrombocytopenia
Gastrointestinal	Anorexia Nausea Vomiting Mucositis Constipation Diarrhea Ulceration Hepatic toxicity
Integumentary	Dermatitis Hyperpigmentation Alopecia Radiation recall
Genitourinary	Cystitis Renal toxicity
Cardiovascular	Cardiac toxicity Venous fibrosis Phlebitis Extravasation
Neurologic	Neurotoxicity Ototoxicity Metabolic encephalopathy Peripheral neuropathy
Pulmonary	Fibrosis Pneumonitis Edema
Reproductive	Infertility Changes in libido Erectile dysfunction
Additional Effects	
Latent effects	Learning disabilities Changes in memory Second malignancies
Mood alterations	Anxiety Depression
Metabolic alterations	Hypocalcemia Hypercalcemia Hypoglycemia Hyperglycemia Hyperphosphatemia Hyperuricemia Hypokalemia Hyperkalemia
Other	Hypersensitivity Fatigue Ocular toxicity

      c. Major toxicities occur in the hematopoietic, integumentary, neurologic, and reproductive systems; also hypersensitivity reactions (see Table 37–2).

    6. Topoisomerase I inhibitors.

      a. Mechanism of action—prevent unwinding of DNA strands by inhibiting the topoisomerase enzyme.

      b. Major toxicities occur in hematopoietic and gastrointestinal systems.

    7. Hormonal agents.

      a. Androgens—alter pituitary function and directly affect malignant cells.

      b. Corticosteroids—lyse lymphoid malignancies and have indirect effects on malignant cells.

      c. Estrogens—suppress testosterone production in males and alter the response of breast cancers to prolactin.

      d. Progestins—promote differentiation of malignant cells.

      e. Estrogen antagonists—compete with estrogens for binding with estrogen receptor sites on malignant cells.

    8. Miscellaneous agents.

      a. Mechanisms of action—poorly understood.

      b. Variety of toxic effects.

IV. Chemoprotective agents.

  A. New agents designed to protect against specific toxic effects of chemotherapy.

    1. Dexrazoxane (Zinecard).

      a. Cardioprotective agent against doxorubicin.

      b. For cumulative dose greater than 300 mg/m^2.

      c. Administer 30 minutes before doxorubicin.

      d. Dose-limiting toxicity: myelosuppression in conjunction with chemotherapy.

    2. Amifostine (Ethyol).

      a. Cytoprotective agent for toxic effects of cisplatin (i.e., myelosuppression and peripheral nervous system toxicity).

      b. Administer 30 minutes before cisplatin.

      c. Side effects.

        (1) Frequent occurrence of transient hypotension.

          (a) Hold antihypertensive agents 24 hours before amifostine administration.

          (b) Frequent assessment of blood pressure: baseline, at least every 5 minutes throughout infusion, and 5 minutes after infusion is completed.

          (c) Stop infusion if systolic blood pressure falls below threshold levels established by manufacturer.

        (2) Nausea, vomiting.

          (a) Administer antiemetics (e.g., serotonin inhibitor and steroid) before amifostine.

V. Routes of administration—advantages of each route, potential complications, and nursing implications are presented in Table 37–3.

Assessment

  I. Pertinent personal and family history.

    A. Type of cancer and phase of cancer trajectory.

TABLE 37–3. **Routes of Administration of Antineoplastic Agents**

Route	Advantages	Disadvantages	Complications	Nursing Implications
Oral	Ease of administration	Inconsistency of absorption	Drug-specific complications	Evaluate compliance with medication schedule
Subcutaneous/ intramuscular	Ease of administration Decreased side effects	Adequate muscle mass and tissue required for absorption	Infection Bleeding	Evaluate platelet count (>50,000) Use smallest gauge needle possible Prepare injection site with an antiseptic solution Assess injection site for signs and symptoms of infection
Intravenous	Consistent absorption Required for vesicants	Sclerosing of veins over time	Infection Phlebitis	Check for IV patency before and after administration of drugs
Intraarterial	Increased doses to tumor with decreased systemic toxic effects	Requires surgical procedure or special radiography for equipment placement	Bleeding Embolism	Monitor for signs/ symptoms of bleeding Monitor prothrombin time (PT), partial thromboplastin time (PTT)
Intrathecal/ intraventricular	More consistent drug levels in cerebrospinal fluid	Requires lumbar puncture or surgical placement of reservoir or implanted pump for drug delivery	Headaches Confusion Lethargy Nausea and vomiting Seizures	Observe site for signs of infection Monitor reservoir or pump functioning
Intraperitoneal	Direct exposure of intraabdominal metastases to drug	Requires placement of Tenckhoff catheter or intraperitoneal port	Abdominal pain Abdominal distention Bleeding Ileus Intestinal perforation Infection	Warm chemotherapy solution to body temperature Check patency of catheter or port Instill solution according to protocol—infuse, dwell, and drain or continuous infusion
Intravesicular	Direct exposure of bladder surfaces to drug	Requires insertion of indwelling catheter	Urinary tract infection Cystitis Bladder contracture Urinary urgency Allergic drug reactions	Maintain sterile technique when inserting indwelling catheter Instill solution, clamp catheter for 1 hr, and unclamp to drain
Intrapleural	Sclerosing of pleural lining to prevent recurrence of effusions	Requires insertion of a thoracotomy tube	Pain Infection	Monitor for complete drainage from pleural cavity before instillation of drug Following instillation, clamp tubing and reposition client every 10–15 min $\times$ 2 hr Attach tubing to suction $\times$ 18 hr Assess client for pain; provide analgesia Assess client for anxiety; provide emotional support

B. Previous cancer therapy and time interval since last therapy.
  1. Attitudes of the client and family toward previous therapy.
  2. Side effects experienced.
  3. Self-care measures used to minimize side effects.
  4. Effectiveness of measures in reducing the incidence and severity of side effects.
C. Dietary intake.
D. Knowledge of rationale for, and goals of, treatment; agents to be given; potential side effects; and relative risks and benefits of treatment.

II. Physical examination.
A. Renal—amount and color of urinary output and patterns of urinary elimination.
B. Gastrointestinal system.
  1. Oral cavity—cleanliness; moisture; and integrity of lips, gums, teeth, oral mucosa, and tongue.
  2. Bowel—presence of bowel sounds; consistency, color and caliber of stool; patterns of bowel elimination.
  3. Rectum—integrity of perirectal and perineal tissue; presence of hemorrhoids, redness, or pain.
C. Hematologic system.
  1. Color of skin and mucous membranes; presence of bruising or petechiae.
  2. Activity intolerance.
  3. Presence of signs and symptoms of infection.
D. Performance status.

III. Psychosocial examination.
A. Previous responses to stressors and effective coping mechanisms used.
B. Level of independence and responsibility, desire, and ability for self-care.
C. Support systems and personnel available to the client and family.

IV. Laboratory data.
A. Hemoglobin, hematocrit, platelet count, and white blood cell count with differential.
B. Liver and renal function test results.
C. Electrolyte levels.

Nursing Diagnoses

  I. Knowledge deficit.
 II. Altered nutrition, less than body requirements.
III. Risk for infection.
IV. Altered oral mucous membrane.
 V. Sexual dysfunction.
VI. Activity intolerance.
VII. Body image disturbance.
VIII. Pain (acute).
IX. Anxiety.

Outcome Identification

I. Client describes the chemotherapy protocol—name of agents, route, method, schedule of administration, and schedule for routine laboratory and physical examination follow-up visits.

II. Client and family list potential immediate and long-term side effects of the antineoplastic agents.

III. Client describes self-care measures to decrease the incidence and severity of complications of therapy.

IV. Client and family list changes that should be reported immediately to the health care team.

    A. Signs and symptoms of infection—temperature greater than 101°F, pain, swelling, redness, or pus.

    B. Nausea or vomiting that persists and is unrelieved by usual methods.

    C. Unusual bleeding or bruising.

    D. Acute changes in mental or emotional status.

    E. Diarrhea or constipation unrelieved by usual control methods.

V. Client and family identify community resources to meet potential demands of treatment and rehabilitation.

VI. Client demonstrates competence in self-care skills demanded by the treatment plan (e.g., care of venous access devices, implanted ports, or intracavity catheters).

Planning and Implementation

I. Interventions to maximize safe administration of chemotherapy to client.

    A. Review orders—compare with formal drug protocol or reference source; check for completeness (e.g., schedule, route, admixture solution).

    B. Determine drug dosage.

        1. Calculate body surface area (BSA).

        2. Recalculate drug dosage and check against order.

    C. Review drugs to be administered and potential side effects and toxicities.

    D. Review and/or obtain orders for other medications (e.g., antiemetics).

    E. Check current laboratory test values.

    F. Verify that informed consent has been obtained if required.

    G. Assess the client.

        1. Previous experience with chemotherapy.

        2. Understanding and acceptance of the treatment plan.

    H. Conduct client and family teaching (e.g., chemotherapy administration procedures, antiemetic schedule, self-care measures for potential side effects).

    I. Prepare drugs, as needed, following safe handling procedures (see Chapter 38).

    J. Double-check chemotherapy order, if required by agency policy.

    K. Obtain appropriate material, emergency equipment, and agents for management of extravasation and/or anaphylaxis as indicated.

    L. Select site for venipuncture, if peripheral administration is to be performed.

        1. Select distal sites before proximal sites.

        2. Evaluate general condition of veins.

        3. Note type of medications to be infused.

        4. Avoid sites where damage to underlying tendons or nerves is more likely to occur—antecubital region, wrist, dorsal surface of the hand, areas with recent venipuncture sites, sclerosed veins, or areas of previous surgery such as skin grafts, side of mastectomy, lumpectomy, node dissection, or partial amputation.

M. Monitor central or peripheral intravenous (IV) administration:
   1. Assess for patency by flushing the line with sterile IV solution. Observe for signs and symptoms of infiltration.
N. Administer pre-chemotherapy hydration, antiemetics, and other preparations, if ordered.
O. Administer chemotherapy drugs according to agency policy, following safe handling procedures (see Chapter 38), and according to the five rights.
   1. Right medication.
   2. Right time.
   3. Right route.
   4. Right dose.
   5. Right client.
P. Assess the client for signs of infiltration (burning, pain, swelling, redness).
Q. Flush the IV with 3 to 10 mL of normal saline solution after administering each agent and at completion of the infusion.
R. Remove the needle or IV catheter or inject heparin into the central line or device as needed.
   1. Apply an adhesive bandage to the peripheral IV site.
   2. Have the client elevate the extremity for 3 to 5 minutes after the needle is withdrawn.
   3. Apply gentle pressure to the site to reduce local bleeding.
S. Document medication administration and client response according to agency policy.

II. Interventions to minimize risk of extravasation.
   A. Obtain appropriate materials and agents for management of extravasation as indicated (Table 37–4).
      1. Extravasation—infiltration or leakage of an IV antineoplastic agent into the local tissues.
         a. Irritants—agents that may produce pain and inflammation at the administration site or along the path of a vein if leakage into subcutaneous tissue occurs (see Table 37–4).
         b. Vesicants—agents that have the potential to cause cellular damage to tissue destruction if leakage into subcutaneous tissue occurs (see Table 37–4).
            (1) Instruct the client to report pain or burning with the infusion.
            (2) Administer vesicants in larger veins of the arm, midway between the wrist and elbow.
            (3) Assess patency every 2 to 3 mL when administering IV push and every 5 minutes for piggyback infusion.
         c. If extravasation occurs or is suspected.
            (1) Discontinue infusion, leaving needle or IV catheter in place.
            (2) Aspirate residual medication and blood from the IV tubing.
            (3) If recommended (see Table 37–4), instill the IV antidote and then remove the needle.
            (4) If no IV antidote is recommended, remove the needle.
               (a) Inject the subcutaneous antidote in a clockwise fashion into the infiltrated area using a 25-gauge needle for each injection.
               (b) Avoid applying pressure to the area to decrease spread of drug infiltrate.
               (c) Apply a sterile, occlusive dressing, heat, or cold as indicated (see Table 37–4).
               (d) Elevate the affected extremity to decrease swelling.
            (5) Notify the physician of extravasation.

TABLE 37–4. **Vesicant and Irritant Chemotherapeutic Agents**

Medications	Description	Local Antidote
Amsacrine (m-AMSA)	Vesicant	None
Carboplatin	Irritant	Unknown
Carmustine (BiCNU, BCNU)	Irritant	Unknown
Cisplatin	Irritant/vesicant	*Vesicant:* if >20 mL of 0.5 mg/mL concentration extravasates, treat with isotonic sodium thiosulfate *Irritant:* no treatment
Dacarbazine (DTIC—Dome)	Irritant	None
Dactinomycin (actinomycin D)	Vesicant	None
Daunomycin	Vesicant	None
Daunorubicin (Cerubidine)	Vesicant	None
Doxorubicin (Adriamycin)	Vesicant	None
Etoposide (VePesid, VP16)	Irritant	Hyaluronidase Treat only if large amount of concentrated solution extravasates
Idarubicin (Idamycin)	Vesicant	None
Ifosfamide	Irritant	Unknown
Mechlorethamine (nitrogen mustard)	Vesicant	Isotonic sodium thiosulfate
Mitomycin-C	Vesicant	None
Mitoxantrone (Novantrone)	Irritant/vesicant	Unknown (ulceration rare unless infiltration of concentrated dose)
Paclitaxel (Taxol)	Vesicant	Hyaluronidase
Plicamycin (Mithramycin)	Vesicant	None
Streptozotocin (Zanosar)	Irritant	Hydrocortisone
Teniposide (VM-26)	Irritant	Hyaluronidase Treat like etoposide
Vinblastine (Velban)	Vesicant	Hyaluronidase
Vincristine (Oncovin)	Vesicant	Hyaluronidase
Vindesine (Eldisine)	Vesicant	Hyaluronidase
Vinorelbine (Navelbine)	Vesicant	Hyaluronidase

Adapted from Powel, L.L. (ed.). (1996). *Cancer Chemotherapy Guidelines and Recommendations for Practice.* Pittsburgh: Oncology Nursing Press, pp. 55–57.

     (6) Document extravasation in medical record to include date, time, needle size and type, site, medications administered, sequence of antineoplastic agents, approximate amount of agent extravasated, subjective symptoms reported by client, nursing assessment of site, nursing interventions, notification of physician and interventions, instructions given to client, follow-up measures, and signature.

III. Interventions to decrease the incidence and severity of complications of chemotherapy.

    A. See the following chapters for interventions for common complications of chemotherapy: fatigue (Chapter 1); anxiety (Chapter 2); alopecia

TABLE 37–5. **Specific Toxicities and Nursing Interventions for Selected Chemotherapeutic Agents**

Chemotherapeutic Agents	Toxicity	Nursing Interventions
Asparaginase (Elspar) Paclitaxel (Taxol) Bleomycin (Blenoxane)	Hypersensitivity	Identify clients at risk—clients with previous allergic reactions to this or other medications Assess for early signs of hypersensitivity—urticaria, pruritus Assess for signs of anaphylactic-type reaction—local or generalized urticaria; angioedema of the face, eyelids, hands, feet; respiratory stridor; hypotension; cyanosis Administer epinephrine in dose of 0.5–0.7 mL (solution strength, 1 : 1000) per physician order ***Paclitaxel*** Premedicate, per physician order, with antihistamine (e.g., diphenhydramine), histamine$_2$-receptor antagonist (e.g., cimetidine, ranitidine), and corticosteroid (e.g., dexamethasone) prior to administration ***Bleomycin*** Administer test dose per physician order before administration of full dose
Bleomycin (Blenoxane)	Pulmonary toxicity presenting as pneumonitis, which may result in pulmonary fibrosis	Monitor cumulative dose, which should not exceed 400 units; doses above this limit significantly increase the risk of pulmonary toxicity Assess for signs of pulmonary toxicity—dry persistent cough, dyspnea, tachypnea, cyanosis, basilar rales Prevent infection by promoting exercise, coughing and deep breathing, and humidification of air
Cisplatin	Renal toxicity	Monitor blood urea nitrogen and creatinine levels, urinary output Monitor other drugs that patient is on that may also be nephrotoxic (e.g., aminoglycoside antibiotics) Provide adequate hydration and diuresis with furosemide or mannitol as ordered by physician

Table continued on following page

TABLE 37–5. **Specific Toxicities and Nursing Interventions for Selected Chemotherapeutic Agents** *Continued*

Chemotherapeutic Agents	Toxicity	Nursing Interventions
		Premedicate, per physician order, with chemoprotective agent, amifostine; monitor for hypotension with administration of this medication
	Ototoxicity	Teach client to report tinnitus Monitor dose levels; risk increases with doses exceeding 60–75 mg/m^2; hearing loss may be cumulative with additional doses and may or may not be reversible Refer client for regular audiograms
Cyclophosphamide (Cytoxan) Ifosfamide (Ifex)	Hemorrhagic cystitis	Ensure adequate fluid intake of 3000 mL/day unless contraindicated Avoid urinary retention by having client void every 2 hr when possible Assess for signs of cystitis, including urinary frequency, pain on urination, cloudy urine, hematuria, low back pain Teach client to report signs of cystitis Administer mesna/continuous bladder irrigation (CBI) as ordered
Daunorubicin (Cerubidine) Doxorubicin (Adriamycin)	Cardiotoxicity manifested by electrocardiographic (ECG) changes, congestive heart failure, cardiomyopathy	Monitor cumulative doses of agents; maximal cumulative dose is 550 mg/m^2; doses above this limit significantly increase the risk of cardiotoxicity; maximal cumulative dose is reduced to 400 mg/m^2 if patient received, or concurrently receiving, radiation therapy to the mediastinum or cyclophosphamide therapy Assess for signs of cardiotoxicity, including ECG changes, signs of congestive heart failure (shortness of breath, hypertension, edema)
Mitoxantrone	Cardiotoxicity	Risk of cardiotoxicity is not as great as with daunorubicin and doxorubicin. Risk appears to increase at 125 mg/m^2 cumulative dose

TABLE 37–5. **Specific Toxicities and Nursing Interventions for Selected Chemotherapeutic Agents** *Continued*

Chemotherapeutic Agents	Toxicity	Nursing Interventions
Etoposide (VePesid)	Hypotension resulting from rapid administration	Administer over 30 to 60 min Monitor blood pressure every 15 min during administration
5-Fluorouracil (5-FU)	Photosensitivity manifested by increased skin pigmentation or erythema	Teach client to avoid prolonged sun exposure or to use sunscreen when exposed to the sun Assess for changes in pigmentation and/or erythema of skin
Ifosfamide (Ifex)	Neurotoxicity	Monitor blood urea nitrogen (BUN) and serum creatinine and albumin levels because elevations in these parameters may be associated with increased risk of neurotoxicity Teach patients and families to report early signs of neurotoxicity
Vincristine (Oncovin)	Neurotoxicity	Assess for numbness of hands and feet, foot drop, tingling of fingertips and toes, decreased fine and gross motor abilities, and slapping gait Monitor bowel function and assess for constipation as a potential early sign of neurotoxicity Teach clients to report symptoms of neurotoxicity

and altered body image (Chapter 3); reproductive issues and sexual dysfunction (Chapter 6); neuropathies and alterations in mental status (Chapter 11); myelosuppression (Chapter 12); anorexia, mucositis, nausea and vomiting, taste alterations, electrolyte imbalances (Chapter 13); pulmonary toxicity, anemia (Chapter 15); and cardiovascular toxicity (Chapter 16).

B. Interventions for specific complications of selected antineoplastic agents are presented in Table 37–5.

Evaluation

The oncology nurse systematically and regularly evaluates the client's and/or family's responses to interventions to determine progress toward the achievement of expected outcomes. Relevant data are collected and actual findings are compared with expected findings. Nursing diagnoses, outcomes, and plans of care are reviewed and revised as necessary.

BIBLIOGRAPHY

Bender, C.M., Yasko, J.M., & Strohl, R.A. (1996). Nursing role in management: Cancer. In S.M. Lewis, I.C. Collier, & M.M. Heitkemper (eds.). *Medical-Surgical Nursing: Assessment and Management of Clinical Problems.* St. Louis: Mosby-Year Book, pp. 261–315.

Cain, J.W., & Bender, C. M. (1995). Ifosfamide-induced neurotoxicity: Associated symptoms and nursing implications. *Oncol Nurs Forum 22*(4), 659–666.

DeVita, V.T., Jr., Hellman, S., & Rosenberg, S.A. (eds.). (1993). *Cancer: Principles and Practice of Oncology* (4th ed.). Philadelphia: J.B. Lippincott.

Galassi, A. (1992). The next generation: New chemotherapy agents for the 1990's. *Semin Oncol Nurs 8*(2), 83–94.

Guy, J.L., & Ingram, B.A. (1996). Medical oncology—the agents. In R. McCorkle, M. Grant, M. Frank-Stromborg, & S.B. Baird (eds.). *Cancer Nursing: A Comprehensive Textbook* (2nd ed.). Philadelphia: W.B. Saunders, pp. 359–394.

Holland, J.F., Frei, E., Bast, R.C., et al. (eds.). (1993). *Cancer Medicine* (3rd ed.). Philadelphia: Lea & Febiger.

Knobf, M.T., & Durivage, H.J. (1993). Chemotherapy: Principles of therapy. In S.L. Groenwald, M. Goodman, M.H. Frogge, & C.H. Yarbro (eds.). *Cancer Nursing: Principles and Practice* (3rd ed.). Boston: Jones & Bartlett, pp. 270–292.

Krakoff, I.H. (1996). Systemic treatment of cancer. *CA Cancer J Clin 46*(3), 134–141.

Miaskowski, C. (1991). Chemotherapy update. *Nurs Clin North Am 26*(2), 331–339.

Powel, L.L. (ed.). (1996). *Cancer Chemotherapy Guidelines and Recommendations for Practice.* Pittsburgh: Oncology Nursing Press.

Quint-Kasner, S., Chisolm, L., de Carvalho, M., & Piemme, J. (1993). Programmed instruction: Cancer chemotherapy. *Cancer Nurs 16*(1), 63–78.

Skeel, R.T., & Lachant, N.A. (1995). *Handbook of Cancer Chemotherapy* (4th ed.). Boston: Little, Brown.

Wheelock, L.D., & Summers, B.L.Y. (1996). New chemotherapy agents in cancer care. *Oncol Nurs Updates 3*(4), 1–12.

Wujcik, D. (1992). Current research in side effects of high-dose chemotherapy. *Semin Oncol Nurs 8*(2), 102–112.

Principles of Preparation, Administration, and Disposal of Antineoplastic Agents

Jan Hawthorne Maxson, RN, MSN, AOCN
Jean Ellsworth Wolk, RN, MS, AOCN

Theory

I. Exposure to antineoplastic agents poses a potential health risk to personnel who prepare, handle, administer, and dispose of these drugs.
  A. Potential routes of exposure.
    1. Direct contact—skin and mucous membrane contact and absorption, inhalation, or ingestion (e.g., contaminated food).
    2. Indirect contact—body fluids and excreta of clients who have received antineoplastic agents within the past 48 hours.
  B. Potential effects of exposure to antineoplastic agents.
    1. Short-term—occur within hours or days after exposure.
      a. Dermatitis.
      b. Hyperpigmentation of skin.
      c. Other reported symptoms not linked conclusively to antineoplastic agent exposure—blurred vision, skin discoloration, sloughing or necrosis of the skin, allergic responses, mucous membrane irritation, dizziness, liver damage, gastrointestinal tract problems, renal problems, and headache.
    2. Long-term—occur within months or years after exposure.
      a. Partial alopecia.
      b. Chromosomal abnormalities.
      c. Increased risk of cancer.
II. Institutional responsibilities with respect to antineoplastic agents.
  A. Define agency policies and procedures about use of antineoplastic agents consistent with professional and federal recommendations to minimize risks to personnel.
  B. Orient all agency personnel who may come in contact with antineoplastic agents about the potential risks of antineoplastic agents and agency policies and procedures.
  C. Review agency policies and procedures about antineoplastic agents at periodic intervals.
  D. Include compliance to policies and procedures as a component of the agency's quality assurance and performance improvement program.

E. Develop a monitoring system for reviewing incident reports involving anti-neoplastic agents.

F. Develop an employment medical surveillance program for monitoring the effects of acute and chronic exposure.

Assessment

I. Previous health history of personnel.
   A. Personal history of cancer.
   B. Family history of cancer.
   C. Personal risk factors for cancer.
   D. Presence of signs and symptoms of site-specific cancers.
II. Physical and psychosocial examination—examination as defined by agency policy.

Outcome Identification

I. Nurse discusses potential risks related to handling antineoplastic agents.
II. Nurse describes procedures designed to minimize exposure to antineoplastic agents.
III. Nurse documents accidental exposure to antineoplastic agents according to agency policy.
IV. Nurse recognizes professional and federal resources for monitoring changes in potential risks from, and recommendations regarding exposure to, antineoplastic agents.

Nursing Diagnosis

I. Risk for injury.

Planning and Implementation

I. Interventions to minimize risk of exposure during preparation. (Drug preparers should be specially trained.)
   A. Follow the manufacturer's recommendations for preparation.
   B. Determine a dedicated environment for drug preparation.
      1. Prepare antineoplastic agents in a centralized area.
      2. Prohibit eating, drinking, smoking, and applying cosmetics in the work area.
   C. Obtain and maintain special equipment for drug preparation.
      1. Prepare antineoplastic agents in a class II, type B biologic safety cabinet with vertical laminar air flow for maximal protection.
         a. Hood should be vented outside if feasible.
         b. Blower should be operated 24 hours a day, 7 days a week.
         c. Hood should be serviced at regular intervals according to manufacturer's recommendations.
      2. Use a disposable, plastic-backed, absorbent pad underneath work area to minimize contamination by droplets or spills.
         a. Pads are changed (at a minimum) at the completion of drug preparation or at the end of the shift.
         b. Pads are changed immediately after a contamination.
      3. Wear protective clothing during preparation of antineoplastic agents.
         a. Disposable, long-sleeved gown made of lint-free, low-permeability fabric with knitted or elastic cuffs and a closed front.

      b. Disposable, surgical latex (0.007 to 0.009 inch), nonpowdered gloves with cuffs long enough to tuck over the cuffs of the gown.
        (1) Gloves should be discarded after each use.
        (2) Gloves should be discarded after puncture, tear, or medication spill.
        (3) Personnel with a latex allergy should consider the use of vinyl or nitrile gloves or glove liners. Double-glove if vinyl gloves are used.
      c. Plastic face shield or splash goggles when splashes, sprays, or aerosols may be generated.
  D. Follow special procedures when preparing drugs.
    1. Wash hands thoroughly before and after preparation of antineoplastic agents.
    2. Use needles, syringes, tubing, and connectors with Luer-Lok attachments.
    3. Use special care when preparing agents packaged in ampules.
      a. Clear all fluid from the neck of the ampule.
      b. Tilt tip of the ampule away from preparer.
      c. Wrap a sterile gauze pad around the neck of the ampule.
      d. Break neck of the ampule away from preparer; use filter straw.
      e. Discard excess solution from ampule into a sealed waste vial or according to agency policy.
    4. Use special care when reconstituting agents packaged in vials.
      a. Employ a multiuse dispensing pin or an 18- or 19-gauge needle with a 0.2 micron hydrophobic filter or dispensing pin.
      b. Create negative pressure in the vial when adding diluent by aspirating a volume of air slightly larger than that of the volume of diluent added.
      c. Add diluent slowly.
      d. Allow diluent to run slowly down the side of the vial.
      e. Withdraw dose of agent into syringe.
      f. Allow air pressure to equalize between the vial and syringe before removing the needle.
    5. Expel air from a syringe or tubing containing antineoplastic agents slowly onto a sterile gauze pad contained in a sealable 4-mL polyethylene bag.
    6. Prime all tubing with intravenous (IV) solution before adding antineoplastic agents if possible.
II. Interventions to minimize exposure to antineoplastic agents during administration.
  A. Wear protective clothing (gloves, gown, mask, and goggles) as indicated by institutional policy when administering antineoplastic agents.
  B. Prepare agents for infusion over an absorbent, plastic-backed pad.
    1. Expulsion of air from syringe or tubing.
    2. Injection into the side arm of a running IV infusion.
    3. Spiking of a bag.
    4. Making Luer-Lok connections from tubing to venous access devices.
  C. Wash hands thoroughly after administering antineoplastic agents.
III. Interventions to minimize exposure to antineoplastic agents during disposal.
  A. Dispose of sharp objects in a puncture-resistant, leak-proof container; needles should not be recapped or clipped.
  B. Dispose of filled containers and contaminated equipment in a sealable 4-mL polyethylene or 2-mL polypropylene bag.
  C. Label all waste containers "Caution: Chemotherapy."

D. Wash hands thoroughly after disposing of antineoplastic agents and equipment.

IV. Interventions to minimize the incidence and severity of exposure to antineoplastic agents.
   A. Direct contact.
      1. Wash exposed areas with copious amounts of water or special solution.
         a. Wash exposed skin thoroughly with soap (nongermicidal) and water.
         b. Flood involved eye while holding the eyelid open with water or an isotonic eye wash for at least 5 minutes.
      2. Seek medical evaluation as soon as possible after an accidental exposure.
      3. Complete an incident report according to institutional policies and procedures.
   B. Accidental spill.
      1. Obtain a spill kit, which is clearly labeled and readily available in all areas where storage, transportation, preparation, and/or administration of chemotherapy occurs. Contents of spill kit include:
         a. Protective clothing—National Institute of Occupational Safety and Health (NIOSH)–approved respirator, splash goggles or safety goggles, two pairs of disposable gloves (inner latex gloves and outer utility gloves), disposable low-permeability coveralls or gown and shoe covers.
         b. Special equipment—two sealable, thick, plastic hazardous waste disposal bags; absorbent, plastic-backed sheets or spill pads; 250-mL and 1-L spill control pillows; small scoop to collect broken glass fragments; disposable toweling; puncture-resistant container.
      2. Wear protective clothing.
      3. Absorb liquids with a spill pad or sheet.
      4. Remove powdered agents with a damp, disposable gauze pad or soft toweling.
      5. Collect glass fragments in scoop.
      6. Dispose of all contaminated materials in a sealed, thick, plastic bag labeled with a chemotherapy warning label.
      7. Wash the contaminated area with detergent three times and rinse with water.
      8. Complete an incident report according to institutional practices and procedures.

V. Interventions to minimize risk of indirect exposure from body fluids of clients who have received antineoplastic agents within the past 48 hours.
   A. Wear protective clothing (gloves minimum) when handling urine, stool, blood, or emesis. Wear gown and goggles if splashing of body fluids is expected.
   B. Avoid splattering body fluids during disposal.
   C. Label all laboratory specimens "Caution: Chemotherapy" or "Biohazard."
   D. Place linen contaminated with body fluids in a specially marked laundry bag placed inside an impervious bag labeled "Caution: Chemotherapy" or "Biohazard."

Evaluation

The oncology nurse systematically and regularly evaluates his/her clinical practice to determine progress toward the achievement of expected outcomes. Relevant data are collected and actual findings are compared with expected findings. Nursing diagnoses, outcomes, and quality monitoring programs are reviewed and revised as necessary.

BIBLIOGRAPHY

Cass, Y., & Musgrave, C.D. (1992). Guidelines for the safe handling of excreta contaminated by cytotoxic agents. *Am J Hosp Pharm 49,* 1957–1958.

Curran, C.F., & Jameson, S.T. (1990). Causes of accidental exposure to antineoplastic agents. *Oncol Nurs Forum 17,* 764–765.

Fuchs, J., Hengstler, J.G., Jung, D., et al. (1995). DNA damage in nurses handling antineoplastic agents. *Mutat Res 342*(1–2), 17–23.

Grajny, A.E., Christie, D., Tichy, A.M., & Talashek, M.L. (1993). Chemotherapy: How safe for the care giver? *Home Healthc Nurs 11*(5), 51–58.

Gullo, S.M. (1988). Safe handling of antineoplastic drugs: Translating the recommendations into practice. *Oncol Nurs Forum 15*(5), 595–601.

Laidlaw, J.L., Cannor, T.H., Theiss, J.C., et al. (1984). Permeability of latex and polyvinyl chloride gloves to 20 antineoplastic drugs. *Am J Hosp Pharm 41*(12), 2618–2623.

McDevitt, J.J., Lees, P.S., & McDiarmid, M.A. (1993). Exposure of hospital pharmacists and nurses to antineoplastic agents. *J Occup Med 35*(1), 57–60.

Mahon, S.M., Caseperson, D.S., Yackzan, S., et al. (1994). Safe handling practices of cytotoxic drugs: The results of a chapter survey. *Oncol Nurs Forum 21*(7), 1157–1165.

Nieweg, R.M., de Boer, M., Dubbleman, R.C., et al. (1994). Safe handling of antineoplastic drugs. Results of a survey. *Cancer Nurs 17*(6), 501–511.

Occupational Safety and Health Administration. (1995). Controlling occupational exposure to hazardous drugs. (OSHA Instruction CPL 2–2.20B). Washington, D.C.: Occupational Safety and Health Administration.

Parillo, V.L. (1994). Documentation forms for monitoring occupational surveillance of health care workers who handle cytotoxic drugs. *Oncol Nurs Forum 21*(1), 115–120.

Powel, L.L. (ed.). (1996). *Cancer Chemotherapy Guidelines and Recommendations for Practice.* Pittsburgh: Oncology Nursing Press.

Sessink, P.J., Van der Kerkhof, M.C., Anzion, R.B., et al. (1994). Environmental contamination and assessment of exposure to antineoplastic agents by determination of cyclophosphamide in urine of exposed pharmacy technicians: Is skin absorption an important exposure route? *Arch Environ Health 49*(3), 165–169.

Tenenbaum, L., Ellsworth-Wolk, J., & Hawthorne, J.L. (1994). Preparation, administration and safe disposal of chemotherapeutic agents. In L. Tenenbaum (ed.). *Cancer Chemotherapy and Biotherapy: A Reference Guide.* Philadelphia: W.B. Saunders, pp. 15–67.

Valanis, B., McNeil, V., & Driscoll, K. (1991). Staff members' compliance with their facility's antineoplastic drug handling policy. *Oncol Nurs Forum 18,* 571–576.

Valanis, B., Vollmer, W.M., Labuhn, K., et al. (1992). Antineoplastic drug handling protection after OSHA guidelines: Comparison by profession, handling activity and work site. *J Occup Med 34,* 149–155.

Wroblewski, S. (1990). Chemotherapy spills on carpet. *Oncol Nurs Forum 17,* 764.

Nursing Implications of Bone Marrow and Stem Cell Transplantation

Teresa Wikle-Shapiro, RN, MSN, CFNP

Theory

I. Principles of bone marrow transplantation.
   A. Many malignancies exhibit a dose-related response to chemotherapy or radiation therapy; increasing the dose raises the number of cells that are destroyed.
      1. The dose of chemotherapy or radiation therapy that can be delivered is limited by the degree of marrow toxicity.
      2. Bone marrow or stem cells from either the client (autograft) or a donor (allograft) are infused and they engraft to "rescue" the client's hematopoietic function from the toxic effects of antineoplastic or radiation therapy. Table 39–1 outlines sources of autografts and allografts.
      3. Therefore, high doses of antineoplastic or radiation therapy may be administered to treat more aggressive, higher-risk diseases.
   B. Process of bone marrow transplantation (Fig. 39–1).
      1. Marrow source is identified (see Table 39–1).
         a. Allografting.
            (1) Allografting involves transplanting marrow, peripheral blood stem cells (PBSC), or umbilical cord blood (UCB) to a recipient who is genetically different.
            (2) Allografting, using a monozygotic twin as a donor, is termed a *syngeneic transplant.*
            (3) The most common and preferred situation is for marrow to be donated by a six-out-of-six antigen, HLA-matched sibling.
            (4) Partially matched family members or matched unrelated donors from a volunteer panel may also be used as donors.
            (5) UCB may be used as a source of allogeneic stem cells in the related, matched sibling as well as in the unrelated donor situation.
            (6) Allografts are indicated for some congenital abnormalities of bone marrow function, or in cases when there is disease involving the marrow not amenable to cure with standard treatment (e.g., leukemias). Table 39–2 shows diseases treated with allogeneic transplantation.

TABLE 39–1. **Sources of Marrow/Stem Cells**

Allografts

Matched Sibling Donor	*Identical Twin Donor*
Bone marrow	Bone marrow
Peripheral blood stem cells	Peripheral blood stem cells
Umbilical cord blood	Umbilical cord blood
Partially Matched Family Member	*Matched Unrelated Donor*
Bone marrow	Bone marrow
Peripheral blood stem cells	Umbilical cord blood
Umbilical cord blood	
Partially Matched Unrelated Donor	
Bone marrow	
Umbilical cord blood	

Autografts

Autologous bone marrow
Peripheral blood stem cells

---

    b. Autografting.
       (1) Autografting involves transplanting marrow or PBSC back into the person from which the blood cells originated.
       (2) Because a marrow or stem cell source for allografting cannot always be found or because it may be too risky, autologous bone marrow or PBSC transplantation is also used as a method for treating a number of malignant disorders.
       (3) Using autologous marrow or PBSCs is not feasible for patients who have a deficiency of their functional bone marrow, as is the case with aplastic anemia, inborn errors of metabolism, and immunodeficiency states.
       (4) May be used in circumstances in which using autologous marrow or PBSCs is preferable to using an allogeneic source of stem cells (e.g., to avoid graft-versus-host disease [GVHD], in situations in which marrow contamination with malignant cells is unlikely, and when there is no evidence of an immunologic antitumor effect ["graft versus leukemia" or something similar] with allogeneic transplant).
       (5) In older clients (older than 50 years of age), autografting may also be considered more desirable because of the high morbidity and mortality associated with allografting and GVHD.
       (6) Most frequently utilized in the setting of high-risk solid tumors in which the chance for cure is relatively low with standard or conventional doses of chemotherapy. In this case, autografting is considered a marrow or stem cell "rescue." Table 39–3 shows diseases treated with autologous transplantation.
       (7) In some autografting situations, it is questioned whether a low (undetectable) level of tumors cells persisting in the infused cells may promote relapse. However, routine purging, even in diseases that involve the marrow, is unproven. Research in this area continues.

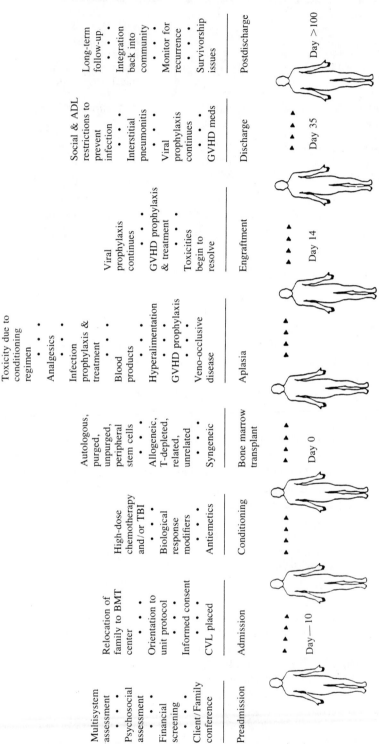

Figure 39–1. Usual stages of the transplant process. (Adapted from Ford, R., & Eisenberg, S. [1990.]. Bone marrow transplant: Recent advances and nursing implications. *Nurs Clin-North Am 25*[2], 406.)

TABLE 39–2. **Diseases Treated With Allografting of Marrow/Blood Cells**

Leukemias—Syndromes	Bone marrow failure
Acute myelogenous leukemia	Severe aplastic anemia
Acute lymphoblastic leukemia	Fanconi's anemia
Chronic myelogenous leukemia	Reticular dysgenesis
Myelodysplastic syndromes	Immunodeficiencies
Acute myelofibrosis	Severe combined immunodeficiency
Lymphoproliferative disorders	Wiskott-Aldrich syndrome
Hodgkin's disease	Miscellaneous immunodeficiencies
Non-Hodgkin's lymphoma	Nonhematologic genetic disorders
Multiple myeloma	Mucopolysaccharidosis
Chronic lymphocytic leukemia	Leukodystrophies
Hematologic disorders	Miscellaneous metabolic disorders
Beta thalassemia	
Sickle cell anemia	
Congenital neutropenias	
Osteopetrosis	

(8) PBSCs are used as an autografting source in cases of prior pelvic irradiation, marrow fibrosis, unacceptable anesthesia risk, or when early engraftment is desired.

c. A bone marrow biopsy is performed on the client to determine if the client is in remission or has malignant cells present.

(1) Optimally, clients are transplanted in the interval as near to complete remission as possible, when their disease is considered "chemoresponsive."

(2) For clients using autologous donation, marrow with malignant cells cannot be harvested; PBSCs may be used instead.

TABLE 39–3. **Diseases Treated With Autografting of Marrow/PBSCs**

Leukemias	Solid tumors
Acute myelogenous leukemia	Neuroblastoma
Acute lymphoblastic leukemia	Ewing's sarcoma
Chronic myelogenous leukemia	Breast cancer
Lymphoproliferative disorders	Testicular cancer
Hodgkin's disease	Melanoma
Non-Hodgkin's lymphoma	Osteosarcoma
Multiple myeloma	Cerebral tumors
Chronic lymphocytic leukemia	Others

d. In the allogeneic patient, histocompatibility testing is done to determine if the client and donor are genetically compatible.
  (1) Human leukocyte antigen (HLA) testing—major histocompatibility complex encoded by genes (one pair from each parent) present on chromosome 6.
    (a) Major loci of importance are HLA-A, HLA-B, and HLA-DR.
    (b) Results of allogeneic transplant are related to the degree of histocompatibility between the donor and recipient.
    (c) Clients without an HLA-matched related donor have approximately a 1 in 20,000 chance of finding an HLA-matched unrelated volunteer donor or donated UCB donor from the National Marrow Donor Registry. Use of such donors is less successful because of higher incidence of GVHD.
  (2) Further deoxyribonucleic acid (DNA) testing of the HLA-DR is also performed to determine the degree of histocompatibility between donor and recipient.
2. Marrow recipient is prepared with dose-intense (marrow ablative) therapy (Figs. 39–2 and 39–3).
  a. Conditioning protocol is established based on the primary disease and type of transplant.
  b. Goals of pretransplant conditioning regimen are to:
    (1) Eradicate remaining malignancy in the recipient.
    (2) Suppress the immune system of the recipient to allow for marrow engraftment (allografts only).
    (3) Open spaces within the marrow compartment for newly infused marrow to engraft.
  c. Conditioning regimen may include high-dose chemotherapy alone or in combination with total lymph node or total body irradiation.
  d. Conditioning regimen is usually completed several days before marrow transplant or infusion.
3. Marrow or PBSC from donor (allogeneic) or client (autologous) is harvested and processed.
  a. Performed under general or regional anesthesia.
  b. Multiple punctures (two to four) are made in the posterior iliac crests bilaterally.
    (1) Approximately 10 mL/kg of the recipient's weight is aspirated.
    (2) Marrow is then filtered to remove bone and fat particles.
    (3) Processed marrow is placed in a blood administration bag for cryopreservation (autologous) or immediate infusion (allogeneic).
    (4) Matched unrelated donor marrow is generally processed at the donor's local hospital and then is transferred to the recipient's transplant center, unless the marrow is T-cell depleted.
  c. Stem cells from an umbilical cord may be utilized if a match is found through the Cord Blood Registry, or if the baby is believed to be a match with a family member who requires an allogeneic transplant.
    (1) Related and unrelated cord blood cells are harvested at birth from volunteer donors and are cryopreserved at a designated cord blood bank.
    (2) The cells are transported to the recipient's transplant center, thawed, and infused on the day of transplant.
    (3) At present, cord blood transplants are generally reserved for patients weighing less than 60 kg.

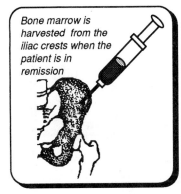

Bone marrow is harvested from the iliac crests when the patient is in remission

MARROW ACQUISITION
or stem cell acquisition

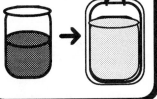

Marrow is filtered to remove fat and bone particles. Marrow may be purged of tumor cells. Processed marrow is placed in a blood bag for cryopreservation.

MARROW PREPARATION

Patient is given high-dose chemotherapy alone or in combination with radiation therapy:

- *to kill remaining cancer cells,*
- *to open spaces within the marrow for donor marrow engraftment.*

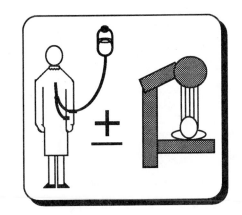

PREPARATION OF AUTOLOGOUS MARROW RECIPIENT

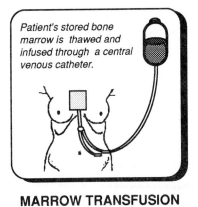

Patient's stored bone marrow is thawed and infused through a central venous catheter.

MARROW TRANSFUSION

Figure 39–2. Preparation of the recipient for an autologous bone marrow transplant.

Recipient is given high-dose chemotherapy alone or in combination with radiation therapy:

- *to kill remaining cancer cells,*
- *to suppress the immune system, and*
- *to open spaces within the marrow for donor marrow engraftment.*

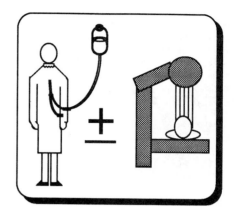

PREPARATION OF ALLOGENEIC MARROW RECIPIENT

Bone marrow is harvested from the iliac crests of the donor.

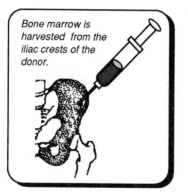

MARROW ACQUISITION
or stem cell or cord blood acquisition

Bone marrow is filtered to remove fat and bone particles. Processed marrow is placed in a blood bag for transfusion.

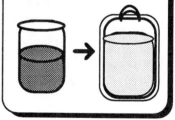

MARROW PREPARATION

Donor bone marrow is infused through a central venous catheter.

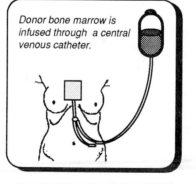

MARROW TRANSFUSION

Figure 39–3. Preparation of the recipient for an allogeneic bone marrow transplant.

    d. If marrow harvesting is not used, peripheral stem cells are thawed and infused into the recipient.
      (1) Cells are collected via a special cell separator and cryopreserved.
      (2) After the patient has completed the conditioning regimen, the cells are thawed and reinfused.
    e. Some centers are using a variety of experimental techniques to purge autologous marrow of possible tumor contaminants.
      (1) Purging may be performed using monoclonal antibodies, chemotherapy, or physical means (centrifugation).
      (2) Purging may damage the marrow, thus increasing the risk of delayed engraftment.
  4. Marrow is infused through a central venous catheter.
    a. With autologous marrow or autologous stem cells transplant, the cells are thawed at the client's bedside and reinfused.
    b. With allogeneic marrow transplant, freshly harvested marrow is brought to the client's room and infused. If allogeneic cord blood is used, the cells are thawed at the client's bedside and reinfused.
  5. Client is supported through the period of aplasia (10–30 days), and preventive measures to decrease potential complications (e.g., infection, graft-versus-host disease) of bone marrow transplantation are instituted. See Table 39–4 for preventive measures for bone marrow transplantation-associated complication control practices.

  II. Role of bone marrow transplantation.
    A. Cure—due to the aggressive nature of the therapy, each client is evaluated with curative intent.
    B. Palliation—few clients are treated to prolong life for a short period of time.
  III. Marrow source.
    A. Type of transplant is based on marrow source (see Table 39–1).
      1. Autologous—client receives own bone marrow or PBSCs that were harvested before the pretransplant conditioning.
      2. Allogeneic—client receives bone marrow, PBSCs, or UCB from a healthy related or unrelated donor.
      3. Syngeneic—client receives bone marrow or PBSCs from a genetically identical twin.
    B. Factors affecting source of donor marrow.
      1. Primary disease to be treated.
      2. Availability of a histocompatible donor.
      3. Age of the patient.

Assessment

  I. Pertinent personal history.
    A. Diagnosis—see Tables 39–2 and 39–3 for conditions commonly treated with bone marrow transplantation.
    B. Clients with malignancies that are at high risk for recurrence after standard therapy are selected for bone marrow transplantation. However, these malignancies must demonstrate a response to either antineoplastic therapy or radiation therapy.
    C. Factors that may increase the incidence of complications of marrow transplantation.
      1. Amount of previous cancer therapy, length of time since last therapy, response to past therapy, and length of disease-free interval.

TABLE 39–4. **Preventive Measures for Bone Marrow Transplantation-Associated Complications**

Complication	Information	Preventive Measures	Nursing Implications
Graft-versus-host disease	Results from engraftment of immunocompetent donor T lymphocytes reacting against immunoincompetent recipient tissues (skin, gastrointestinal tract, and liver) Occurs in 30 to 60% of allogeneic bone marrow transplant recipients Risk is increased when donor is not a 6/6 HLA antigen match or when a matched unrelated donor is used Can be either acute or chronic	Depletion of T cells from marrow Preventive immunosuppressive agents Cyclosporine A High-dose steroids Antithymocyte globulin Muromonab-CD3 (OKT-3) Azathioprine (Imuran) Thalidomide Monoclonal antibodies Irradiate all blood products	Monitor for delayed marrow engraftment Monitor for prolonged lymphopenia and neutropenia Evaluate cyclosporine levels and notify practitioner of significant abnormalities Monitor for side effects of immunosuppressive agents Monitor for signs of infection Maintain skin integrity Maintain client's functional capacity
Pulmonary interstitial pneumonitis	Occurs most frequently in clients >30 years of age, with history of chest irradiation or previous bleomycin therapy; and CMV-positive Causative agents: Cytomegalovirus 50% *Aspergillus* 30% *Pneumocystis carinii* 5% Other 15%	Use of cytomegalovirus (CMV)-seronegative blood products when donor and recipient are CMV-seronegative Use of filtered air system Antimicrobial therapy Ganciclovir Foscarnet Intravenous immunoglobulin Trimethoprim and sulfamethoxazole (Septra) Aerosolized pentamidine Ribavirin	Monitor for side effects of antimicrobial therapy Implement turn, cough, and deep-breathe routine Encourage activity

2. Underlying kidney, lung, liver, or cardiac dysfunction.
3. Previous infections and response to therapy.
4. Age—older clients (>17 years) are more likely to develop transplant-related complications.
5. Psychosocial dysfunction.

II. Physical examination.
  A. Pulmonary—respiratory rate, depth, and rhythm; lung expansion; adventitious breath sounds.
  B. Renal—color and odor of urine and urinary output.
  C. Mobility—muscle strength and endurance, range of motion, gait, and activity level.
  D. Nutrition—weight, skin turgor; amount, content, and patterns of nutritional intake.
  E. Comfort level.
  F. Cardiovascular—heart rate and rhythm, heart sounds, blood pressure.
  G. Gastrointestinal—color, consistency, and caliber of stool.
  H. Genitourinary—color of urine, suppleness of bladder, condition of perineum.
  I. Integumentary—color and intactness of skin, condition of oral mucous membranes, dental evaluation, condition of perineum and rectum.
  J. Neurologic—mental status, orientation, sensation, and reflexes.

III. Psychosocial examination.
  A. Psychological evaluation.
    1. Feelings on decision to have bone marrow transplant.
    2. Understanding of aggressiveness of treatment, goals of therapy, and chances of survival.
    3. Number, type, effectiveness of coping mechanisms used in past stressful situations by client and family members.
    4. Perceptions of client and family about isolation, prolonged hospitalization, living will, use of life-support technology, and potential death or survival.
  B. Social evaluation.
    1. Previous roles and responsibilities within the family and community.
    2. Type, number, and history of use of support systems within the family and community.
    3. Financial status—employment, insurance coverage, and resources for daily living needs.
    4. Eligibility for community resources.

IV. Critical laboratory and diagnostic data unique to marrow transplantation.
  A. Hematologic—complete blood count, differential, platelet count, coagulation studies, type and crossmatch with marrow donor.
  B. Hepatic—lactic acid dehydrogenase (LDH) and bilirubin levels.
  C. Renal—electrolyte, blood urea nitrogen (BUN), creatinine, cyclosporine A levels, tacrolimus (FK-506) levels.
  D. Cardiovascular—electrocardiogram and cardiac ejection fraction.
  E. Pulmonary—chest x-ray examination, pulmonary function tests; arterial blood gases, oxygen saturation (pulse oximetry).
  F. Immune—antibody titers for cytomegalovirus (CMV), herpesviruses, Epstein-Barr virus, toxoplasmosis, hepatitis B surface antigen, immunoglobulin levels, human immunodeficiency virus antibody.
  G. Infectious disease—blood cultures for bacteria and fungi; urine and stool cultures for bacteria, fungi, and viruses; blood for buffy coat; respiratory and sputum cultures for bacteria, fungi, viruses, *Legionella,* acid-fast bacilli (AFB), stool and urine for electron microscopy.

Nursing Diagnoses

I. Anxiety.

II. Risk for infection.

III. Acute pain.

IV. Diarrhea.

V. Diversional activity deficit.

VI. Altered growth and development.

Outcome Identification

I. Client and family describe the rationale for bone marrow transplantation.

II. Client participates in self-care strategies to decrease the risk and severity of predictable side effects of bone marrow transplantation on health.

III. Client and family describe recommended changes in self-care, lifestyle, and social interactions to minimize the effects of bone marrow transplantation on health.

IV. Client and family discuss strategies to maintain valued roles and relationships during the transplant and posttransplant periods.

V. Client and family list community resources available for assistance and support.

VI. Client and family discuss the rationale, schedule, and procedures required for continued follow-up care after bone marrow transplantation.

Planning and Implementation

I. Interventions to maximize safety for the client and family.
  A. Maintain aseptic techniques and the level of protective isolation as identified by the bone marrow transplantation program. (See Table 39–4 for general guidelines.)
  B. Implement the conditioning regimen as ordered by the physician.
  C. Teach the client and family strategies to decrease risk of infection, bleeding, and injury during period of aplasia following bone marrow or stem cell or cord blood infusion.

II. Interventions to decrease the incidence and severity of complications unique to bone marrow transplantation.
  A. Anxiety.
    1. Assess changes in and perceived contributing factors to anxiety levels in client and family.
    2. Provide a thorough orientation to the bone marrow transplant unit and procedures common to bone marrow transplantation.
    3. Implement strategies to encourage the client and family to express concerns about bone marrow transplantation demands.
    4. Consult with the occupational therapist to develop a plan for diversional activities during isolation.
    5. Teach new anxiety-relieving strategies as desired or needed by client and family.
  B. Risk for infection (see Chapter 12). Table 39–5 outlines common opportunistic infections and their time of occurrence posttransplant.
    1. Notify the physician of initial temperature greater than 101.0°F (38.3°C) or other symptoms indicative of infection.
    2. Teach the client and family strategies to decrease the risk of endogenous infections.
      a. Meticulous handwashing (Table 39–6).
      b. Routine oral and perineal care.
      c. Skin care.

TABLE 39–5. Infectious Complications and Occurrence in BMT Recipients

Organism	Common Site
First Month Post-Transplant	
Viral	
Herpes simplex virus (HSV)	Oral, esophageal, skin, GI tract, and genital
Respiratory syncytial virus (RSV)	Sinopulmonary
Epstein-Barr virus (EBV)	Oral, esophageal, skin, GI tract
Bacterial	
Gram-positives (*Staphylococcus epidermidis, S. aureus,* streptococci)	Skin, blood, sinopulmonary
Gram-negatives (*E. coli, Pseudomonas aeruginosa, Klebsiella*)	GI, blood, oral, perirectal
Fungal	
Candida species (*C. albicans, glabratta, krusei*)	Oral, esophageal, skin
Aspergillus (*A. fumigatus, flavus*)	Sinopulmonary
1–4 Months Post-Transplant	
Viral	
Cytomegalovirus (CMV)	Pulmonary, hepatic, GI
Enteric viruses (rotavirus, coxsackievirus, adenovirus)	Pulmonary, urinary, GI, hepatic Sinopulmonary
RSV	Pulmonary
Parainfluenza virus	
Bacterial	
Gram-positives	Sinopulmonary and skin
Fungal	
Candida species	Oral, hepatosplenic, integument
Aspergillus species	Sinopulmonary, CNS
Mucormycosis	Sinopulmonary
Coccidioidomycosis	Sinopulmonary
Cryptococcus neoformans	Pulmonary, CNS
Protozoa	
Pneumocystis carinii	Pulmonary
Toxoplasma gondii	Pulmonary, CNS
4–12 Months Post-Transplant	
Viral	
CMV, echoviruses, RSV, varicella-zoster virus (VZV)	Integument, pulmonary, hepatic
Bacterial	
Gram-positives (*Streptococcus pneumoniae, Haemophilus influenzae,* pneumococci)	Sinopulmonary and blood Sinopulmonary
Fungal	
Aspergillosis	Sinopulmonary
Coccidioidomycosis	Sinopulmonary
Protozoa	
Pneumocystis carinii	Pulmonary
Toxoplasma gondii	Pulmonary, CNS
Greater Than 12 Months Post-Transplant	
Viral	
VZV	Integument
Bacterial	
Gram-positives (streptococci, *H. influenzae,* encapsulated bacteria)	Sinopulmonary and blood

Data from Chaplin, R.E., & Gale, R.P. (1984). The early complications of bone marrow transplantation. *Semin Hematol 21*(2), 101–108; Hertz, M.I., Englund, J.A., Snover, D., et al. (1989). Respiratory syncytial virus-induced acute lung injury in adult patients with bone marrow transplants: A clinical approach and review of the literature. *Medicine 68*(5), 269–281; Saral, R. (1985). Viral infections in bone marrow transplantation recipients. *Plasma Ther Transfus Technol 6,* 275–284; Tutschka, P.J. (1988). Infections and immunodeficiency in bone marrow transplantation. *Pediatr Infect Dis J 7*(Suppl), 22–29; Ezzone, S., & Camp-Sorrell, D. (eds.). (1995). *Manual for Bone Marrow Transplant Nursing: Recommendations for Practice and Education.* Pittsburgh: Oncology Nursing Press.

TABLE 39–6. **Centers for Disease Control Recommendations for Handwashing**

Handwashing Indications

1. In the absence of a true emergency, personnel should *always* wash their hands
   a. **Before** performing invasive procedures
   b. **Before** taking care of particularly susceptible patients, such as those who are severely immunocompromised and newborns
   c. **Before** and **after** touching wounds, whether surgical, traumatic, or associated with an invasive device
   d. **After** situations during which microbial contamination of hands is likely to occur, especially those involving contact with mucous membranes, blood or body fluids, secretions, or excretions
   e. **After** touching inanimate sources that are likely to be contaminated with virulent or epidemiologically important microorganisms; these sources include urine-measuring devices or secretion-collection apparatuses
   f. **After** taking care of an infected patient or one who is likely to be colonized with microorganisms of special clinical or epidemiologic significance, for example, multiple-drug resistant bacteria
   g. **Between** contact with different patients
2. Most routine, brief patient-care activities involving *direct* patient contact other than that discussed above (e.g., taking a blood pressure) do not require handwashing except in high-risk units such as bone marrow transplant units
3. Most routine hospital activities involving indirect patient content (e.g., handing a patient medications, food, or other objects) do not require handwashing

Handwashing Technique

For routine handwashing, a vigorous rubbing together of all surfaces of lathered hands for at least 10 seconds, followed by thorough rinsing under a stream of water, is recommended

Handwashing with Plain Soap

1. Plain soap should be used for handwashing unless otherwise indicated
2. If bar soap is used, it should be kept on racks that allow drainage of water
3. If liquid soap is used, the dispenser should be replaced or cleaned and filled with fresh product when empty; liquids should not be added to a partially full dispenser

Handwashing with Antimicrobial-Containing Products (Health-Care Personnel Handwashes)

1. Antimicrobial handwashing products should be used for handwashing before personnel care for newborns and when otherwise indicated during their care, between patients in high-risk units, and before personnel take care of severely immunocompromised patients
2. Antimicrobial-containing products that do not require water for use, such as foams or rinses, can be used in areas where no sinks are available

Handwashing Facilities

1. Handwashing facilities should be conveniently located throughout the hospital
2. A sink should be located in or just outside every patient room; more than one sink per room may be necessary if a large room is used for several patients
3. Handwashing facilities should be located in or adjacent to rooms where diagnostic or invasive procedures that require handwashing are performed (e.g., cardiac catheterization, bronchoscopy, sigmoidoscopy)

From the Centers for Disease Control and Prevention (1985). *Guidelines: Nosocomial Infections in Handwashing and Hospital Environmental Control.* Washington, D.C.: Author.

   3. Teach the client and family strategies to decrease risk of exogenous infections.
      a. Restrict visitors with suspected or known infections.
      b. Limit visitation of children (especially school-aged children).
      c. Place the client on a sterile or low microbial diet.
      d. Avoid invasive procedures (e.g., peripheral intravenous catheter, intramuscular injections, urinary catheterization, rectal examinations, rectal temperatures).
   4. Administer prophylactic antimicrobial therapy as ordered.
      a. Fluconazole, itraconazole, clortrimazole, or nystatin to prevent fungal infection.
      b. Trimethoprim-sulfamethoxazole (Septra/Bactrim) or pentamidine for prevention of *Pneumocystis carinii* pneumonia.
      c. Acyclovir for prevention of herpesvirus infection and CMV.
      d. Ganciclovir or foscarnet for prevention of CMV infection.
      e. Intravenous immunoglobulin for prevention of CMV infection.
      f. Oral nonabsorbable antibiotics or ciprofloxacin for decontamination of the gastrointestinal tract of endogenous bacteria.
   5. Perform routine surveillance cultures for bacteria, fungi, and viruses.
   6. Transfuse CMV seronegative blood products or leukopoor-filtered blood products to clients who are seronegative for CMV.
C. Risk for injury.
   1. For clients receiving high-dose cyclophosphamide, hemorrhagic cystitis is a potential complication.
      a. Administer continuous bladder irrigation (CBI) as ordered.
      b. If CBI is not used, administer hydration, push oral fluids, and have the patient void every hour for 6 hours following cyclophosphamide administration.
      c. Administer mesna, a uroprotectorant, as ordered.
      d. Administer antispasmodics and analgesics as ordered.
D. Alteration in comfort related to keratitis (corneal irritation).
   1. Provide sunglasses and darken the room to relieve discomfort.
   2. Discourage the client from rubbing eyes—use mittens.
   3. Administer artificial tears, steroid eye drops, and analgesics as ordered.
E. Altered oral mucous membrane (see Chapter 13).
III. Interventions to monitor for unique complications of bone marrow transplantation.
A. Graft-versus-host disease (Table 39–7).
   1. Monitor condition of skin (erythema or rash) especially on the palms of hands and soles of feet.
   2. Evaluate changes in liver function study results.
   3. Monitor the amount, consistency, frequency, and color of stool.
B. Hepatic veno-occlusive disease.
   1. Weigh the client every day; notify the medical practitioner of weight gain greater than 5 pounds.
   2. Monitor location of pain (right upper quadrant).
   3. Evaluate for elevation in serum bilirubin.
   4. Evaluate changes in mental status.
   5. Measure abdominal girth every day if other parameters (1–3) indicate possible veno-occlusive disease.

TABLE 39–7. **Clinical Staging and Grading of Acute GVHD**

Staging by Organ

Organ	Stage	Parameters
		Rash
Skin	I	<25% BSA
	II	25–50% BSA
	III	Generalized erythroderma
	IV	Bullae and desquamation
		Total Bilirubin (mg/dL)
Liver	I	2.0–3.5
	II	3.5–8.0
	III	8.0–15.0
	IV	>15.0
		Volume of Diarrhea (mL/24hr)
Gut	I	Adult: 500–1000 mL/d
		Pediatric: 10–15 mL/kg/d
	II	Adult: 1000–1500 mL/d
		Pediatric: 15–20 mL/kg/d
	III	Adult: 1500–2000 mL/d
		Pediatric: 20–30 mL/kg/d
	IV	Adult: >2000 mL/d
		Pediatric: >30 mL/kg/d

Overall Clinical Grade

Grade	Description
0	Stage I clinical skin GVHD
I	Stage II clinical skin GVHD
II	Stage II–III clinical skin GVHD and stage II–IV clinical liver and/or gut GVHD. Only one system stage III or greater
III	Stage II–IV clinical skin GVHD (with ≥grade 2 histology) and stage II–IV clinical liver and/or gut GVHD. Only one system stage III or greater
IV	Stage II–IV clinical skin GVHD (with ≥grade 2 histology) and stage II–IV clinical liver and/or gut GVHD. Two or >systems stage III or greater

BSA = body surface area; GVHD = graft-versus-host disease.

   C. Pulmonary interstitial pneumonitis.
     1. Monitor temperature.
     2. Assess for presence of cough, chest pain, or adventitious breath sounds.
     3. Evaluate activity tolerance.
IV. Interventions to enhance adaptation and rehabilitation.
   A. Implement a program of range of motion and isometric exercises during the isolation period.
   B. Initiate client and family teaching about care of the central venous catheter early in the course of hospitalization.
   C. Encourage the client, donor, and significant other to express concerns related to the transplant experience.
   D. Discuss potential changes in lifestyle and social interaction required immediately after discharge from the hospital.

Evaluation

The oncology nurse systematically and regularly evaluates the client's and/or family's responses to interventions to determine progress toward the achievement of expected outcomes. Relevant data are collected and actual findings are compared with expected findings. Nursing diagnoses, outcomes, and plans of care are reviewed and revised as necessary.

BIBLIOGRAPHY

Beatty, P.G. (1991). The use of unrelated donors for bone marrow transplantation. *Marrow Transplantation Rev 1*(1), 1–7.

Ezzone, S., & Camp-Sorrell, D. (eds.). (1994). *Manual for Bone Marrow Transplant Nursing: Recommendations for Practice and Education.* Pittsburgh: Oncology Nursing Press.

Ford, R., & Ballard, B. (1988). Acute complication after bone marrow transplantation. *Semin Oncol Nurs 4*(1), 15–24.

Ford, R., & Eisenberg, S. (1990). Bone marrow transplant: Recent advances and nursing implications. *Nurs Clin North Am 25*(2), 405–422.

Hagglund, H., Bostrom, L., & Remberger, M. (1995). Risk factors for acute graft versus host disease in 291 consecutive HLA identical bone marrow transplant recipients. *Bone Marrow Transplant 16*(6), 747–754.

Hartsell, W. F., Czyzewski, E.A., Ghalie, R., & Kaizer, H. (1995). Pulmonary complications of bone marrow transplantation: A comparison of total body irradiation and cyclophosphamide to busulfan and cyclophosphamide. *Int J Radiat Oncol Biol Phys 32*(1), 69–73.

Holmes, W. (1993). Cyclosporin immunosuppression: Clinical practice issues. *Curr Issues Cancer Nurs Pract 1*(10), 1–7.

Kanfer, E. (1995). Graft versus host disease. In J. Treleaven & P. Wiernik (eds.). *Color Atlas & Text of Bone Marrow Transplantation.* St. Louis: Mosby-Year Book, pp. 143–153.

Kaplan, E.B., Wodell, R.A., Wilmott, R.W., et al. (1994). Late effects of bone marrow transplantation on pulmonary function in children. *Bone Marrow Transplant 14,* 613–621.

Quabeck, K. (1994). The lung as a critical organ in marrow transplantation. *Bone Marrow Transplant 14,* 519–528.

Sanford, J.P., Gilbert, D.N., Gerberding, J.L., & Sande, M.A. (eds.). (1996). *The Sanford Guide to Antimicrobial Therapy* (24th ed.). Dallas: Antimicrobial Therapy, Inc.

Sparano, J.A., Ciobanu, N., & Gucalp, R. (1995). Solid tumors. In J. Treleaven & P. Wiernik (eds.). *Color Atlas & Text of Bone Marrow Transplantation.* St. Louis: Mosby-Year Book, pp. 77–100.

Treleaven, J., & Wiernik, P. (eds.). (1995). *Color Atlas & Text of Bone Marrow Transplantation.* St. Louis: Mosby-Year Book.

Whedon, M.B., & Wujik, D. (eds.). (1997). *Bone Marrow and Stem Cell Transplantation: Principles, Practice, and Nursing Insights* (2nd ed.). Boston: Jones & Bartlett.

Wikle-Shapiro, T.J. (1997). Cardiopulmonary complications of bone marrow transplantation. In M.B. Whedon & D. Wujik D (eds.). *Bone Marrow Transplantation: Principles, Practice, and Nursing Insights* (2nd ed.). Boston: Jones & Bartlett, pp. 266–297.

Wujcik, D. (1994). Overview of colony-stimulating factors: Focus on the neutrophil. In R.M. Carroll-Johnson (ed.). *A Case Management Approach to Patients Receiving G-CSF.* Pittsburgh: Oncology Nursing Press.

PART SEVEN

Health Promotion

40

Prevention of Cancer

Sharon J. Olsen, RN, MS, AOCN
Candis H. Morrison, PhD, CANP
Barbara W. Ashley, RN, MSN, CANP

Theory

I. Definitions
  A. Primary prevention.
    1. Involves reducing the risk of cancer in individuals and groups generally considered both physically and emotionally healthy through client behaviors related to:
      a. Eliminating or limiting exposure to causative factors.
      b. Promoting protective factors (including health-promoting activities).
  B. Secondary prevention.
    1. Activities include defining and identifying high-risk groups and groups with precursor stages of cancer, early diagnosis or detection, and screening (see Chapter 41).
  C. Risk—the likelihood that exposure to a certain factor will influence the chance of developing a particular cancer based on the national average.
    1. Types of risk.
      a. Absolute risk—a measure of cancer occurrence in terms of cancer incidence and mortality.
      b. Relative risk—an estimate of increased probability of developing a certain cancer based on amount of exposure to the associated risk factor(s). The higher the relative risk, the greater the risk of developing that specific cancer.
        (1) Example—the relative risk (RR) for lung cancer among uranium miners exposed to radon and to tobacco smoke ranges from 6.4 to 52.0, depending on the level of exposure and number of cigarettes smoked per day. The RR for lung cancer for the nonexposed nonsmoker is 1.0.
      c. Attributable risk—the arithmetic difference in cancer rates between the group exposed to the factor and the unexposed group factor.
        (1) Example—suppose the mortality rate among heavy smokers subject to low doses of industrial ionizing radiation is 2.7 per 1000 men, and the mortality rate among nonsmokers with the same dose of ionizing radiation is 0.23 per 1000 men. The attributable risk is 2.5, meaning that an additional 2.5 deaths per 1000 men occurred that were attributable to smoking. These excess deaths would not have occurred if the person had not smoked heavily.

    D. Risk factor—an element of personal behavior, genetic makeup or exposure that is statistically associated with an increased frequency of disease, disability, or death.

    E. Risk assessment—procedure by which the probability of a person's development of disease, disability, or death is predicted through analysis of individual characteristics known as risk factors.

      1. Purpose.

        a. Assist in diagnosis.

        b. Help establish patterns of inheritance.

        c. Assist in identification of persons at risk.

        d. Contribute to the biologic understanding of cancer.

        e. Alter or change risk factors to result in a decrease in new cases of cancer.

II. Theoretical principles.

    A. Prevention strategies continue to gain importance as evidence suggests that as much as 50% or more of cancer incidence (new cases) can be prevented through smoking cessation and changed dietary habits.

    B. Recognizing risk factors identifies individuals at higher risk for cancer.

    C. Changes in lifestyle have the potential to reduce cancer risks.

    D. Reduction of exposure to carcinogens may reduce cancer risk.

      1. Cancer results from the accumulation of discrete genome changes that occur over time, perhaps 10 to 30 years.

      2. Cancer results from initiating and promoting factors.

      3. Promotion can be reversed.

      4. Avoiding synergistic exposures (alcohol and tobacco, asbestos and tobacco) may decrease cancer incidence.

    E. Cancer risk factors.

      1. Mechanisms of carcinogenesis predict that individual susceptibility to cancer may result from several factors, including:

        a. Differences in the metabolism of carcinogenic chemicals (uptake, activation, and detoxification).

        b. Deoxyribonucleic acid (DNA) repair.

        c. Inherited or acquired alterations in protooncogenes or tumor suppressor genes.

        d. Nutritional status.

        e. Hormonal factors.

        f. Immunologic factors.

        g. Occupational and environmental exposures.

Assessment

I. Identify lifestyle risk factors (Table 40–1).

    A. Tobacco use.

      1. Accounts for at least 30% of cancer deaths.

      2. Single major cause of cancer mortality in the United States (US).

      3. Strongly linked to lung cancer (risk is 10 times greater by middle age for smokers versus lifelong nonsmokers).

      4. Associated cancers—bladder, pancreas, cervix, uterus, esophagus, oral cavity, stomach.

      5. Cigarettes are most important cause of tobacco-related cancer. Other forms of tobacco, notably chewing tobacco and snuff, are also established carcinogens.

(*Text continued on page 687*)

TABLE 40–1. **Cancer Risk Factors and Associated Familial Syndromes**

Cancer	Epidemiologic or Etiologic Factors and Relative Risk (RR)	Associated Familial Syndromes

Breast[1, 4]	Age >60 (4.0–5.0)
	Family/Personal History
	  Previous history of breast cancer in 1 breast (2.0–4.0)
	  Family history
	    1 First-degree relative (2.0–4.0)
	    ≥Two first-degree relatives (4.0–6.0)
	  Fibrocystic disease
	    Any (1.1–2.0)
	    Proliferative (2.0–4.0)
	    Atypical hyperplasia (>4.0)
	Reproductive/Hormonal
	  Age at menarche <12 (1.1–2.0)
	  Age at first full-term pregnancy >30 (1.1–2.0)
	  Age at menopause >55 (1.1–2.0)
	  Estrogen replacement therapy >6 years (1.1–2.0)
	  Oral contraceptive use, >10 yrs increases risk for early
	    onset, age <45, breast cancer (1.0–2.0)
	Diet
	  Obesity, 90th percentile (1.1–2.0)
	  High-fat diet, >38% calories from fat (no association to
	    1.5)
	  Alcohol, 1 drink/day (1.1–2.0)
	Environment/Occupational
	  Radiation
	    Atomic bomb (1 Gy) (2.0–4.0)
	    Repeat fluoroscopy (1.2–2.0)
	Protective Factors
	  Dietary fiber
	  Physical activity
	  Lactation
		Li-Fraumeni
		
		Early-onset breast, ovarian
		
		Hereditary nonpolyposis
		  colorectal cancer
		  (HNPCC)?
		Ataxia-telangiectasia (AT)

Ovarian[1, 2, 3]	Geographic and Socioeconomic
	  Northern European and American (1–5)
	    >Age 55 (3.5)
	  Caucasian (RR 1.5)
	    Income and education, higher levels (1.5–2)
	Hormonal
	  Never used oral contraceptives (1.5)
	Genetics
	  Family history (first- or second-degree relative) (2–3)
	  Cancer family syndromes (5–35)
	Reproductive
	  Nulliparity and/or infertility (1.5–2)
	Chronic talc exposure (2.0)
	Protective Factors
	  More than one full-term pregnancy
	  Oral contraceptive use (more than 5 years of use may
	    reduce risk by 37%)
		HNPCC?
		
		Three patterns of familial
		  ovarian cancer
		  Site-specific ovarian cancer
		  Breast and ovarian
		  Cancer family syndrome

Cervix[1, 2, 3, 5]	Geographic and Socioeconomic
	  Latin American, Asian, African (2.0–6.0)
	  Rural (1.0–3.0)
	  African American (2.0)
	  Lower income and education level (2.0–3.0)
	Age >65 yrs old (2.0–3.0)
	Hormonal
	  Long-term use of oral contraceptives (1.5–2.0)
		None identified

Table continued on following page

TABLE 40–1. **Cancer Risk Factors and Associated Familial Syndromes** (*Continued*)

Cancer	Epidemiologic or Etiologic Factors and Relative Risk (RR)	Associated Familial Syndromes

	Reproductive History
	  Multiparity (2.0–4.0)
	  Early age (<16 yr) intercourse (2.0)
	  ≥Three sexual partners (2.0–3.0)
	  Sexually transmitted disease (2.0–10.0)
	    Human papillomavirus (HPV) types 16, 18
	    HSV-2, HHV-6
	    HIV
	No Prior Pap Smear Screening (2.0–6.0)
	Long-term Cigarette Smoking (2.0–4.0)
	Diet
	  Low in beta carotene and vitamin C (2.0–3.0)	

Prostate[1, 6–8, 10]	Hormonal
	  Testosterone
	Age >65 yr
	Geographic and Socioeconomic
	  African American
	Genetics
	  Father and/or brothers:
	    One (2.0)
	    Two (5.0)
	  Father/brother or grandfather/uncle
	    One (1.5)
	    Two (2.3)
	Diet
	  High-fat diet
	Occupational Exposure
	  >10-year exposure to cadmium and zinc
		Autosomal dominant
		  inheritance pattern[9]

Bladder[1, 7]	Occupational Exposures
	  Aniline dyes (textile workers)
	  Benzidine
	  2-naphthylamine
	  Aromatic amines (rubber workers)
	  4-aminobiphenyl
	  Parachloro-orthotoluidine
	  Aluminum production workers
	  Coal gasification workers
	  Coke production workers
	  Exhaust exposure (railroad workers, truck and bus drivers,
	    and dockers)
	  Leather workers
	Radiation Exposure
	  Atomic bomb survivors
	  Spondylitis patients with history of radiation to spine
	Cigarette Smoking
	Genetics
	  Family history of bladder cancer (2.0)
	Certain Drug Exposures
	  Phenacetin-containing analgesics
	  Alkylating agents (cyclophosphamide)
	Protective Factors
	  Vitamin A
	  Beta carotene
	  Vitamin C
	  Vitamin E
		HNPCC

TABLE 40–1. **Cancer Risk Factors and Associated Familial Syndromes** (*Continued*)

Cancer	Epidemiologic or Etiologic Factors and Relative Risk (RR)	Associated Familial Syndromes

Kidney[1, 7]	Cigarette Smoking
	Abuse of Certain Drugs
	  Diuretics
	  Phenacetin
	Occupational Exposures
	  Cadmium
	  Asbestos
	  Rubber workers
	  Leather dusts
	  Organic solvents
	  Coke oven workers
	  Insulators
	  Gasoline station attendants
	Radiation Exposure
	  Atomic bomb survivors
	  Spondylitis patients with history of radiation to spine
		von Hippel-Lindau
		  syndrome
		Hereditary papillary renal
		  cell cancer
		
		Wilms' tumor
		Beckwith-Wiedemann
		  syndrome

Lung[1, 11]	Cigarette Smoking
	Occupational Exposures
	  Asbestos
	  Radon
	Factors That May Act Synergistically With Cigarette
	    Smoking
	  Family history of lung cancer (5.0)
	  Asbestos exposure
	  Indoor radon exposure
	  Dietary deficiency of Vitamin A
	Side-stream Smoke Exposure
		Li-Fraumeni

Colorectal[1, 12]	Diet
	  High-fat diet
	  Low-fiber diet
	  Obesity
	Age >50 years
	Inflammatory bowel disease
	  Chronic ulcerative colitis
	  Chronic granulomatous colitis
	Genetics
	  Family history of colorectal adenomas
	  Family history of colorectal cancer
	  Personal history:
	    Colorectal adenomas
	    Colorectal cancer
	    Breast, ovarian, uterine cancer
	Protective Factors
	  High-fiber diet
	  Calcium
	  Vitamins C and A
	  Selenium
		HNPCC
		
		Familial adenomatous
		  polyposis (FAP)
		
		Gardner's syndrome
		
		Peutz-Jeghers syndrome
		
		Juvenile polyposis
		
		Turcot's syndrome
		
		Oldfield's syndrome

Pancreatic[13]	Diet
	  High carbohydrate intake
	Occupational Exposures
	  Heterocyclic amines
	  Methylene chloride
	  Solvents	

Gastric[1, 14]	Geographic
	  Japan (8.0)
	Helicobacter pylori Infection
	Diet
	  Highly salted foods
	  Nitrates
	  Smoked meats
	  Pickled vegetables	

Table continued on following page

TABLE 40–1. **Cancer Risk Factors and Associated Familial Syndromes** (*Continued*)

Cancer	Epidemiologic or Etiologic Factors and Relative Risk (RR)	Associated Familial Syndromes

Non-Hodgkin's lymphoma[1, 15]	Immunosuppression
	  Genetic
	  Iatrogenic (transplant)
	  AIDS
	Viral Cofactors
	  EBV
	  ? HHV-6
	  HTLV-I
	Occupational Exposures
	  Benzene
	  Pesticides, herbicides
	  Aromatic amines and solvents in rubber industry workers
	Hair Dyes (dark dyes, >20 yrs)
	Bacterial Cofactors
	  Helicobacter pylori associated with low grade
	  B-cell gastric lymphoma of mucosa-associated lymphoid
	  tissue (MALT)
		Genetic Immunodeficiency
		  Syndromes
		Wiskott-Aldrich
		Severe combined
		  immunodeficiency
		  (adenosine deaminase)
		Common variable
		  immunodeficiency
		
		Ataxia-telangiectasia

Melanoma[1, 15]	Geographic
	  Australia
	  Proximity to equator
	  Higher socioeconomic status
	Age >30 years
	Host Factors
	  Family history of melanoma (2.0–8.0)
	  Caucasian
	  Tendency to sunburn rather than tan
	  History of severe (blistering) sunburn especially before age
	  20
	  History of congenital melanocytic nevi
	Sunlight Exposure
	  UVA (sun lamp is important source)
	  UVB
		Cutaneous malignant
		  melanoma/dysplastic
		  nevi syndrome
		
		Xeroderma pigmentosum

BSE = breast self-examination, CBE = clinical breast examination, CRCs = chlorofluorocarbons, FOBT = fecal occult blood test, HNPCC = hereditary nonpolyposis colorectal cancer, HHV-6 = human herpesvirus 6, HIV = human immunodeficiency virus, HPV = human papillomavirus, HSV = herpes simplex virus, PSA = prostate-specific antigen, RR = relative risk, UVA = ultraviolet A, UVB = ultraviolet B.

Data from 1. The Subcommittee to Evaluate the National Cancer Program. (Sept. 1994). *Cancer at a crossroads: A report to the congress for the nation.* Bethesda, MD: National Cancer Institute. 2. NIH. (1994). *Consensus development conference statement: Ovarian cancer: Screening, treatment and follow-up.* Bethesda, MD: NIH. 3. Daly, M.B., Bookman, M.A., & Lerman, C.E. (1995). Female reproductive tract: Cervix, endometrium, ovary. In P. Greenwald, B.S. Kramer, & D.L. Weed (eds.). *Cancer Prevention and Control.* New York: Marcel Dekker, pp. 585–610. 4. Helzlsouer, K.J. (1995). Early detection and prevention of breast cancer. In P. Greenwald, B.S. Kramer, & D.L. Weed (eds.). *Cancer Prevention and Control.* New York: Marcel Dekker, pp. 509–535. 5. Report of the U.S. Preventive Services Task Force. (1996). *Guide to clinical preventive services.* Alexandria, VA: International Medical Publishing. 6. Mettlin, C., et al. (1993). Defining and updating the American Cancer Society guidelines for the cancer-related checkup: Prostate and endometrial cancers. *CA Cancer J Clin 43*, 42–46. 7. Madajewicz, S. (1995). Genitourinary cancer. In P. Greenwald, B.S. Kramer, & D.L. Weed (eds.). *Cancer Prevention and Control.* New York: Marcel Dekker, pp. 659–671. 8. Walsh, P.C., & Worthington, J.F. (1995). *The Prostate: A Guide for Men and the Women Who Love Them.* Baltimore: The Johns Hopkins University Press. 9. Carter, B.S., Beaty, T.H., Steinberg, G.D., et al. (1992). Mendelian inheritance of familial prostate cancer. *Proc Natl Acad Sci U S A 89,* 3367–3371. 10. Giovannucci, E., Ascherio, A., Rimm, E.B., et al. (1995). Intake of carotinoids and retinol in relation to risk of prostate cancer. *J Natl Cancer Inst 87*(23), 1767–1776. 11. Samet, J.M. (1995). Lung cancer. In P. Greenwald, B.S. Kramer, & D.L. Weed (eds.). *Cancer Prevention and Control.* New York: Marcel Dekker, pp. 561–583. 12. Winawer, S.J., & Shike, M. (1995). Prevention and control of colorectal cancer. In P. Greenwald, B.S. Kramer, & D.L. Weed (eds.). *Cancer Prevention and Control.* New York: Marcel Dekker, pp. 537–559. 13. Howe, G.R. (1995). Metaanalysis. In P. Greenwald, B.S. Kramer, & D.L. Weed (eds.). *Cancer Prevention and Control.* New York: Marcel Dekker, pp. 279–280. 14. Kramer, B.S., & Johnson, K.A. (1995). Other gastrointestinal cancers: stomach, liver. In P. Greenwald, B.S. Kramer, & D.L. Weed (eds.). *Cancer Prevention and Control.* New York: Marcel Dekker, pp. 673–694. 15. Koh, H.K., & Lew, R.A. (1995). Skin cancer: Prevention and control. In P. Greenwald, B.S. Kramer, & D.L. Weed (eds.). *Cancer Prevention and Control.* New York: Marcel Dekker, pp. 611–640.

6. Environmental tobacco smoke (sidestream smoke).
    a. Approximately 30% of all lung cancers caused by factors other than smoking are attributable to exposure to environmental tobacco smoke.
    b. Known impact on children—increased risk of bronchitis, pneumonia, fluid in middle ear, asthma attacks, respiratory tract irritation, and reduced lung function.
7. Synergistic effect with alcohol; increased risk of cancers of the mouth, throat, larynx, and esophagus.
8. Primary prevention strategies available to reduce smoking prevalence.
B. Alcohol consumption.
    1. Contributes to about 3% of cancer mortality.
    2. Contributes to cancer of the esophagus, liver, and pharynx.
    3. Synergistic effect with tobacco.
    4. As few as one to two drinks a day may contribute to breast and perhaps colon and rectal cancer.
C. Diet and nutritional factors (Table 40–2).
    1. Accounts for about 20 to 42% of cancer deaths.
    2. Animal (saturated) fat in general and red meat in particular are associated with cancers of the colon, rectum, and prostate.
    3. Dietary fat and breast cancer association is controversial.
    4. Obesity—associated with increased risk of cancers of the colon, rectum, prostate, gallbladder, biliary tract, breast, cervix, endometrium, and ovary.
    5. Micronutrients (Table 40–3).
        a. Selenium—low levels are associated with risk of colon and rectal cancers.
        b. Vitamin A and retinoids—data concerning their role in prostate cancer is inconsistent; protective effect with some squamous cell cancers.
        c. Beta carotene appears to increase the risk for lung cancer in smokers.

TABLE 40–2. **Estimates of Cancer Deaths Avoidable by Dietary Change**

Types of Cancer	Percent Avoidable		
	Doll-Peto (1981)	*Willett (1994)*	*Range (1994)*
Lung	20	20	10–30
Colon/rectum	90	70	50–80
Breast	50	50	20–80
Prostate	(with other)	75	20–80
Pancreas	50	50	10–50
Stomach	35	35	30–70
Endometrium	50	50	50–80
Gallbladder	50	50	50–80
Larynx, bladder, cervix, mouth, pharynx, esophagus	20	20	10–30
Other types	10	10	———
Overall estimate	35	32	20–42

From Nelson, N.J. (1996). Is chemoprevention overrated or underfunded? *J Natl Cancer Inst* 88(14), 948.

TABLE 40–3. **Micronutrients and Relationship to Cancer**

Micronutrient	Causative Relationship	Protective Relationship
Vitamin A and synthetic retinoids		Bladder cancer Lung cancer Suppresses oral leukoplakia Reduced risk for second primaries of head and neck Cervical dysplasia regression
Beta carotenes		Bladder cancer
Vitamin C	Low plasma levels may increase risk for colon cancer	Bladder cancer Lung cancer Decreases rectal polyps
Vitamin E	Low plasma levels may increase risk for colon cancer	Inhibits bladder cancer
Selenium	Low serum levels may increase cancer risk for all sites	Lung cancer
Calcium		May reduce hyperproliferation of colonic mucosa cells.

6. Contaminants—the bacterial contaminant *Helicobacter pylori* is linked to gastric cancer; aflatoxin combined with chronic hepatitis B virus infection may increase the risk for liver cancer.
7. High-fiber diet (in particular, one high in fruits and vegetables) appears protective for cancers of the lung, colon, rectum, bladder, oral cavity, stomach, cervix, and esophagus.
II. Identify occupational and physical environmental risks.
   A. Occupational cancer risks.
      1. Accounts for about 4% of cancers.
      2. Asbestos—single most important known occupational carcinogen. Asbestos-related lung cancer and mesothelioma peaked during the middle to late 1980s because of extensive occupational exposure in shipyards during World War II.
      3. Occupational exposures to asbestos fibers, environmental smoke, and/or radon have a synergistic role in elevated risk of smoking-related lung cancer.
      4. Carcinogenic substances of concern—certain metals, solvents, dyes, asbestos, organic and inorganic dusts, pesticides and herbicides.
      5. Special population concerns.
         a. African Americans—discriminatory work assignments have historically resulted in placement in more hazardous jobs: steel, rubber, and chemical industries.
         b. Blue collar workers—tend to have higher smoking rates that increase risks associated with occupational exposures.
         c. Steel workers—increased lung cancer rates.
         d. Rubber workers—increased prostate cancer rates.

      e. Chemical workers—increased bladder cancer rates.

      f. Miners—increased exposure to uranium and radon with a subsequent increase in gastric cancer and birth defects.

  B. Environmental risk factors.

    1. Contributes to about 2% of cancer deaths.

    2. Ultraviolet light (sunlight; in particular UVB) contributes to about 90% of skin cancers, including melanoma.

    3. Electromagnetic field (EMF) exposures—relationship to carcinogenesis is inconclusive thus far; some evidence for contribution to childhood leukemia.

    4. Contribution of cellular telephones, microwave, and other wireless systems to cancer is not proven.

III. Identify biologic risk factors.

  A. Viral exposures.

    1. Associated with 15% of cancers.

    2. Hepatocellular carcinoma of the liver accounts for about 80% of virus-linked cancers to date.

    3. Human immunodeficiency virus (HIV) infection results in immunosuppression that increases risk of Kaposi's sarcoma and B-cell lymphomas.

    4. Epstein-Barr virus (EBV)—linked to Burkitt's lymphoma and nasopharyngeal cancers.

    5. Human papilloma virus (HPV) causally related to cervical cancer.

    6. Evidence supports causal relationship between human T-cell lymphotropic virus-1 (HTLV-1) and certain T-cell leukemias.

  B. Familial and genetic contributions.

    1. Inherited genetic mutations account for 5 to 10% of cancers.

      a. Associated features—early age of onset; bilaterality of tumors; multiple primary lesions; multiple family members with cancer.

    2. Certain cancers are product of genetic and environmental interaction (Amos, 1994).

IV. Identify iatrogenic risks.

  A. Hormonal agents.

    1. Estrogen therapy in menopausal women is associated with endometrial cancer.

    2. Estrogen exposure in the fetus (from diethylstilbestrol) is associated with vaginal cancer in adulthood.

    3. Contraceptives may be associated with liver cancer and possibly premenopausal breast cancer (data inconclusive).

    4. Anabolic steroids may be associated with liver cancer.

    5. Tamoxifen use may increase the risk for endometrial cancer.

    6. Certain fertility drugs (i.e., menotropins [Pergonal]) may increase the risk for ovarian cancer.

    7. Growth hormones given to children may increase the risk for leukemia.

  B. Immunosuppressive agents (for organ recipients) increase the risk of non-Hodgkin's lymphoma.

  C. Antineoplastic agents (especially alkylating agents) increase the risk of secondary cancers.

V. Assess combination risk factors to identify subpopulations at greatest risk.

  A. Synergistic effects of carcinogens (e.g., alcohol and tobacco).

  B. Hereditary predisposition and lifestyle choices (e.g., pigmented nevi syndrome and sun exposure).

VI. Assess other contributing factors.
   A. Socioeconomic status.
      1. Poverty—underrecognized factor that contributes significantly to cancer (Table 40–4).
         a. Illiteracy compromises access to health education messages that recommend prevention, screening, and early detection.
         b. Unemployment, poor or substandard housing, inadequate or substandard nutritional status may place day-to-day survival priorities over prevention, screening, and early detection.
         c. Inadequate or substandard housing and diets modify immune status and increase exposures to risk factors.
         d. Inadequate access to health care compromises access to high-quality and consistent screening, early detection, and follow-up care, which often results in detection of cancers too advanced for optimal outcomes.
   B. Motivation for preventive behavior (health belief model).
      1. Perceived susceptibility to cancer—evidence indicates that individuals at risk often are unaware of their risks (ask "How likely do you feel you are to develop cancer?").
      2. Perceived severity of cancer (ask "How serious do you feel cancer is?").
      3. Perceived benefits of preventive behavior (ask "Do you think you can decrease your risk for cancer by not smoking [or the habit in question]?").
         a. Prevention may not be valued in certain cultures with a fatalistic view of cancer.
      4. Perceived barriers to preventive action (ask "What problems do you think you may have lowering the fat content in your diet [or the behavior in question]?").
         a. Deleterious effects of risk behaviors may not become manifest for years (latency); therefore, present-versus-future orientation may be a barrier.
         b. Lack of motivation to change lifestyle may be related to addictive nature of the habit in question (e.g., smoking, alcohol consumption).
         c. Costs and limited access to care may result in knowledge or resource deficits.

TABLE 40–4. **Abbreviated Demographic Profile, 1991, 50 States and the District of Columbia**

Cultural/Ethnic Group	Number of People (in thousands)	Median Age in Years	Percent 65 Years and Older	Percent of Persons Living in Poverty
Whites	210,341	33.9	12.9	10.7
African Americans	30,977	28.0	4.2	31.9
Mexican Americans	14,628	24.6	4.2	30.1
Puerto Rican Americans	2402	26.9	5.8	36.5
Cuban Americans	1071	43.6	20.4	18.1
Central and South American origin	3052	28.6	3.9	26.7
American Indians and Alaska natives	1900	23.4		30.9

From US Bureau of the Census, Public Inquiry, 1991, Washington, D.C.

Nursing Diagnosis

I. Knowledge deficit.

Outcome Identification

I. Client identifies cancer risk factors associated with lifestyle, occupation, genetics, and the environment.
II. Client lists strategies for reducing or eliminating exposure to cancer risk factors.
III. Client identifies barriers and facilitators to adopting cancer prevention strategies.
IV. Client develops a plan for behavior change.
V. Client identifies resources and programs for cancer prevention.
VI. Client adopts behavioral strategies for reducing cancer risk(s).

Planning and Implementation

I. Identify and personalize cancer risks.
   A. Risk assessment.
      1. Health risk appraisal.
         a. Definition—an educational tool utilizing selected biomedical measures, combined with a self-report behavioral inventory, to generate a computerized client health profile.
         b. Actuarial estimates, epidemiologic findings, and medical opinion used to calculate probability of the client dying of selected causes in the next 10 years.
         c. Fundamental assumption—rational information about personal risk factor levels and the potential health benefit of their reduction should motivate the client to adopt lifestyle change.
         d. Recommended use—mass screening programs, public marketing campaigns, health fairs.
         e. Weaknesses.
            (1) Often based on outdated statistics.
            (2) Generally no opportunity to assess adherence to recommendations.
            (3) No opportunity to clarify myths, misconceptions.
      2. Comprehensive cancer risk survey.
         a. Often developed by clinician or investigator to meet clinical agency and/or population needs.
         b. Generally identifies cancer risks (e.g., personal, genetic) to plan and develop personalized interventions and recommendations.
         c. Strengths.
            (1) May be computerized for aggregate data analysis and outcome data analysis.
         d. Limitations.
            (1) Self-report potential based on literacy level.
            (2) Must protect confidentiality.
            (3) Reliability and validity seldom assessed.
      3. Occupational and environmental survey.
         a. Provides for systematic assessment of occupational and environmental risks for appropriate referral and intervention.

   b. Precautions.
      (1) Must maintain confidentiality.
      (2) Adverse client consequences from employer possible if work-related exposures are not being appropriately managed.
II. Facilitate lifestyle change.
   A. Smoking cessation (as proposed by the Agency for Health Care Policy and Research, 1996).
      1. Act as a role model by not smoking.
      2. Ask about and record the tobacco-use status of every patient.
      3. Advise every smoker to quit.
         a. Be clear. (Say, "I think it is important for you to quit smoking now, and I will help you.")
         b. Speak strongly. (Say, "As your clinician, I need you to know that quitting smoking is the most important thing you can do to protect your current and future health.")
         c. Personalize your advice. (Say, "You've already had one heart attack.") Mention the impact of smoking on children or others in the household. (Say, "You know your children need you.")
      4. Assist the client with a quit plan.
         a. Advise the smoker to:
            (1) Set a quit date, ideally within 2 weeks.
            (2) Inform friends, family, and coworkers of plans to quit, and ask for support.
            (3) Remove cigarettes from home, car, and workplace, and avoid smoking in these places.
            (4) Review previous quit attempts—what helped, what led to relapse.
            (5) Anticipate challenges, particularly during the critical first few weeks, including nicotine withdrawal.
         b. Give advice on successful quitting.
            (1) Total abstinence is essential—not even a single puff.
            (2) Drinking alcohol is strongly associated with relapse.
            (3) Having other smokers in the household hinders successful quitting.
         c. Encourage use of nicotine replacement therapy.
            (1) Both the nicotine patch and nicotine gum are effective pharmacotherapies for smoking cessation.
            (2) Nicotine patch may be easier to use than the gum in most clinical settings.
         d. Keep culturally and educationally appropriate materials on cessation techniques readily available.
      5. Follow-up.
         a. Counsel for relapse.
         b. Reinforce abstinence.
   B. Avoidance of sun exposure.
      1. Limit sun exposure (especially between the hours of 10:00 AM and 3:00 PM).
      2. Avoid tanning facilities.
      3. Wear protective clothing (long-sleeve shirts and wide-brim hats).
      4. Apply sunscreen with a sun protection factor (SPF) of at least 15.
   C. Diet and weight control.
      1. Maintain a desirable body weight.

2. Eat a balanced diet.
   a. Daily recommendations (as proposed by the US Department of Agriculture, US Department of Health and Human Services, 1990).
      (1) Fruit—two to four servings per day.
      (2) Vegetables—three to five servings per day (e.g., cruciferous, dark green, and deep yellow and orange vegetables).
      (3) Bread, cereal, rice, and pasta—6 to 11 servings per day.
      (4) Milk, yogurt, cheese—two to three servings per day.
      (5) Lean meat, skinless poultry, fish and alternatives—two to three servings per day.
      (6) Fats—three to six servings per day.
      (7) Avoid sweets. Moderate alcohol (one to two drinks/week) intake.
      (8) Limit consumption of salt-cured, smoked, and nitrite-preserved foods.
D. Prevent HIV exposure.
   1. Advocate for abstinence or monogamy.
   2. Encourage safe-sex and condom use.
   3. Counsel against intravenous (IV) drug use or educate about and facilitate access to sterile needle and syringe programs.
   4. Advocate that preventing pregnancy in infected women avoids exposure to the fetus.
E. Avoid occupational carcinogen exposures.
   1. Recognize and avoid workplace carcinogen exposure.
   2. Use protective clothing and/or devices and follow safety procedures when exposure is mandatory.
F. Exercise.
   1. Association between physical activity and lower incidence of colon cancer may be due to reduced transit time with an associated decrease in temporal exposure of the colonic mucosa to bile acids.
   2. For hormonally regulated cancers (e.g., breast, endometrial, and ovarian) strenuous physical exercise as a young adult may be protective if it delays onset of regular ovulatory cycles or results in secondary amenorrhea.
   3. Regular exercise has been shown to be associated with many health benefits, such as:
      a. Reductions in coronary artery disease, hypertension, noninsulin-dependent diabetes mellitus, stress, anxiety, depression, weight, bone loss associated with osteoporosis.
      b. Increases in longevity, high-density lipoprotein (HDL) ("good") cholesterol, immune function, self-image, and quality of life.
   4. Aerobic exercise promotes physical fitness.
G. Participation in chemoprevention trials.
   1. Chemoprevention involves administration of natural or synthetic chemical agents that reverse, suppress, arrest, or prevent carcinogenesis before the development of invasive malignancy.
   2. Potential agents include phenolic antioxidants, retinoids, prostaglandin inhibitors, indole, dehydroepiandrosterone analogue, and pharmaceuticals (finasteride, tamoxifen, sulindac, aspirin).
   3. Primary targets—colorectal, prostate, lung, breast, bladder, oral, and cervical cancers.

    4. Examples.
        a. The Breast Cancer Prevention Trial—a randomized, placebo-controlled clinical trial to determine the worth of tamoxifen for preventing breast cancer.
        b. The Prostate Cancer Prevention Trial—a phase III randomized, double-blind, placebo-controlled study of finasteride (Proscar) for the chemoprevention of prostate cancer.

III. Revise plan based on feedback.

Evaluation

The oncology nurse systematically and regularly evaluates the client's and/or family's responses to interventions to determine progress toward the achievement of expected outcomes. Relevant data are collected and actual findings are compared with expected findings. Nursing diagnoses, outcomes, and plans of care are reviewed and revised as necessary.

BIBLIOGRAPHY

Agency for Health Care Policy and Research. (1996). *Smoking Cessation: Information for Specialists.* Publication #96-0694, No. 18. Rockville, MD: USDHHS, PHS, AHCPR, CDCP.

American Nurses Association. (1995). *Managing Genetic Information: Implications for Nursing Practice.* Washington, D.C.: American Nurses Association.

Amos, C.I. (1994). Identifying gene-environment interactions in cancer etiology. *Cancer Bull 46*(3), p. 6.

Environmental Protection Agency. (August, 1993). *Respiratory Health Effects of Passive Smoking: Lung Cancer and Other Disorders.* NIH Publication No. 93–3605. Bethesda, MD: USDHHS, PHS, NIH.

Frank-Stromborg, M., & Olsen, S.J. (eds.). (1993). *Cancer Prevention in Minority Populations: Cultural Implications for Health Care Professionals.* St. Louis: C.V. Mosby.

Greenwald, P., Kramer, B.S., & Weed, D.L. (1995). *Cancer Prevention and Control.* New York: Marcel Dekker.

Heath, C.W. (1996). Electromagnetic field exposure and cancer: A review of epidemiologic evidence. *CA Cancer J Clin 46,* 29–44.

Institute of Medicine. (1995). *Nursing, Health, and the Environment.* Washington, D.C.: National Academy Press.

Mittendorf, R., Longnecker, M.P., Newcomb, P.A., et al. (1995). Strenuous physical activity in young adulthood and risk of breast cancer (United States). *Cancer Causes Control 6,* 347–353.

National Cancer Advisory Board. (September, 1994). *Cancer at a Crossroads: A Report to Congress for the Nation.* Bethesda, MD: NCI, NIH.

National Center for Health Statistics. (1995). *Healthy People 2000: Review 1994.* Hyattsville, MD: Public Health Service.

Stellman, J.M., & Stellman, S.D. (1996). Cancer and the workplace. *CA Cancer J Clin 46,* 71–91.

U.S. Department of Health and Human Services. (January, 1994). *Tobacco and the Clinician.* NIH Publication No. 94–3693. Bethesda, MD: PHS, NIH.

White, E., Jacobs, E.J., & Daling, J.R. (1996). Physical activity in relation to colon cancer in middle-aged men and women. *Am J Epidemiol 144,* 42–50.

Wingo, P.A., Bolden, S., Tong, T., et al. (1996). Cancer statistics for African Americans, 1996. *CA Cancer J Clin 46,* 123–125.

Screening and Early Detection of Cancer

Candis H. Morrison, PhD, CANP
Sharon J. Olsen, RN, MS, AOCN
Barbara W. Ashley, RN, MSN, CANP

Theory

I. Rationale.
  A. The best and most effective treatment for cancer is prevention. Early detection of cancer and effective therapy can result in decreased morbidity and mortality.
  B. Development of risk profiles and screening guidelines enhances screening efficacy and decreases costs.
II. Definition of terms.
  A. Secondary prevention.
    1. Early detection of the potential for development of a disease or condition, or existence of a disease, while an individual is asymptomatic. Allows positive interference to prevent, postpone, or attenuate the symptomatic clinical state.
    2. Emphasizes early diagnosis (via application of screening and diagnostic examinations and tests) and prompt treatment to halt the pathologic process, thereby shortening its duration and severity, and enabling the person to return to a former state of health at the earliest time possible.
    3. Employs use of selective screening strategies to detect preclinical disease in the asymptomatic person at a time when the disease is presumed to be localized, for the purpose of decreasing morbidity and mortality.
  B. Surveillance.
    1. The regular ongoing monitoring of people who have already been identified as being at high risk.
    2. Based on established guidelines.
  C. Risk—the likelihood that exposure to a certain factor will influence the chance of developing a particular cancer, based on the national average. (See also Chapter 40.)
    1. Relative risk—an estimation of increased probability of development of a certain cancer, based on the amount of exposure to the associated risk factor(s). The higher the relative risk factor, the greater the risk of development of that cancer.
    2. Attributable risk—the amount of preventable disease, allowing for a calculation of incidence of the disease likely to occur in the absence of all identified risk factors.

   D. Diagnosis.
      1. The clinical problem-solving process applied to symptomatic clients or those asymptomatic clients with abnormal screening tests.
III. Epidemiology—the study of distribution and determinants of disease in population groups. Assists in development of population-based risk profiles.
   A. Incidence—number of new cases of cancer during a specified time period in a defined population. Incidence rates estimate the probability of developing a disease and provide valuable measures of temporal or geographic differences. For example, in the United States (US) in 1995, there were an estimated 182,000 new cases of breast cancer diagnosed.
   B. Prevalence—the number of cancer cases, both old and new, present at a point in time in a defined population. Prevalence rates provide an estimate of the burden of disease in a defined population. For example, in the US, 30% of men age 60 to 69 years will have prostate cancer at any point in time.
   C. Mortality—number of deaths attributed to cancer during a specified time period in a defined population. For example, in the US in 1995, an estimated 46,000 deaths occurred from breast cancer in women.
   D. Case-fatality—number of persons among all those who have a form of cancer who die of it during a specified period of time. This provides a measure of the aggressiveness of cancer or of the success of medical intervention. For example, lung cancer accounts for 33% of the cancer deaths in men, or the overall five-year survival rate for lung cancer is 10 to 15%.
   E. Minority statistics—development of risk profiles require racial considerations. There are differences in both incidence and mortality based on race (see Chapter 4, Tables 4–1 and 4–2).
   F. Other demographic variables.
      1. Age—incidence of most cancer increases with age.
      2. Sex—cancer is more common in males than females.
      3. Geography.
         a. Major incidence and mortality differences exist in different locations.
         b. Migratory data demonstrate adoption of the cancer pattern of the area to which migration occurs, suggesting lifestyle and behavioral factors as well as environmental ones as causative or exacerbating.
      4. Socioeconomic status (SES).
         a. Increased tobacco use among poorer populations.
         b. Low SES groups avail themselves of screening services less often.
         c. More advanced disease presentations are evident in rural and lower SES groups.
         d. Urbanization and pollution are associated with increased incidences of disease.
IV. Screening.
   A. Principles of screening tests.
      1. Utility—screening tests are used to:
         a. Identify asymptomatic persons with risk factors for disease.
         b. Detect occult disease and permit early treatment.
         c. Reassure patients found free of disease, with or without risk factors.
         d. Direct clients to genetic counseling in familial conditions when appropriate.
      2. Attributes of screening tests.
         a. Sensitivity—a measure of the probability that a test result will be *positive* if the disease being investigated is present.

  b. Specificity—a measure of the probability that a test result will be *negative* if the disease being investigated is not present.
  c. Predictive value—positive and negative.
     (1) Positive predictive value—the percentage of persons with a positive screening test result who actually have the disease.
     (2) Negative predictive value—the percentage of persons with a negative screening test result who clearly do not have the disease.
  d. Ease of administration.
  e. Acceptability to patients. The following test characteristics serve to enhance compliance and utilization, and minimize short- or long-term side effects.
     (1) Safe, has few potential complications.
     (2) Convenient (preferably readily available during health care visits).
     (3) Acceptable to the public.
     (4) Relatively low cost.
3. Characteristics of disease—to warrant risks and costs associated with any screening program.
  a. Sufficiently common to justify the effort to detect it.
  b. Causes—sufficient morbidity and mortality if untreated.
  c. Effective treatment is available (and acceptable) to alter its natural history.
  d. There is a presymptomatic, or preinvasive, period during which detection and treatment may occur.
  e. Presymptomatic treatment yields better results.
4. Characteristics of the population.
  a. Sufficiently high prevalence of disease.
  b. Accessible to screening.
  c. Likely to comply with subsequently recommended diagnostic tests and treatment.
5. Types of screening bias. These three biases invalidate comparisons of stage distribution or survival between series of asymptomatic screen-detected and symptomatic screen-detected disease. Well-designed, randomized trials generally control for these biases.
  a. Lead-time bias—occurs when disease is detected earlier but the detection does not affect mortality. Survival time appears to be longer but actually is not. The appearance of improved survival in screen-detected cases that results from moving the diagnosis forward by screening, merely lengthens the interval from diagnosis to death rather than lengthening life. This bias is most notable when short follow-up periods, such as 5-year survival rates, are used. Lead-time bias is determined by the sensitivity of the test, testing interval, and duration of the preclinical stage.
  b. Length bias—at any point in time, a population consists of persons with aggressive and symptomatic disease and symptomatic less aggressive disease. Screening identifies both but, because a greater proportion have less aggressive disease, it appears that survival is lengthened because the average lifespan observed increases. The improved survival in the screened population derives, at least in part, from the growth properties of the tumor rather than from the benefits of the screening.

c. Selection bias—can occur if patients undergoing screening have better health habits than the general population or have lower mortality or longer survival because they are more resistant to the disease or more compliant with therapy.

6. Outcome measures in cancer screening.
   a. Short-term measures.
      (1) Number of individuals in the target population offered screening.
      (2) Number and proportion of individuals in the target population who received screening.
      (3) Number and proportion of the target population examined by multiple screens.
      (4) Number or prevalence of preclinical cancers detected in abnormal screenees brought to definitive diagnosis or follow-up.
      (5) Cost per cancer detected.
      (6) Sensitivity and specificity of the screening test.
      (7) Positive and negative predictive values of the screening test.
   b. Long-term measures.
      (1) Stage distribution of detected cancers.
      (2) Case-fatality rate of screened individuals.
      (3) Site-specific cancer mortality rate of screened target population.
      (4) Total costs.
      (5) Impact of early detection on quality of life (positive and negative, e.g., prostate-specific antigen [PSA] and prostate cancer controversy).

B. Types of screening.
   1. Mass screening—screen an entire population (e.g., for phenylketonuria [PKU]).
   2. Selective or prescriptive screening—high-risk populations, looking for a specific problem or condition (e.g., for BRCA-1 gene, Tay-Sachs disease, sickle cell anemia, myelomeningocele).
   3. Single screening—for a single defect or condition (e.g., for hypertension).
   4. Multiple screening—two or more defects or conditions (e.g., school vision and hearing screening).
   5. Multiphasic screening—profile over time (e.g., Denver Developmental Screening Test).
   6. May have combinations.
      a. Multiple or mass screening (e.g., health fairs for height, weight, blood pressure, hematocrit level).
      b. Selective and mass screening (e.g., vision or hearing).
      c. Selective and single screening (e.g., sickle cell anemia).
      d. Multiphasic and mass screening (e.g., Denver Developmental Screening Test).
      e. Multiphasic and selective screening (e.g., vision).

C. Recommendations for cancer screening (Table 41–1).

Assessment

I. Components necessary for development of a client's individual risk profile.
   A. History.
      1. Demographic—age, sex, race, date and place of birth, occupation, insurance coverage.

TABLE 41–1. **American Cancer Society Recommendations for the Early Detection of Cancer in Asymptomatic People**

Test or Procedure	Sex	Age	Frequency
Breast self-examination	F	20 & over	Every month.
Clinical breast examination	F	20–40 Over 40	Every 3 years Every year
Mammography*	F	40–49 Over 50	Every 1–2 years Every year
Pap test	F	All women who are or who have been sexually active, or have reached age 18, should have an annual Pap test and pelvic examination. After a woman has had 3 or more consecutive satisfactory normal annual examinations, the Pap test may be performed less frequently at the discretion of her provider.	
Pelvic examination	F	18–40 Over 40	Every 1–3 years with Pap test Every year
Endometrial tissue sample	F	At menopause if high risk[†]	At menopause and thereafter at the discretion of the physician.
Sigmoidoscopy, preferably flexible	M & F	50 and over	Every 3–5 years
Fecal occult blood test	M & F	50 and over	Every year
Digital rectal examination	M & F	40 and over	Every year
Prostate examination[‡]	M	50 and over	Every year
Health counseling and cancer checkup[§]	M & F	Over 20 Over 40	Every 3 years Every year

*Screening mammography should begin by age 40.
[†]History of infertility, obesity, failure to ovulate, abnormal uterine bleeding, or unopposed estrogen or tamoxifen therapy.
[‡]Annual digital rectal examination and prostate-specific antigen should be performed on men age 50 and older. If either is abnormal, further evaluation should be considered.
[§]To include examination for cancers of the thyroid, testicles, ovaries, lymph nodes, oral region, and skin.
From Mettlin, C., Jones, G., Averette, H., et al. (1993). Defining and updating the American Cancer Society guidelines for the cancer-related checkup: Prostate and endometrial cancers. *CA Cancer J Clin 43,* 45.

2. Chief complaint—reason for seeking examination. If related to a symptom, a complete symptom analysis is mandatory.
3. History of present illness.
   a. Onset of symptom.
   b. Location of pain.
   c. Duration.
   d. Characteristics.
   e. Aggravating factors.
   f. Relieving factors.
   g. Timing.
4. Allergies, current medications.
5. Past medical history—previous state of health, previous cancer and/or cancer treatment, chronic illnesses, surgeries, hospitalizations.
6. Family history—medical and cancer history in relatives.

    7. Occupational history (see Chapter 40).

    8. Social history (e.g., smoking, drinking, drug use, sexual habits, exercise).

    9. Review of systems.

       a. Weight—present, usual, recent gain or loss.

       b. Performance status—previous and present level of activity; note any weakness, fatigue, malaise.

       c. Skin—changes in warts or moles; bleeding; change in sensation, any new lesions.

       d. Head and neck—pain; tenderness; difficulty swallowing or chewing; hoarseness; discharge from eyes, ears, nose.

       e. Lymphatic—lymphadenopathy, lymph node tenderness.

       f. Respiratory—cough, pain, dyspnea, hemoptysis, shortness of breath.

       g. Cardiac—hypertension, dyspnea, orthopnea, chest pain.

       h. Gastrointestinal—change in appetite, pain, nausea, vomiting, change in bowel pattern.

       i. Genitourinary—change in urinary pattern, hematuria, change in force or caliber of stream, pain.

       j. Gynecologic—discharge, nonmenstrual or intermenstrual bleeding, bloating, enlarged abdominal girth.

       k. Endocrine—flushing, sweating, tachycardia, palpitations, polyuria, polydipsia, appetite disturbance.

       l. Hematologic—bruising, anemia, petechiae, purpura, bleeding disorder, night sweats.

       m. Musculoskeletal—pain, stiffness, limitation of movement.

       n. Neurologic—headache; vertigo; seizures; visual disturbances; sensory, motor, or cognitive deficits.

       o. Immune system—fever, chills, frequent infections (particularly respiratory).

  B. Risk factors (see Chapter 40).

II. Cancer-directed physical examination (see Table 41–1 for screening recommendations).

  A. Even in the absence of symptoms, the complete procedure should include examination of the skin, mouth, lymph nodes, breasts, cervix, pelvis, testicles, rectum, and prostate.

  B. Cancer checkup every 3 years in asymptomatic individuals under 40 years of age.

  C. Annual checkups for those over 40 years of age.

  D. Remaining examination is directed by presence of abnormal findings.

  E. Specific foci.

    1. Skin.

       a. Inspection of all cutaneous and mucous membrane surfaces.

       b. Sun-exposed areas such as face, chest, back, arms, legs, scalp, interdigital webs, and axillae; palms of hands and soles of feet deserve particular attention.

       c. Distribution of nevi noted and description of size, symmetry of border, regularity of color and surface, scaling, or bleeding.

    2. Oral cavity.

       a. Inspection for color and integrity of mucous membranes, tongue, lesions or plaques. Include area under tongue.

       b. Palpation for masses, tenderness.

    3. Breasts—clinical breast examination consists of systematic steps.

       a. Inspection for asymmetry, dimpling, skin changes, irregular venous pattern, nipple direction, nipple discharge.

   b. Palpation for supraclavicular and infraclavicular nodes, and for axillary tenderness, masses, nodules.
4. Female genitalia.
   a. Inspection for masses, asymmetry, lesions, discharge, bleeding.
   b. External palpation for masses, tenderness, shape and consistency of abdominal organs, including uterus, ovaries, colon.
   c. Pelvic examination—note mucosal integrity and color; presence of lesions, bleeding or friability; discharge; constriction; nodules; masses.
   d. Rectal examination—note external lesions, sphincter tone, masses, tenderness, bleeding.
   e. Stool for occult blood.
5. Male genitalia with digital rectal examination (DRE).
   a. Inspection for masses, shape of scrotum, cutaneous lesions or nodules.
   b. Palpation for tenderness, masses, consistency, contour, scrotal contents (testes, epididymis), inguinal adenopathy.
   c. Palpation of prostate gland for nodules, masses, tenderness, size, texture, and firmness.
   d. Rectal examination—note external lesions, masses, sphincter tone, constriction, masses, tenderness, bleeding.
   e. Stool for occult blood.
III. Screening and diagnostic laboratory tests and tumor markers (Table 41–2).

Nursing Diagnoses

   I. Knowledge deficit.
  II. Anxiety.
 III. Health-seeking behaviors deficit.

Outcome Identification

   I. Client and family discuss recommendations for screening and early detection.
  II. Client describes self-examination procedures and recommendations.
 III. Client identifies personal risk factors.

Planning and Implementation

   I. Lessen perceived and actual barriers.
      A. Target high-risk groups (e.g., elderly, socioeconomically disadvantaged) within respective community.
      B. Personalize risk by using health history and risk profiles.
      C. Maximize quality control of screening tests (low false-negative results and low false-positive results).
      D. Use media resources to publicize benefits of early detection.
      E. Collect data to evaluate quality control of screening.
         1. Number screened.
         2. Proportion of population screened once, twice, or more.
         3. Detected prevalence of preclinical disease.
         4. Cost per case.
         5. Proportion of positive findings brought to diagnosis and treatment.
         6. Predictive value of positive test results (proportion found to have cancer).
         7. Costs of follow-up of false-positive findings.

(*Text continued on page 706*)

TABLE 41–2. **Screening and Diagnostic Tests**

Test	Classification	Significance
Screening Tests		
Mammography	Breast radiography	Screening mammography plays an important role in the early detection of breast cancer Large randomized clinical trials and demonstration projects have shown a significant reduction in mortality from breast cancer when mammography was included in the screening examination
Pap smear	Tissue sample from uterine cervix	In the majority of women, carcinoma in situ (CIS) persists in a detectable state for an extended period of time before becoming invasive cancer of the cervix (ICC) However, in some younger women there may be an etiologically distinct subgroup of lesions that have rapid progression time. This has contributed to the debate on recommended frequency of this test
Fecal occult blood tests (FOBT)*	Fecal smear	Blood in the stool can result from a wide variety of both benign and malignant conditions. FOBT is not specific for cancer, but evidence suggests that stool blood testing in asymptomatic individuals can detect cancer or polyps Approximately 50% of cancers lie beyond the reach of standard sigmoidoscopes. There has been a recent phenomenon of cancer shifting toward the right side of the colon, therefore FOBT is an acceptable screen. The American Cancer Society (ACS) has recommended dietary preparations for the stool blood test to increase sensitivity and specificity*
Sigmoidoscopy	Endoscopic procedure	Demonstrated to decrease colon cancer mortality through early detection and removal of polyps. The more comfortable flexible scopes may increase public and clinician acceptance of sigmoidoscopy. The benefit-risk ratio of sigmoidoscopy supports its inclusion in the periodic cancer-related checkup. The initiation of sigmoidoscopic examination of average-risk persons at age 50 has been determined by the age-specific incidence rates of the disease

*ACS Dietary Guidelines for FOBT. Guidelines should be initiated at least 48 hours prior to the collection of the first stool sample and continued until the final stool sample has been collected.

Do not take vitamin C supplements

Do not take oral iron medication

Do not take multivitamins containing vitamin C or iron

Avoid foods with high peroxidase activity, such as broccoli, turnips, cantaloupes, cauliflower, radishes, horseradish, and parsnips

Do not eat red meat. Well-cooked poultry and fish may be eaten; also bran, peanuts, popcorn and cooked fruits and vegetables

Do not take aspirin (ASA) or nonsteroidal anti-inflammatory drugs. Aspirin substitutes such as acetaminophen may be used

TABLE 41–2. **Screening and Diagnostic Tests** *Continued*

Test	Reference Range	Significance
Confirmatory Tests		
Prostatic biopsy	Tissue for cytopathology	Needle biopsy of suspicious prostatic tissue with or without ultrasound guidance
Skin biopsies	Tissue for cytopathology	Because tissue is the gold standard for cancer diagnosis, skin biopsies are recommended for any suspicious lesions. Techniques such as punch biopsies make this a simple office procedure. Small lesions are excised; large lesions require punch or incisional biopsy for tissue diagnosis
Serum Tumor Markers		
Prostate specific antigen (PSA)	0.0–4.0 ng/mL	PSA is a glycoprotein produced by most prostatic carcinomas, by normal prostatic tissue, in benign prostatic hypertrophy (BPH), and prostatitis. Elevations are related to an increase in the size of the gland, either malignant or benign. The test is used to screen for prostate cancer in conjunction with digital rectal examinations, for identification of patients at increased risk for occult cancer when used in conjunction with transrectal ultrasound, for posttherapeutic evaluation of prostate cancer therapy, and for predicting treatment failure in patients undergoing radiation therapy for prostate cancer
Alkaline phosphatase	4–13 U/dL	Increased in metastatic cancer of bone and liver, osteogenic sarcoma, myeloma, and Hodgkin's lymphoma with bony involvement
Serum alpha fetoprotein (AFP)	<30 ng/mL	Increased in 70% of hepatocellular cancers, and in choriocarcinoma, teratoma, embryonal cell tumors of the testis and ovary, some pancreatic, stomach, colon, and lung tumors
Human chorionic gonadotropin (β-hCG)	<5.0 IU/L in males and nonpregnant females	Increased in hydatidiform mole, choriocarcinoma, testicular teratoma; ectopic hCG production by some cancers of the pituitary gland, stomach, pancreas, lung, colon, and liver
Carcinoembryonic antigen (CEA)	Nonsmokers: 0–5 ng/mL Smokers: <5.0 ng/mL	Increased in 70% of colon cancer patients Useful in following patients who have been treated for colon cancer to judge the effectiveness of treatment and to determine prognosis. May be used to assist in confirmation of the diagnosis of pancreatic cancer
CA 125	<35 U/mL	Helpful in monitoring patients with nonmucinous epithelial ovarian cancer Elevated CA 125 levels can also be found in liver disease and in tumors of the breast, pulmonary tree, or GI tract

Table continued on following page

TABLE 41–2. **Screening and Diagnostic Tests** *Continued*

Test	Reference Range	Significance
Serum Hormonal Assay		
Adrenocorticotropic hormone (ACTH)	Subject to diurnal variation. Lowest in evening, highest in morning <70 pg/mL at 8:00 AM	Increased in ectopic ACTH-producing tumors (lung, particularly small cell; adrenal carcinoma, adenoma)
Androstenedione	Male: 107 ± 25 ng/dL Female: 151 ± 38 ng/dL	Increased in ectopic ACTH-producing tumors, ovarian tumors
Antidiuretic hormone (ADH)		Increased in primary or secondary brain tumors; increased in systemic malignancies with ectopic ADH production
Calcitonin	Male: <100 pg/mL Female: <25 pg/mL (fasting)	Increased in medullar carcinoma of the thyroid, some lung and breast tumors, carcinoids, colon cancer, and GI malignancies
Estrogens (total)	Adult male: 40–115 pg/L Adult female: 61–350 pg/L	Increased in estrogen-producing ovarian tumors, some testicular tumors, and adrenocortical tumors
Glucagon	50–100 pg/mL (fasting)	Decreased in some pancreatic neoplasms
Growth hormone (hGH)	Male: <2 ng/mL Female: <10 ng/mL	Increased in ectopic secretion by some stomach and lung tumors
Parathyroid hormone (hPTH)	<1.5 pmol/L	Increased in squamous cell or epidermoid lung cancers and renal cell cancers producing an ectopic hyperparathyroidism
Progesterone	Male: 0.12–0.03 ng/mL Nonpregnant female: 0–30 ng/mL	Increased in some ovarian tumors, molar pregnancy
Testosterone	Adult male: 572 ± 135 ng/dL Nonpregnant female: 37 ± 10 ng/dL	Increased in some adrenocortical tumors, gonadotropin-producing extragonadal tumors
Urine Hormonal Assay		
17-ketogenic steroids	24-hour acidified urine Male: 5–23 mg/d Female: 3–15 mg/d	Increased in adrenal adenoma and carcinoma, ectopic adrenocorticotropic hormone (ACTH) syndrome
17-ketosteroids	24-hour urine Male: 8–22 Female: 6–15	Increased in adrenal tumors, testicular tumors, interstitial cell tumors, androgenic ovarian tumors
Tissue Hormonal Assay		
Estrogen (estradiol) receptor assay	Negative: <3.0 fmol/mg protein Borderline: 3–10 fmol/mg protein Positive: >10 fmol/mg protein	60% of breast cancers are characterized by estrogen receptors. Useful for identifying breast tumors most likely to respond to endocrine manipulation

TABLE 41–2. **Screening and Diagnostic Tests** *Continued*

Test	Reference Range	Significance
Tissue Hormonal Assay		
Progesterone receptor assay	Normal: ≤5 fmol/mg protein Positive: >10 fmol/mg protein	May be useful in predicting tumors likely to respond to endocrine manipulation
Serum Chemistries		
Calcium	Adult: 8.4–10.2 mg/dL (fasting)	Increased in 9% of malignancies with bone involvement (mainly breast, lung, and kidney) Also in multiple myeloma; lymphoma; leukemia; squamous cell carcinoma of the lung; cancers of the kidney, esophagus, pancreas, liver, and bladder
Cholesterol	Adults: 140–210 mg/dL Fasting ≥12 hour	Decreased in 16% of malignancies with bone involvement. Increased in some prostatic, liver, and pancreatic malignancies
Ferritin	Male: 15–200 mg/dL Female: 12–150 mg/dL	Increased in acute myeloblastic and lymphoblastic leukemias, some Hodgkin's lymphomas, and breast cancers
Glucose	70–105 mg/dL	Increased in pheochromocytoma, glucagonoma; pancreatic malignancies. May also be increased in the presence of islet cell tumor, carcinoma of the adrenal gland, stomach, and fibrosarcoma
Uric acid	Male: 4.2–8 mg/dL Female: 3.2–7.3 mg/dL	Increased in some disseminated malignancies Decreased in some neoplasms, including Hodgkin's lymphoma, multiple myeloma, and bronchogenic carcinoma
Serum Enzymes		
Amylase	Adult: 56–190 IU/L	Increased in some lung and ovarian tumors
Lactic dehydrogenase (LDH) and LDH isoenzymes	Ranges are highly method-dependent, i.e.: 1. Pyruvate to lactate (210–420) 2. Lactate to pyruvate (45–90)	Increased in extensive carcinomatosis and malignant processes. Increased in 90% of patients with acute leukemia. Increased with massive platelet destruction and in lymphomas and lymphocytic leukemias. May be increased in prostatic cancer
Leucine aminopeptidase (LAP)	Male: 80–200 U/mL Female: 75–185 U/mL	Increased in 60% of patients with pancreatic carcinoma with liver metastases
Lysozyme	4.0–13.0 mg/L	Increased in monocytic or myelomonocytic leukemia and chronic myeloid leukemia
Serum gamma glutamyl transpeptidase (AST)	Males: 6–37 mU/mL Females: 4–24 mU/mL	Increased in some cases of renal cell carcinoma and liver metastases
Serum glutamic oxaloacetic transaminase (ALT)	5–40 U/mL	Increased in about 50% of patients with liver metastases or infiltration
Serum glutamic pyruvic transaminase (SGPT)	5–35 U/mL	Increased in some liver carcinomas

Table continued on following page

TABLE 41–2. **Screening and Diagnostic Tests** *Continued*

Test	Reference Range	Significance
Serum Proteins		
Immunoglobulins are produced by lymphocytes and plasma cells. They are fractionated into major components by electrophoresis		
Immunoglobulin A (IgA)	Adult: 60–330 mg/dL	Slight polyclonal increase in some malignancies of breast, and a monoclonal increase in IgA myeloma
Immunoglobulin D (IgD)	Adult: 0–15 mg/dL	Slight monoclonal increase in IgD myeloma
Immunoglobulin E (IgE)	Adult: 0.01–0.04 mg/dL	Slight monoclonal increase in IgE myeloma / Slight increase in certain advanced stage neoplasms
Immunoglobulin G (IgG)	Adult: 550–1900 mg/dL	Slight monoclonal increase in IgG myeloma
Immunoglobulin M (IgM)	Adult: 45–145 mg/dL	Accounts for approximately 10% of immunoglobulins / Is the first antibody to respond to bacteria and bacterial toxins / Elevated monoclonally in Waldenstrom's macroglobulinemia
Haptoglobin (Hp)	Adult: 30–160/dL	May be increased in cancer, particularly with metastases, and in lymphomas
Hematology		
White blood cell (WBC) count	Adult male: 3900–10,600/mm³ / Adult female: 3500–11,000/mm³	WBC count increased in hematologic malignancies and myeloproliferative disorders
Differential count	Neutrophils (%) Segmented: 56 Bands: 3 Lymphocytes: 34 Monocytes: 4 Eosinophils: 2.5 Basophils: 0.5	Components increased in a wide range of myeloproliferative disorders and leukemias / May be increased in widespread malignancies, and decreased in aplastic anemia
Hematocrit (Hct) and hemoglobin (Hgb)	Adult males: 42–52% (Hct) 13.5–17.5 g/dL (Hgb) / Adult females: 37–47% (Hct) 12.0–16.0 g/dL (Hgb)	Decreased in anemia that is associated with many processes, and in leukemias
Platelet count	150,000–400,000/mm³	Increased in myeloproliferative disorders / May be increased in advanced malignancies / May be decreased in leukemias and tumors metastatic to bone marrow

Based on Davis, M. (1993). Secondary prevention in oncology nursing practice. In J.C. Clark & R.F. McGee (eds.). *Core Curriculum for Oncology Nursing* (2nd ed.). Philadelphia: W.B. Saunders, pp. 47–53.

II. Implement patient education.
    A. Teach screening recommendations and monitor compliance.
    B. Initiate public education on early detection in schools and workplaces.
    C. Teach and monitor self-examination procedures.
        1. Breast (see Fig. 41–1).
        2. Testicular (see Fig. 41–2).
        3. Skin (see Fig. 41–3).

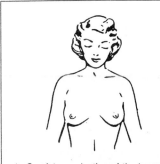
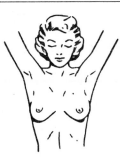
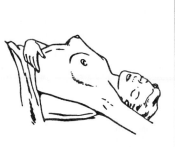

1. Careful examination of the breasts before a mirror for symmetry in size and shape, noting any puckering or dimpling of the skin or retraction of the nipple.

2. Arms raised over head, again studying the breasts in the mirror for the same signs.

3. Reclining on bed with flat pillow or folded bath towel under the shoulder on the same side as breast to be examined.

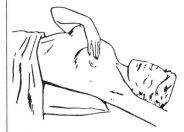
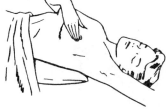
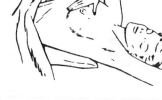

4. To examine the inner half of the breast the arm is raised over the head. Beginning at the breastbone and, in a series of steps, the inner half of the breast is palpated.

5. The area over the nipple is carefully palpated with the flat part of the fingers.

6. Examination of the lower inner half of the breast is completed.

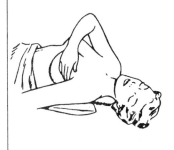
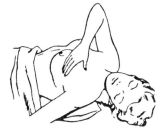
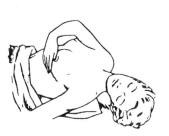

7. With arm down at side self examination of breasts continues by carefully feeling the tissues which extend to the armpit.

8. The upper outer quadrant of the breast is examined with the flat part of the fingers.

9. The lower outer quadrant of breast is examined in successive stages with flat part of the fingers.

Figure 41–1. Breast self-examination. (From American Cancer Society.)

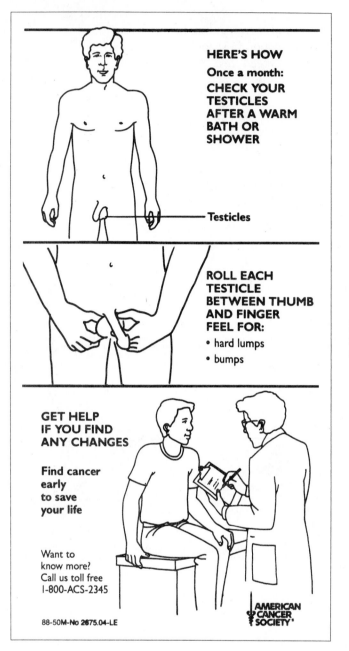

HERE'S HOW

Once a month:
CHECK YOUR TESTICLES AFTER A WARM BATH OR SHOWER

Testicles

ROLL EACH TESTICLE BETWEEN THUMB AND FINGER FEEL FOR:

• hard lumps
• bumps

GET HELP IF YOU FIND ANY CHANGES

Find cancer early to save your life

Want to know more? Call us toll free 1-800-ACS-2345

88-50M-No 2675.04-LE

AMERICAN CANCER SOCIETY®

Figure 41–2. Testicular self-examination. (From American Cancer Society.)

D. Teach "Seven Warning Signals of Cancer" mnemonic *CAUTION:*
   1. *C*hange in bowel or bladder habits.
   2. *A* sore that does not heal.
   3. *U*nusual bleeding or discharge.
   4. *T*hickening or lump in breast or elsewhere.
   5. *I*ndigestion or difficulty swallowing.
   6. *O*bvious change in wart or mole.
   7. *N*agging cough or hoarseness.

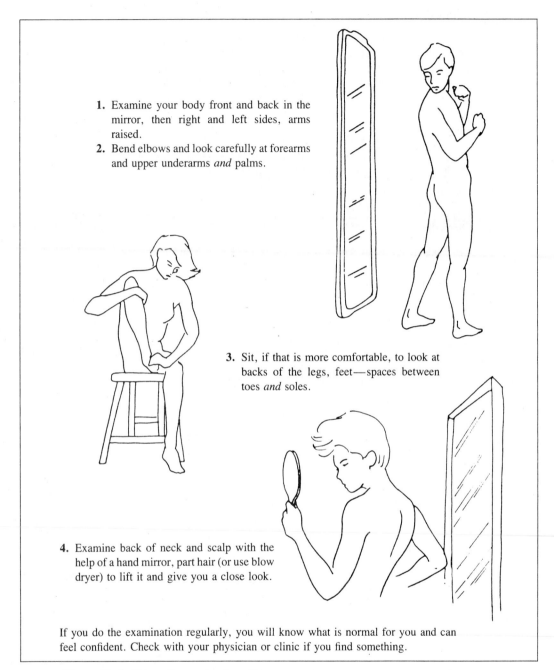

1. Examine your body front and back in the mirror, then right and left sides, arms raised.
2. Bend elbows and look carefully at forearms and upper underarms *and* palms.

3. Sit, if that is more comfortable, to look at backs of the legs, feet—spaces between toes *and* soles.

4. Examine back of neck and scalp with the help of a hand mirror, part hair (or use blow dryer) to lift it and give you a close look.

If you do the examination regularly, you will know what is normal for you and can feel confident. Check with your physician or clinic if you find something.

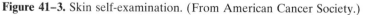

Figure 41–3. Skin self-examination. (From American Cancer Society.)

III. Provide education and follow-up care for clients with positive screening test results.
   A. Identify resources for cancer education and information.
   B. Facilitate referral for further evaluation.
   C. Reinforce importance of timely evaluation.
   D. Discuss implications of positive screening test results and describe confirmatory evaluation.

Evaluation

The oncology nurse systematically and regularly evaluates the client's and/or family's responses to interventions to determine progress toward the achievement of expected outcomes. Relevant data are collected and actual findings are compared with expected findings. Nursing diagnoses, outcomes, and plans of care are reviewed and revised as necessary.

BIBLIOGRAPHY

Davis, M. (1992). Secondary prevention in oncology nursing practice. In J.C. Clark & R.F. McGee (eds.). *Core Curriculum for Oncology Nursing* (2nd ed.). Philadelphia: W.B. Saunders, pp. 43–61.

Mettlin, C., Jones, G., Averette, H., et al. (1993). Defining and updating the American Cancer Society guidelines for the cancer-related checkup: Prostate and endometrial cancers. *CA Cancer J Clin* 43(1), 42–56.

Reintgen, D.S., & Clark, R.A. (eds.). (1996). *Cancer Screening.* St. Louis: Mosby-Year Book.

Tilkian, S.M., Conover, M.B., & Tilkian, A.B. (eds.). (1995). *Clinical and Nursing Implications of Laboratory Tests.* St. Louis: Mosby-Year Book.

Weiss, G.R. (ed.). (1996). *Clinical Oncology.* Norwalk, CT: Appleton & Lange.

PART EIGHT

Professional Performance

42

Application of the Standards of Practice and Education

Deborah Lowe Volker, RN, MA, OCN

Theory

I. Oncology Nursing Society (ONS)/American Nurses' Association (ANA) standards of oncology nursing practice.
   A. Definitions.
      1. Standard—authoritative statement that is enunciated and promulgated by the profession by which the quality of practice, service, or education can be judged.
      2. Client—the individual, family, group, or community for whom the nurse provides specifically planned services.
   B. Components of each standard.
      1. Standard statement.
      2. Rationale—explanation of the underlying reason for the standard.
      3. Measurement criteria—relevant, measurable indicators that demonstrate compliance with the standard.
   C. Standards of care (Table 42–1).
      1. Standards of care encompass professional nursing activities demonstrated by the oncology nurse, and include:
         a. Assessment.
         b. Diagnosis.
         c. Outcome identification.
         d. Planning.
         e. Implementation.
         f. Evaluation.
      2. The standards of care are focused on the 11 high-incidence problem areas common to clients cared for by oncology nurses.
         a. Prevention and early detection.
            (1) Personal risk factors.
            (2) Early detection practices.
            (3) Cultural and social factors.
         b. Information—includes the client's:
            (1) Developmental level.
            (2) Current knowledge of diagnosis, treatment, resources, and potential problems and side effects.
            (3) Participation in care (e.g., financial matters, availability of caregivers, cultural factors, current health-related practices, and hospice use).
            (4) Knowledge/perceptions of advance directives.

TABLE 42–1. **Standards of Care**

Standard I. Assessment
The oncology nurse systematically and continually collects data regarding the health status of the client.

Standard II. Diagnosis
The oncology nurse analyzes assessment data in determining nursing diagnoses.

Standard III. Outcome Identification
The oncology nurse identifies expected outcomes individualized to the client.

Standard IV. Planning
The oncology nurse develops an individualized and holistic plan of care that prescribes interventions to attain expected outcomes.

Standard V. Implementation
The oncology nurse implements the plan of care to achieve the identified expected outcomes for the client.

Standard VI. Evaluation
The oncology nurse systematically and regularly evaluates the client's responses to interventions in order to determine progress toward achievement of expected outcomes.

From Oncology Nursing Society & American Nurses' Association (1996). *Statement on the Scope and Standards of Oncology Nursing Practice.* Washington, D.C.: American Nurses' Association.

    c. Coping.
      (1) Past and present coping mechanisms.
      (2) Present concerns (e.g., spiritual concerns, role changes, and employment changes).
      (3) Present and potential support systems.
      (4) Current ability and availability to mobilize resources.
      (5) Alternative coping strategies during all phases of care.
    d. Comfort.
      (1) Source and degree of comfort.
      (2) Method of pain and symptom management, including cultural and folk remedies.
      (3) Impact of fatigue on daily living.
      (4) Effects of disease and treatment on lifestyle.
      (5) Outcomes of interventions to alleviate discomfort.
    e. Nutrition.
      (1) Current nutritional status.
      (2) Effects of disease and treatment.
      (3) Estimated time that the patient is at risk for being nutritionally impaired.
      (4) Past and present nutritional patterns and beliefs.
      (5) Function of gastrointestinal tract versus need of alternative route.
    f. Protective mechanisms.
      (1) Immune function.
      (2) Hematopoietic function.
      (3) Integumentary function.
      (4) Sensory and motor function, including level of consciousness and thought processes.
    g. Mobility.
      (1) Level of mobility.
      (2) Ability to perform activities of daily living.

        (3) Actual and potential disease and treatment risk factors that can alter mobility.

        (4) Potential for rehabilitation and recovery.

        (5) Impact of mobility on overall cancer survivorship.

   h. Elimination.

        (1) Past and present patterns of elimination.

        (2) Effects of disease and treatment.

   i. Sexuality.

        (1) Effects of disease and treatment on body image (e.g., alopecia, mastectomy, and ostomy).

        (2) Effects of disease and treatment on sexual functioning (e.g., infertility, impotence, early menopause, and dry mucous membranes).

        (3) Psychosocial responses of client and significant other to disease and treatment.

        (4) Past and present sexual patterns and functioning.

   j. Ventilation.

        (1) Level of respiratory status.

        (2) Alterations in gas exchange related to disease and treatment.

        (3) History of exposure to respiratory contaminants.

   k. Circulation.

        (1) Alterations in tissue perfusion.

        (2) Alterations in cardiac output.

3. Purpose of standards of care in oncology nursing.

   a. For the nurse generalist.

        (1) Serves as a guide to provide quality care by applying the nursing process to ensure that:

           (a) Data collection is systematic, culturally competent, continuous, collected from multiple sources, documented, and communicated with members of the multidisciplinary cancer care team.

           (b) Nursing diagnoses are derived from interpretation of presenting data and reflect the client's actual or potential health problems.

           (c) Identified outcomes are derived from the nursing diagnoses and are individualized to the client's needs.

           (d) The plan of care is derived from current knowledge of the nursing, biologic, social, behavioral, cultural, and physical sciences.

           (e) The plan of care reflects the client's priorities and prescribed nursing strategies to achieve health promotion, maintenance, and restoration.

           (f) Client participation does occur.

           (g) Client progress is assessed jointly by the nurse and client.

           (h) Client evaluation of outcomes directs reassessment and revision of the plan of care.

        (2) Facilitates professional development by:

           (a) Identifying gaps in the knowledge base.

           (b) Determining range of practice for which one is prepared.

   b. For oncology nursing practice, standards of care promote development by:

        (1) Providing a basis for the development of performance evaluation instruments.

(2) Providing a basis for quality assurance.

(3) Providing the basis and impetus for peer review.

(4) Generating research questions.

(5) Stimulating research to validate practice.

(6) Providing a basis for program evaluation.

(7) Promoting intradisciplinary and interdisciplinary collaboration.

   c. For the client, standards ensure:

(1) Participation in health restoration, promotion, and maintenance.

(2) Quality of care consistent with existing standards.

D. Standards of professional performance (Table 42–2) are related to:

1. Quality of care.

2. Performance appraisal.

3. Education.

4. Collegiality.

5. Ethics.

6. Collaboration.

7. Research.

8. Resource utilization.

E. Examples of methods by which oncology nurses apply standards of care and professional performance standards in clinical settings.

1. Application of standard of care III (outcome identification) to guide development of institution-specific plans of care for the 11 high-incidence problem areas.

TABLE 42–2. **Standards of Professional Performance**

Standard I. Quality of Care
The oncology nurse systematically evaluates the quality of care and effectiveness of oncology nursing practice.

Standard II. Performance Appraisal
The oncology nurse evaluates his/her own practice in relation to professional practice standards and relevant statutes and regulations.

Standard III. Education
The oncology nurse acquires and maintains current knowledge in oncology nursing practice.

Standard IV. Collegiality
The oncology nurse contributes to the professional development of peers, colleagues, and others.

Standard V. Ethics
The oncology nurse's decisions and actions on behalf of clients are determined in an ethical manner.

Standard VI. Collaboration
The oncology nurse collaborates with the client, significant others, and multidisciplinary cancer care team in providing client care.

Standard VII. Research
The oncology nurse contributes to the scientific base of nursing practice and the field of oncology through the review and application of research.

Standard VIII. Resource Utilization
The oncology nurse considers factors related to safety, effectiveness, and cost in planning and delivering client care.

From Oncology Nursing Society & American Nurses' Association (1996). *Statement on the Scope and Standards of Oncology Nursing Practice.* Washington, D.C.: American Nurses' Association.

a. For example: impaired skin integrity related to radiation therapy (Table 42–3). (Pertains to protective mechanisms.)

b. Relevant measurement criteria. The client:

   (1) Lists measures to prevent or minimize skin breakdown.

   (2) Identifies the signs and symptoms of skin breakdown and infection.

   (3) Identifies an appropriate cancer care team member to contact if initial signs and symptoms of skin breakdown or infection occur.

   (4) Describes self-care measures to manage skin breakdown and infection.

2. Application of professional performance standard I (quality of care) as a framework for an institutional quality assurance program. (See Table 42–4 for an example.)

   a. Use the measurement criteria of each standard of care as statements of acceptable practice.

   b. Use the 11 high-incidence problems as an outline for identification of potential indicators (well-defined, measurable dimensions of the quality and appropriateness of an important aspect of the client's care, which can include measurable care processes, clinical events, complications, or outcomes) that can be used to monitor oncology nursing care.

   c. Determine a threshold (a preestablished aggregate level of performance that should be achieved) for action.

   d. Collect data that monitor the quality and effectiveness of oncology nursing care.

   e. Analyze data to identify areas for improvement of care.

   f. Formulate recommendations to improve client outcomes and satisfaction with care.

   g. Implement recommendations and evaluate effectiveness.

3. Application of standards of care and professional performance to education.

   a. Use the standards to form a curricular outline for generalist oncology nursing education, staff development, and continuing education programs.

   b. Use the measurement criteria as learner objectives for both nurses and clients, as appropriate (Table 42–5).

4. Application of standards of care and professional performance to management.

   a. Both the standards of care and professional performance standards can be used as a framework for development of staff performance evaluation instruments (Table 42–6).

   b. Resource justification. Use the resource utilization standard (VIII) to address resources required for the practice of oncology nursing.

5. Application of professional performance standards VII, research, and VIII, research utilization, to formulate an institution's oncology nursing research program.

   a. Use the measurement criteria for standard VII to outline the staff nurse role and responsibilities.

   b. Use the measurement criteria for standard VIII to outline core activities within a research utilization program.

6. Identification of possible research questions.

   a. Which nursing interventions promote optimal patient outcomes?

      (1) Some of the high-incidence areas (e.g., prevention and early detec-

TABLE 42–3. **Institution-Specific Care Plan
for the Client With Alteration in Protective Mechanisms**

Standard. Impaired Skin Integrity Related to Radiation Therapy.

Expected Outcomes
1. Patient/caregiver verbalizes rationale for potential or actual impairment of skin integrity.
2. Patient/caregiver identifies/demonstrates measures to control or correct impaired skin integrity.

Nursing Interventions
1. Assess irradiated skin for color, dryness, moisture, scaling, temperature, tenderness, or itching and note high-risk area, such as skinfolds (e.g., perineum, axilla), ostomies, tracheostomy.
2. Assess areas of wet desquamation for signs of infection.
3. For dry desquamation, the following measures should be used unless otherwise ordered:
    a. Use only water-based, topical ointments (e.g., hydrous lanolin, Aquaphor, aloe vera) as ordered to control tenderness/dryness of skin.
    b. Do not use metal-based ointments (e.g., zinc oxide).
    c. Remove all ointment prior to radiation therapy.
4. For wet desquamation, the following measures should be used unless otherwise ordered:
    a. Cleanse area with water or saline. Pat dry.
    b. A 1:2 mixture of hydrogen peroxide and saline may be used for odor control.
    c. Avoid powders.
    d. Keep area moist to promote healing (e.g., moisture-permeable dressings, hydrocolloids, hydrogels).
5. Promote comfort by using:
    a. Bed cradles to keep linen off body.
    b. The prevention mode on the Hill-Rom 2000 bed; if Hill-Rom bed is not available, use overlay mattress of choice.
    c. Body positioning and supports; avoid friction when moving patient.
    d. Systemic analgesics as ordered.
6. Implement and teach hygienic/protective measures:
    a. No lotion, soap, cream, deodorant, perfume, hot or cold water or application, etc. is used in the treatment area unless prescribed by physician.
    b. Tepid water is permitted to trickle over the treatment area, but the area is not soaked or scrubbed.
    c. Avoid rubbing or friction to the area (i.e., wear soft, cotton, nonrestrictive clothing; do not scratch, use a patting motion or hair dryer set on cool setting if the area must be dried.
    d. Avoid activities that cause perspiration.
    e. Expose area to air as much as possible.
    f. Use an electric razor. Do not use pre- or post-shaving cream.
    g. Avoid shampooing the treated area.
    h. Protect markings. Verify with physician or technologist unmarked treatment areas that need to be protected.
7. Consult with enterostomal therapist regarding management of ostomies or skin care in the radiation field.
8. Explain rationale and measures to maintain adequate nutritional and fluid status.
9. Teach patient/caregiver:
    a. Signs and symptoms of infection.
    b. Rationale for radiation therapy-related side effects.
    c. Signs/symptoms of skin changes, including those reportable to health care team (e.g., erythema, tenderness, moist desquamation).
    d. Appropriate skin care regimen.
    e. To avoid sun exposure to the treated area for a lifetime.
    f. Post-therapy, to wear sunscreen with an SPF greater than or equal to 15.
    g. Drugs may potentiate radiosensitivity; discuss with physician potential for interaction with current medication.

From The University of Texas, M.D. Anderson Cancer Center, Division of Nursing, Houston, Texas, 1993.

TABLE 42–4. **Quality Improvement Project: Self-Care of Central Venous Access Devices (CVAD)**

Standard (statement of acceptable practice)
The client describes self-care measures and appropriate actions for highly predictable problems, oncologic emergencies, and side effects related to disease or therapy (Standard III. Outcome Identification, Measurement Criteria for Information).

Indicator
Before discharge with CVAD, 100% of clients (e.g., patient or designated caregiver) demonstrate ability to manage care of the CVAD independently, including:
a. Performance of heparin flush.
b. Changing heparin cap.
c. Changing dressing.
d. Verbalization of problems that must be reported to the health care team.
e. Verbalization of the phone number to call in the event of a problem.

Threshold for Action
Less than 100%.

Monitoring for Occurrences
For a 1-month period, all patients discharged with a CVAD will be assessed on the above items (a. through e.) within 24 hours before discharge and reassessed during first return visit to the ambulatory clinic. Results of the assessment will be documented on the CVAD Patient Education Monitoring Tool by the infusion therapy clinical nurse specialist.

Analysis of Findings
Data will be compiled and analyzed, and submitted to the interdisciplinary Infusion Therapy Practice Council for review. In the event the threshold for action is reached, a report of the problem analysis, plan for corrective action, and plan for remonitoring will be submitted to the institution interdisciplinary Quality Council.

TABLE 42–5. **Application of Measurement Criteria to Patient Education**

Use of Standards of Care III measurement criteria for teaching the client with an alteration in nutrition related to nausea and vomiting

Goal
The client will manage nutrition in a way that meets his or her goal of maximizing health maintenance and restoration during chemotherapy treatment.

Learning Objectives
The client will:
1. Identify foods that are tolerated and those that cause discomfort or are distasteful and unappealing.
2. Describe measures that enhance food intake and retention.
3. Select appropriate dietary alternatives to provide sufficient nutrients when foods that were part of the customary diet no longer are tolerated.
4. Describe methods of modifying consistency, flavor, or amounts of nutrients to ensure adequate nutrient intake.
5. Describe modifications in environment and eating habits that enhance oral intake.
6. Describe dietary modifications compatible with his/her cultural, social, and ethnic practices.
7. Describe interventions to relieve symptoms (nausea and vomiting) that interfere with nutritional intake.
8. Identify an appropriate cancer care team member to contact if dietary intake is inadequate.

Modified from Oncology Nursing Society & American Nurses' Association (1996). *Statement on the Scope and Standards of Oncology Nursing Practice.* Washington, D.C.: American Nurses' Association, pp. 14, 17, 18.

TABLE 42–6. **Excerpts from an Oncology Staff Nurse Performance Evaluation Tool**

Professional Performance Standard III. Education: The oncology nurse acquires and maintains current knowledge in oncology nursing practice.

Criteria	Rating* 1	2	3
1. Participates in ongoing educational activities (including inservices, continuing education, formal education, and experiential learning) to expand oncology knowledge of professional issues.			
2. Updates his or her own knowledge of political, cultural, spiritual, social, health care reimbursement, and ethical issues related to oncology care and the practice setting.			
3. Seeks experiences to develop and maintain clinical skills.			
4. Seeks knowledge and skills appropriate to the practice setting.			
5. Utilizes oncology nursing colleagues as resources.			

*Rating scale: 1, performance below standard; 2, meets standard; 3, exceeds standard.
From Oncology Nursing Society & American Nurses' Association (1996). *Statement on the Scope and Standards of Oncology Nursing Practice.* Washington, D.C.: American Nurses' Association, pp. 26, 27.

tion, comfort, and protective mechanisms) have been targeted by nurse researchers.

(2) Most of the measurement criteria, however, have not been validated.

 b. Are the highest priority areas for cancer nursing research (listed below) consistent with the standards?

  (1) Pain (included in the "comfort" high-incidence problem area).

  (2) Prevention (designated as a high-incidence problem area).

  (3) Quality of life (crosscuts all of the high-incidence problem areas).

  (4) Risk reduction/screening (designated as a high-incidence problem area).

  (5) Ethical issues (reflected in the ethics professional performance standard).

 c. Do measurement instruments exist for research related to the standards? Although ongoing development is critical, numerous instruments exist that measure a variety of phenomena associated with the high-incidence problems,

  (1) Instruments for assessing health and function (e.g., functional status, mental status and level of consciousness, coping, spirituality, hope, sexuality, information-seeking behaviors, quality of life).

  (2) Instruments for assessing clinical problems (pain, nausea and vomiting, dyspnea, skin integrity, elimination).

II. Standards of oncology education: Patient/family and public.

 A. Definitions.

  1. Education—the process of inducing measurable changes in knowledge, skills, and attitudes through planned learning activities.

  2. Standards—a norm that expresses an agreed-upon level of practice that has been developed to characterize, measure, and provide guidance for achieving excellence.

3. Family—persons who are related or who represent a significant support group for the person at risk for or experiencing cancer.
4. Public—the people of an organized community.
5. Domains of learning.
    a. Cognitive—knowledge and intellectual abilities.
    b. Psychomotor—physical skills.
    c. Affective—attitudes, values.
B. Purpose and intended outcomes of the standards.
    1. Purposes are to provide comprehensive guidelines for nurses to:
        a. Develop, implement, and evaluate formal and informal patient/family teaching.
        b. Develop, implement, and evaluate formal and informal public education programs.
    2. Intended outcomes are to:
        a. Enhance the quality of patient teaching.
        b. Exemplify the scope of teaching in all phases of cancer care, including prevention, early detection, rehabilitation, and supportive care.
        c. Improve health promotion and care for the public.
C. Format of the standards—descriptive statements, with defining criteria designed to guide the achievement of quality education for the patient/family and public. The standards address the following components:
    1. Nurse.
    2. Resources.
    3. Curriculum.
    4. Teaching-learning process.
    5. Learner.
D. Statement of standards of oncology education.
    1. Patient/family education (Table 42–7).
    2. Public education (Table 42–8).
E. Examples of application of standards of oncology education to clinical practice.
    1. Use the standards to guide development of standardized patient teaching plans. Table 42–9 presents an example that uses criteria from standards IV and V.
    2. Use the standards as a framework for quality assurance programs to monitor quality of patient/public educational activities.
        a. Monitoring project described in Table 42–4 also illustrates aspects of standard V of the standards of oncology education—the patient/family apply knowledge, skills, and attitudes to management of actual or potential human responses to the cancer experience.
        b. Relevant criteria for the monitoring project—the patient/family.
            (1) Demonstrate psychomotor and coping skills required for self-care (catheter care, criterion 4).
            (2) Describe signs and symptoms that should be reported to the interdisciplinary health care team (criterion 6).
F. Examples of application of standards of oncology education to professional education.
    1. Use the standards to form curricular outlines for generalist oncology nursing education, staff development, and continuing education programs. Table 42–10 provides an example of a lesson plan for teaching the public about prevention and early detection of skin cancers.
    2. Use the standards and criteria as learner objectives for cancer nursing education programs.

TABLE 42–7. **Patient/Family Education**

Standard I. Oncology Nurse
The oncology nurse at both the generalist and advanced practice levels is responsible for patient/family education related to cancer.

Standard II. Resources
Adequate resources to achieve the objectives of patient/family education related to cancer care are available and appropriate.

Standard III. Curriculum
Knowledge, skills, and attitudes related to the management of human responses to cancer are reflected in the educational activity for the patient/family experiencing cancer.

Standard IV. Teaching-Learning Process
Teaching-learning theories are applied to the development, implementation, and evaluation of learning experiences related to cancer care.

Standard V. Learner: The Patient/Family
The patient/family apply knowledge, skills, and attitudes to management of actual or potential human responses to the cancer experience.

From Oncology Nursing Society (1995). *Standards of Oncology Education: Patient/Family and Public.* Pittsburgh, PA: The Society, pp. 4–8.

TABLE 42–8. **Public Education**

Standard I. Oncology Nurse
The oncology nurse provides formal and informal cancer-related public education commensurate with personal education and experience.

Standard II. Resources
Adequate resources for public education related to cancer prevention, detection, treatment, and care are current and appropriate to achieve education objectives.

Standard III. Curriculum
Knowledge, skills, and attitudes related to the physical and psychosocial aspects of cancer prevention, early detection, treatment, and care are included in public education activities.

Standard IV. Teaching-Learning Process
Teaching-learning theories are applied to the development, implementation, and evaluation of learning experiences related to cancer education for the public.

Standard V. Learner: The Public
Personal behaviors and public policy related to cancer prevention, detection, treatment, rehabilitation, and supportive care are influenced by formal and informal cancer public education.

From Oncology Nursing Society (1995). *Standards of Oncology Education: Patient/Family and Public.* Pittsburgh, PA: The Society, pp. 9–13.

TABLE 42–9. **Teaching Plan for the Patient Who Experiences Thrombocytopenia Secondary to Myelosuppressive Chemotherapy**

RELEVANT STANDARDS: Teaching-learning theories are applied to the development, implementation, and evaluation of learning experiences related to cancer care (Standard IV); the patient/family apply knowledge, skills, and attitudes to management of actual or potential human responses to the cancer experience (Standard V).

Teaching Goal
The patient will demonstrate ability to describe the effect of chemotherapy on platelet production, self-care actions to prevent or diminish bleeding, and signs/symptoms to report to the health care team.

Teaching Plan	Relevant Standard Criteria
1. Assess level of education and ability and readiness of patient to learn.	The nurse collects data systematically from the patient/family and other sources to assess learning needs, readiness to learn, and situational and psychosocial factors influencing learning (Standard IV, Criterion 1).
2. Assess cognitive, affective, and psychomotor learning needs relevant to thrombocytopenia.	Analyzes assessment data to identify cognitive, psychomotor, and affective learning needs (Standard IV, Criterion 2).

3. In collaboration with patient, develop teaching plan based on identified need.
a. Behavioral objectives.
  (1) Explain the production and function of platelets.
  (2) Describe effect of chemotherapy on platelet production.
  (3) Explain the relationship between platelet count and risk of bleeding.
  (4) List signs/symptoms of bleeding that should be reported.
  (5) Describe measures to prevent/control bleeding.
	Develops a teaching plan in collaboration with the patient/family that includes behavioral objectives based on identified learning needs (Standard IV, Criterion 3.1).

b. Content (select as appropriate):
  (1) Normal bone marrow function.
    (a) Platelet production.
    (b) Platelet function.
  (2) Impact of chemotherapy.
    (a) Myelosuppression.
    (b) Recovery of cell production.
  (3) Relationship between platelet count and risk of bleeding.
  (4) Signs/symptoms of bleeding:
    Bleeding gums or nose.
    Spontaneous bruising, petechiae.
    Blood in urine or stool.
    Excessive bleeding after venipuncture.
    Hematemesis.
    Hemoptysis.
    Heachache, blurred vision.
    Vaginal bleeding.
    Rectal bleeding.
  (5) Measures to prevent bleeding:
    Prolonged pressure at puncture sites.
    No intramuscular injections.
    No medications that contain aspirin.
    Electric razor instead of straight-edged razor.
    No tampons, suppositories, rectal medications or temperatures.
    Extreme caution during manicure or pedicure.
	Content meets identified objectives (Standard IV, Criterion 3.2).

Table continued on following page

TABLE 42–9. **Teaching Plan for the Patient Who Experiences Thrombocytopenia Secondary to Myelosuppressive Chemotherapy** (*Continued*)

Teaching Plan	Relevant Standard Criteria
c. Suggested teaching strategies (select as appropriate): (1) One-to-one discussion. (2) Printed booklets. (3) Videotapes. (4) Chemotherapy class.	Teaching strategies and learning experiences promote active participation by the patient/family (Standard IV, Criterion 3.3).
d. Teaching/learning environment: provide environment free of interruption/distraction that promotes patient participation.	Environmental adaptations promote learning (Standard IV, Criterion 3.4).
e. Evaluation criteria (select as appropriate): evaluation methods include verbalization and demonstration. Upon completion, patient will demonstrate ability to: (1) Explain normal platelet function. (2) Describe the relationship between bone marrow function, platelet count, risk of bleeding. (3) List signs/symptoms of bleeding to report. (4) Demonstrate/describe self-care measures for prevention, detection, and control of bleeding.	Methods and criteria for evaluation (Standard IV, Criterion 3.5). The patient/family describes behaviors that promote a level of independence appropriate to learning ability (Standard V, Criterion 3) and describes signs and symptoms that should be reported to the health care team (Standard V, Criterion 6).
4. Implement teaching plan.	Implements the teaching plan in an environment conducive to learning (Standard IV, Criterion 4).
5. Evaluate ability of patient to meet the selected evaluation criteria via: a. Verbalization. b. Return demonstration.	Collects data from the patient/family and other sources to evaluate achievement of learning objectives, effectiveness and efficiency of instruction, and the need to revise the teaching plan (Standard IV, Criterion 5).
6. Modify plan; reinforce teaching as necessary (e.g., use of written instructions) to reinforce learning, teaching a family member to serve as a resource for the patient.	Modifies teaching-learning process based on evaluation data (Standard IV, Criterion 6).

From Oncology Nursing Society (1995). *Standards of Oncology Education: Patient/Family and Public.* Pittsburgh, PA: The Society, pp. 7–8.

G. Examples of application of standards on oncology education to management.
  1. The standards and criteria can be incorporated into staff performance evaluation instruments (educator component of the role). See Table 42–11 for an example.
  2. Resource justification. Use standard criteria to:
     a. Address the resources and environment required for patient/family and public education activities.
     b. Support the need for time, funding, systems, and personnel required for education in accordance with the standards.
H. Examples of application of standards of oncology education to research—suggested areas for investigation. Clinical testing of specific criteria for each standard.

TABLE 42–10. **Content Outline for Public Education Program on Prevention and Early Detection of Skin Cancers**

RELEVANT STANDARD: Knowledge, skills, and attitudes related to the physical and psychosocial aspects of cancer prevention, early detection, treatment, and care are included in public education activities (Standard III).

Content Outline	Relevant Criteria
I. Overview of skin cancers: carcinogenesis (how skin cancers arise).	Public education program includes:

II. Risk factors.
A. Fair, freckled complexion.
B. Sun exposure.
  1. Recreational.
  2. Occupational.
C. Chemical exposure.
D. Radiation exposure.
E. Scars from previous burns.
	Accurate and current information about principles of carcinogenesis, and genetic, environmental, and lifestyle risks for cancer (Criterion 1).

III. Signs and symptoms. A. Changes in moles; sore that does not heal. B. Persistent lump/swelling. C. Bleeding from mole, birthmark, freckle.	Signs and symptoms of common cancers (Criterion 4).
IV. Early detection A. Skin self-examination techniques (National Cancer Institute booklet). B. Community agencies for follow-up.	Community resources for health promotion and cancer-related information and services (Criterion 8).

V. Prevention.
A. Minimization of sun exposure.
  1. Avoid sunbathing and use of tanning booths.
  2. Use sunscreens.
  3. Wear protective clothing.
B. Occupational precautions.
	Methods to modify health behaviors and practices for cancer prevention and health promotion (Criterion 2).

From Oncology Nursing Society (1995). *Standards of Oncology Education: Patient/Family and Public.* Pittsburgh, PA: The Society, p. 11.

1. Investigation of various teaching methods and the impact on patient learning outcomes (e.g., does the use of interactive videodisc teaching modules improve the ability of the patient to perform self-care activities?).
2. Investigation of optimal approaches to teaching people with low literacy skills (e.g., what is the effect of using group classroom learning activities versus one-to-one teaching of self-care activities in the low-literacy population?).
3. Investigation of the impact of public education programs on the practice of lifestyle choices that minimize personal risks for cancer (e.g., what is the effect of public education programs on the use of sunscreen products?).
4. Investigation of the influence of religious, cultural, and ethnic practices on the teaching-learning process (e.g., what cultural characteristics influence the teaching-learning process in the Latino population?).

TABLE 42–11. **Excerpt from an Oncology Staff Nurse Performance Evaluation Tool**

Standard	Rating* 1	2	3
STANDARD IV: Teaching-learning theories are applied to the development, implementation, and evaluation of learning experiences related to cancer education for the public. **Criteria—The nurse:** 1. Collects data systematically from the patient/family and other sources to assess learning needs, readiness to learn, and situational and psychosocial factors influencing learning.			
2. Analyzes assessment data to identify cognitive, psychomotor, and affective learning needs.			
3. Develops a teaching plan in collaboration with the patient/family that includes: a. Behavioral objectives based on identified learning needs. b. Content to meet identified objectives. c. Teaching strategies and learning experiences that promote active participation by the patient/family. d. Environmental adaptations to promote learning. e. Methods and criteria for evaluation of patient/family outcomes.			
4. Implements the teaching plan in an environment conducive to learning.			
5. Collects data from the patient/family and other sources to evaluate achievement of learning objectives, effectiveness and efficiency of instruction, and the need to revise the teaching plan.			
6. Modifies teaching-learning process based on evaluation data.			

*Rating scale: 1, performance below standard; 2, performance meets standard; 3, performance exceeds standard.
From Oncology Nursing Society (1995). *Standards of Oncology Education: Patient/Family and Public.* Pittsburgh, PA: The Society, p. 7.

BIBLIOGRAPHY

Dorsett, D.S. (1993). Quality of care. In S.L. Groenwald, M.H. Frogge, M. Goodman, & C. Yarbro (eds.). *Cancer Nursing: Principles and Practice* (3rd ed.). Boston: Jones & Bartlett, pp. 1453–1484.

Fitch, M., & Thompson, L. (1996). Fostering the growth of research-based oncology nursing practice. *Oncol Nurs Forum 23,* 631–637.

Frank-Stromborg, M. (1988). *Instruments for Clinical Nursing Research.* Norwalk, CT: Appleton & Lange.

Iwamoto, R., Rumsey, K., & Summers, B. (1996). *Statement on the Scope and Standards of Oncology Nursing Practice.* Washington, D.C.: American Nurses Publishing.

Miaskowski, C., & Rostad, M. (1990). Implementing the ANA/ONS standards of oncology nursing practice. *J Nurs Qual Assur 4*(3), 15–23.

Oncology Nursing Society. (1995). *Standards of Oncology Education: Patient/Family and Public.* Pittsburgh, PA: Oncology Nursing Society.

Patton, M.D. (1993). Action research and the process of continual quality improvement in a cancer center. *Oncol Nurs Forum 20,* 751–755.

Stetz, K, Haberman, M., Holcombe, J., & Jones, L. (1995). 1994 Oncology Nursing Society research priorities survey. *Oncol Nurs Forum 22,* 785–789.

43

The Education Process

Mary B. Johnson, RN, PhD, OCN, HNC
Judith (Judi) L. Johnson, RN, PhD, FAAN

Theory

I. Education of the community, the client and family facing cancer, and the health professionals providing care involves three types of education—health education, client education, and staff education.

   A. *Health education*—the process of assisting individuals, acting separately and collectively, to make informed decisions on matters affecting individual, family, and community health. The World Health Organization (WHO) defines health education as any combination of planned activities leading to a situation in which people want to be healthy, know how to obtain health information, do what they individually and collectively can, and seek help when needed.

   B. *Client education*—a series of structured or nonstructured experiences designed to help clients and families:
      1. Cope with the crisis responses to the diagnosis of cancer.
      2. Cope with long-term adjustments to disease and treatment.
      3. Cope with symptoms.
      4. Gain information about sources of prevention, diagnosis, and care.
      5. Develop needed self-care skills.
      6. Develop attitudes that facilitate the healing process.
      7. Explore resources that promote a sense of wholeness and well-being.

   C. *Staff education*—activities and experiences aimed at expanding and improving professional performance to improve client, family, and community health outcomes; often employer-sponsored but may be individually sought via continuing education programs, ONS programs, others.

II. Rationale for education of persons at risk for or living with a diagnosis of cancer and those who provide care.

   A. Education is an integral part of adaptation and is part of total health care.

   B. Planned educational experiences ensure that important health-related information is available and is presented in a consistent manner.

   C. Education empowers clients, families, and communities for active participation in decision-making and self-care.

   D. Staff education provides an avenue for bringing together practitioners with differing perspectives and centralizing efforts to provide innovative approaches for teaching clients, families, and communities.

E. Educational experiences give clients, families, communities, and health care professionals the opportunity to exchange ideas, discuss problems, and develop solutions with each other.

F. Educational experiences strengthen the concept of partnership among clients, families, communities, and health care providers.

III. Theoretical principles of teaching and learning.
   A. Human factors.
      1. Learning occurs when people perceive a need to ascertain something.
         a. Needs identified by health care providers may not be consistent with needs identified by the community, client, or family.
         b. Learner-identified needs should receive priority.
         c. Motivation for learning comes when a gap exists between what people know and what they want to know.
         d. Learning should be problem-centered not subject-centered.
      2. Learning is influenced by accumulated life experiences.
      3. Learning is influenced by trust, mutual respect, acceptance of differences, and freedom of expression.
      4. Learning needs to be reinforced; it does not necessarily occur because the teaching has been done.
      5. Opportunities for practice, repetition, and feedback need to be included in a teaching plan.
   B. Organizational factors.
      1. Client, family, and community education is a component of the job description of registered nurses in cancer care.
      2. Client, family, and community education programs are supported and recognized by all parties responsible for the delivery of health care.
      3. Staff is responsible for learning new and innovative approaches to client education with a focus on outcomes.
      4. The educational process consists of assessment, diagnosis, planning, implementing, and evaluation.
   C. Physical factors.
      1. The learning environment facilitates learning by providing privacy, adequate space, comfortable seating, adequate lighting, and minimal distractions.
      2. Adequate time and appropriate equipment are required to facilitate learning.
   D. Educational materials and methods factor.
      1. Selected materials are appropriate for the developmental, educational, and socioeconomic status, as well as to cultural and spiritual values of the community or client and family.
      2. Methods used in education engage individuals and groups in the learning process.
         a. Teaching-learning requires human interaction.
         b. People learn better when more than one of their senses are stimulated.
      3. Materials and methods are selected based on the objectives of the learning experience and the learning styles of the community or client and family.

Assessment

I. Client and family—pertinent personal history.
   A. Developmental level—physical, intellectual, and emotional changes associated with aging, and past life experiences.
   B. Sociocultural background—values, customs, beliefs, communication patterns, and roles.

    C. Socioeconomic status—lifestyle, work situation, and use of leisure time.

    D. Intellectual status—vocabulary and language skills, extent of formal education, concrete and abstract thinking skills, and problem-solving skills.

    E. Spiritual orientation—beliefs in a higher being and roles of the higher being in the lives of individuals.

    F. Social support systems—types, patterns of use, adequacy, and value to individual.

  II. Client and family—responses to disease and treatment.

    A. Physical responses—presence of alterations in comfort levels can result in a decrease in motivation and receptiveness to learning.

      1. Presence of fever, sleep deprivation, weakness, fatigue, nausea, vomiting, and pain.

      2. Physical and mental changes resulting from medications used to control physical responses.

    B. Emotional responses—intense positive or negative responses can result in a decrease in receptiveness to learning.

      1. Presence of anxiety, depression, anger, fear, and distrust.

      2. Emotional changes resulting from medications used to control disease as well as physical responses to disease and treatment.

    C. Stages of adaptation—responses such as disbelief, developing awareness, reorganization, resolution, and identity changes may influence the content, timing, and methods used for education.

  III. Community needs assessment—the community needs to be involved with the assessment of particular community needs as well as with planning, implementation, and evaluation.

  IV. Staff needs assessment—Joint Commission on the Accreditation of Healthcare Organizations (JCAHO) standards addressing client education and discharge planning need to be addressed with a focus on methods, resources, and documentation.

Nursing Diagnoses

  I. The cancer experience can be viewed as a series of phases, each creating unique concerns and problems for the client and family and each requiring particular nursing diagnoses. Because effective learning is facilitated when information is problem-centered and timely, nursing diagnoses for clients and families are suggested for each phase of the cancer experience. Community and staff education departments may use these phases in more comprehensive educational programs. Table 43–1 provides a complete list of potential nursing diagnoses seen with these phases and the education process.

  II. The most commonly used nursing diagnosis for the education process itself is: Knowledge deficit.

Outcome Identification

  I. Oncology Nursing Society Standards of Oncology Education.

    A. Client and family describe the illness, goals and plan of therapy, potential risks and benefits, and available treatment options.

    B. Client and family assume an active role in decision-making and identification of needs with respect to the development, implementation, and evaluation of the plan of care.

    C. Client and family describe behaviors that promote a level of independence appropriate to age, development stage, learning ability, resources, personal preference, prognosis, and physical ability.

TABLE 43–1. **Potential Nursing Diagnoses Through the Phases of the Cancer Experience and the Education Process**

Phase	Focus	Potential Nursing Diagnoses
Prediagnostic	The focus of client, family, and community education is to influence health behavior—a set of activities in which an individual engages to maximize wellness, avoid risks, participate in cancer screening measures, and build a knowledge base of the signs and symptoms of possible malignancies	Health-seeking behaviors (cancer prevention) Knowledge deficit (cancer screening and early detection strategies) Potential for enhanced community coping Potential for growth: family coping
Diagnostic	The focus is on diagnostic workup measures and supporting the client and family in understanding and coping with the diagnosis	Impaired verbal communication Anxiety Ineffective individual coping Ineffective family coping: compromised or disabling Anticipatory grieving Hopelessness
Treatment	The focus is on treatment options and strategies for coping with the side effects of treatment. Nursing diagnoses from the Diagnostic Phase may continue to be pertinent	Knowledge deficit (new diagnosis, treatment, managing side effects) Decisional conflict Altered role performance Family therapeutic regimen: Effective or ineffective management Individual therapeutic regimen: Effective or ineffective management Energy field disturbance
Surveillance	The focus is on compliance with follow-up testing and lifestyle change to promote wellness. This phase may extend throughout a person's life as a permanent phase of cancer survival. The previous nursing diagnoses may continue to be pertinent	Noncompliance (missed appointments for follow-up testing) Knowledge deficit (complementary therapies, support groups) Altered family processes Potential for enhancement of spiritual well-being Personal identity disturbance
Recurrence	The focus is on the reality of further disease, and the possibility of a decline in health must now be faced. There is a possibility of more intense grief over a longer period of time. Nursing diagnoses identified earlier in the cancer experience need to be reevaluated, updated, and refined to more specifically address the educational needs of the client and family at this phase	Impaired adjustment Powerlessness Knowledge deficit (control and palliation issues) Defensive coping Spiritual distress Situational low self-esteem Acute pain Altered nutrition, less than body requirements
Dying	The focus is on the irreversible progression of the client's disease process. Nursing diagnoses in this phase are influenced by the client's dying trajectory and may include several previously identified in other phases	Fear Fatigue Anticipatory and/or dysfunctional grieving Risk for loneliness Relocation stress syndrome Impaired adjustment Caregiver role strain
Bereavement	The focus is on validating the death of a loved one, acknowledging grief and loss, giving and receiving emotional support among family and friends	Posttrauma response Potential for growth, family coping Social isolation Impaired adjustment

D. Client and family demonstrate psychomotor and coping skills required for self-care.

E. Client and family describe methods to modify behaviors for health promotion and cancer prevention, detection, treatment, and care.

F. Client and family describe signs and symptoms that should be reported to the interdisciplinary health care team.

G. Client and family discuss interpersonal responses to cancer treatment and care.

H. Client and family identify community resources available for health promotion and cancer care.

II. Oncology Nursing Society Standards of Oncology Education.

A. Community demonstrates realistic attitudes about cancer.

B. Community describes lifestyle choices that minimize personal risks for cancer and promote health.

C. Community participates in appropriate or recommended cancer screening activities.

D. Community identifies a course of action for early detection when signs and symptoms of cancer are discovered.

E. Community identifies sources of cancer information, care, rehabilitation, and supportive care in the community.

F. Community describes the political process for accomplishing social change to minimize environmental and lifestyle risks for cancer and to benefit individuals experiencing cancer.

G. Community demonstrates support and acknowledgment of cancer survivors.

III. Standards of Oncology Nursing Education.

A. Nurse applies theoretical concepts as a basis for critical thinking in oncology nursing practice.

B. Nurse utilizes the nursing process systematically to develop an outcome-oriented care plan that is individualized, holistic, culturally sensitive, cost-effective, incorporating cancer prevention, detection, treatment, rehabilitation, and supportive care.

C. Nurse communicates assessment data and responses to appropriate members of the oncology health care team.

D. Nurse assumes responsibility for personal professional development in oncology nursing.

E. Nurse contributes to the professional growth of others.

F. Nurse collaborates with the multidisciplinary team to assess, plan, implement, and evaluate across all levels of health care need.

G. Nurse participates in peer review and multidisciplinary program evaluation to assure that quality oncology nursing care is provided.

H. Nurse uses appropriate documents, such as the ANA Code for Nurses, A Patient's Bill of Rights, and ONS position papers as guides for ethical decision-making in oncology nursing practice.

I. Nurse participates in oncology nursing research problem identification, implementation, and/or application to cancer care.

J. Nurse practices health behaviors consistent with health promotion as a role model for the public.

Planning and Implementation

I. Develop outcome goals for the educational experience.

A. Include the learners in goal development.

B. Identify goals that are congruent with the interdisciplinary treatment plan and the specific phase of the cancer experience in which the learners currently dwell.

    C. State goals in realistic and measurable terms.

    D. Prioritize goals in collaboration with the learners and health care providers.

    E. Assign a time period for achievement of goals.

II. Determine content and experiences that contribute to goal achievement.

    A. Review current literature related to the knowledge, skills, or attitudes that are a part of the established goals.

    B. Review literature related to the experiences that are most effective in assisting the learner to achieve established goals.

    C. Develop a content outline for each teaching session.

III. Select materials and methods to guide the learner to goal achievement.

    A. Obtain and review educational materials specific to the established goals.

        1. Resources for community, family, and client cancer education are available from:

            a. American Cancer Society.

            b. American Lung Association.

            c. Cancer Information Service (1-800-4-CANCER).

            d. Hospital equipment companies.

            e. Leukemia Society of America.

            f. Mechanical device companies (e.g., venous access devices).

            g. National Cancer Institute.

            h. National Coalition for Cancer Survivorship.

            i. Pharmaceutical companies.

        2. Printed materials may be developed using the following guidelines:

            a. Identify target audience for content and literacy.

            b. Organize information in a logical way.

            b. Use short words, sentences, and paragraphs.

            c. Select descriptive nouns and active verbs for headings.

            d. Incorporate developmental and cultural considerations.

            e. Use illustrations to complement copy.

            f. Write a caption for each illustration.

            g. Avoid unfamiliar jargon.

    B. Select materials appropriate to the intellectual status, reading level, and cultural and socioeconomic backgrounds of the learner.

    C. Select methods and strategies determined to be the most effective in teaching specific content, skills, or attitudes within the specific phase of the cancer experience.

IV. Develop a plan for evaluating the effectiveness of the teaching and learning.

    A. Determine the level of measurement to evaluate achievement of the goal such as accuracy, increasing approximations to the behavior, number of behaviors, persistence, or originality.

    B. Define the methods to use to evaluate achievement: direct observation of behavior, oral questioning, written tests, chart audits, and self-reports.

    C. Determine the methods for evaluating the efficacy of teaching style and methods and the appropriateness of content.

    D. Establish the time frames for evaluation.

    E. Define the process for documentation of achievement of outcomes, provision of feedback to learners, and revision of the teaching-learning plans based on evaluation data.

Evaluation

    The oncology nurse systematically and regularly evaluates the client's and/or family's responses to interventions to determine progress toward the achievement

of expected outcomes. Relevant data are collected and actual findings are compared with expected findings. Nursing diagnoses, outcomes, and plans of care are reviewed and revised as necessary.

BIBLIOGRAPHY

Babcock, D., & Miller, M. (1994). *Client Education: Theory and Practice.* St. Louis: C.V. Mosby.

Bandman, E.L., & Bandman, B. (1995). *Critical Thinking in Nursing* (2nd ed.). Norwalk, CT: Appleton & Lange.

Blumberg, B.D., & Johnson, J. (1993). Teaching strategies: The patient. In S.L. Groenwald, M.H. Frogge, M. Goodman, & C.H. Yarbro (eds.). *Cancer Nursing: Principles and Practice* (3rd ed.). Boston: Jones & Bartlett, pp. 1576–1586.

Brookfield, SD. (1990). *The Skillful Teacher.* San Francisco: Jossey-Bass.

Doak, C., Doak, L., & Root, J. (1995). *Teaching Patients With Low Literary Skills* (2nd ed.). Philadelphia: J.B. Lippincott.

Fernsler, J.I., & Ades, T.B. (1996). Developing strategies for public education in cancer. In R. McCorkle, M. Grant, M. Frank-Stromborg, & S.B. Baird (eds.). *Cancer Nusing: A Comprehensive Textbook* (2nd ed.). Philadelphia: W.B. Saunders, pp. 1235–1246.

Iwamoto, R.R., Rumsey, K.A., & Summers, B.L.Y. (1996). *Statement on the Scope and Standards of Oncology Nursing Practice.* Washington, D.C.: American Nurses Publishing.

Johnson, J., & Klein, L. (1994). *I Can Cope: Staying Healthy With Cancer* (2nd ed.). Minneapolis: Cronimed Publishing.

Joint Commission on the Accreditation of Healthcare Organizations. (1995). Education of the patient: Standards and scoring guidelines. In *1995 Comprehensive Accreditation Manual for Hospitals.* Chicago: Joint Commission on the Accreditation of Healthcare Organizations.

Lee, P.R., & Estes, C.L. (1994). *The Nation's Health* (4th ed.). Boston: Jones & Bartlett.

McCorkle, R., Grant, M., Frank-Stromborg, M., & Baird, S.B. (eds.). (1996). *Cancer Nursing: A Comprehensive Textbook.* Philadelphia: W.B. Saunders.

Oncology Nursing Society. (1995). *Standards of Oncology Education: Patient/Family and Public.* Pittsburgh: Oncology Nursing Press.

Oncology Nursing Society. (1995). *Standards of Oncology Nursing Education: Generalist and Advanced Practice Levels.* Pittsburgh: Oncology Nursing Press.

Pender, N. (1995). *Health Promotion in Nursing Practice* (3d ed.). Stamford, CT: Appleton & Lange.

Rankin, S., & Stallings, K. (1996). *Patient Education: Issues, Principles, and Practices* (3d ed.). Philadelphia: J.B. Lippincott.

Redman, B. (1993). *The Process of Patient Education* (7th ed.). St. Louis: Mosby-Year Book.

Senge, P.M. (1990). *The Fifth Discipline: The Art and Practice of the Learning Organization.* New York: Currency Doubleday.

U.S. Department of Health and Human Services. (1994). *Update: Healthy People 2000.* June–July, 1994. Washington D.C.: U.S. Department of Health and Human Services.

Vaill, P.B. (1996). *Learning as a Way of Being: Strategies for Survival in a World of Permanent White Water.* San Francisco: Jossey-Bass.

Yoder Wise, P. (1995). *Leading and Managing in Nursing.* St. Louis: Mosby-Year Book.

RESOURCES FOR SPECIFIC EDUCATIONAL PROGRAMS

Cancer Practice: A Multidisciplinary Journal of Cancer Care
Cancer Nursing
Cancer Educational Journal
Cope: Oncology Forum and News for Professionals
Journal of Continuing Education in Nursing
Journal of Nursing Quality Assurance
Journal of Nursing Staff Development
Oncology Nursing Forum. Official Journal of the Oncology Nursing Society
Patient Education and Counseling
Seminars in Oncology Nursing

44

Legal Issues Influencing Cancer Care

Mary Magee Gullatte, RN, MN, ANP, AOCN

I. Definition: pertaining to a law, conformity with a given law, or statute.

II. Primary sources of law affecting health-related issues include:
   A. Statutes—written laws enacted by legislatures that encompass the rules of society and are signed by a president or governor.
   B. Common law—court-made law that serves as the basis for most malpractice litigation.
   C. Administrative law—law made by administrative agencies appointed by the executive branch of government.

III. Purposes—concern over legal issues in the area of health care result from a need to:
   A. Protect the rights of citizens, both the public and professionals.
   B. Delineate the responsibilities of recipients and providers of health care.
   C. Delineate the scope of practice for health care professionals and institutions.
   D. Ensure the provision of reasonable and customary health care.

IV. Sources used in legal decision-making relevant to oncology nursing practice.
   A. Professional documents used to establish minimal acceptable standards of practice and health care:
      1. Nurse practice acts:
         a. Provide definition and role of nursing by state.
         b. Regulate the practice of nursing.
         c. Delineate requirements and specifications of licensure.
         d. Establish a board of nursing.
         e. Provide a mechanism for due process and penalties.
      2. Professional standards of practice.
         a. *ANA Standards of Nursing Practice.*
         b. *ONS/ANA Standards of Oncology Nursing Practice.*
         c. *ONS Standards for Oncology Education: Patient/Family and the Public.*
         d. *ONS Standards of Oncology Nursing Education: Generalist and Advanced Practice Levels.*
   B. Agency or institutional policies and procedures:
      1. Regulations override institutional policies.
      2. Statutes override regulations.

    C. Requirements of accrediting or governing agencies:
1. Joint Commission on Accreditation of Healthcare Organizations (JCAHO).
2. American College of Surgeons.
3. Occupational Safety and Health Administration (OSHA)—safety standards.
4. Centers for Disease Control and Prevention—infection control standards.
5. Department of Health and Human Services.

    D. Client rights (Table 44–1).
1. American Hospital Association (AHA)—Patient's Bill of Rights.
2. JCAHO—standards of care related to client rights.
3. Right of self-determination.
4. Informed consent documents.

    E. Client and proxy agreements.
1. Living wills.
2. Directives for organ and tissue donation.
3. Directives for withholding or withdrawing life-support measures.
4. Durable Power of Attorney.
5. Advance Directives for Medical Care.

V. Individual and professional nurse accountability.
    A. Individual nurse is responsible for professional nursing practice.
    B. "Respondent superior" renders employer liable and responsible for the actions of the employee.

VI. Liability.
    A. Negligence—deviation from the acceptable standard of care that a reasonable person would use in a specific situation.
    B. Malpractice—deviation from a professional standard of care.
    C. Duty—care relationship between client and provider.
    D. Breach of duty—failure to meet an acceptable standard of care.

VII. Litigations involving oncology nurses include:
    A. Medication errors by omission or commission.
    B. Failure to follow acceptable standard of care, resulting in client harm.
    C. Incomplete or absent documentation in medical record.
    D. Inadequate referral or follow-up.
    E. Lack of teaching.
    F. Insufficient discharge planning.
    G. Failure to follow through on assessed client need.

VIII. Potential actions resulting from legal allegations.
    A. Out-of-court settlement, which may include monetary or other restitution.
    B. Trial by jury resulting in monetary restitution, imprisonment, public service payback, or loss of licensure if found guilty; admissible evidence includes medical records, sworn testimony, and expert witness.
    C. Agency or institutional sanctions.
    D. Professional sanctions by state board of nursing.

IX. Prudent action by nurses to ensure "reasonable or customary care" is rendered to the client and is documented in the medical record.
    A. Demonstrate knowledge of and adherence to professional standards and procedures as determined by self-evaluation and peer review.
    B. Participate in policy review and revisions within the agency, private practice, and professional organizations.

TABLE 44–1. **Patient Rights Organizations**

Organization	Goals/Objectives	National Office
American Civil Liberties Union (ACLU)	Actively protects the Constitutional rights of citizens Rights to privacy, equal protection, confidentiality, access to records, and equal access to care	ACLU 132 W. 43rd Street New York, NY 10036
American Society of Law and Medicine	Professional continuing education related to current trends in health law Journals: *Law, Medicine and Health Care* *American Journal of Law and Medicine*	American Society of Law and Medicine 765 Commonwealth Avenue Boston, MA 02215
Children in Hospitals, Inc.	Helps parents stay with and support their children during hospitalization Publishes a newsletter	Children in Hospitals, Inc. 31 Wilshire Park Needham, MA 02192
Citizen Advocacy Center (CAC)	A support program for public members who serve on health care regulatory boards and governing bodies as representatives of the consumer interest. Provides research, training, technical support, and networking opportunities for public members	CAC 1424 Sixteenth Street Suite 105 Washington, DC 20036
Concern for Dying and Society for the Right to Die (formerly the Euthanasia Educational Council)	Provides information and support for those interested in exercising their rights as patients, especially the right to refuse medical treatment Developed the living will *Right to Die:* an annual updated collection of all state living will laws	Concern for Dying 250 W. 57th Street New York, NY 10107 Society for the Right to Die (same address)
The Hemlock Society	Promotes legislation to legalize physician-assisted suicide and distributes literature on the subject	The Hemlock Society P.O. Box 11830 Eugene, OR 97440
Law, Medicine and Ethics Program	Education, research, and advocacy in health law, with emphasis on patient rights, health care regulation, and medical ethics	Law, Medicine and Ethics Program Boston University Schools of Medicine and Public Health 80 E. Concord Street Boston, MA 02118
The National Hospice Organization	Information center about hospices Publishes a national directory and provides information	The National Hospice Organization 1901 North Fort Myer Drive Suite 902 Arlington, VA 22209
National Health Law Program	Legal services and back-up center, specializing in health law, Medicaid, and access issues for the poor Publishes a newsletter	National Health Law Program 26396 South LaCienega Blvd. Los Angeles, CA 90034

TABLE 44–1. **Patient Rights Organizations** *Continued*

Organization	Goals/Objectives	National Office
People's Medical Society	Provides information on issues regarding patient rights Membership organization for consumers of medical services	People's Medical Society 14 East Minor Street Emmaus, PA 18049
Pew Health Professions Commissions	Established in 1984, and administered by the University of California at San Francisco Center for Health Professionals, workforce policymakers and educational institutions in responding to the challenges of the changing health care system	Pew Health Professions Commission UCSF Center for the Health Profession 1388 Sutter Street Suite 805 San Francisco, CA 94109
Public Citizen Health Research Group	Ralph Nader–affiliated consumer advocacy group Concerned with issues of medical care, drug, safety, medical device safety, physician competence, and consumer health care issues	Public Citizen Health Research Group 2000 P Street N.W. Suite 708 Washington, DC 20036

Annas, G.J. (1992). The Rights of Patients: The Basic ACLU Guide to Patients Rights (2nd rev. ed.). Totowa, NJ: Humana Press.

    C. Maintain current knowledge of personal and institutional liability.
    D. Maintain adequate individual and agency liability insurance coverage.
    E. Keep diligent records with respect to:
       1. Accuracy of entries.
       2. Timeliness of charting.
       3. Accurate and timely filing of incident reports according to agency policy.
       4. Referrals and follow-up care.
 X. Cancer legislation—current legislative issues related to cancer care focus on:
    A. Prevention and early detection of disease.
    B. Research and clinical trials.
    C. Evaluation of alternative treatments.
    D. Investigation using human subjects.
    E. Minority health issues.
    F. Treatment of economically disadvantaged clients, including the poor, elderly, homeless, and refugees of all races and all ethnic groups.
    G. Health issues of women.
    H. Environmental hazards.
     I. Occupational hazards.
    J. Access to health care.
    K. Economics of cancer.
    L. Research ethics.
    M. Research funding.
XI. Issues pertinent to oncology nursing practice.
    A. Ownership of human cells and tissues.
    B. Right to self-determination and autonomy.

C. Withholding care to terminally ill clients.

D. Withdrawing medical treatment.

E. Occupational and environmental hazards.

F. Smoking among oncology nurses.

G. Human subject research.

H. Alternative treatments.

I. Chemical dependency among health care workers.

J. Informed consent—explicit versus implied.

K. Advance directives.

L. Quality of life and survivorship.

M. Political reform related to access to health care for all.

XII. Nurse managers—a wide range of legal issues confront the nurse manager, including:

A. The reduction of professional nursing staff and the issue of liability; recommendations to reduce liability include the following responsibilities:

1. Communicate inadequate number of professional nursing staff.

2. Define the system to objectively measure acuity.

3. Define the number and skill mix of staff needed to provide safe client care.

4. Identify equipment and supply needs.

5. Initiate client care standards.

6. Document the impact of an inadequate number of professional nursing staff on client care.

7. Ensure that "reasonable" efforts have been taken to address the staffing problem.

8. Define job description and competency for use of unlicensed assistive personnel (UAP).

B. Temporary staff and agency nurse liability—ostensible agency or apparent authority (client believes a health care worker is an employee of the health care agency); recommendations to reduce liability of the health care agency with respect to acts of independent contractors include the following responsibilities:

1. Verify credentials such as nursing licensure, malpractice insurance, and cardiopulmonary resuscitation.

2. Orient to hospital and care unit.

3. Review health care agency policies and procedures.

4. Validate competency.

5. Identify professional as a contract nurse.

6. Evaluate care given.

7. Contract with a limited number of reputable per diem agencies.

C. Labor relations—collective bargaining is becoming more pervasive in the health care system.

1. Taft-Hartley Act exempted nonprofit hospitals from jurisdiction of the National Labor Relations Board (NLRB).

2. Hospitals became subject to the NLRB after 1974.

3. Solicitation for union member—a "no solicitation" rule is often in effect to inhibit union solicitation within the health care agency.

4. Recommendations for maintaining a "union-free" workplace include:

a. Fair labor practices.

b. Wide range of benefits.

c. Avoidance of discrimination on basis of sex, race, color, creed, national origin, physical challenge, or lifestyle.

    d. Equitable hiring and promotion practices.

    e. Fair and competitive wages.

    f. Open line of communications between management and labor.

D. Impaired health care professionals (chemical dependency).

    1. State boards of nursing report chemical dependency as the leading cause of disciplinary action; the number of addicted nurses is reported at 10 to 12%.

    2. Factors contributing to chemical dependency among nurses—job-related stress, easy access to controlled substances, inadequate narcotic control on nursing unit, financial concerns, home situations, failure of colleagues to report suspicious behaviors.

    3. Management responsibilities.

        a. Establish policy on impaired professionals.

        b. Investigate suspected abuse promptly.

        c. Protect client and health care agency from harm and liability.

        d. Notify board of nursing and document actions.

        e. Offer support through peer or employee assistance programs.

        f. Provide reentry support.

        g. Investigate State Nursing Association Peer Assistance options.

BIBLIOGRAPHY

Annas, G.J. (1992). *The Rights of Patients: The Basic ACLU Guide to Patient Rights* (2nd rev. ed.). Totowa, NJ: Humana Press.

Barhamand, B.A. (1996). Documentation issues in cancer nursing. In R. McCorkle, M. Grant, M.F. Stromborg, & S. Baird (eds.). *Cancer Nursing: A Comprehensive Textbook* (2nd ed.). Philadelphia: W.B. Saunders, pp. 1356–1365.

Cassel, C.K. (1989). Care of the dying: The limits of law, the limits of ethics. *Law Med Health Care 17,* 232–233.

Childress, J.F. (1989). Dying patients: Who's in control? *Law Med Health Care 17,* 227–231.

Cohen, A. (1989). The management rights clause in collective bargaining. *Nurs Manage 20,* 24–26, 28–30, 34.

Dimond, M. (1989). Health care and the aging population. *Nurs Outlook 37,* 76–77.

Fiesta, J. (1983). *The Law and Liability: A Guide for Nurses.* New York: John Wiley & Sons.

Fiesta, J. (1990). Agency nurses—Whose liability? *Nurs Manage 21,* 16–17.

Fiesta, J. (1990). The impaired nurse—Who is liable? *Nurs Manage 21,* 20, 22.

Fiesta, J. (1991). Law for the nurse manager. QA and risk management: Reducing liability exposure. *Nurs Manage 22,* 14–15.

Fowler, M.D. (1989). Slow code, limited code. *Heart Lung 18,* 533–534.

Goldsmith, M.F. (1988). Health decisions for the American people subject of new national bioethical policy group. *JAMA 260,* 14–5.

Hall, J.K. (1996). *Nursing Ethics and Law.* Philadelphia: W.B. Saunders.

Hoefler, J.M. (1994). *Deathright: Culture, Medicine, Politics, and the Right to Die.* Boulder, CO: Westview Press.

Humber, J.M., Almeder, R.F., & Kasting, G.A. (1993). *Physician-assisted Death.* Totowa, NJ: Humana Press.

McCabe, M.S., & Piemme, J.A. (1996). Cancer legislation. In R. McCorkle, M. Grant, M.F. Stromborg, & S. Baird (eds.). *Cancer Nursing: A Comprehensive Textbook* (2nd ed.). Philadelphia: W.B. Saunders, pp. 1409–1424.

Majewski, J. (1993). Local government. In D.J. Mason, S.W. Talbott, & J.K. Leavitt (eds.). *Policy and Politics for Nurses* (2nd ed.). Philadelphia: W.B. Saunders, pp. 421–432.

Meisel, A. (1989). Refusing treatment, refusing to talk, and refusing to let go: On whose terms will death occur? *Law Med Health Care 17,* 221–226.

Pabst, B.M. (1994). *The Least Worst Death: Essays in Bioethics on the End of Life.* New York: Oxford University Press.

Reynolds, J.J. (1989). Love, medicine, and money: Issues of access, use, and advocacy. *Health Soc Work 14,* 6–7.

Rizzo, R.F. (1989). The living will: Does it protect the rights of the terminally ill? *N Y State J Med 89,* 72–79.

Salladay, S.A., & McDonnell, M.M. (1989). Spiritual care, ethical choices, and patient advocacy. *Nurs Clin North Am 24,* 543–549.

Scanlon, C., & Fibison, W. (1995). *Managing Genetic Information: Implications for Nursing Practice.* Washington, D.C.: American Nurses Publishing.

Scanlon, C., & Fleming, C. (1989). Ethical issues in caring for the patient with advanced cancer. *Nurs Clin North Am 24,* 977–986.

Schulmeister, L. (1987). Litigation involving oncology nurses. *Oncol Nurs Forum 14,* 25–28.

Stromborg, M.F., & Chamorro, T. (1996). Legal responsibilities of the nurse. In R. McCorkle, M. Grant, M.F. Stromborg, & S. Baird (eds.). *Cancer Nursing: A Comprehensive Textbook* (2nd ed.). Philadelphia: W.B. Saunders, pp. 1388–1408.

Taylor, I. (1988). Patients' rights and clinical research. *Lancet 2,* 1370.

White, G.B., & O'Connor, K.W. (1990). Rights, duties, and commercial interests: John Moore versus the regents of the University of California. *Cancer Invest 8,* 65–70.

Zweibel, N.R., & Cassel, C.K. (1989). Treatment choices at the end of life: A comparison of decision by older patients and their physician-selected proxies. *Gerontologist 29,* 615–621.

Selected Ethical Issues in Cancer Care

Robin R. Gwin, RN, MN, FNP
Joan Exparza Richters, RN, MN, CRNH

I. Informed consent.
  A. Definition—a decision made freely by the client or a legally authorized representative after full knowledge and understanding of risks, benefits, and available options about various treatment alternatives are obtained.
  B. Purpose.
    1. Enable autonomous choice.
    2. Protect client against harm.
    3. Ensure responsible medical and nursing professional actions.
    4. Avoid exploitation.
  C. Situations requiring consent.
    1. Treatment with potential for altering patient health.
    2. Clinical trials.
    3. Research.
  D. Components of informed consent.
    1. Disclosure—explanation of the purpose, expected duration, and description of the procedure, which includes known risks, discomforts, benefits, and alternative treatment.
    2. Understanding—ability to comprehend and apply judgment.
    3. Voluntariness—ability to act freely without restraint or coercion.
    4. Competence—mental, physical, and legal ability to make a personal choice as a means to a desired goal.
    5. Capacity—ability to understand and appreciate the nature and consequences of a health care decision.
      a. Mental capacity—ability to reason without psychological or cognitive deficits.
      b. Physical capacity—ability to reason with psychomotor deficits present.
      c. Legal capacity—ability of a person of legal age to make decisions independent of others.
    6. Consent—approval or acceptance of an act proposed or performed by another.
  E. Factors inappropriate in obtaining informed consent.
    1. Coercion—influencing a person to act against his or her will.

2. Captivity—restraint of a person without consent.
3. Deception—misrepresentation of information.
4. Paternalism—assumption of decision-making responsibilities for another person.
5. Unvalidated understanding—no proof of comprehension of knowledge by the person receiving treatment.
6. Language barriers—incongruent languages, illiteracy, and/or incomprehensible language without an interpreter or intermediary.
7. Sensory impairment—sight, hearing, and/or speech deficits.
8. Altered level of consciousness—confusion, disorientation, medication side effects, disease processes, coexisting disease processes.
9. Medication influences—altered thought processes resulting from effects of medication.
10. Vulnerability or powerlessness—feelings of loss of control, loss of power, and/or helplessness.
11. Quackery—unproven treatment modalities.

F. Guidelines for the consent process.
1. Ensuring that the components of informed consent—including understanding, voluntariness, and competence—are met.
2. Medical explanation of the condition warranting treatment.
3. Explanation of the purpose of the treatment or procedure.
4. Description of the treatment or procedure.
5. Explanation of known risks, benefits, alternatives, or consequences of not accepting treatment.
6. Explanation of right to refuse consent or withdraw consent at any time.

G. Situations in which complete disclosure is not required.
1. Therapeutic privilege.
   a. The individual may elect not to be informed.
   b. The individual may have prior knowledge of the treatment or procedure.
   c. The physician may anticipate that harm may come to the individual if the information is disclosed.
   d. In emergency situations, consent is inferred.
2. Therapeutic use of placebos when used for the welfare of the client.
3. Incomplete disclosure with research subjects when full knowledge would affect results (randomization, double-blind experiments, and other methods used to compensate for bias).

H. The role of the nurse in informed consent.
1. Disclosure. (Physicians are responsible for explaining medical treatments and procedures.)
   a. Reinforce and clarify information presented.
   b. Notify physician if unable to validate understanding.
   c. Inform physician of possible medication administration that may interfere with comprehension.
   d. Ascertain documentation of informed consent on the medical record.
2. Client advocacy.
   a. Respect the right of the client to choose.
   b. Encourage the client to ask questions and actively participate in decision-making.
   c. Assess and report anxiety and/or ambivalence related to the procedure or treatment.

II. Clinical trials.
   A. Definition—method consisting of four phases used in research or in evaluation of an investigational drug or intervention that may have therapeutic implications for clients.
      1. Phase I—determination of safe drug levels and/or schedules of a new drug using human subjects.
      2. Phase II—determination of therapeutic efficacy when applied to clients with various diagnoses.
      3. Phase III—once efficacy is established, comparison of the drug to an existing, effective, standard therapy for the same diagnosis.
      4. Phase IV—utilization as standard therapy to determine optimal use of the drug with large client populations.
   B. Ethical principles.
      1. Justice—the investigator treats the client fairly.
      2. Autonomy—the right of a person to make independent decisions.
      3. Beneficence—obligation of health care workers to do good for clients.
      4. Nonmaleficence—obligation of health care workers to do no harm.
      5. Veracity—obligation of health care workers to tell the truth.
   C. Obligations of the researcher.
      1. Obtain investigational review board approval for most educational and health care agencies and all institutions receiving Department of Health and Human Resources funds.
      2. Maintain separation between practice and research.
      3. Obtain informed consent.
      4. Ensure confidentiality.
      5. Ensure anonymity when appropriate to the research design.
      6. Ensure that client selection is congruent with phase criteria.
   D. Role of the nurse in clinical trials.
      1. Ensure that informed consent is obtained and documented.
      2. Assess and document the response to the treatment or intervention.
      3. Manage symptoms related to the treatment or intervention.
      4. Provide physical and psychosocial care.
      5. Collaborate with the research team.
      6. Maintain current knowledge of the treatment or interventions.
      7. Encourage client autonomy throughout the research period.
III. Advance directives.
   A. Definition—a means for competent individuals to influence treatment decisions in the event of serious illness and subsequent loss of competency (e.g., withdrawal of life-sustaining interventions [do not resuscitate—DNR], durable power of attorney for health care, and living will).
      1. Purpose—a method to communicate an individual's desires concerning medical treatment.
      2. Specific advance directive considerations.
         a. Withdrawal of life-sustaining interventions.
         b. Antiinfective therapy.
         c. Blood products.
         d. Nourishment.
         e. Hydration.
         f. Hospitalization.
         g. Continuance of antineoplastic treatment.
         h. Pain management.

B. Do not resuscitate (DNR)—a decision made by the client or his or her legal representative not to perform cardiopulmonary resuscitation in the event that pulse and respirations cease.
   1. Purpose—to validate agreement between the client, family, and health care team regarding right to die without resuscitation.
      a. Potential indications—brain death; poor prognosis; in accordance with client wishes.
      b. Contraindications—any client or family ambivalence regarding code status.
   2. Role of the nurse.
      a. Ensure that a clear understanding exists between the physician and client and family members regarding resuscitation orders.
      b. Promote independent decision-making throughout treatment by encouraging the client and family members to communicate openly with the health care team.
      c. Ensure proper documentation and appropriate renewal procedures of resuscitation orders according to institutional policies.
      d. Respect cultural values regarding death and dying.
      e. Validate emotional responses of the client and family to the resuscitation orders.
      f. Respect the right of the client and family to choose or deny resuscitation orders.
      g. Refer the client and family to other appropriate resources (support groups, pastoral care, clinical nurse specialist, nurse practitioner, psychiatrist, social services).
      h. Act as a client and family advocate.
C. Durable power of attorney for health care—a legally designated individual (health care surrogate) responsible for making health care decisions on behalf of a person who is no longer competent.
   1. Purpose—to understand and uphold the client's wishes and communicate with caregivers to choose the appropriate treatment or nontreatment options.
      a. Indications—appropriate at any stage along the health care continuum.
      b. Requirements—mutually agreed on by the client and health care surrogate, legally recognized.
   2. Role of the nurse.
      a. Educate the client and family regarding the opportunity to establish durable power of attorney for health care.
      b. Refer the client to appropriate resource to initiate the necessary legal documents.
      c. Promote communication between the health care team and the person holding durable power of attorney.
D. Living will—defines health care decisions during the terminal phase of a client's illness.
   1. Purpose—to understand and uphold the client's wishes regarding treatment at the end of the health care continuum.
   2. Limitations.
      a. Applicable only during the terminal phases of illness.
      b. State-specific recognition of the document.
      c. Limited to the specifications outlined in the document
   3. Role of the nurse.
      a. Educate the client and family regarding the use of a living will.
      b. Refer the client to an appropriate resource to initiate a living will.
      c. Ensure that the health care team is aware of the existence and content of the living will.

BIBLIOGRAPHY

Berry, D.L., Dodd, M.J., Hinds, P.S., & Ferrell, B.R. (1996). Informed consent: Process and clinical issues. *Oncol Nurs Forum 23*(3), 507–512.

Carroll-Johnson, R.M. (ed.). (1993). Ethics and oncology nursing: Report of the ethics task force. *Oncol Nurs Forum 20*(10):suppl (entire issue).

Fry, S. T. (1991). Ethics and cancer care. In S.B. Baird, R. McCorkle, & M. Grant (eds.). *Cancer Nursing: A Comprehensive Textbook.* Philadelphia: W.B. Saunders, pp. 31–37.

Grafius, L.C. (1995). *Ethics for Everyone: A Practical Guide to Interdisciplinary Biomedical Ethics Education.* Chicago: American Hospital Publishing.

Holly, C.M. (1993). The ethical quandaries of acute care nursing practice. *J Prof Nurs 9*(2), 110–115.

Martinez, J., & Wagner, S. (1993). Hospice care. In S.L. Groenwald, M.H. Frogge, M. Goodman, & C.H. Yarbro (eds.). *Cancer Nursing: Principles and Practice* (3rd ed.). Boston: Jones & Bartlett, pp. 1432–1450.

Milner, S. (1993). An ethical nursing practice model. *J Nurs Adm 23*(3), 22–25.

Thomasma, D.C. (1993). Ethical issues in cancer nursing practice. In S.L. Groenwald, M.H. Frogge, M. Goodman, & C.H. Yarbro (eds.). *Cancer Nursing: Principles and Practice* (3rd ed.). Boston: Jones & Bartlett, pp. 1520–1535.

46

Cancer Economics and Health Care Reform

Mary Ann Crouch, RN, MSN

I. The national health care and cancer care dilemma.
   A. By the year 2000, it is estimated that United States (US) health care spending will reach $1.6 trillion, or 16.4% of the nation's gross domestic product.
   B. It is currently estimated that approximately 40 million people in the US have no medical insurance (13 million of these are children).
   C. At the state level, Medicaid expenditures have risen to over $140 billion, with states paying about $40 billion.
   D. By the year 2000, the American population will be older, with the greatest increase in those over the age of 85.
   E. Each year over 1 million Americans are diagnosed with cancer and 500,000 die from this disease.
   F. By the year 2000, cancer will overtake heart disease as the leading cause of death, which will capture greater than 20% of health care expenditures.
   G. The National Cancer Institute (NCI) reported the overall cost of cancer to be $104 billion (10% of the total cost of disease in the US).
      1. Direct costs = $37 billion.
      2. Cost of lost productivity = $12 billion.
      3. Mortality costs = $57 billion.
   H. Age continues to be the greatest risk factor for developing cancer; 50% of all cancers occur after age 65 years; 60% of all cancer deaths occur after age 65 years.
   I. Despite increasing resources spent on cancer care, there has been no corresponding change in quality or quantity of life for the majority of cancer patients.
   J. End-of-life care is expensive for cancer patients.
      1. Average intensive care unit (ICU) costs are $82,900 to gain 1 year of life; 79% spend fewer than 3 months at home after discharge.
      2. The last year of life for a cancer patient costs as much as 75% of total lifetime health care costs.
      3. 46% of reported Medicare costs are spent in the last 60 days of life.
II. The emergence of "managing" health care.
   A. Managed care definition—a linkage of payers, providers, and purchasers in systems and activities that controls the costs and utilization of care, while maintaining high quality and access.
      1. Managed care insurance plans are replacing traditional indemnity plans.

2. In 1994 there were more than 50 million enrollees (20% of the national population) in health maintenance organizations (HMOs).

3. There is increasing evidence of the growth of Medicaid and Medicare managed care plans.

B. Indemnity insurance, coverage in which the insured is reimbursed by the insurance carrier for medical expenses, allows open choice of physician and hospital. Generally the insurance carrier uses fee-for-service (FFS) payment practices, which is payment for each service provided to a patient that corresponds to a fee paid to the provider.

C. Types of managed care plans.

1. HMO—a prepaid health plan that provides or arranges health services for its members.

2. Independent practice association (IPA)—an HMO that contracts directly with physicians in independent practice.

3. Physician hospital organization (PHO)—an entity sponsored and jointly governed by a hospital and medical staff to negotiate and service managed care contracts.

4. Preferred provider organization (PPO)—blend between managed care and indemnity plan that provides FFS payment at established rates. Economic incentives encourage PPO members to use the preferred providers of the plan for health care services.

5. Exclusive provider organization (EPO)—a rigid type of PPO that requires the use of designated providers or reimbursement is sacrificed.

6. Point of service (POS)—blends indemnity and HMO plans. At the time of service the insured can elect to receive service from a network provider (HMO) at a discount or no out-of-pocket cost or from a non-network provider for a higher patient cost.

D. Comparison of nonmanaged and managed care (Table 46–1).

E. Managed care reimbursement—there are varying degrees of financial risk from the FFS (previously described) to the fully capitated payment system.

1. Discounts—hospitals and physicians agree to a percentage reduction from charges as payment in full.

2. Per diem—fixed amount paid per day regardless of amount of ancillary services provided.
   a. Creates incentive to reduce ancillary services.
   b. Rate independent of actual costs.
   c. May create incentive for increased length of stay.

3. Per case—fixed reimbursement per stay regardless of length of stay.
   a. Creates incentive to decrease use of ancillary services and length of stay.
   b. Aggressive utilization review process may decrease length of stay and thus allow for increased profit.

4. Global case rate—amount of reimbursement is all-inclusive for both institutional and professional services.

5. Capitation—providers receive a fixed amount for each person eligible to receive services, regardless of services used by any specific individual.
   a. Often referred to as premium paid per member per month.
   b. Creates incentive to reduce frequency of hospital admissions, length of stay, and ancillary use.

TABLE 46–1. **Comparison of Nonmanaged and Managed Care**

	Nonmanaged Care	**Managed Care**
Health Service Delivery		
Focus	Episodic treatment	Prevention and continuity of care
Provider autonomy	Liberal	Routinely uses standard practice guidelines, care maps, clinical pathways, other methods
Referrals	Unlimited	Strict control
Physician usage	Multiple physician groups	Selected group of physicians
Market Factors		
Type of competing providers	Independent	Networks
Ancillary service use	High numbers	Lower numbers
Inpatient hospitalization rates/ days	Higher	Lower
Information Systems		
Characteristics	Fragmented, episodic and financially focused	Mature managed market has well-developed patient-focused information systems. May include computerized medical record. Data are outcome driven from financial, utilization, and clinical perspectives
Reimbursement		
Effect on volume	Uses fee-for-service system that provides incentive to increase or maintain high volume of services provided	Uses provider risk-sharing strategies to create an incentive to control volume
Type of reimbursement	Open ended reimbursement; emphasizes productivity	Limited reimbursement with focus on efficiency
Type of care	Emphasizes specialty care	Uses primary care model
Market share	Defined by number of inpatient admissions and/or clinic visits	Defined by number of covered lives for which it is liable to provide services if needed

    c. May span the spectrum from capitation separate for primary care, specialty care, hospital services, to a full-capitation plan that covers all services.

    d. Premium is often prepaid on a monthly basis; the challenge to providers is to manage costs for the entire group in need of services.

    e. Various methods exist to determine capitation calculation methods.
      (1) Flat fee per member per month.
      (2) Percentage amount paid of total premium.
      (3) Amount adjusted for age and sex of covered members.
III. Managed care system evolution.
    A. Event-driven cost avoidance.
      1. Focus on price, decrease hospitalization days, use of specialists, discounting of care.
      2. Strategies—preadmission review, concurrent review, use of physician extenders.
      3. Low HMO penetration rate (10%).
      4. Competition in service; technology-focused.
      5. Primary pricing FFS.
    B. Value improvement.
      1. Goal to control use and intensity of resources; improve delivery of care, increase customer satisfaction.
      2. Pricing per diem, capitation of specialists per case.
      3. Strategies—care delivery redesign, use of clinical pathways, outcome measurement, cost control, ICU care, drugs, laboratory services, procedures, information system development, increased multidisciplinary collaborative practice.
      4. HMO penetration increasing, development of structured networks; emergence of integrated systems.
    C. Health improvement.
      1. Population-based health status focus; goal is to reduce total health services cost.
      2. HMO penetration 70 to 80%.
      3. Strategies—increased capitation; formal care management models, targeted interventions for at-risk individuals, groups; case management.
    D. Mature market characteristics include:
      1. Provider willingness to assume and manage risk for a population.
      2. Formal physician/hospital/health system structures/linkages across the continuum of care.
      3. Reconfiguration of delivery system to focus on patient needs.
      4. Provider and community partnerships developed to target health care needs of the group.
IV. Legislative strategies developed to manage health care costs at the state and national level.
    A. Diagnosis related group (DRG)—a system of Medicare classification for inpatient hospital services based on primary and secondary diagnoses, procedures, age, sex, and complications. Used as a financing mechanism to reimburse hospitals and providers for services rendered.
    B. Employer-mandated insurance—requires employers to offer and pay for a portion of workers' health insurance coverage.
    C. Medicaid expansion—by relaxing requirements, expands coverage to individuals who otherwise would not qualify for benefits.
    D. Single-payer or regulated multiple-payer systems.
      1. In a single-payer system, state government collects premiums and administers health care benefits for everyone in the state.
      2. In a multiple-payer system, the state government regulates reimbursement levels.

E. Managed competition—health care providers and insurance companies create health plans that compete with other health plans for large groups of customers. Providers are organized into networks and compete for business.

1. Minnesota is instituting a regulated all-payer system for low-income and uninsured people that reimburses for care on a rate-regulated fee schedule.

2. Florida is in the process of implementing a voluntary universal-access health plan version.

3. Washington is adding premium caps to a managed competition model. The plan controls growth in spending by establishing maximal premiums. Increases in premiums would be regulated in accordance with growth in per-capita income.

F. Small group purchasing alliances—allow small employers to combine resources, spread the risk of premiums, and use increased leverage in negotiating discounts from providers of health care.

G. Group insurance reform—laws designed to make health insurance more accessible and affordable to small employers. Some features include guaranteed renewal, portability, and guaranteed issue.

1. Connecticut was one of the first states to establish a medical risk pool designed to insure people with medical conditions such as cancer.

H. Cost controls—include various efforts such as expenditure targets and caps, targets for rate increases, total budgets for health care services, and uniform payment systems for ambulatory care and physicians.

I. HMOs and PPOs—regulation at the state level of primarily utilization review laws.

J. Health service planning—includes legislation concerning the certificate of need process, development of statewide health information systems, bulk purchasing agreements, and standardization of forms and processes to reduce administrative costs.

K. Malpractice litigation reform—caps set for pain and suffering, limits on attorney fees, limits on liability.

L. Provider availability—identifies strategy for rural community access to health services. Focuses on scholarship, loan repayment programs, as well as restructuring medical education in favor of primary care.

M. Scope of practice—grants prescriptive privileges to health professionals other than physicians. Expands practice of nurses and physician assistants.

N. Pharmaceutical practice—broadened access and cost containment programs, especially to mail order and managed care pharmacies; some implementing technology to track prescription purchases.

O. Medicaid reform—changes in the structure of the system to a managed care format.

V. Future of oncology care in an economically challenged environment.

A. Cancer issues of interest to economists.

1. A great deal of knowledge exists about the cause of premature death due to cancer, but the development and implementation of national health policies to address these risks is slow.

2. Variations in the treatment of cancer patients exist, and there is little agreement about the appropriateness of treatment.

3. A great need has emerged to gather information about the cost-effectiveness of cancer screening and treatment interventions.

4. Clinical trials often enroll small numbers, affecting results; cost and overall quality of life are not evaluated.

B. Technologic innovation in oncology will produce many new advances in cancer care; yet the new techniques will require evaluation. Managed plans often challenge new advances and do not provide coverage for such care; such a scenario may hinder advances in oncology care.
   1. Diagnostic technologies.
      a. Magnetic resonance imaging (MRI).
      b. Computed tomography (CT).
      c. Positron emission tomography (PET).
      d. Teleradiology.
      e. Stereotactic biopsy systems.
      f. Tumor markers—prostate specific antigen; cancer antigens; alpha-fetoprotein; interleukin-2 receptor; may allow for earlier detection or diagnosis of cancer.
      g. Radiolabeled monoclonal antibodies—may be used as a diagnostic and treatment tool; potentially useful to identify location and degree of metastasis.
   2. Treatment technologies.
      a. Chemotherapy.
         (1) New drug development.
         (2) Increase use of high-dose therapy.
      b. Radiation therapy—advances may minimize harm to surrounding tissues.
         (1) Proton beam therapy.
         (2) Intraoperative electron beam therapy.
         (3) Brachytherapy.
         (4) Conformal therapy.
         (5) Multileaf collimator.
         (6) Stereotactic radiosurgery.
      c. Immunologic therapies—modification of immune responses to enhance adjunctive therapies or assist with hematopoietic recovery.
         (1) Monoclonal antibodies.
         (2) Cytokines.
         (3) Hematopoietic growth and colony stimulating factors.
         (4) Interleukins.
         (5) Interferons.
         (6) Tumor antigen vaccines.
   3. Genetic technologies.
      a. Deoxyribonucleic acid (DNA) probe test—may be able to predict individual or familial risk of predisposition to certain cancers.
      b. Polymerase chain reaction—identifies changes in DNA that indicate the onset or recurrence of certain cancers.
      c. Oncogene inhibitors—developed to attack and prevent triggering of an oncogene before the onset of cancer.
C. The current NCI position is that payers should pay for the cost of patient care delivered in a bona fide NCI-sponsored trial, but not for associated research costs.
D. The American Society of Clinical Oncologists adopted a policy statement on reimbursement for clinical trials.
   1. Treatment provided must be of therapeutic intent.
   2. Treatment is provided in a trial approved by the NCI, cooperative groups, community clinical oncology programs, the Food and Drug Administra-

tion (FDA), Department of Veterans Affairs, or nongovernmental agencies, as identified in the guidelines for NCI cancer center support grants.

3. Trial has been reviewed and approved by a qualified institutional review board.
4. Facility and personnel providing treatment are capable of doing so by virtue of their experience and training.
5. No noninvestigational therapy is clearly superior to the protocol treatment.
6. Available clinical or preclinical data provide a reasonable expectation that the treatment will be at least as efficacious as noninvestigational therapy.

VI. The role of the oncology nurse.
  A. Standards of practice as developed by the Oncology Nursing Society are maintained with special emphasis on:
    1. Quality care.
    2. Education.
    3. Ethics.
    4. Collaboration.
    5. Research.
    6. Resource utilization.
  B. Understand managed care and the continually changing environment.
  C. Proactivity versus reactivity; look for new solutions; new care delivery strategies—be a change agent.
  D. Understand personal strengths and weaknesses; continually build on or improve.
  E. Build multidisciplinary collaborative relationships.
  F. Enact or affect local, regional, national efforts to influence health care policy development and implementation.
  G. Establish comfort level with role ambiguity and health care changes.
  H. New role opportunities for nurses.
    1. Primary care provider.
    2. Case manager.
    3. Educator.
    4. Triage coordinator.
    5. Quality improvement/assurance.
    6. Risk manager.
    7. Benefit interpreter.
    8. Provider liaison.
    9. Utilization management.

BIBLIOGRAPHY

Antman, K. (1993). Reimbursement issues facing patients, providers, and payers. *Cancer 72*(Suppl), 2842–2845.

Antman, K. (1995). Presidential address, thirty-first annual meeting of the American Society of Clinical Oncology. *J Clin Oncol 13,* 2980–2989.

Antman, K., Berkman, B.J., Huber, S.L., et al.(1993). The economic impact of therapy on cancer patients. *Cancer 72* (Suppl), 2862–2864.

Berkman, B.J., & Sampson, S.E. (1993). Psychosocial effects of cancer economics on patients and their families. *Cancer 72* (Suppl), 2846–2849.

Brown, M.L., & Fireman, B. (1995). Evaluation of direct medical costs related to cancer. *J Natl Cancer Inst 87,* 399–400.

Coile, R.C. (1992). Health care outlook 1995: Strategic directions for oncology. *J Oncol Manage 1*(5), 31–33.

Coopers & Lybrand, Health Decision Support Group. (1994). Health care reform: Innovations at the state level. *Nurs Manage 25*(4), 30–42.
Goldsmith, J.C., Goran, M.J., & Nackel, J.G. (1995). Managed care comes of age. *Health Care Forum J 38*(5), 14–24.
Health Care Advisory Board. (1994). *The Future for Oncology: New Technologies and Their Impact on the Competitive Marketplace.* Washington, D.C.: The Advisory Board Company.
Jenks, S. (1995). Some HMO's embrace clinical trials. *J Natl Cancer Inst 87,* 1104.
Kennedy, B.J. (1994). Oncology issues in health care reform. *Cancer Invest 12,* 249–256.
Leake, A.R. (1995). The economic impact of cancer. *Nurse Pract Forum 6,* 207–214.
Smith, T.J., Hilner, B.E., & Desch, C.E. (1993). Efficacy and cost-effectiveness of cancer treatment: Rational allocation of resources based on decision analysis. *J Natl Cancer Inst 85,* 1460–1474.

47

Changes in Oncology Health Care Settings

Ellen Carr, RN, MSN, AOCN

I. Decision-making regarding care settings.
   A. Decision makers vary.
      1. Client and family decisions affected by:
         a. Health care coverage.
         b. Treatment modality.
         c. Plan of care.
      2. Members of the health care team collaborate and consult in areas of expertise.
         a. Physician—diagnosis, treatment, follow-up of disease; disease progression; iatrogenic responses; complications; side effects.
         b. Nurse—diagnosis and treatment of human responses to actual or potential health problems; education; resource development; coordination of care (between primary in-hospital and office or home health nurses).
         c. Case manager and/or discharge planner—coordination of care, especially focused on client's health care coverage and benefits.
         d. Social worker—evaluation of resources; discharge planning; utilization review; family support; coordination of outpatient care and equipment.
         e. Pharmacist, radiation technologist—provide treatment product (e.g., chemotherapy, radiation treatment).
         f. Dietitian—diet education; diet enhancement.
         g. Chaplain/minister—spiritual care; community support.
         h. Rehabilitation specialist—coordinates care of client after treatment course completed.
      3. Client/family treated as unit of care—encouraged to remain autonomous, independent, and interdependent in making decisions.
         a. Choices in care settings are more and more limited because of the need to make care delivery cost-effective.
   B. Decision-making process should be flexible.
      1. Collaboration facilitates comprehensive approach.
         a. Health care team is adjunctive to the primary care provider.
         b. Client and family are included in care planning.

2. Ongoing—revised as changes occur and needs arise.
3. Proactive—includes anticipated needs of client/family; is sensitive, creative, and adapted to changing needs of clients/families within rapidly changing inpatient or community health care systems.
C. Decision-making process is systematic, involving:
  1. Data collection.
    a. Assessment of client needs.
      (1) Begins with the presenting problem of the client in any setting.
      (2) Includes (but is not limited to) physiologic needs (disease state, treatment demands, symptom management) stated in the Oncology Nursing Society (ONS) Practice Standards.
        (a) Prevention and early detection.
        (b) Current knowledge and information needs.
        (c) Coping strategies affecting health.
        (d) Comfort/discomfort and management.
        (e) Current nutritional status.
        (f) Functioning of protective mechanisms.
        (g) Level of mobility.
        (h) Elimination patterns (past/present).
        (i) Sexual patterns and current functioning.
        (j) Ventilation/current respiratory status.
        (k) Circulation (adequate tissue perfusion).
      (3) Encompasses social needs (relating to family and community—including coping with the disease and physical changes).
      (4) Includes emotional and spiritual needs (dealing with sense of self and meaning of cancer experience).
      (5) Involves determination of socioeconomic and vocational needs (work and financial responsibilities).
    b. Assessment of family and/or significant other's needs.
      (1) Elicit past experiences with illness.
      (2) Assess strengths gained from past illnesses.
      (3) Assess unresolved losses or maladaptive responses to previous losses.
      (4) Determine meaning of cancer and treatment for client and family members.
      (5) Explore ways that family may participate in therapy.
      (6) Identify any sense of loss or fears family may be experiencing (e.g., client suffering, anticipated role changes, fear of unknown, difficulty getting information).
      (7) Evaluate family composition, roles, availability for care.
    c. Assessment of care setting.
      (1) Determine source of health care insurance coverage; establish the impact of client's coverage on treatment plan and care setting.
      (2) Determine options of care setting.
      (3) Evaluate adequacy in meeting the needs of the client/family.
      (4) Identify the primary care provider.
      (5) Verify availability of appropriate support persons, equipment, medications, and resources.
      (6) Determine accountability for ongoing assessment or care and follow-up.

(7) Consider home the preferred setting whenever possible.

(8) Begin discharge planning and/or follow-up with client/family upon diagnosis or admission to care setting or physician's service.

  d. Additional assessment concerns (after treatment plan and health insurance plan established).

(1) Determine client/family eligibility for resources from community agencies.

(2) Assess availability of resource people, supportive services, and health delivery agencies within the community and beyond (call local American Cancer Society [ACS] or develop a catalogue of resources).

(3) Evaluate services, criteria for admission, costs, and goals.

(4) Assess client's/family's usual resources for skills, services, and funds.

(5) Develop a database for referral (National Cancer Institute [NCI], university hospitals) when access to care is limited within home community.

  2. Evaluation of alternatives.

    a. Assessment of perceived obstacles to selecting an appropriate care setting.

(1) Change in socioeconomic status (e.g., loss of job, decreased income).

(2) Insurance coverage: limits and allowances.

(3) Disagreement among client/family and health care providers about choice of care setting.

    b. Weight of relative benefits among alternative settings.

D. Consider special care issues affecting the selection.

  1. Persons with human immunodeficiency virus (HIV)-related illnesses.

  2. Socioeconomically disadvantaged populations.

  3. Ethnic minorities.

  4. The elderly.

  5. Persons undergoing nontraditional therapies or early-phase research protocols.

  6. Treatment using radioisotopes or radioactive implants.

  7. Bone marrow and peripheral stem cell transplantation—preoperative and postoperative care, insurance coverage.

  8. Terminally ill children.

  9. Families geographically distant or psychologically impaired.

  10. Families culturally different from the mainstream.

  11. Illiteracy and patient education issues.

  12. The following is an example of consideration of special care needs of the client with HIV-related illnesses.

    a. Confronting the care needs of persons with HIV-related illnesses has become a tremendous challenge to nursing today.

(1) Reminiscent of the cancer problem 20 to 30 years ago.

(2) Services and therapy for persons with cancer have improved over the last several years, which can in turn have a positive effect on the care environments of persons with HIV-related illnesses.

    b. Caring for persons with HIV-related illnesses involves four areas of concern: occupational risks, infection control, professional competence, and reexamination of personal values and prejudices.

(1) With appropriate education and support, all health care professionals can safely assume responsibility for care of persons with HIV-related illnesses.

        (2) Given experience with immunocompromised patients, oncology nurses are especially well prepared to care for these patients.

        (3) The oncology unit may be the setting of choice for inpatient care of same.

    c. With incorporation of universal blood/body fluid precautions (Center for Disease Control [CDC] recommendations and guidelines; see Chapter 29), persons with HIV-related diseases and persons immunocompromised because of cancer and cancer therapy can be housed safely on the same unit; in using universal precautions, all clients are treated as potentially infectious, thereby eliminating the need to differentiate HIV-infected persons from others.

    d. Persons with HIV-related disorders often have a clinical disease course of remissions interspersed with acute exacerbations, ending with a variable period of terminal illness. Factors that complicate the choice of care setting include:

        (1) Social isolation and disapproval of lifestyle.

        (2) Nontraditional or limited support systems.

        (3) Limited or expended financial resources.

        (4) High incidence of neuropsychiatric problems.

        (5) Poor prognosis and limited community services.

        (6) Uncertainty, leading to helplessness and hopelessness.

        (7) Need for specialty care (e.g., infectious diseases).

    e. Decentralized and outpatient community liaison services for persons with HIV-related illnesses enhance services available outside metropolitan acquired immunodeficiency syndrome (AIDS) centers.

    f. Persons with HIV-related illnesses receive care in varied settings—hospitals, homes, clinics (general or AIDS/HIV primary care), physicians' offices, schools, public health centers, drug treatment facilities, mental health centers, residential care facilities, nursing homes, hospices, and others.

        (1) Case management and primary care are recommended to promote continuity of care.

        (2) Sensitive, comprehensive approach is warranted for meeting many levels of needs through the disease trajectory.

  E. Care settings to consider in planning and implementation.

    1. Inpatient care.

    2. Ambulatory care.

    3. Home care.

    4. Skilled nursing or subacute care.

    5. Hospice care.

II. Planning care in inpatient settings.

  A. The oncology unit.

    1. Definition—a designated hospital area that facilitates the team approach to comprehensive cancer care by bringing into close proximity personnel and facilities necessary for such care; provides not only for the physical needs of the cancer client, but also for the ongoing emotional, social, and spiritual support of the client and his or her family or significant others.

    2. Inpatient oncology units are primarily concerned with providing care for clients requiring critical care, bone marrow transplant (BMT), or high-dose investigational therapy.

    3. Ideally, the following conditions are required for an oncology unit:

      a. A physical setting with ample room for nurses to work and conduct conferences and for client/family comfort (including private space, kitchen facilities, and sleeping facilities for family).

b. Professional nursing staff to meet the specific needs of cancer clients as determined by a client-classification system (regarding client acuity and nursing hours).

c. Policies and procedures for unit operation using a multidisciplinary treatment approach.

d. A philosophy of nursing that focuses on the client/family unit and incorporates the importance of service, education, and research.

e. A nurturing work environment in which staff is actively supported through:

    (1) Specialty orientation.

    (2) Ongoing staff development.

    (3) Stress management.

    (4) Individualized reward systems.

f. An excellence of practice that is marked by continuous evaluation of quality of care.

4. Advantages of an oncology unit.

a. Specialized needs of persons with catastrophic and sometimes life-threatening diseases addressed by specialty nursing personnel.

b. Technical proficiency combined with sensitivity to cancer as a disease affecting the whole family.

c. "High touch in a high-tech environment."

d. High degree of trust and individual attention of clients/families and nurses well known to each other.

5. Disadvantages of oncology unit: professional burnout—related to the continuous close contact with cancer clients; major factors are:

a. Staffing shortages or skill mix.

b. Frustrating client/family demands.

c. Personal psychological strains.

6. Over the next 10 years, the number of inpatient oncology units is expected to decline by 20 to 30%.

B. The scattered-bed unit.

1. Definition—mixed medical-surgical or nononcology specialty unit in hospitals in which cancer admissions do not justify an organized oncology unit or in which administrative support for such a unit is lacking.

2. Advantages of a scattered-bed unit.

a. Even with a substantial number of cancer admissions, a scattered-bed approach may be considered more cost-effective.

b. Cancer-specific skilled nursing care is still possible with:

    (1) An oncology clinical nurse specialist, oncology nurse educator, or designee to update staff's oncology knowledge base.

    (2) Ongoing continuing education programs specific to the needs of clients with cancer.

    (3) Oncology transition service and case management.

    (4) Collaboration with nurses in oncology office practices.

3. Disadvantages of scattered-bed unit.

a. Difficult to maintain oncology knowledge base of nursing staff and to establish ongoing oncology competency.

b. Continuity of care can suffer; families need special consideration when confronted by different nurses on every hospital admission.

c. Family-centered nursing may not be the orientation of the unit.

d. Subtle changes in client's status may be missed or thought unimpor-

tant because of unfamiliarity with the disease process or client's history.
e. Client education may be more generic rather than individualized or specific to current status or treatment regimen.
III. Planning care in ambulatory settings.
  A. Oncology office or clinic practice setting.
    1. Definition—associated office or clinic practices that may include any or all of the following oncology specialties:
      a. Surgery and gynecology.
      b. Medical oncology (including hematology).
      c. Immunology and infectious diseases.
      d. Pediatric oncology.
      e. Radiation oncology.
      f. Cancer risk assessment, screening, and diagnosis.
      g. Psychosocial oncology.
    2. Often affiliated with regional cancer centers and other large hospitals but also found in smaller communities.
    3. Disease- and treatment-related sequelae monitored frequently to avoid unnecessary discomfort or toxicity.
    4. The role of oncology office or clinic nurse is instrumental in the success of therapy for clients in at least four areas:
      a. Direct care (e.g., chemotherapy, comfort, symptom management).
      b. Information exchange (e.g., education, interpretation of reports).
      c. Client/family support (e.g., support groups, phone follow-up, and counseling).
      d. Coordination of care/case management.
    5. Advantages.
      a. Reimbursement and cost-efficiencies in an outpatient setting fuel growth.
      b. Expert, specialized care.
      c. Hospitalizations minimized, with problems managed in ambulatory setting whenever possible. (1997 estimates: 80–90% of all oncology clients are treated in outpatient setting.)
      d. Accessibility of research programs to enhance treatment options.
      e. Frequently, physician-nurse team assumes primary responsibility for care, adding to trust and confidence of client and family; clients and families are encouraged to call the office to manage symptoms or to clarify instructions.
      f. Less hospital-like setting (e.g., easy chairs, cozy rooms).
    6. Disadvantages.
      a. Professional stress related to:
        (1) High patient volume-to-time ratios.
        (2) Time-consuming functional tasks, including insurance authorizations for client's treatments.
        (3) Inadequate staffing ratios, long hours.
      b. Because of urgency (related to above points), client and family may not feel a part of the treatment-planning process.
      c. Time required for consultation, physician visits, and treatment often frustrating for all involved.
      d. Need for patient education increases, although time and resources to provide patient education can be limited.

B. General/primary practice setting.
   1. Definition—client-care system wherein all or most of the problems of the client are managed by one physician or physician group (e.g., general surgeon, family practitioner, internist).
   2. Often, in rural settings with few physicians, the same physician who assessed the initial symptomatology may proceed with surgery and later oversee follow-up.
   3. In more settings with managed care predominating, a primary care physician (gatekeeper) is an integral part of the care team; the primary care physician may consult with specialists but retain primary responsibility for workup and management of presumed malignancy.
   4. Requires that office or clinic staff (physician and nurse) be both generalist and specialist.
   5. Advantages.
      a. Allows client to remain in home community to receive therapy.
      b. High level of trust and commitment already established between client/family and physician/nurse.
   6. Disadvantages.
      a. Tremendous challenge to physician and nurse to provide optimal cancer-related care, depending on resources such as:
         (1) Professional cancer journals and textbooks.
         (2) Affiliation with cancer centers and organizations.
         (3) Regional or national specialty seminars or inservices.
         (4) Teleconferencing.
      b. Lack of case volume to develop expertise in managing more obscure diagnoses or complications or to participate in clinical trials.
      c. Ethical dilemma of whether client is receiving optimal care.
C. Employee health service.
   1. Definition—personnel assistance program providing routine examinations, follow-up laboratory studies, and even chemotherapy in the workplace as incentive to clients to remain actively involved in the workforce.
   2. Advantages.
      a. Cost-effective and time-efficient to employer and employee.
      b. Especially important to persons who are presently cancer free but have some risks.
         (1) Several years after diagnosis and/or treatment.
         (2) No longer under the supervision of an oncologist.
         (3) Cancer prone—strong family history of cancer or lifestyle promoting cancer risk (e.g., smoking, obesity, alcoholism).
      c. Can be instrumental in enhancing health promotion activities or lifestyle changes because of employer support.
   3. Disadvantages.
      a. Workup may not be comprehensive.
      b. Physician-nurse team may not be current on cancer-related symptomatology or even risk factor management.
      c. Focus is returning employee to workforce; therefore, some complaints may not be evaluated thoroughly.
      d. Very dependent on the employer health belief system and on-site health benefits provided; varies among employers.
IV. Planning care for home settings.
   A. Home nursing agencies and home health care agencies.
      1. Definition—according to the Department of Health and Human Services, home health care is "that component of a continuum of compre-

hensive health care whereby health services are provided to individuals and families in their places of residence for the purpose of promoting, maintaining or restoring health, or of maximizing the level of independence, while minimizing the effects of disability and illness, including terminal illness."
2. Home health agencies provide assistance by:
   a. Providing treatment and/or monitoring activity.
   b. Dealing with client problems such as symptom distress (e.g., pain, nausea, pressure sores), poor nutrition, elimination disturbances, fatigue, emotional strain, high technology equipment.
   c. Engaging other family or community members to assist in client care, thereby extending the stay at home.
   d. Offering respite for primary care providers to support the client's choice to stay in the home.
   e. Cooperating as partners with client's primary physician-nurse team in providing comprehensive care.
3. The client may contract with home health agency for varied services from care providers, including:
   a. Home care nurses and home health aides.
   b. Social workers and chaplains.
   c. Physical and occupational therapists.
   d. Pharmacists and medical equipment vendors.
   e. Respiratory therapists.
   f. Dietitians.
   g. Home maintenance.
   h. Speech and language therapists.
   i. Other services.
4. High-acuity support services, available through home care, are options for clients who have an ongoing need for:
   a. Intravenous (IV) therapy and/or parenteral nutrition.
   b. Chemotherapy (IV, arterial infusion pump, intrathecal, peritoneal).
   c. Antibiotic therapy.
   d. Analgesic infusion pump therapy.
   e. Specimen sampling for laboratory studies.
5. Caregiver support.
   a. Sensitivity toward, and support of, the caregiver is essential.
   b. Need exists for continual assessment of options available to:
      (1) Support care in the home (usually client's choice).
      (2) Build family confidence and expertise.
      (3) Allay anxieties while offering services and resources.
      (4) Maintain communication and documentation when patient is transferred (e.g., to day care, ICU).
6. Advantages of the home care setting.
   a. High level of care in the comfort of home; all other care settings coordinate with home care.
   b. Increased self-sufficiency of client/family unit; home is client's natural social environment.
   c. Reduction in frequency and number of hospitalizations.
   d. Reduction in the incidence of infections (especially pulmonary).
   e. Prevention and/or recognition of potentially life-threatening complications and implementation of appropriate actions by home care team.

      f. Restoration and maintenance of optimal performance of activities of daily living.

      g. Promotion of compliance with the medical regimen.

    7. Disadvantages of the home care setting.

      a. Occasional conflicting goals among client/family members (e.g., client wants to stay in home; family prefers the security of institutional care).

      b. High level of stress for home care provider.

        (1) In some cases, clients/families may have the option of institutional care over home if a feeling of burden or inability to provide client comfort or safety exists.

        (2) Home care provider maintains major role as first-line observer of changes in client's health and comfort status, which may be anxiety-provoking and difficult to continue over time. With increased patient acuity comes increased stress for the care provider.

        (3) Home care provider must contend with multiple roles, requiring new skills and the need to delegate tasks (which may be difficult).

      c. Burnout of home care provider—requires respite intervention (either institutional care or recruiting helpers).

      d. Home care services may not be covered financially. Reimbursement may be complicated.

V. Planning care in nursing home, subacute, or residential settings (also called "skilled nursing").

  A. Definition—according to the Social Security Act, "posthospital extended care for continuation of necessary medical treatment in an institution that provides a level of care distinguished from the intensive care ordinarily furnished by a hospital," including either:

    1. Licensed (RN, LVN, LPN) nursing services.

    2. Intermediate care (health services for persons needing institutional care but not skilled nursing).

  B. Occasionally clients or families initiate hospitalization and/or skilled nursing placement in response to a home care crisis; these admissions may be painful if seen by families as a failure to meet the client's needs at home.

  C. If the client and family still prefer home care, that option should be restored if at all possible; temporary or permanent skilled nursing placement may be considered as an alternative if other resource avenues have been exhausted.

  D. Advantages of skilled nursing facility placement.

    1. A care option for clients who no longer require hospitalization but do not have the resources needed at home or an available home care provider.

    2. An opportunity for respite for the primary caregiver at home even when home nursing support is available but not adequate at present for a caregiver under stress.

    3. For elderly clients, specialty care geared toward needs and concerns of senior adults.

  E. Disadvantages of skilled nursing facility placement.

    1. Stigma attached by many clients/families and rejection of care option by same.

2. Client-staff ratios and staffing composition that differ from those of hospital to facility (possible disruptions in care).
3. Philosophies of care (i.e., pain management protocols) may differ, thereby affecting continuity of care.
4. Complications of cancer therapies, as well as symptom management, may not be familiar to skilled facility staff; thus, detection and intervention may differ.
5. Accountability issue (who will assume primary care responsibility).

VI. Planning for hospice care. (See also Chapter 7.)
   A. Hospice care.
      1. Definition—specialized, holistic, and multidisciplinary care that provides support and assistance to clients with a terminal illness and their families.
      2. A concept or philosophy of care that concentrates on rehumanizing the experience of dying and joins sophisticated methods of pain and symptom control and sensitive, respectful, noninvasive caring; with hospice support, clients who choose to die at home usually can.
      3. On November 1, 1983, legislation provided funding for certified hospices to care for Medicare-eligible clients. Legislation encouraged other third-party payors to provide a hospice benefit.
      4. Hospices provide many rewards for nurses, yet the care is demanding and support services are needed to alleviate stress and prevent burnout.
   B. Types of hospice care settings and approaches.
      1. Community-based program.
         a. No facility other than an office.
         b. A multidisciplinary team.
         c. Home care is the focus; goal is to provide comfort, autonomy, and emotional and physical support to the client/family.
         d. Clients may continue in cancer therapy.
         e. Hospice team collaborates with cancer treatment team to provide optimal cross-coverage and continuity of care.
      2. Inpatient-based program.
         a. May be an inpatient program and/or inpatient-based home care program.
         b. Inpatient program allows, for example, for hospital admission for respite care or new pain management protocol.
         c. Inpatient-based home care program may have partial or full hospital backing from a hospice interdisciplinary team or consultants from various departments.
      3. Inpatient-based hospice team.
         a. May also be called the palliative care team.
         b. Clients are received through in-hospital referral or consultation.
         c. The team physician may become the client's primary physician or the referring physician may remain, working in concert with the hospice team.
         d. Inpatient beds may be allocated for hospice care or clients may be seen throughout the hospital.
         e. The hospice team makes rounds each day, making recommendations as needed.
      4. Freestanding hospice.
         a. A freestanding facility, usually with a home care program.
         b. If unable to maintain care in the home, the client or family may elect admission to the hospice facility.

        c. Hospice care is uninterrupted because the same team members facilitate transition between home and hospice facility.

        d. Cancer therapy usually has been discontinued, and the primary physician may have relinquished all care responsibility to the hospice physician.

  C. Advantages of the hospice care setting (also criteria for hospice care).

    1. The client and family comprise the unit of care.

    2. Care includes around-the-clock care commitment (staff available on premises or are on call 24 hours per day).

    3. Care is focused.

    4. Communication is facilitated by interdisciplinary team planning and family input.

    5. Volunteers are recruited actively and used as members of care team.

    6. A physician is an integral part of the team, usually as the medical director.

    7. Accepting and nonjudgmental attitudes persist among members of the care team.

    8. Pain or symptom control is highly emphasized, but commitment also is made to psychosocial, emotional, and spiritual needs of client and family.

    9. Hospice care continues with the family after the client's death through bereavement follow-up.

   10. Care minimizes trips to physician office, inpatient facilities.

  D. Disadvantages of hospice care setting and approach.

    1. Hospice programs vary widely from community to community; client and family must assess services available to them.

    2. Stigma is associated with hospice for some who focus on the terminal care component of program.

    3. Stress level is high for staff and primary caregiver during the time when the client's condition deteriorates; support for both hospice staff and family is essential.

VII. Trends in cancer care related to settings.

  A. Cost-effective care delivery—provided safely and optimized by technology (e.g., treatments, IV access, monitoring systems).

  B. Ambulatory care settings are becoming the treatment site choice of clients; care planning is more proactive than reactive, exploring creative means of delivering care to clients who prefer the comfort of home.

    1. The phone is a vital link in ambulatory care, and nurses in all settings can optimize care through phone triage.

    2. Phone conversations between client/family and nurse promote early problem-solving and curtail complications.

    3. Documentation of problems and nursing actions promotes continuity and legal record of practice.

  C. Alliances among all health care providers (acute, subacute, outpatient, hospice, others).

    1. Continuity of care is focus of processes and systems.

    2. According to Beddar and Aikin, key components of continuity of care are:

        a. Interdisciplinary approach to care.

        b. Comprehensive client and family assessment for needs and strengths.

      c. Client and family education and decision-making.
      d. Development of measurable goals and care plans.
      e. Identification of supplemental resources.
      f. Integrated care through transitions.
      g. Evaluation.
   3. Communication, collaboration, and documentation are essential elements of health care delivery.
   4. Technology (computers, faxes, other devices) reduce administrative inefficiencies.
  D. Because clients and families are voicing concerns and preferences in cancer care, health care providers are responding.
   1. Task forces, comprised of professionals and community representatives, can help in establishing programs focused on the client and family.
   2. Support groups, first started by clients, are available (e.g., Reach to Recovery, United Ostomy Association).
  E. Hospice care has become a model for holistic care.
   1. Hospice philosophy has influenced caregivers at stages of the life cycle other than dying.
   2. Models for multidisciplinary care that support a continuum of physical, psychosocial, and spiritual need have been developed.
  F. Primary nursing has become a model of care that:
   1. Promotes continuity and quality of care through 24-hour accountability.
   2. May be implemented best through nurse-physician teams.
   3. In oncology nursing, allows the primary nurse to be a clinician, teacher, care manager, consultant, and/or researcher.
   4. May not always be possible, due to licensed personnel cutbacks (i.e., decreased full time equivalents [FTEs]).
  G. Qualified nurses are practicing independently.
   1. In a joint or collaborative practice in which the care of a client population is shared with a physician and other health care professionals.
   2. In a direct contract with clients and families.
      a. The client or family may request education or a specific service.
      b. The nurse may provide a wide range of services as defined by the nurse practice act of the respective state; service may include:
         (1) Physical assessment.
         (2) Family and client education.
         (3) Family and client counseling and psychotherapy.
         (4) Coordination of contracted services (social services, nutritional counseling, physical therapy, and home nursing services).
      c. As the case manager, bringing all elements and resources together for better outcomes.
VIII. Cancer rehabilitation—an approach to care across settings. (See also Chapter 8.)
  A. Definition—preventive, restorative, supportive, and palliative activities engaged to improve the quality of life for maximal productivity with minimal dependence, regardless of life expectancy and within the limits imposed by disease and treatment.
  B. More than 50% of clients diagnosed with cancer today will be alive in 5 years.
   1. Cancer rehabilitation begins at the time of diagnosis.
      a. From diagnosis, cancer clients should be considered survivors, not victims.

        b. This perception and commitment to wellness and healing influence quality of life.

   2. Cancer can create dependency, and the goal of cancer rehabilitation is to promote independence through the coordinated efforts of the rehabilitation team, including:

        a. Nurses, physicians, case managers.

        b. Occupational, physical, and recreational therapists.

        c. Art and music therapists.

        d. Chaplains, counselors, and social workers.

        e. Appliance fitters.

        f. Speech therapists.

        g. Community liaisons.

        h. Employment counselors.

C. Rehabilitation is a process that must occur in all care settings (Table 47–1).

   1. Prescriptions for rehabilitation can be completed through a hospital, a freestanding cancer facility, or office practices.

   2. The ambulatory care setting can be the most natural and least disruptive for clients and families engaging in a rehabilitation program.

TABLE 47–1. **Rehabilitation Issues Associated With Specific Cancer Sites**

Cancer Site	Rehabilitation Issues
Head and neck cancers	Maintenance of optimal nutrition and deglutition Shoulder dysfunction rehabilitation Neck dysfunction rehabilitation Self-care considerations Speech/communication Restoring acceptable appearance and function
Breast cancer	Physical restoration of affected arm Psychosocial rehabilitation regarding loss, body image alterations, and sexuality Cosmetic rehabilitation with form, prosthesis, or reconstruction
Bone and soft-tissue malignancies	Restore near-normal function through prostheses, appliances, and aids to ambulation Restore acceptable appearance Vocational rehabilitation Psychosocial restoration
Lung cancer	Preoperative rehabilitation emphasizes breathing retraining Pulmonary disability prevention after radiation or surgery
Colorectal and bladder malignancies resulting in ostomies	Self-concept adjustment Elimination control and ostomy adjustment Self-care considerations Psychosocial rehabilitation Effective skin care
Central nervous system	Preventing unnecessary loss of function and diminished quality of life Cognitive function evaluation Mobility modifications Retraining for activities of daily living Bowel and bladder management

Modified from DeLisa, J.A., Miller, R.M., Melnick, R.R., Gerber, L.H., & Hillel, A.B. (1989). Rehabilitation of the cancer patient. In V.T. DeVita, S. Hellman, & S.A. Rosenberg (eds.). *Cancer: Principles and Practice.* Philadelphia: J.B. Lippincott.

D. Clients and families also seek rehabilitation services through self-help and other support services.
   1. I Can Cope—an educational program sponsored by the ACS.
   2. We Can Weekend—a guided family experience with individual and group activities geared toward enhancing family communication and coping with cancer.
   3. WIN—a unique physical conditioning and rehabilitation program for women cancer survivors (similar to Outward Bound).
   4. National Coalition for Cancer Survivorship—a network of independent organizations and individuals working in cancer survivorship and support to generate a nationwide awareness of survivorship as a vibrant productive life after the diagnosis of cancer.
      a. Cancer survivors speak on their own behalf to address educational, employment, and social needs.
      b. The focus is health enhancement, risk prevention, and promotion of care settings committed to careful follow-up and support of health-protective activities.
         (1) Y-Me: National Organization for Breast Cancer Information and Support, Inc.
         (2) Look Good, Feel Better: Joint venture of ACS and Cosmetic, Toiletry, and Fragrance Association.
         (3) Reach to Recovery: Support effort, providing emotional and practical information to women with breast cancer.
         (4) International Association of Laryngectomees: Support and education for laryngectomy clients.
E. In some communities, comprehensive cancer rehabilitation services may be minimal; reasons for the deficit may include:
   1. A persistent and common view that cancer is a terminal rather than a curable or chronic illness.
   2. Lack of third-party reimbursement for such services.
   3. Perceived hierarchy of needs for limited services in which resources are concentrated on acute care versus rehabilitation.
   4. Lack of awareness of rehabilitative needs and demands by the public for services.
F. Improved diagnostic and treatment regimens have resulted in longer and healthier lives among individuals with cancer and have made cancer rehabilitation an integral part of the treatment plan.
IX. Evaluation of desired outcomes.
A. Clients and families report the availability of professional assistance needed to:
   1. Seek a health restorative process.
   2. Maintain an adapted health status.
   3. Cope with an end-stage or a terminal phase of cancer.
B. Nurses actively assess services available in the community and identify areas that need enhancement.
C. Nursing research supports changes in care delivery.
   1. Nurses collaborate with physicians and other colleagues to identify gaps in care.
   2. Nurses use research to validate clinical assumptions about nursing needs of clients with cancer. Four needs with respect to cancer nursing have been identified:

       a. 24-hour accessibility and availability.

       b. Effective communication skills.

       c. Accepting and nonjudgmental attitudes.

       d. Practitioner competence.

    3. Nurses secure financial support for research through pharmaceutical companies, the ACS, and cancer nursing organizations.

D. Initial treatment services support continuity of care through:

    1. Interdisciplinary communication between the client, family, and treatment team and involvement in decision-making related to therapeutic modalities.

    2. Early discharge planning and follow-up care.

E. Transition services are available to coordinate care between inpatient and outpatient settings to enhance ease of setting change and accessibility.

    1. Types of available assistance include hospital services under titles such as "Continuity of Care" or "Managed Care," nursing agencies, physicians' offices, employee health departments, and liaison personnel.

    2. The nurse in transition services:

       a. Supports the client and family as educator and advocate.

       b. Provides a communication link between client/family and the community health care system.

       c. Facilitates personalized, cost-effective care planning and comfort for the client, family, and public.

F. Support services are available for the dying client and primary caregiver.

    1. Respite care, support groups, use of volunteers, and appropriate staffing and coverage are facilitated in community oncology care services.

    2. An option for home death within personal surroundings with family members present is valued and supported in the community.

G. Oncology nurses manifest active involvement in the challenge of maintaining quality care to increasing numbers of ill clients in all health care settings.

BIBLIOGRAPHY

Alkire, K., & Shelton, B.K. (1994). Creating critical care oncology beds. *Semin Oncol Nurs 10*(3), 208–221.

Baldwin, P.D. (1994). Caring of the indigent patient: Resources to improve care. *Semin Oncol Nurs 10*(2), 130–138.

Beddar, S.M., & Aikin, J.L. (1994). Continuity of care: A challenge for ambulatory oncology nursing. *Semin Oncol Nurs 10*(4), 254–263.

Berry, D.E., Boughton, L., & McNamee, F. (1994). Patient and physician characteristics affecting the choice of home based hospice, acute care inpatient hospice facility, or hospitals as last site of care for patients with cancer of the lung. *Hosp J 9*(4), 21–38.

Boyle, D.M. (1994). New identities: The changing profile of patients with cancer, their families and their professional caregivers. *Oncol Nurs Forum 21*(1), 55–61.

Cooley, M.E., Lin, E.M., & Hunter, S.W. (1994). The ambulatory oncology nurse's role. *Semin Oncol Nurs 10*(4), 245–253.

Dudgeon, D.J., Raubertas, R.F., Doerner, K., et al. (1995). When does palliative care begin? A needs assessment of cancer patients with recurrent disease. *J Palliat Care 11*(1), 5–9.

Evangelista, M. (1995). Critical path network. Transferable pathway benefits hospital, hospice. *Hosp Case Manage 3*(5), 75–78.

Harvey, C. (1994). New systems: The restructuring of cancer care delivery and economics. *Oncol Nurs Forum 21*(1), 72–77.

Hoyer, K. (1994). Collaboration between institutions improves patient care. *Oncol Nurs Forum 21*(7), 1249.

Lamkin, L. (1994). Outpatient oncology settings: A variety of services. *Semin Oncol Nurs 19*(4), 229–236.

Otte, D. (1993). Ambulatory care. In S.L. Groenwald, M.H. Frogge, M. Goodman, C.H. Yarbro (eds.). *Cancer Nursing: Principles and Practice* (3rd ed.). Boston: Jones & Barlett, pp. 1371–1402.

Porter, H. (1993). Part 1, The effect of ambulatory oncology nursing practice models on health resource utilization; Part 2, Different practice models—different use of health resources? *J Nurs Adm* 25(2), 15–22.

Shelton, B. (1994). Cancer critical care: Past, present and future. *Semin Oncol Nurs 10*(3), 146–155.

Stephens Mills, D. (1992). Changes in oncology health care settings. In J. Clark, & R. McGee (eds.). *Core Curriculum for Oncology Nursing* (2nd ed.). Philadelphia: W.B. Saunders, pp. 205–220.

Varricchio, C. (1994). Human and indirect costs of home care . . . for cancer patients. *Nurs Outlook 42*(4), 151–157.

Walter, J. (1994). Nursing care delivery models in ambulatory oncology. *Semin Oncol Nurs 10*(4), 237–244.

48

Professional Issues in Cancer Care

Coni Ellis, RN, MS, OCN, C, CETN, CS

Professional Development

I. Professional mandates related to professional development.
   A. American Nurses' Association (ANA)/Oncology Nursing Society (ONS) Standards of Oncology Nursing Practice, Standards of Professional Performance:
      1. Standard III: Education—the oncology nurse acquires and maintains current knowledge in oncology nursing practice.
      2. Standard IV: Collegiality—the oncology nurse contributes to the professional development of peers, colleagues, and others.
   B. ONS Standards of Oncology Nursing Education: Generalist and Advanced Practice levels.
      1. Standard V: learner—the oncology nurse generalist:
         a. Assumes responsibility for personal professional development in oncology nursing.
         b. Contributes to the professional growth of others.
      2. Standard V: learner—the advanced practice oncology nurse:
         a. Assumes responsibility for personal professional development.
         b. Contributes to the development of nursing theory, research, and practice.
         c. Disseminates nursing knowledge.
   C. Joint Commission of Accreditation of Healthcare Organizations (JCAHO).
      1. Nursing care chapter from the 1991 Accreditation Manual for Hospitals, Standard NC 2: all members of the nursing staff are competent to fulfill their assigned responsibilities.
         a. Required characteristic NC 2.1: each member of the nursing staff is assigned clinical and/or managerial responsibilities based on educational preparation, applicable licensing laws and regulations, and assessment of current competence.
         b. Required characteristic NC 2.3: nursing staff members participate in orientation, regularly scheduled staff meetings, and ongoing education designed to improve their competence.
II. Professional development strategies.
   A. Identification of professional development needs.
      1. Conduct self-assessment of learning needs; differentiate between "real educational needs," wherein there is a lack of specific understanding,

skills, or attitudes, and "felt" needs—needs that are perceived by the learner. (These provide the greatest motivation for learning.)

2. Determine priorities and establish goals.
3. Assess personal resources.
4. Initiate independent learning activities (e.g., reading professional literature, participating in professional organizations, identifying resource staff, participating in professional support groups, joining clubs and study groups, and using self-directed learning modules).
5. Participate in continuing education activities.
6. Seek experience to develop and maintain clinical skills.
7. Maintain an awareness of personal beliefs, values, biases, and traditions that influence client care.

B. Professional certification.
1. Certification acknowledges nurses' additional education or experience.
2. Rationale for certification—enables a profession to define and articulate for its members the new knowledge required for practice.
3. Rationale for recertification—enables a profession to validate the competency changes over time as knowledge and technology changes.

C. Continued professional competency—the National Council of State Boards of Nursing, Inc., in studying competency from several aspects (entry level, reentry level for either disciplinary reasons or personal choice, and renewal) has identified six methods to ensure continued competency*:
1. Peer review.
2. Continuing education.
3. Client review.
4. Periodic refresher courses.
5. Competency examinations.
6. Minimal practice requirements.

III. Outcomes of professional development.
A. Enhancement of the development of the profession.
B. Beneficial to individual professional.
C. Beneficial to recipients of care.
D. Fulfillment of the characteristics of a profession.
1. Specialized knowledge—profession is based on specialized knowledge that is passed to new practitioners through education and demonstration.
2. Commitment—implies career orientation; concerned not only with present work performance but also with improving standards and the status of the profession.
3. Vital service—provides a service of critical importance to society.
4. Autonomy—self-regulating or self-governing; responsible for developing standards that govern practice and performance; accountable.
5. Authority—the power to act independently because of competency.

IV. Ten major forecasts for cancer in the 21st century will affect professional development and survival of oncology nurses.
A. Client and family profile—tomorrow's consumers of cancer care will be dramatically different from those of today, predominated by people of advanced age and diverse ethnic backgrounds, by people living in poverty, and by those willing to assume a greater role in health care–related decision-making.

---

* Sheets, V. Personal communication, April 16, 1996.

B. Social support—social support dilemmas will be addressed by family mobilization and by unique intervention programs.
C. Oncology nurse profiles—new "hybrids" of oncology nurses will emerge, evidenced by where and how they practice.
D. Client subgroups—cancer prevention, diagnosis, treatment, and follow-up or survivorship will be customized for, and targeted to, select client subgroups.
E. Therapeutic paradigm—cancer management will be characterized by rapid technology transfer, emphasis on prevention, and aggressive multimodality treatment.
F. Mind-body renaissance—the "self-care movement" will drive a reintegration of a holistic healing and recovery orientation into cancer care.
G. Influence of ethics—ethical responsibilities will become an accentuated component of oncology nursing.
H. Cancer care economics—the hallmarks of cancer care economics will be universal access, fewer payors, rationing of care, and salaried professionals.
I. Practice setting—team-directed cancer care will be delivered in multiple community-based sites.
J. Language reorientation—cancer care will be articulated through novel communication technologies and governed intensively by quality and cost outcomes.
V. Five goals of transformational leadership agenda for oncology nurses as they plan for the future and foster innovation.
A. Develop a transformational consciousness—encourage fundamental shifts in work ethics, designs, and outcomes.
B. Reconfigure the system—understand that viability is influenced by questioning and challenging evolving service demands.
C. Manage complexity—creatively address technology's demands and its application to life's myriad experiences.
D. Focus on relationships—foster nurses "owning" their practice settings and recognize the value of knowledge—workers within the system.
E. Build coalitions and networks—acknowledge the power of dynamic, synergistic, collaborative interactions.

Multidisciplinary Collaboration

I. Professional mandates related to multidisciplinary collaboration.
A. ANA/ONS Standards of Oncology Nursing Practice, Standards of Professional Performance, Standard VI: Collaboration—the oncology nurse collaborates with the client, significant others, and multidisciplinary cancer care team in providing client care.
1. Rationale: the complexity of oncology care requires coordinated, ongoing interaction among the client, significant others, and the multidisciplinary cancer care team. Through the collaborative process, health care providers use their diverse abilities to assess, plan, implement, and evaluate oncology care.
2. The oncology nurse collaborates with the client, significant others, and multidisciplinary cancer care team to formulate desired outcomes of care, the treatment plan, an evaluation of quality of care, and other decisions related to client care, and nursing's role in the delivery of oncology services when possible.

3. The oncology nurse consults with other health care providers and makes appropriate referrals, including provisions for continuity of care, such as rehabilitation, home care, and hospice, as appropriate.
4. The oncology nurse collaborates with other health care providers in educational programs, consultation, management, and research endeavors as opportunities arise.

B. ONS Standards of Oncology Nursing Education: Generalist and Advanced Practice Levels.
1. Standard V: learner—oncology nurse generalist—collaborates with the multidisciplinary team to assess, plan, implement, and evaluate across all levels of health care need.
2. Standard V: learner—advanced practice oncology nurse—initiates collaboration with individuals and groups to minimize cancer risks and to promote health.

C. Joint Commission of Accreditation of Health Care Organizations: nursing staff members collaborate, as appropriate, with physicians and other clinical disciplines in making decisions regarding each client's need for nursing care.

D. Five essential factors of National Joint Practice Commission Model for collaborative practice between nurses and physicians.
1. Communication.
2. Competence.
3. Accountability.
4. Trust.
5. Administrative support.

E. Association of Community Cancer Centers (ACCC), Standard 1: there is a multidisciplinary team approach to planning, implementing, and evaluating the care of cancer clients and families.

F. ANA Nursing, A Social Policy Statement: collaboration among health care professionals involves recognition of the expertise of others within and outside of one's (nursing) profession and referral to those providers when appropriate collaboration also involves some shared functions and a common focus on the same overall mission.

G. Society: society's emphasis on health care requires health care planning rather than fragmentation into disciplines such as medical care, nursing care, physical therapy services; the very nature of health care mandates involvement of more than a single health care provider.

II. Types of working relationships.
A. Slave-master relationships—person with power gives a command that another individual obeys; assumes that the responding individual has little knowledge, few skills, and little or no judgment or initiative.
B. Detente—recognized power among individuals; a recognition and acceptance of separate spheres of activity and responsibility; mutuality of interests and commonality of goals.
C. Collaboration—a true partnership in which the power on both sides is valued by both, with recognition and acceptance of separate and combined spheres of activity and responsibility, mutual safeguarding of the legitimate interests of each party, commonality of goals that is recognized by both parties; individuals in a true partnership believe that collaboration provides synergism of talents and efforts.

III. Barriers to the development of collaborative relationships.
A. Lack of identification with one's own profession.
B. Tendency to regard professional expertise as bias.
C. Discomfort with responsibility.

       D. Felt discrimination in relationships.

       E. Failure of others to value one's profession.

       F. Competency inconsistencies within one's profession because of lack of uniform preparation.

       G. Lack of clearly defined, distinct domain of influence.

       H. Lack of understanding for another's perception.

       I. Overlapping and changing domains of practice that produce competition.

       J. Perceived threats to autonomy.

       K. Lack of administrative support for collaborative relationships.

       L. Lack of recognition for knowledge and expertise.

       M. Role confusion (role extension versus role expansion) within or among professions.

IV. Opportunities for collaboration.

       A. Potential for collaboration among health care providers/agencies exists wherever and with whomever the client and family have contact. Although emphasis is often placed on physician-nurse collaboration, nurses have the potential for collaborative relationships with any member of the multidisciplinary health care team.

       B. Nurse-to-nurse collaboration may be influenced by the following:

          1. Role—clinician, educator, researcher, administrator (clinician-researcher collaboration in the identification of a clinical problem and evaluation of applicable research findings to address the problem; educator-administrator-clinician collaboration in the development, implementation, and evaluation of staff nurse orientation; clinician-administrator-researcher collaboration in the development and testing of a client acuity classification system).

          2. Domain of responsibility such as shift and performance standards (day, evening, and night shift nurses collaborate on developing change-of-shift report guidelines; primary nurse and associate nurse collaborate on the nursing process).

          3. Specialization (collaboration among nurses with a specialty [e.g., oncology, critical care, intraoperative care] in planning for continuity of care for the client diagnosed with lung cancer undergoing a thoracotomy).

          4. Subspecialization (collaboration among nurses with a subspecialty [e.g., medical oncology, surgical oncology, radiation oncology, biotherapy] in the development of a cancer care orientation packet for clients and families).

          5. Practice setting—acute care, outpatient, home care and hospice, ambulatory cancer treatment center, community hospital, rural community (collaboration among nurses from a variety of practice settings to develop a chronic pain protocol).

       C. Collaborative relationships may extend beyond direct care health care providers to members of voluntary agencies and organizations (e.g., nurse, Leukemia Society volunteer, and client collaborate in the development and implementation of a client and family support group).

       D. The future of oncology nurses is dependent on critical collaborative partnerships being formed within clinical practice arenas as well as the different roles in which the nurse may practice. For the first time, forming collaborative partnerships with industry will be a high priority (Fig. 48–1).

V. Benefits of collaborative relationships.

       A. Maximizes the unique skills of each person.

       B. Assumes shared responsibility.

       C. Delineates shared and individual responsibilities and accountability.

       D. Expedites planned action.

EDUCATION

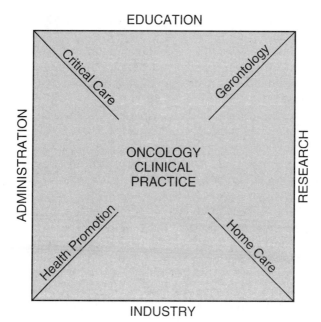

Figure 48–1. Collaborative partnerships critical to survival in 2000 and beyond.

E. Enhances communication.
F. Creates and modifies norms.
G. Facilitates role clarification by revealing the uniqueness of each professional domain.
H. Benefits recipients of service.

Research

I. Professional mandates related to research.
   A. ANA/ONS Standards of Oncology Nursing Practice, Standards of Professional Performance, Standard VII—Research—the oncology nurse contributes to the scientific base of nursing practice and the field of oncology through the review and application of research.
   B. ONS Standards of Oncology Nursing Education: Generalist and Advanced Practice Levels.
      1. Oncology Nurse Generalist Standard III: the curriculum includes:
         a. Application of research findings to oncology nursing practice.
         b. Delineation of the role of the nurse in cancer care, education, research, and public policy.
      2. Oncology Nurse Generalist Standard V: learner—oncology nurse generalist participates in oncology nursing research problem identification, implementation, and/or application to cancer care.
      3. Advanced Practice Standard III: the curriculum includes:
         a. Application of theories and research to the practice of oncology nursing at the advanced practice level.
         b. Opportunities to develop skills as a consumer of research and a beginning researcher.

    4. Advanced Practice Standard V: learner—the advanced level oncology nurse:

      a. Applies the scientific method to initiate, evaluate, and apply nursing research within the scope of advanced practice.

      b. Contributes to the development of nursing theory, research, and practice.

      c. Assumes responsibility for personal professional development.

II. Research roles of nurses by level of education.

  A. ANA Cabinet on Nursing Research developed a hierarchy of research roles based on research preparation by level of education.

  B. Research roles of nurses for the five levels of research preparation include:

    1. Associate degree.

      a. Identify clinical problems.

      b. Assist in data collection.

      c. Collaborate in using research in clinical practice.

    2. Baccalaureate degree.

      a. Evaluate research reports.

      b. Understand ethical principles in research.

      c. Assist investigations in accessing research subjects.

      d. Provide input about data collection methods.

      e. Use research findings in clinical practice.

    3. Master's degree.

      a. Provide clinical expertise for the research process.

      b. Evaluate clinical relevance of research findings.

      c. Ensure integration of research into practice.

      d. Generate a clinical practice environment supportive to conducting research.

    4. Doctorate degree.

      a. Conduct independent investigations in collaboration with other scientists and clinicians.

      b. Acquire external research funding.

      c. Disseminate research findings.

    5. Postdoctoral education—develop research programs.

III. Implementation of the research role of the oncology nurse generalist.

  A. Research role of the oncology nurse generalist includes:

    1. Identification of practice problems through observation of client populations and quality assurance activities; focus of the practice problem may include:

      a. Developing and testing interventions designed to improve client outcomes, such as the ability to perform central venous catheter care after one-to-one teaching compared with the effect of group teaching, or the impact of oral care protocol after the administration of mucosa toxic chemotherapy.

      b. Identifying variables associated with specific client problems or needs, such as pattern of diarrhea and perineal skin breakdown after the administration of high-dose cytosine arabinoside (Ara-C).

      c. Describing the characteristics of a given situation, such as non-nursing tasks assigned to nurses in the outpatient clinic or content of change-of-shift reports.

      d. Testing methods of delivering nursing care, such as time and motion studies of nursing activities to determine whether to administer intra-

venous intermittent antibiotic therapy via intravenous piggyback or multichanneled pumps.
2. Participation in evaluation of existing research.
3. Collaboration in identifying the solution to a clinical problem.
    a. Incorporate applicable research into clinical practice.
    b. Identify the need for research study.
4. Participation in research activities under the guidance of a qualified researcher.
    a. Conceptualization and design of a research study.
        (1) Establish the clinical significance of the problem.
        (2) Identify important clinical variables and client eligibility criteria.
        (3) Assess the feasibility of the methods and procedures proposed for the study.
    b. Implementation of the research protocol.
        (1) Client accrual.
        (2) Implementing physician orders as described in the protocol.
        (3) Observing client responses and toxicities.
        (4) Collecting data.
        (5) Educating the client's caregiver and other health care team members.
5. Participation in clinical trials.
    a. Phase I clinical trials determine the maximal tolerated dose (MTD) and drug toxicities.
    b. Phase II trials focus on the specific tumor types for which the treatment appears promising.
    c. Phase III trials determine:
        (1) The effects of treatment relative to the natural history of the disease.
        (2) Whether a new treatment is as effective as a standard therapy but is associated with less morbidity.
    d. Phase I studies are restricted to National Cancer Institute (NCI)-designated centers; phase II and III studies may be conducted at institutions with cooperative arrangements with NCI-designated centers.
B. Characteristics of employer support of research role of oncology nurse generalist.
    1. Values nursing research as evidenced by:
        a. Inclusion of a research role in job description and performance standards.
        b. Maintenance of a nursing research committee.
    2. Supports research activities with time, money, resources, and recognition.
    3. Provides opportunities for the nurse to participate in research activities.
    4. Values expertise of nurse generalist in identifying research problem.
    5. Provides resource staff to assist the nurse in:
        a. Research critique.
        b. Incorporation of research findings into practice.
        c. Evaluation of outcomes of incorporating research findings into practice.
    6. Research utilization program in place with:
        a. Clinical nursing director.
        b. Nurse researcher to direct program.

      c. Research associates.

      d. Advanced practice nurse role models.

      e. Health sciences library.

      f. Staff nurse participants.

      g. Secretarial and technologic support.

      h. Statistician access.

      i. Scientific manuscript personnel access.

      j. Recognition program.

IV. Guidelines for evaluating research reports.

  A. Areas fundamental to research reports include:

    1. Problem and purpose.

      a. Statement of the research problem includes:

        (1) Generalized discussion of the problem.

        (2) Introduction to the area of study.

        (3) Statement of the importance of the subject.

        (4) Summarization of the related facts and theories.

      b. Statement of the purpose includes:

        (1) Focus of the study.

        (2) Specific variables.

        (3) Data collection methods.

        (4) Setting.

        (5) Nature of the sample.

      c. Statement of the purpose can be written as:

        (1) Question.

        (2) Statement.

        (3) Hypothesis.

    2. Theoretical framework—support of hypothesis, research statement, or question by a clear and concise review of relevant research, literature, and conceptual framework or scientific theory.

    3. Methodology.

      a. Description of how the investigator plans to seek answer to the research question.

      b. Types of research designs—qualitative and quantitative.

        (1) Qualitative research.

          (a) Purpose—to describe and explore phenomena or to gain understanding.

          (b) Characteristics—process focused, subjective, and not generalizable.

          (c) Types—descriptive, surveys, phenomenology, and content analysis.

        (2) Quantitative research.

          (a) Purpose—to describe relationships and cause and effect and to identify facts.

          (b) Characteristics—outcome-focused, objective, generalizable.

          (c) Types—quasi-experimental, experimental, and correlational.

      c. Research design selection depends on:

        (1) Current knowledge about the problem.

        (2) Setting.

        (3) Ethics.

        (4) Skills of the researcher.

        (5) Time.

        (6) Resources (Table 48–1).

        (7) Funding (Table 48–1).

TABLE 48–1. **Research Funding Resources and Agencies**

Bauer, D. (1988). The Computer Grants Sourcebook for Nursing and Health. New York: American Council on Education and MacMillan Publishing.

> Provides profiles on federal, corporate, and foundation support of nursing research activities. For each funding source, author details the following: program title and address, purpose, areas of interest, types of assistance, examples of funding recipients, funding restrictions, financial profile, application process, and review process/selection criteria. Explains preparation of grant applications and provides examples.

Catalogue of Federal Domestic Assistance (CFDA)

> Provides extensive information of federal programs and sources of research funding.

> c/o Superintendent of Documents
> U.S. Government Printing Office
> Washington, DC 20402

Foundation Centers

> Publications provide regional details of the philanthropic industry and support of research. Resource book: Haile, S. (1991). *Foundation Grants to Individuals.* New York: The Foundation Center. ISBN 0-87954-387-6

Northeast	*Midwest*	*East*
Foundation Center	Foundation Center	Foundation Center
79 Fifth Ave. 8th Flr.	Kent H. Smith Library	1001 Connecticut Ave. NW
New York, NY 10003	1422 Euclid Ave.	Washington, DC 20036
(212)620-4230	Cleveland, OH 44115	(202)331-1400
	(216)861-1933	

West	*South*
Foundation Center	Foundation Center
312 Sutter St., Rm. 312	Suite 150
San Francisco, CA 94108	Hurt Building
(415)397-0902	Atlanta, GA 30303
	(404)880-0094

National Institutes of Health (NIH) Guide for Grants and Contracts: NIH home page on World Wide Web (1996) or call for National Center of Nursing Research (NCNR) fact sheet and publication list.

- Contains program announcements and requests for applications detailing specific research areas of interest to NIH institutes, centers and divisions and information on types of award mechanisms and updates on existing programs and policies.
- Explains the types of research and research training supported by the NCNR and the NIH mechanisms available to provide this support.

> Office of Information and Legislative Affairs
> National Center for Nursing Research
> National Institutes of Health
> Building 31, Room 5B13
> Bethesda, MD 20892
> (301)496-0207

- NCNR within the NIH was created in 1986. With the creation of NCNR, many new opportunities exist to obtain funding for nursing research, research training, and career development. Patricia A. Grady, RN, PhD, is the director of NCNR.

> National Center for Nursing Research
> National Institutes of Health/Public Health Service
> Building 31, Room 5B13
> Bethesda, MD 20892
> (301)496-0207

Table continued on following page

TABLE 48–1. **Research Funding Resources and Agencies** *Continued*

Sigma Theta Tau International Honor Society of Nursing

Information and grant applications can be obtained from the following address:

Sigma Theta Tau
Attention: Program Department
550 West North Street
Indianapolis, IN 46202
317-634-8171

American Nurses' Foundation

The American Nurses' Foundation of the American Nurses' Association underwrites 20 grants each year. Information and grant applications can be obtained from the following address:

American Nurses' Foundation
600 Maryland Ave. SW
Suite 100 West
Washington, DC 20024-2571
1-800-284-2378 ext. 7227

Oncology Nursing Society and the Oncology Nursing Foundation Research Grants

Information and grant applications can be obtained from the following address:

Oncology Nursing Society
501 Holiday Drive
Pittsburgh, PA 15220
412-921-7373

American Association for Critical Care Nurses

Information can be obtained from the following address:

American Association for Critical Care Nurses
101 Columbia
Aliso Viejo, CA 92656-1491
(714)644-9310

    d. Description of the sample.
       (1) Method of sample selection.
       (2) Representiveness of sample to larger population.
    e. Methods to collect data.
       (1) Discussion of the data collection instrument(s).
       (2) Rationale for data collection instrument(s) selection.
    f. Instrument(s) development.
       (1) Instrument(s) reliability.
       (2) Instrument(s) validity.
    g. Analysis of the data.
       (1) Description of the sample.
       (2) Description of statistics applied to the data.
       (3) Statistical procedures determined by research question and study design and the level of measurement of the variables.
          (a) Research question.
             (i) Description of phenomena—descriptive statistics such as the frequencies, means, and standard deviation.
             (ii) Prediction of differences and relationships—inferential statistics such as t-test, analysis of variance (ANOVA), or chi square (x^2).

    (b) Level of measurement.
        (i) Application of descriptive or inferential statistics de-
            pends on the types of variables measured—nominal,
            ordinal, interval, or ratio.
        (ii) The higher the level of measurement, the more powerful
            the statistical test applied and the greater the degree
            of certainty that the results are factual rather than
            chance occurrences.
4. Interpretation and conclusions.
    a. Presentation of the findings—discussions of statistically significant
        findings and probable explanation for both significant and nonsig-
        nificant findings.
    b. Conclusion.
        (1) Integration of the research findings with previous literature, re-
            search, and theory.
        (2) Identification of practical and statistical significance.
        (3) Application of findings to nursing practice.
        (4) Suggestions for further research.
B. Questions asked before implementation of research findings into nursing
    practice.
    1. Are the resources and institutional support adequate to implement
        the findings?
    2. Are the results clinically significant?
    3. Can the results be generalized?
    4. Are the implementation strategies discussed by the researcher desirable
        and feasible in practice?
    5. Can the outcome of implementing the findings be measured?
V. In the future, research priorities may stay in the same areas of interest, but
    priority of one over another or the means by which the research is conducted
    may change.
    A. National Center for Nursing Research (1990).
        1. Low birth weight—mothers and infants.
        2. Human immunodeficiency virus (HIV) infection—prevention and care.
        3. Long-term care for older adults.
        4. Symptom management.
        5. Information systems.
        6. Health promotion for children and adolescents.
        7. Technology dependency across the life span.
    B. Research priorities identified by ONS (1991).
        1. Quality of life.
        2. Symptom management.
        3. Pain control and management.
        4. Prevention and early detection.
        5. Cancer rehabilitation.
        6. Economic influence on oncology.
        7. Outcome measures for interventions.
        8. Cancer survivorship.
        9. Cost containment.
        10. Research utilization.

Work-Related Stress

I. Professional mandates related to work-related stress.
    A. ANA/ONS Standards for Oncology Nursing Practice, Standards of Profes-
        sional Performance, Standard III: Education—the oncology nurse acquires
        and maintains current knowledge in oncology nursing practice, and Stan-

dard IV: Collegiality—contributes to the professional development of peers, colleagues, and others.

    1. Structure criteria—a mechanism is in place to provide staff development and continuing education opportunities informing staff about legal aspects of oncology nursing, stress management for oncology nursing, and occupational hazards.

    2. Outcome criteria—the oncology nurse maintains his or her physical, mental, and emotional health.

  B. ONS Standards of Oncology Nursing Education: Generalist and Advanced Practice Levels, Standard V: learner (oncology nurse generalist and advanced practice oncology nurse) practices health behaviors consistent with health promotion as a role model for the public.

II. Stress and burnout concepts.

  A. Definitions of stress.

    1. Stress is necessary for life.

    2. Stress requires or signals that a change is needed: adaptational change—physical, emotional, intellectual, spiritual, intuitive, and social.

    3. Stress involves a transaction between an individual and the environment.

    4. The individual is the focal mediator between the stress stimulus and the response.

    5. Individual judgment and evaluation of the stimulus influence perception of the stimulus and the nature of the response.

    6. Stress is the perceived imbalance between demands and abilities or resources.

  B. Stress becomes problematic when the level of stress exceeds one's ability to respond effectively and when the adaptation becomes growth-inhibiting rather than growth-promoting.

  C. The cost of failing to effectively cope with stress effectively can be high and may include compromised client care, job burnout, and even physical and psychological deterioration.

  D. Professional stress demands adaptation in the performance of one's professional role.

  E. The impact of stress is intensified by:

    1. Suddenness of onset.

    2. Chronicity of stressors.

    3. High degree of intensity.

    4. Significance of the stressor to the individual.

    5. Vulnerability of the individual.

    6. Occurrence of multiple stressors.

  F. Definition of burnout.

    1. Burnout is exhaustion caused by excessive demands on energy, strength, or resources.

    2. Burnout is insidious, cumulative, and progressive.

  G. Professional burnout is the deterioration of professional performance that is directly related to the demand for adaptational change brought on by perceived stressors in the work environment.

  H. Chronic stress contributes to job dissatisfaction, turnover, impaired job performance, and lack of productivity.

III. Stressors affecting oncology nurses—work-related stress in oncology nursing is multidimensional, involving:

A. Characteristics of the individual nurse.
  1. Overly dedicated and committed.
  2. High need to control.
  3. Overidentification with clients and families.
  4. Strong dependency needs.
  5. Perfectionism.
  6. Unrealistic goals and self-expectations.
  7. Diffuse personal boundaries.
  8. Idealistic.
  9. Home and personal conflict.
  10. Faced with society's devaluing of caring "women's work."
B. Characteristics of cancer client population and nature of care.
  1. Elusive cause.
  2. Heterogeneity of malignancies.
  3. Variability of prognosis.
  4. Unpredictability of health-illness trajectory.
  5. Confrontation with disfigurements, disability, pain, and death.
  6. Social stigma of working with people diagnosed with cancer.
  7. Knowledge base constantly in a state of growth.
  8. Labile emotions of clients, families, and staff.
  9. Inability to restore health.
  10. Repeated sense of failure if cure orientated.
  11. Prolonged involvement with client and family.
  12. Lack of consensus of treatment goals.
C. Characteristics within the work setting.
  1. Inadequate nurse-client ratio.
  2. Limited opportunity to participate in decision-making.
  3. Limited recognition and rewards for work performance.
  4. Limited autonomy and authority.
  5. Unclear role expectations; role ambiguity, role conflict, role overboard.
  6. Conflicts between professional goals and organizational goals.
  7. Inadequate psychological support from peers.
  8. Deficient administrative support or lack of feedback.
  9. Competitive rather than collaborative relationships.
  10. Limited upward mobility.
  11. Limited open and honest communications with peers, managers, and physicians.
  12. Inappropriate discharges.
  13. Work overload.
  14. Organizational change (care delivery system change).
  15. Increased use of nurse registries and unlicensed personnel.
  16. Pay inequities.
  17. Overcrowded units, noise, poor lighting, poor ventilation, and malfunctioning equipment.
IV. Stress responses (Table 48–2).
V. Stress management strategies.
  A. Goals of stress management strategies include:
    1. Eliminating those stressors that can be eliminated.
    2. Mastering stress that cannot be eliminated.
    3. Developing techniques for recognition and modification of stress responses.

TABLE 48–2. **Stress Responses**

Physical Responses	Emotional Responses	Intellectual Responses
Constant state of fatigue	Angry outbursts	Forgetfulness
Sleep disturbances	Irritability	Preoccupation
Change in food, alcohol, drug, and/or cigarette consumption	Feelings of worthlessness	Mathematical and grammatical errors
	Feelings of helplessness	Lack of concentration
Changes in physical appearance	Depression	Lack of attention to details
	Isolation of self from others	Denial
Repetitive accidents	Self-criticism	Assuming responsibility for behavior or feelings of others
Change in sexual behavior	Feelings of guilt	
Exacerbation of physical illness	Inability to identify and express feelings	Indecisiveness
	Difficulty forming and maintaining intimate relationships	Difficulty setting limits
Muscular pain (e.g., neck and lower back)		Lying when telling the truth would be easier
	Martyrdom	Past, rather than present or future orientation
	Numbing feelings through addictions	Diminished productivity
	Cynical and negative feelings toward clients, families, and coworkers	Impaired problem solving
		Resistance to change
	Whining	Change to abstract and analytic thinking
		Feelings of powerlessness
		Breakdown in effective communication
		Strict adherence to rules rather than consideration of the uniqueness of others
		Objectifying clients (e.g., "the new leukemic")
		Pessimism
		Uncooperativeness
		Tardiness or absenteeism

B. Stress management strategies include:
   1. Legitimizing one's own needs by commitment to self-care.
   2. Conducting a self-assessment, including:
      a. Needs.
      b. Motivations.
      c. Goals.
      d. Support systems—work and social.
      e. Stress responses.
         (1) Physical.
         (2) Emotional.
         (3) Intellectual.
      f. Communication style.
      g. Time management ability.

      h. Conflict resolution skills.

      i. Sources of stress.

   3. Asking for help from leadership, coworkers, or a professional counselor.

C. Concrete strategies for coping with stress include:

   1. Reappraisal of goals.

   2. Time management.

   3. Acknowledging vulnerabilities.

   4. Compartmentalizing life and work.

   5. Self-reinforcement.

   6. Change in attitudes.

   7. Creating balance.

   8. Accentuating the positive.

   9. Adopting a wellness philosophy.

  10. Relaxation.

  11. Establishing a sense of control over one's practice.

D. Based on self-evaluation, strategies for self-care and stress management may include:

   1. Increasing physical activity.

   2. Engaging in social activity.

   3. Becoming open to emotionally intimate relationships.

   4. Establishing realistic goals and expectations.

   5. Identifying and working to eliminate irrational beliefs.

   6. Seeking professional counseling.

   7. Practicing relaxation techniques.

   8. Maintaining a personal journal to record and analyze feelings and thoughts.

   9. Taking responsibility when appropriate; delegating when appropriate.

  10. Acquiring new skills through continuing education courses (time management, dealing with difficult people, conflict resolution techniques).

  11. Balancing home and work life.

  12. Positive self-talk and cognitive restructuring.

  13. Allowing for decompression time.

  14. Creating balance in caring with a blend of compassion and objectivity or detached concern.

  15. Advocating the following in the work setting:

      a. Development of support groups.

      b. Balanced nurse-client ratios that support the provision of quality care.

      c. Employee benefit packages that provide for vacations, mental health days, and reimbursement for professional counseling and continuing education.

      d. Recognition and financial incentives that reward quality performance.

      e. Establishment of an ethics committee.

      f. Participation in decision-making.

      g. Agency philosophy that supports multidisciplinary collaboration.

      h. "Time-out" activities for breaks or lunch, or "time out" from difficult assignment.

      i. Development of a "workteam" approach to foster a sense of belonging and common goals and mutual support.

      j. Implementation of sexual harassment policies and procedures.

  k. Implementation of a "Stop the Violence" program at work.

  l. Acquisition of the "Ten Basic Rights for Health Care Professionals": the right to be treated with respect; to a reasonable workload; to an equitable wage; to determine your own priorities; to ask for what you want; to refuse without making excuses or feeling guilty; to make mistakes and be responsible for them; to give and receive information as a professional; to act in the best interest of the client; to be human.

Quality Improvement

I. Professional mandates related to quality improvement.

 A. ANA/ONS Standards of Oncology Nursing Practice, Standards of Professional Performance, Standard I: Quality of Care—the oncology nurse systematically evaluates the quality of care and effectiveness of oncology nursing practice.

  1. Rationale: the complex and dynamic nature of the health care environment and the increasing body of oncology nursing knowledge and research provide both the impetus and the means for the oncology nurse to be competent in clinical practice, to continue professional development, to maintain competency in clinical practice, and to improve the quality of client care.

  2. Continuing peer review, interdisciplinary program evaluation, management, nursing quality assurance programs, and nursing research are used in this endeavor.

 B. ANA Nursing, A Social Policy Statement: each nurse remains accountable for the quality of her or his practice within the full scope of nursing practice. Nursing practice demands professional intention and commitment carried out in accordance with the ANA *Standards of Nursing Practice* and its ethical code. All nurses are ethically and legally accountable for actions taken in the course of nursing practice as well as for actions delegated by the nurse to others assisting in the delivery of nursing care. Such accountability may be accomplished through the regulatory mechanisms of licensure, through criminal and civil laws, through the code of ethics of the profession, and through peer evaluation.

 C. ANA Code.

  1. The nurse acts to safeguard the client/public when care and safety are affected by incompetent, unethical, or illegal conduct of any person.

  2. The nurse participates in the profession's efforts to implement and improve standards of nursing.

  3. The nurse participates in activities that contribute to the ongoing development of the profession's body of knowledge.

  4. The nurse maintains competence in nursing.

  5. The nurse exercises informal judgment and uses individual competence and qualifications as criteria in seeking consultation, accepting responsibilities, and delegating nursing activities to others.

II. General statements about quality assurance.

 A. Society gives professional bodies the privilege to govern their concerns, empowering professions to manage their own functions; in return, professionals are accountable to society for their actions.

 B. Self-regulation to assure quality in performance and products is a hallmark of a profession.

C. Nurses have a professional responsibility to assure quality control and improvement.

D. Nursing has the right and professional responsibility to define and control its own practice.

E. In that nursing is a major component of health care, quality assurance in nursing is essential to guarantee the overall quality of health care.

F. Professional and practice standards provide a mechanism to assure and evaluate quality care.
  1. Practice standards pertain to theory, data collection, diagnosis, planning, intervention, and evaluation.
  2. Professional standards pertain to professional behavior—professional development, interdisciplinary collaboration, quality assurance, ethics, and research.

G. Professional and practice standards may be found in the following:
  1. State nurse practice acts.
  2. Published standards of professional organizations such as:
     a. ANA Standards of Nursing Practice.
     b. ANA/ONS Standards of Oncology Nursing Practice.
     c. ONS Standards of Oncology Nursing Education: Generalist and Advanced Practice Levels.
     d. ONS Standards of Oncology Education: Patient/Family and Public.
     e. ONS Standards of Advanced Practice in Oncology Nursing.
  3. Federal agencies guidelines and regulations (e.g., Joint Commission on Accreditation of Health Care Organization [JCAHO], Social Security Administration).
  4. Hospital or agency policy and procedure manuals.
  5. Job description and performance evaluation criteria.
  6. Professional organizations publications (ANA Nursing: A Social Policy Statement; ANA: A Code for Nurses).
  7. Professional literature.

H. No one source is sufficient to describe quality of care or performance.

I. Professional quality assurance strategies may include:
  1. Mandatory licensure.
  2. Peer review.
  3. Development and implementation of quality assurance programs.
  4. Professional certification.
  5. Certification of education programs and continuing education programs.
  6. Risk management.

III. Peer review.
  A. Peer review is a process in which professional nurses appraise the quality of care provided by professional nurse(s) in accordance with established standards.
  B. Peer review process includes both appraisal of nursing care delivered by a group of nurses and the appraisal of an individual nurse.
    1. Nursing Professional Standards Review: review of nursing care provided by a group of nurses. Purposes of Nursing Professional Standards Review include:
       a. Evaluation of the quality of nursing care to identify the extent of consistency to established standard.
       b. Identification of strengths and weaknesses in nursing care.
       c. Justification of recommendations for new or revised policies, procedures, and standards to improve nursing care.
       d. Identification of practice areas in which knowledge is needed.

2. Nursing Performance Review: review of nursing care provided by an individual nurse. Purposes of Nursing Performance Review include:
   a. Provision of assistance for the nurse in improving the quality of practice.
   b. Provision of commendation and/or constructive criticism of an individual nurse's performance when applicable.
   c. Protection of the nurse from ill-founded and unjust accusations.
   d. Appraisal of how the practice of the nurse maintains or deviates from accepted practice and professional standards.
3. Data collected from Nursing Performance Review may be used to make recommendations to a certification board and/or to provide input into the performance evaluation that qualifies the nurse for clinical advancement or salary increases.

IV. The Joint Commission on Accreditation of Healthcare Organization promotes the use of any problem-solving process that evaluates quality of care. Two examples of the problem-solving process are described in Table 48–3.

V. Practice acts.
   A. The Nurse Practice Act is the state law that governs the practice of nursing.
   B. The Board of Nursing is the administrative agency that implements the statutes, with power granted by the state legislature.
   C. Basic components of nurse practice acts include:
      1. Definition of professional nursing.
      2. Requirements for licensure.
      3. Provision for endorsements or sanctioning of persons licensed in another state.
      4. Specifications of exemptions from licensure.
      5. Grounds for disciplinary actions, which may include:
         a. Improper procurement of a license.
         b. Conviction for a felony.
         c. Physical or mental incapacity.
         d. Unprofessional conduct.
         e. Incompetence, negligence, and malpractice.
         f. Substance abuse.
      6. Provisions for the board of nursing with an outline of their responsibilities.
      7. Penalties for practicing without a license or substance abuse.

VI. Certification.
   A. Certification is a process by which a nongovernmental agency or association certifies that an individual licensed to practice a profession has met certain predetermined standards specified by that profession for specialty practice; its application to nursing means that a nurse has achieved competence in a field of specialty within the profession.
   B. Certification enables a profession to define and articulate for its members the new knowledge required to practice.
   C. Purposes of certification include:
      1. Protection of the public.
      2. Recognition of an expert practitioner.

Client Advocacy and Empowerment

I. Nursing literature has used the term "advocacy" to denote a variety of nursing roles, each derived from a specific set of beliefs and values. "Advocate" as a term has been used to represent several related and sometimes conflicting concepts:

TABLE 48–3. Quality Assurance Problem-Solving Process Examples

Ten-Step Model for Quality Improvement

1. Assign responsibility for monitoring and evaluation activities
2. Delineate the scope of care provided, including a description of the following:
   a. Types of clients served
   b. Treatments or activities performed
   c. Basic clinical activities required
   d. Types of practitioners providing care
3. Identify important aspects of care—essential elements of activities that constitute nursing care
4. Identify indicators for monitoring the important aspects of care that are measurable variables relating to the structure, process, or outcomes of care.
   a. Structure criteria describe organizational, financial, and physical attributes of the agency and provider characteristics (agency philosophy, nurse-client ratio, qualifications of staff, equipment, environment, educational preparation of professional staff [e.g., annual continuing education requirements, certification], client classification system used to determine staffing needs).
   b. Process criteria describe actions and behaviors that focus on the nature of activities, interventions, and sequence of events in the delivery of nursing care (job descriptions, performance standards, procedures, protocols, implementation strategies of nursing care plans).
   c. Outcome criteria describe expected end results of nursing care such as measurable changes in the health status of the client (health knowledge, improved health status [physiologic, psychological, and/or functional], satisfaction)
5. Establish the thresholds for evaluation for the indicators—a threshold for evaluation is an established level or point in the cumulative data that will trigger an intensive evaluation of care (e.g., aspect of care—vesicant extravasation; indicator—number of clients who experience a vesicant extravasation; threshold for evaluation—0%; intensive evaluation—any vesicant extravasation).
6. Monitor the important aspects of care by collecting and organizing measurements needed to determine whether or not standards are attained—data collection methods may include concurrent and retrospective audit, direct observation of nurse or client performance, questionnaire, interview, knowledge testing
7. Evaluate care when thresholds for the indicators are reached to identify problems or opportunities for improvement
8. Develop and implement a plan of action to correct identified problems or improve care; the plan may include:
   a. Description of the problem
   b. Who or what is expected to change or improve
   c. What resources are needed
   d. Who is responsible for implementing action
   e. What action is appropriate in view of cause (insufficient knowledge, defects in systems, deficient behavior or performance), scope, and severity
   f. When change is expected to occur
   g. When reevaluation will occur
   h. Who is responsible for evaluation of the plan
9. Evaluate the effectiveness of the actions and document the improvement in care
10. Communicate the results of the monitoring and evaluation process to relevant individuals, departments, and to the organization-wide quality assurance program

Performance Improvement

1. Plan
2. Design
3. Measure
4. Assess
5. Improve

    A. Beneficence—the principle of doing good.

    B. Nonmaleficence—the principle of doing no harm.

    C. Unitary—transformative paradigm—a perspective that views human beings as unitary, self-organizing energy fields interacting with a larger environmental energy field.

    D. Utilitarianism—an ethical doctrine in which actions are focused on accomplishing the greatest good for the greatest number of people.

II. Types of advocacy.

    A. Simplistic advocacy—one who pleads the cause of another.

    B. Paternalistic advocacy—doing something for or to another without that person's consent and on the premise that it serves the person's own good.

    C. Consumer advocacy—nurse is required to provide the client with information to make a decision and then withdraw so as to not unclearly bias the client.

    D. Consumer-centric advocacy—nurse provides information and then supports clients in their decision.

    E. Existential advocacy and human advocacy—the nurse's active participation with the client in determining the unique meaning that the experience of health, illness, suffering, or dying is for that individual.

    F. Human advocacy—when the whole nurse nurses, the whole person can be nursed; nurse discloses her views to the client.

III. Empowerment—refers to a liberating pedagogy that reverses the dehumanization and objectification of oppressed people through development of their own critical consciousness and simultaneous action.

    A. Client is active and equal participant in his or her own empowerment.

    B. Empowerment is an enabling process that enhances personal control.

    C. An awareness and commitment to change problematic social and cultural contexts.

    D. Regarding the other as a subject, rather than object, and as capable of transforming his or her own realities.

IV. Several authors (cited in bibliography) have used the term "advocacy" to describe a variety of nursing roles quoted earlier. Rafael finds these roles to be congruent with the concept of empowerment and with caring in the human health experience.

V. Caring is a process of mutuality and creative unfolding.

VI. Existential advocacy and human advocacy complement each other and are congruent with a unitary-transformative approach to caring.

VII. The client relationship common to both advocacy and caring are consistent with conditions in which empowerment can occur.

BIBLIOGRAPHY

Abruzzese, R. (1996). Nursing staff development/strategies for success. In P. Yoder Wise (ed.). *Learning Needs Assessment.* St. Louis: Mosby-Year Book, pp. 188–207.

Abruzzese, R. (1996). Nursing staff development/strategies for success. In Katz, J.M. (ed.). *Managing the Deal Dimension of Quality.* St. Louis: Mosby-Year Book, pp. 302–324.

Abruzzese, R. (1996). Nursing staff development/strategies for success. In C.A. Mottola (ed.). *Research in Nursing Staff Development.* St. Louis: Mosby-Year Book, pp. 326–344.

Al-Assaf, A.F., & Schmelel, J.A. (1993). *The Textbook of Total Quality in Healthcare.* Delray Beach, FL: St. Lucie Press.

American Nurses' Association. (1993). The American Nurses' Association position statement on registered nurse utilization of unlicensed assistive personnel. *Am Nurs* February, 6–8.

American Nurses' Association. (1995). *Nursing, a Social Policy Statement.* Washington D.C.: American Nurses' Association.

Barriball, K.C., & While, A.E. (1996). Participation in continuing professional education in nursing: Findings of an interview study. *J Adv Nurs 23*(5), 999–1007.

Baumgart, A. (1996). Promoting nursing practice through nursing research. *Int Nurs Rev 43*(2), 45–48, 57.

Bean, C.A., & Holcombe, J.K. (1993). Personality types of oncology nurses. *Cancer Nurs 16*(6), 479–485.

Belcher, A., & Shurpin, K.M. (1995). Education of the advanced practice nurse in oncology. *Oncol Nurs Forum 22*(8), 19–24.

Burns, N., & Grove, S.K. (1993). *The Practice of Nursing Research Conduct and Critique and Utilization* (2nd ed.). Philadelphia, W.B. Saunders.

Cloud, H. (1996). Finding healthy relationships. *Single-Parent Fam,* Feb, 6–10.

Curtin, L. (1996). What everybody knows. *Nurs Manage 27*(1), 7–8.

Engelking, C. (1994). New approaches: Innovations in cancer prevention, diagnosis, treatment, and support. *Oncol Nurs Forum 21*(1), 62–71.

Esterhuizer, P. (1996). Is the professional code still the cornerstone of clinical nursing practice? *J Adv Nurs 23*(1), 25–31.

Fitzpatrick, M.J. (1994). Performance improvement through quality improvement teamwork. *J Nurs Adm 24*(12): 20–27.

Gaydon, J.E., West, P., Galloway, S., et al. (1993). Bridging the gap between research and clinical practice: A collaborative approach. *Oncol Nurs Forum 20*(6), 953–957.

Greco, K.E. (1995). Regulation of advanced nursing practice part one—second licensure. *Oncol Nurs Forum 22*(8), 35–42.

Harvey, C. (1994). New systems: The restructuring of cancer care delivery and economics. *Oncol Nurs Forum 21*(1), 72–76.

Harwood, K. (1994). Speciality focus: Oncology nursing. *Adv Pract Nurs* Fall/Winter, 54–57.

Hogston, R. (1995). Nurses' perceptions of the impact of continuing professional education on the quality of nursing care. *J Adv Nurs 22*(3), 86–93.

Holzemer, W. (1996). The impact of multiskilling on quality of care. *Int Nurs Rev 43*(1), 21–25.

Iwamoto, R.R., Rumsey, K.A., & Summers, B.L.Y. (1996). *Statement on the Scope and Standards of Oncology Nursing Practice.* Washington, D.C.: American Nurses Publishing.

Joint Commission on Accreditation of Healthcare Organizations. (1996). *Accredition Manual for Hospitals.* Chicago: Joint Commission on Accreditation of Healthcare Organizations.

Kirchholl, K.T., & Mateo, M.M. (1996). Roles and responsibilities of clinical nurse researchers. *J Prof Nurs 12*(2), 86–90.

McCaffrey Boyle, D. (1994). New identities: The changing profile of patients with cancer, their families, and their professional caregivers. *Oncol Nurs Forum 21*(1), 55–60.

McCaffrey Boyle, D., Engelking, C., & Harvey, C. (1994). Making a difference in the 21st century: Are oncology nurses ready? *Oncol Nurs Forum 21*(1), 53–55.

McCaffrey Boyle, D., Engelking, C., & Harvey, C. (1994). Taking command of the future: Getting ready now for the 21st century. *Oncol Nurs Forum 21*(1), 77–79.

McGuire, D.F., Walczak, J.R., & Krum, S.L. (1994). Development of a nursing research utilization program in a clinical oncology setting: Organization, implementation, and evaluation. *Oncol Nurs Forum 21*(4), 704–709.

Manion, J. (1995). Understanding the seven stages of change. *AJN 95*(6), 41–43.

Mateo, M.A., & Kirchhoff, K.T. (1995). Productivity of nurse researchers employed in clinical settings. *J Nurs Adm 25*(10), 37–42.

Noer, D. (1993). *Healing the Wounds.* San Francisco: Jossey-Bass.

Oncology Nursing Society. (1995). *Standards of Oncology Nursing Education. Generalist and Advanced Practice.* Pittsburgh: Oncology Nursing Society.

Patton, M.D. (1993). Action research and the process of continual quality improvement in a cancer center. *Oncol Nurs Forum 20*(5), 751–755.

Polit, D.F., & Hungler, B.P. (1995). *Nursing Research: Principles and Methods* (5th ed.). Philadelphia: J.B. Lippincott, pp. 624–654.

Pritchett, P., & Pound, R. (1995). *A Survival Guide to the Stress of Organizational Change.* Dallas: Pritchett and Associates.

Rafael, A. (1995). Advocacy and empowerment: Dichotomous or synchromous concepts? *Adv Nurs Sci 18*(2), 25–32.

Reiley, P., Seibert, C.P., Miller, N.E., et al. (1994). Implementation of a collaborative quality assessment program. *J Nurs Adm 24*(5), 65–71.

Sheets, V. (1996). Director of Public Policy, Nursing Practice, Education. National Council of State Boards of Nursing, Inc. Personal communication.

Silva, M. (1995). *Ethical Guidelines in the Conduct, Dissemination, and Implementation of Nursing Research.* Washington D.C.: American Nurses Publishing.

Triolo, P., Allgeier, P., & Schwarts, C. (1995). Layoff survivor sickness. *J Nurs Adm 25*(3), 56–63.

Young, W., Minnick, A., & Marcantonio, R. (1996). How wide is the gap in defining quality care? Comparison of patient and nurse perceptions of important aspects of patient care. *J Nurs Adm 26*(5), 15–20.

49

Issues and Challenges: Alternative Therapies

Paul J. Ross, RN, MA

Theory

I. Definition—alternative therapies are considered outside the realm of conventional (allopathic, orthodox) medicine, yet they claim physiologic benefits ranging from cancer cure to symptom relief. Alternatives are used both independently and in conjunction with biomedical interventions, the latter referred to as complementary.

II. Features.
   A. Mechanism of action is proposed in common sense terms.
      1. Often highlight cancer as a symptom of body imbalance.
   B. Stress self-healing, psychosocial as well as physical needs, "natural" and "nontoxic" interventions, egalitarian relationship between healer and patient.
   C. Provided in home settings (e.g., folk medicines), retreats, unregulated clinics often outside the United States (e.g., Tijuana, Mexico), and/or with formal hospital approval (e.g., music therapy).
   D. Advocated by popular media, social networks, and practitioners such as folk healers, "experts" with esoteric "diplomas," some physicians and nurses.
   E. Promise positive outcomes.
      1. Evidence of efficacy is often anecdotal.
      2. Practices are not routinely subject to scientific scrutiny (i.e., tested and reviewed in reputable journals).
      3. Lack of acceptance by biomedicine may be dismissed as evidence of conspiracy and bureaucratic inefficiency.
   F. Used by ever-increasing numbers of cancer patients.
      1. Primarily as an adjunct to biomedical regimens.
      2. Resulting in more attention from biomedicine; a growing focus of nursing and medical school courses, journals, and research institutions (e.g., National Institutes of Health [NIH]).

III. Diverse approaches.
   A. Dietary regimens.
      1. Rationale—if diet can reduce risk of or prevent cancer, it also can cure.
      2. Include both familiar and exotic foods, single supplements (e.g., "pharmafoods" such as garlic), and complete diets (e.g., macrobiotic).
   B. Mind-body techniques.
      1. Rationale—assume that the client's emotions influence the course of disease.

2. Range from practices that aim to reduce stress and disease risk (e.g., yoga, biofeedback) to those suggesting cure (e.g., visualizations of white blood cells engulfing cancer cells).
C. Traditional and folk medicines.
   1. Rationale—there are valid understandings of pathology and physiology that differ from biomedical paradigms.
   2. Include well-integrated, classical systems (e.g., Chinese, Ayurveda) and others fostered by cultural and ethnic identity (e.g., Hawaiian lomilomi).
D. Pharmacologic and biologic treatments.
   1. Rationale often borrowed piecemeal from biomedicine.
   2. Highly controversial approaches that target the immune system (e.g., antineoplaston, enzyme and amino acid infusions, immunoaugmentative therapy) or aim to purge body "toxins" (e.g., through colonic irrigations, coffee enemas, laetrile, and shark cartilage infusions).
E. Herbal or plant medicines.
   1. Include elements of medical traditions (e.g., Arabic, Native American) as well as isolated "natural" products (e.g., Essiac, iscador) that claim to boost the immune system.
F. Manipulative methods.
   1. Range from osteopathy and chiropractic to the therapeutic and/or healing touch practices taught by nurses.

Assessment

I. Relevant client history.
   A. Demographics—education, residence, economic status, ethnic and cultural identity.
      1. Alternative practices appeal to well-educated, urban, middle-class patients.
      2. For some cultural groups, alternative practices are an integral part of their health values and beliefs.
   B. Perspective on disease etiology and treatment.
      1. Ethnic and cultural identity helps shape care decisions.
      2. Contrasting experience of biomedicine.
         a. Value of holistic, personal care—with a focus on quality of life, an emphasis on the "client" and not just the "tumor"—as an alternative to the reductionistic perspective of biomedicine.
         b. Intimidation by, or fear of, conventional (likely iatrogenic) therapy; attracted to the "natural," "low tech," and easily explained.
         c. Distrust of "established medicine," bureaucracies, and obstructive regulations.
         d. Dissatisfaction with effectiveness.
            (1) Use of alternatives is not directly related to stage of disease progression or prognosis.
            (2) Biomedicine does not target all symptoms.
            (3) Discussions of statistical probabilities confuse clients.

Nursing Diagnoses

   I. Knowledge deficit.
  II. Decisional conflict.
 III. Health-seeking behaviors.

Outcome Identification

I. Nurses identify and discuss the therapeutic objectives of health care professionals *and* clients.

II. Nurses describe criteria and methods used to evaluate the efficacy of cancer
therapies.

III. Nurses document uses of all alternative therapies.

IV. Nurses report client-perceived side effects to the health care team.

Planning and Implementation

I. Interventions to provide for an optimally informed client.
   A. Encourage open communication about biomedical options and alternative
   or complementary therapies.
      1. Support an informal dialogue initiated by nurses, clients, and/or their fam-
      ilies.
         a. Success depends on building rapport, ensuring a culturally sensitive and
         nonjudgmental milieu.
         b. Recognize that quick dismissals of alternatives may shut down further
         communication.
      2. Explain biomedical options so that they are accessible.
         a. The attraction of alternatives is that they are easily conveyed, are com-
         prehensible and persuasive.
      3. Seek to comprehend why biomedicine may not satisfy clients (e.g., lack
      of psychosocial support? poor symptom control?).
      4. Emphasize and support the client's right to choose from among therapeu-
      tic options.
   B. Support the need for a well-informed health care team.
      1. Familiar with professional and popular literature.
      2. Able to recognize that clients are important sources of information con-
      cerning alternatives.
      3. Aware that alternatives may reflect cultural preferences and provide an
      integral component of a client's family and social identification.
      4. Recognize that clients may deny use of alternatives out of fear of losing
      biomedical services.
      5. Capable of effectively discussing alternatives from a biomedical perspec-
      tive that includes consideration of theory and tested outcomes.
   C. Differentiate alternatives that interfere with biomedicine from those that
   complement biomedicine.
      1. Practices that should be given primary attention include those that risk
      harm (e.g., provide antagonistic biophysical results, cause delay or termina-
      tion of biomedical treatment).
      2. Include popular features of alternative therapies such as more personal
      care and greater access to providers into more conventional regimens.
         a. Identifying why alternatives are sought may suggest more effective
         conventional interventions.

Evaluation

The oncology nurse systematically and regularly evaluates the client's and/or
family's responses to interventions to determine progress toward the achievement
of expected outcomes. Relevant data are collected and actual findings are compared

with expected findings. Nursing diagnoses, outcomes, and plans of care are reviewed and revised as necessary.

BIBLIOGRAPHY

Cassidy, C. (1996). Cultural context of complementary and alternative medicine systems. In M.S. Micozzi (ed.). *Fundamentals of Complementary and Alternative Medicine.* New York: Churchill Livingstone, pp. 9–34.

Cassileth, B.R., & Chapman, C.C. (1996). Alternative and complementary cancer therapies. *Cancer 77*(6), 1026–1034.

Engebretson, J. (1996). Comparison of nurses and alternative healers. *Image 28*(2), 95–99.

Ford, S., Fallowfield, L., & Lewis, S. (1996). Doctor-patient interactions in oncology. *Soc Sci Med 42*(11), 1511–1519.

Hildenbrand, G., Hildenbrand, L.C., Bradford, K., et al. (1995). Five-year survival rates of melanoma patients treated by diet therapy after the manner of Gerson: A retrospective review. *Alternative Ther 1*(4), 29–37.

Lane, I.W., & Comac, L. (1996). *Sharks Still Don't Get Cancer.* Garden City Park: Avery Publishing Group.

Montbriand, M.J. (1995). Decision tree model describing alternate health care choices made by oncology patients. *Cancer Nurs 18*(2), 104–117.

Moss, R.W. (1995). *Cancer Therapy.* New York: Equinox Press.

Moss, R.W. (1997). *The Cancer Chronicles* [On-Line], Available: http://www.ralphmoss.com/

Nwoga, I.A. (1994). Traditional healers and perceptions of the causes and treatment of cancer. *Cancer Nurs 17*(6), 470–478.

Sawyer, M.G., Gannoni, A.F., Toogood, I.R., et al. (1994). The use of alternative therapies by children with cancer. *Med J Aust 160*(21 March), 320–322.

Todd, A.D. (1994). *Double Vision.* Hanover: Wesleyan University Press.

University of Pennsylvania Cancer Center (1997). *Oncolink.* [On-Line], Available: http://www.onco-link.upenn.edu/

University of Texas, Houston Health Science Center (1997). *Center for Alternative Medicine Research in Cancer.* [On-Line], Available: http://www.sph/uth.tmc.edu/www/utsph/utcam/index.htm

Zaloznik, A.J. (1994). Unproven (unorthodox) cancer treatments. *Cancer Pract 2*(1), 19–24.

Index

Note: Page numbers in *italics* refer to illustrations; page numbers followed by t refer to tables.